# 1 MONTH OF
# FREE
# READING

## at
## www.ForgottenBooks.com

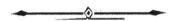

By purchasing this book you are eligible for one month membership to ForgottenBooks.com, giving you unlimited access to our entire collection of over 1,000,000 titles via our web site and mobile apps.

To claim your free month visit:

www.forgottenbooks.com/free787378

ISBN 978-0-483-03783-0
PIBN 10787378

# Long Island Medical Journal

EDITED BY

## HENRY GOODWIN WEBSTER, A.B., M.D.

OF BROOKLYN-NEW YORK

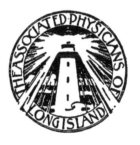

VOLUME VII.

JANUARY-DECEMBER, 1913

THE OFFICIAL ORGAN OF THE

ASSOCIATED PHYSICIANS OF LONG ISLAND

364 WASHINGTON AVENUE, BROOKLYN, N. Y., U. S. A.

Published Monthly by the

# Associated Physicians of Long Island

SAMUEL HENDRICKSON
President

JAMES P. WARBASSE          GUY H. TURRELL
DUDLEY D. ROBERTS
Vice-Presidents

JAMES COLE HANCOCK          EDWIN S. MOORE
Secretary          Treasurer

Publication Committee

WILLIAM H. ROSS
Chairman

FRANK F. DeLANO     WILLARD G. REYNOLDS     HENRY G. WEBSTER
ROGER DURHAM          JAMES C. HANCOCK
SAMUEL HENDRICKSON

# LONG ISLAND MEDICAL JOURNAL

# INDEX TO VOLUME VII

# 1913

# INDEX TO AUTHORS

# BOOK REVIEWS.

# NECROLOGY.

**A**

ALLEN, EMMA T. P., 487.

**B**

BAKER, CLARENCE ALBERT, 74.
BIRDSALL, ALFRED THORNTON, 487.
BRISTOW, ALGERNON THOMAS, 194.
BRUNDAGE, JOHN DUTTON, 488.
BUNN, REV. ALBERT CARRIER, 74.

**C**

CALLAN, WILLIAM JAMES, 154.
CARHART, EDWARD WILLIAM, 367.
CARNEY, JAMES LESTER, 367.
CAROLAN, EUGENE JOSEPH, 282.
CLOWMINZER, WILLIAM HENRY, 367.

**D**

DROGE, JOHN HERMAN, 283.
DRURY, GEORGE, 487.
DUDLEY, WILLIAM FREDERICK, 73.
DUFFIGG, BERNARD ALOYSIUS, 368.

**G**

GANSTER, WILLIAM FOSTER, 154.
GOODMAN, ALEXANDER MANSFIELD, 282.

**H**

HENRY, JESSE WILLIAMS, 367.
HIRSEMAN, GOTTHARD, 488.
HISS, PHILIP HANSON, 195.
HUBER, S. S., 488.
HYDE, OVID ALLEN, 366.

**I**

IRELAND, TREADWELL LEWIS, 153.

**J**

JACHES, JOSEPH J., 73.
JEFFERY, GEORGE CLINTON, 153.

**L**

LELAND, MATTHEW JOHN, 368.
LITTLE, FRANK, 283.
LITTLE, WILLIAM ARTHUR, 154.

**Mc**

McLENATHAN, WILLIAM H., 366.

**M**

MANATON, WILLIAM P., 366.
MEHRENLENDER, ALBERT NOCHIM, 73.
MITCHELL, WILLIAM ANDERSON, 488.
MOORE, ROBERT EMORY, 486.

**O**

OATMAN, EDWARD LEROY, 75.
O'BRIEN, KERAN, 75.

**P**

PALMER, ERNEST, 153.

**R**

REX, WILLIAM FREDERICK, 73.

**S**

SHAY, DANIEL ALOYSIUS, 487.
SMALL, GEORGE HENRY, 74.
STANLEY, GRANT, 283.
STIVERS, JOHN RANDALL, 486.

**T**

TREZISE, JOHN DAVIES, 282.
TURNER, HENRY CUSHMAN, 487.

**W**

WATT, JAMES LEWIS, 366.
WELLS, CHARLES E., 74.
WELTON, ROBERT BRADLEE, 75.
WESTBROOK, GEORGE RANSOM, 368.
WILLICH, CARL, 488.

# LONG ISLAND
# MEDICAL JOURNAL

VOL. VII.        JANUARY, 1913        No. 1

## ⚓riginal Articles.

### MEDICAL BOOKS OF OTHER DAYS AND SOME REASONS WHY WE CHERISH AND PRESERVE THEM.*

By Lewis Stephen Pilcher, M.D., LL.D.,

of Brooklyn, N. Y.

THE literature of Medicine has engaged the services of the ablest men. Said Holmes, "What glorifies a town like a cathedral? What dignifies a province like a University? What illuminates a country like its scholarship, and what is the nest that hatches scholars but a library?" Then he continues, "The physician, some may say, is a practical man and has little use for all this book learning. Every student has heard Sydenham's reply to Sir Richard Blackmore's question as to what works he should read, meaning medical works. 'Read Don Quixote,' was his famous answer. But Sydenham himself made medical books, and may be presumed to have thought *those* at least worth reading. Descartes was asked where was his library, and in reply held up the dissected body of an animal. But Descartes made books, great books, and a great many of them. A physician of common sense without erudition is better than a learned one without common sense, but the thorough master of his profession must have learning added to his natural gifts."

Said Weir Mitchell:

"Show us the books he loves and I shall know
The man far better than through mortal friends."

By books and by literature I do not mean medical journals and medical text books, vade mecums, and manuals. These are important and invaluable in their place. They are the daily bread and the working tools of the physician, and are to be kept in constant use. Their value is a present but ephemeral value—those of yesterday are supplanted by those of today, and these in turn will give place to those of tomorrow. These alone would be of supreme interest to physicians, if medicine was a mere trade, the mastery of which consisted in learning to do a few things in a certain way, and continuing to do those things in the same way day after day *ad infinitum*. As a learned profession, however, it has a literature

* Read before the Medical Library Association of Brooklyn, March 31, 1912.

which contributes to culture, and familiarity with which exerts an elevating influence on the reader. The elements of this literature have a wide and permanent influence. They are books of today, yes, sometimes, but more frequently of the past, and often of the distant past. In the fields of history and biography, in discussions of medical life and ideals, in essays, even in poetry and romance, they are to be found, and wherever found they awaken lofty sentiment, they broaden views of life, they introduce a more correct perspective into one's estimates as to the value of present things, and they tend to create in the student a mental attitude which makes him more worthy to be classed as a member of a learned profession rather than the mere practitioner of a useful trade.

There are certain great works and writings which mark in a special manner the progress of medicine. These have a permanent interest not only as historical records of the development of medical knowledge, but still more as memorials more enduring than brass, which remind us of the great men and the great achievements of the past. No man can be considered a medical scholar who does not know about them, their place in literature, and the part which their writers played in the evolution of medicine, although he may not read in detail the books themselves. Such are the books of Hippocrates, of Celsus and Galen among the ancients; of Avenzoar and of Avicenna among the Arabians; of Mundinus and Guy de Chauliac, marking the close of the Dark Ages and the beginning of the Renaissance in anatomy and in surgery; of the Regimen Sanitatis Salerni, preserving the memory of the great mediæval medical school at Salernum; of Benivieni, the morning star of pathology; of Berengarius da Carpi, who first demonstrated the practical use of illustrations in anatomical treaties; of Vesalius, the Flemish knight errant of anatomy who revolutionized that department of medicine and made his name immortal before he was thirty years of age; of Paracelsus, the medical iconoclast; of Paré, the practical thinker and wise constructor in surgery; of Harvey, the devoted Royalist, who first grasped the idea and demonstrated the fact of the perpetual circuit of the blood; of Sydenham, the grim Puritan, the English Hippocrates; of Boerhaave, whose aphorisms, and of Albinus, whose plates, marked the high point of the Dutch school at the close of the seventeenth and beginning of the eighteenth century; the books of Cheselden, of Monro, and of Hunter, signalling the rise of the English school at the close of the eighteenth century.

These are by no means all the names worthy of being mentioned in this connection, but I content myself with these few as examples of what I mean now to enforce. These are great mountain peaks of the medical world that stand out the more clearly as a wider historical horizon is attained.

There has recently come into my possession a list of the books contained in the library left by the great Boerhaave, the illustrious scholar and teacher of Leyden, whom you will have noted I have included among the highest peaks of medicine. I have been interested to look this list over, and see what Boerhaave thought of the place that should be given to the ancients. Foremost I find to stand Hippocrates, of whose works, either entire or in portions, he had on his shelves twenty editions. Of Galen there was the great *editio princeps* of 1525 from the Aldine Press, and the succeeding edition of 1538. For Celsus and Avicenna room was given for but one edition each, but of Vesalius, there were collected no less than fourteen editions, from the great folio of 1543 and the tiny duodecimo of 1552 that appeared during the life of the great anatomist, to the magnificent folio volumes of the complete works issued by Albinus and Boerhaave himself in 1725. The school of Salernum, Mundinus, Carpus, and Paracelsus, all were included. William Harvey also seems to have elicited the special interest of the great Dutchman, for in this library he had assembled four editions of the *De Motu Cordis,* and three editions of the *Exercitationes de Generatione Animalium.* It was in the companion-ship of such books and in the spirit engendered by them that Boerhaave gathered the inspiration that made him in his time the first physician in Christendom.

It is true that none of us are Boerhaaves, but it is equally true that there is no one of us who would not be the better man and physician if he were more familiar with the literature and history of his chosen profession, of the lofty and magnificent character of whose traditions and chronicles we have but an inadequate con-ception.

In the earlier years of my own residence in New York, I used to frequently visit the Library of the New York Hospital which through the generosity of that institution was thrown open to the general medical public. In the hallway at the head of the stairs as we ascended from the vestibule to the floor above, where the books were, were cases filled with the folios and quartos of the old masters of medicine. They always spoke to me as I entered and welcomed me as if they held the key to the arcana of medicine which they were glad to open to any earnest seeker after truth. Years after I became intimate with the late Dr. George Jackson Fisher, of Sing Sing, N. Y., who, though a typical country doctor, had accumulated the finest private collection of the medical classics that has yet been formed in this country. Guided by him I became more familiar with the treasures of the past and learned somewhat of the art of collecting them for myself. As I sit in my library now and pen these lines, the room is full of the stir of these companions chosen from all the ages. In the magnificent folios which bear the imprint of Aldus, or Oporinus, or Stephanus, or Plantin, or in dainty duodecimos issued by the Elzevirs, or in quartos and octavos from the presses of Leyden, Venice, Lyons, Basle or Frankfort, their voices are contained, ready to speak whenever I am ready to hear. The lives, the work, the character of these authors are part of the precious heritage to which each century is adding and which is being handed down freely to whoever will accept it.

It is not possible for every physician to have a copy of an *editio princeps* of the various worthies of the past whose special labors or illustrious characters may most command his personal admiration. Whenever, however, such an opportunity does pre-sent itself, it should be taken advantage of, and such a book esteemed as the particular ornament of the library, to be venerated quite in the spirit which the Chinaman worships his ancestral tablets. What an influence for culture of mind, for nobility of character and elevation of thought, for purity of purpose, what a corrective for the rampant commercial tendencies of the day would a wide knowledge of the work and the ideals of the great men of the past have upon the workers of the present!

One of the most important functions of a library such as that which has become housed within these walls is that it may bring these liberalizing influences in a more extended and important degree to all the physicians of the community by assembling on its shelves many examples of these great classics and by calling frequent and importunate attention to them. Such accumulations of books as those now to be found in the Library of the Surgeon-General's Office at Washington, in the buildings of the Boston Medical Library, of the Medical and Chirurgical Faculty of Maryland, of the College of Physicians of Philadelphia, of the Academy of Medicine of New York, and last but by no means least, of the Medical Society of the County of Kings, in Brooklyn, have already done and will continue to do much to foster a spirit of the highest professional quality in the physicians of this country.

A peculiar interest to us attaches to the disposition of the unique library of ancient authors accumulated by Dr. George Jackson Fisher, to which I have already alluded. When an untimely death snatched him away, his library was acquired by a hospital situated in one of the interior cities of our state, whose trustees were moved to purchase it by the enthusiasm of their Medical Superintendent who appreciated its worth.

A most charming and every way fitting building to contain them was constructed, and it seemed as if in this beautiful building overlooking the Hudson River this unusual collection of medical classics had obtained a fitting and a permanent home beyond our reach, except as we might from time to time make hasty pilgrimages to visit it. But strange are the changes which time brings about! With the lapse of years new men came into the Board of Trustees of the hospital whose choicest jewel was this grand collection of books. A new superintendent occupied the chair of the former one. With the new men came a new spirit. They could see no value in a lot of old books; they could make better use of the space and the building which they occupied, and lo, this really priceless collection was again announced for sale. A movement was started which culminated in securing for the Library of the Medical Society of the County of Kings this most desirable collection, and here they are today, in what it is hoped will be their permanent home. What the presence of these books upon the shelves of our own library means to us I have tried to faintly indicate in what I have already said.

There are more than a score of them which bear the dates of the fifteenth century and count as typographical *incunabula*, valuable not merely as samples of early printing in general, but even more so to us as examples of the earliest printed medical works. Of the books of the sixteenth century, a period during which many of the noblest books ever manufactured were produced, there are nearly two hundred and fifty examples.

What wanderings, what changes have these books witnessed since they left the primitive presses that printed them! I know how Fisher treasured them, idealized them, and cared for them. It is growing increasingly difficult to get together such works as the years go on. Their number in the nature of things is decreasing, for they are of perishable materials and the number of those who value them and seek for them is increasing. To me, one of those ancient tomes, with its thick white paper, its Gothic letter columns, its rubricated capitals, its illuminated title page, its sides of solid oak, its cover of embossed hogskin, and its clasps of brass, is as instructive, as attractive, and as precious as is a cathedral to an architect, a great bridge to an engineer, or a cataract or mountain peak to a lover of nature.

### Early Medical Books.

It will be remembered that the date of the first use of movable type for printing was about 1455. The earliest medical books printed began to appear fifteen years later, 1470, in which year there appears to have been printed four medical books.

First, that which is of especial interest to Anglo-Saxon scholars, because it was from the press of William Caxton, the first English printer while he was still living in Cologne, and because it was by an English author, was the book of Glanville (Bartholomæus de Glanvilla Anglicus), an English monk. This book was known by the title "De Proprietatibus Rerum," which are the first few words of the descriptive title, *viz*: "The Properties of Things Very Useful and Profitable to the Human Body, that is to say, the virtues and properties of artificial waters, of herbs, of the nativity of men and women according to the signs of the zodiac, and many receipts against disease. Also a remedial ointment against the pestilential fever and other material approved by many doctors of medicine. Also, there is added at the end a very useful medicine, called 'The Medicine of Horses and Other Beasts.'"

This book was many times reprinted during the succeeding twenty-five years. It was translated into English and printed by Wynkyn de Worde, and was one of the first books printed upon paper made in England. At the end of this English translation occurs the following reference to the first edition:
"and also of your charyte call to remembraunce the soule of William Caxton first pryter of this boke in laten tong at Coleyn hyself to avance that every well disposed man may thereon loke."

Before the year 1,500 there were thirty-three editions of this book issued.

The second book was the "Arzneybuch" of Ortolff von Bayrlandt, printed at Augsburg by Gunter Zainer.

The third was a treatise on the Plague by Valescus de Tarenta, of which several editions followed in quick succession. There is in the Kings County Library a copy of the book of de Glanville, of the edition of 1485.

The fourth of these earliest books printed was upon the art of dying well: "Ars Bene Moriendi," "Tractatus brevis ac valde utilis de arte & scientia bene morient." The author is not known, but one of the earlier editions bears the name of Mathieu of Cracovie, Bishop of Worms. In several editions translated in Italian, the book is accredited to Dominique de Capranica, Cardinal and Bishop of Fermo, but it is probable that this Italian prelate was only the translator. About the first printed edition known was issued at Strasburg in 1470. Of this there is a copy in the Kings County Library, being the earliest printed book in that collection.

In general medicine the Arabic authors were among the first

to be put into type. The year 1471 witnessed the printing of the books of Albucasis, Rhazes, Mesne, and Maimonides, in 1472, Avicenna, and in 1473 Serapion. The wonderful vogue of Avicenna is shown by the fact that before the end of the century forty-three editions of the book had been printed. Fifteenth century copies of all of these authors excepting Maimonides are in the Kings County Library.

Shortly following the appearance of the first editions of these Arabic authors appeared an immense folio by a professor of medicine in the University of Ferrara, Giovanni Michele Savanarola, treating of "all of the diseases of the human body from the head to the feet." This was published in 1486, and is a most interesting example of early typography and binding. A fine copy of it is in this Library. In its teachings it followed closely the Arabic authors.

Of the great classical authors, Hippocrates, Galen, and Celsus, the latter first was put into print in 1478. A copy of this edition is in my own personal library. A second edition appeared in 1481, and of this there is a copy in the Kings County Library. Fragments of Hippocrates and of Galen began to appear in the eighties, but it was not until 1525 for Galen, and 1526 for Hippocrates, that the Venetian house of Aldus gave to the world the magnificent *editio princeps* of these two authors. The Aldine Galen of 1525 is one of the treasures of the County Library.

In anatomy, the book of Mundinus, which had been circulated in manuscript since it was written, in 1326, was first put into type in 1478. A copy of an edition of Mundinus of about 1483 is in the Library. Other editions of Mundinus quickly followed. One of the most celebrated is that which appeared in the collection published by Johannus de Ketham, which is of special note for the reason that it is the first book in which any attempt at anatomical illustration was contained. A de Ketham of the year 1500 is in the Library.

In surgery, the books of William of Saliceto, Peter Argelata and of Guy de Chauliac received early printing, de Chauliac in 1473, Saliceto in 1474, and Argelata in 1480. Of these de Chauliac had the greater vogue, some twenty-three editions, of which were printed in various languages before the close of the century. Among the manuscripts which were early reproduced in type, none was more sought for than the "Regimen Sanitatis Salerni." The first edition of this appears to have been published in 1472. Then followed in quick succession many others, so that the total number before the end of the century had reached fifty-five known editions. It is said that in the course of years more than 250 editions of this little book have been published, and of these, more than 100 are in the Library of the Medical Society of the County of Kings.

# THE VALUE OF BLOOD CULTURE IN THE DIAGNOSIS OF INFECTIOUS DISEASE.

## By Francis A. Hulst, A.M., M.D.

Pathologist to the Brooklyn Hospital, St. Mary's and St. Catherine's Hospitals, Brooklyn, N. Y.

THE bacteriology of the blood in infectious disease was one of the early fields of investigation in the realms of germ pathology, and the presence of certain bacteria in the circulation was demonstrated soon after the discovery of pathogenic micro-organisms. The isolated cases of this earlier period were rare and the failures were many, which led to the belief that a bacteræmia was a comparatively rare phenomenon. This view is attributable to an imperfect technique which has been gradually improved until we are approaching a degree of accuracy which renders blood cultures one of the most reliable methods of diagnosis, and is teaching us that bacteræmia is not a rare phenomenon, but the rule in many infectious diseases, especially early in their course.

In taking up the discussion of this subject, I make no claim of adding anything material to what is already known. It is rather my intention to present a summary of the work done in this field and point out the present status of the blood culture in diagnosis as established by those who have made elaborate studies in a variety of cases, and to emphasize its value as a routine in clinical pathology. While there are doubtless errors of technic and a lack of uniformity of methods still existing, results are becoming more constant and the value of these examinations cannot be ignored by the clinician, not only as important diagnostic aids, but also of therapeutic significance. There can no longer be any doubt of the efficacy of bacterial vaccines in certain classes of infectious diseases. The discovery of the infecting organism in the blood of the patient indicates the nature of the stock vaccine to be given in case the severity of the infection precludes an autogenous vaccine because of the time required in its preparation, or gives a pure culture from which an autogenous one may be made.

*Sepsis.*—It is in the diseases caused by the usual pyogenic cocci in cases, where general sepsis has intervened, that blood cultures have been most used. It is also in this class of cases that there is a great divergence of results as obtained by different men. Spassokukotzki (1) reporting from work done in a St. Petersburg hospital in 1910 finds in bacteriological examination in 81 cases of surgical infections characterized by local infective processes that a bacteræmia is the rule. He finds that acute osteomyelitis is a general infection with localization in the bone marrow. Staphylococcus was found in the blood in each of 23 cases examined. Erysipelas is a general infection with localization in the skin and subcutaneous tissue, bacteræmia soon subsiding. Streptococci were found in all but 2 of 29 cases examined by blood culture and in these two the staphylococcus was found. Cannon (2) in 1893, finds 40 per cent. positive out of 70 cases of sepsis, pyræmia and osteomyelitis, when the blood was taken a few hours post mortem, and 11 out of 17 cases when taken during life.

In contrast with these are the findings of Kraus (2) who reports 88 cases in which streptococci and staphylococci were found only 17 times. In another series of 104 cases in which the blood was drawn directly into the medium, 12 positive results were obtained. Kunnau (2) taking 10 cc. of blood from a vein through a cannula directly into the medium reports only 6 positive out of 121 cases. Blood obtained by the older method of finger puncture gave a considerably higher percentage of positive results for staphylococci. Czerniewski (2) in 1888, made 370 blood cultures in 37 cases of puerperal sepsis in which but 15 tubes in 10 cases showed any growth. White (4) in 1889 studied 18 cases and made 37 blood cultures of which only 4 were positive, 3 of streptococcus and one of staphylococcus. All positive cultures were late and earlier attempts were failures. He believes that the value of blood cultures in the diagnosis of "cryptogenetic sepsis" has been much over estimated. Positive results are interesting and remove suspicion that surrounds autopsy findings because of the possible agonal or terminal infections.

Such a difference of results and opinions as shown here is significant only of men and methods. The more uniform results of later workers cannot help but emphasize this point. A great variety of methods have been attempted both in the drawing of the blood and in the manner of innoculating the media. One fault in the earlier work was the small dilution of the blood in cultures. As an instance of the later results, Van Eisenberg (3) in 156 cases of sepsis finds bacteria in the blood before death in 77 cases. The organisms encountered were streptococcus, straphylococcus, pneumococcus, gonococcus and bacillus coli communis. Others in small series of cases report from 70 per cent. to 100 per cent. positive results.

Puerperal sepsis is still sufficiently common to deserve a special word in this connection. While infection during the lying-in period is pretty well guarded by modern aseptic precautions, when such a misfortune does occur, it is a matter of great concern to both the patient and the physician. It is important to know the source, extent and nature of the infection. It may be difficult from the symptoms to tell whether the woman is suffering from a severe toxemia from a purely local infection, or from a bacteriemia, or from both. The combined examination of the blood and the endometrium by carefully taken cultures are reliable in ascertaining these facts which in themselves make your diagnosis, and, as has been pointed out, may suggest the treatment by vaccines.

Evans (6) reports a series of 90 cases of postpartum pyrexis studied by blood culture and otherwise. Fifty-two of these cases were attended by a bacteriemia, and in these 94 per cent. gave positive cultures on the first examination, and the others became positive on subsequent examination, making 100 per cent. positive results. In 8 of these cases, the cultures showed Bacillus typhosus, surely an important bit of information to be learned as early as possible. In other cases studied which gave negative results from the blood, definite causes were found for the febrile disturbances such as malaria, scarlet fever, stitch abscess, breast abscess, or other local inflammation determined by clinical manifestations or by intrauterine and vaginal cultures.

It has been questioned whether or not the staphylococci can be found in the blood before death. Some claim that when it is found in the cultures, it is due to a contamination from the skin. Libman (7) gives a report of 23 cases in which the staphylococcus pyogenes aureus was isolated from the blood in cultures which were proved to be specific by identification of the same organisms either post mortem or in other lesions during life. Of these cases, 13 were osteomyelitis, 3 general sepsis, 1 carbuncle, 1 cellulitis, 2 endocarditis and 3 abscesses. In

330 other cases, he never found a colony of aureus. The same writer gives a review of 700 blood cultures in a very complete and interesting paper well worth the study of all clinicians (8). In speaking of the findings in some surgical conditions, he notes that there is high percentage of positive results in the diseases of the pelvic organs, especially in obstetric cases, in which the organism usually present is the streptococcus. Of intra-abdominal infections, viz., cholecystitis, appendicitis (including anærobic cultures), and peritonitis all blood cultures were negative.

*Pneumonia.*—Some interesting reports are found in the literature on the results of blood cultures in the course of lobar pneumonia. Straus and Clough (9) report 25 cases, of which 14 showed the pneumococcus in the cultures. Of the positive cases, 7 were repeated after the crisis or during lysis and all were negative. Of the 11 negative cases, 4 were taken the day of the crisis and 3 the day before the crisis; 2 were unusually mild and 2 others were even more severe than any of those which gave positive cultures. Fluid media was used such as broth, milk and Wein's "10 per cent. peptone and 2 per cent. glucose water." As soon as growths were observed transfers were made to solid media. Growth was usually evident in 18 hours. Dilutions were made 1 to 10 and 1 to 75. Rosenow (10) found 91 per cent. positive in a series of 175 cases. He used broth diluting the blood 1 to 50 or 1 to 75. He found positive results 12 hours after the initial chill before there were any symptoms in the lungs. Kingsley (11) finds 12 per cent. when mixing 8 or 9 cc. of blood with 50 cc. of bouillon, and 76 per cent. positive, when diluting the blood 1 to 20. Cole (12) in 1901 found, but nine cases positive out of 30 and all these were fatal cases. He used higher dilutions of the blood in litmus milk. Prochaska (13) reports 100 per cent. positive in 40 cases examined. Wolf (14) finds that in 16 cases that were positive before the crisis that 6 were also positive after the crisis. Of these 3 were in uncomplicated cases, and 3 in cases of delayed resolution, 7, 16, and 17 days after the fall of the temperature. White (4) made 32 cultures in 19 cases and found but 3 positive and all of these were late in the disease.

It seems to be the experience of most of the observers that pneumonia is characterized by a bacteriemia early in the disease which afterwards disappears, but may remain in severe or complicated cases.

*Typhoid Fever.*—Some of the most interesting work, as well as most valuable from the standpoint of diagnosis is that of the blood culture in relation to typhoid fever. What we were taught in the text books regarding the rarity with which typhoid bacilli reach the blood has been proven to be quite erroneous. A bacillemia is the rule, and probably is present in all cases but may not persist after the second week. It is most marked in the first week. The bacilli are recovered from the blood with comparative ease. The blood does not require large dilution and the organisms grow readily on most media. However, some special media have been introduced and claims have been been made for their superiority in the cultivation of bacillus typhosus. There are two bile media, one introduced by Conradi consisting of ox-gall, glycerine and peptone, the other introduced by Kayser consisting of pure ox-gall. Epstein (15) introduces another medium. On the ground that the principal advantage of the bile is to prevent clotting of the blood, he has tried with equally good results a solution of sodium chlorid and ammonium oxylate in distilled water. Blood to the amount of 10 cc. is taken in a test tube or flask with an equal amount of the saline solution, shaken well and incubated. In bile cultures, the method has been to add 2.5 cc. of blood to 5 cc. of the medium and shake well. In a limited experience with the bile mixtures, I have found little advantage over broth media, except that in using the clot from a Widal tube or blood taken from the finger instead of the vein, the bile has a tendency to control contaminations.

Coleman and Buxton (16) have reviewed 1602 cases including 123 of their own and find that 75 per cent. gave positive results. This percentage does not fully indicate the value of the test for diagnostic purposes. The highest percentages will always be found in the first week, when the Widal reaction is negative, or positive in only a small per cent. of the cases. As will be seen from some of the reports which will be reviewed, the two methods of diagnosis of typhoid fever, viz., the Widal reaction and the blood culture complement each other and may be made simultaneously.

In the 1602 cases of Coleman and Buxton referred to, 89 per cent. were positive in the first week, 73 per cent. in the second week, 60 in the third week and 39 in the fourth week. From this they diminish in frequency giving 26 per cent. in all cases after the fourth week. Epstein (17) reports 158 cases using 11 different kinds of media, with a view of determining their relative efficiency. He finds the highest percentage of positive results in his ammonium oxylate mixture (92 per cent.), the next highest in glucose bouillon (81.4 per cent.), and the next in plain bouillon (75 per cent.) He gets less than 60 per cent. positive on either of the bile media. He also finds that the first week shows 88.6 per cent. positive cultures and 28.5 per cent. positive Widals, the second week 88.5 per cent. positive cultures and 63.5 per cent. positive Widals, the third week 60 per cent. positive cultures and 86 per cent. positive Widals, and so on through subsequent weeks, the percentage of cultures drops as the percentage of Widals rises. Joslin and Overlander (18) using bile media find 21 positive out of 30 cases, 100 per cent. positive in tht first week and rapidly dropping from that. Kayser (19) has divided his cases, according to their severity and tried to show that a higher per cent. of positive results were obtained in the very severe cases, viz., 78 per cent., that what he calls severe cases, 76 per cent. positive and medium 61 per cent. and mild 42 per cent. Peabody (20) in two series of cases aggregating 115 cases reports the same general results, finding 100 per cent. positive in the first week. He also reports positive results in 4 cases of relapse. Todd (21) in 23 cases and Ruchland (22) in 49 cases report similar findings. Lyons (23) has used the clot from Widal tubes placing it in a bile medium, and finds 100 per cent. positive, all of which were also positive by the ordinary method. Others have reported gratifying results from this simple method. My own experience with this procedure in the few cases in which I have tried it has tended to discourage its use.

The value of the foregoing work may be more readily appreciated when summarized in tables as follows:

Review of 1412 cases showing cultures by week.

| | Cases. | Positive Culture. | | |
|---|---|---|---|---|
| 1st Week .......... | 276 | 247 | or | 89.5 P. C. |
| 2d Week ........... | 630 | 466 | or | 74 |
| 3d Week .......... | 371 | 234 | or | 63 |
| 4th Week .......... | 135 | 32 | or | 25 |
| | 1412 | 979 | · | 69.3 P. C. |

Review of 333 cases, showing relation of positive cultures to positive Widals.

| | Cases. | Positive Widal. | Positive Culture. |
|---|---|---|---|
| 1st Week ...... | 52 | 19 or 36.5 P. C. | 47 or 90.4 P. C. |
| 2d Week ...... | 146 | 104 or 71.2 | 113 or 78.8 |
| 3d Week ...... | 103 | 81 or 78.6 | 56 or 54.3 |
| 4th Week ...... | 32 | 25 or 78.1 | 17 or 53.1 |
| | 333 | 229    68.7 P. C. | 233    70.0 P. C. |

During the past few months, I have been called upon to make 79 blood cultures in the course of routine laboratory work.* The method employed is to take from 5 to 10 cc. of blood from a superficial vein and mix thoroughly with a broth medium immediately. There are two ways by which this has been accomplished, one by a syringe and the other by drawing the blood directly into the medium. For the latter the broth is sterilized in a filtering flask which has a small side neck to which a catheter rubber is attached. A suitable needle is attached to the other end of the rubber and covered with a small test tube. The mouth of the flask is properly stoppered. Such a flask may be kept several days and is always ready for use. After the needle has entered the vein, suction may be made at the mouth of the flask to accelerate the flow. A disadvantage of this is that the amount of blood drawn is but roughly estimated. In using the syringe one may draw a definite amount of blood and divide it into such media as he sees fit. For collecting blood outside of the hosptal, I have found it convenient to draw the blood into a large tube containing an equal amount of ammonium oxylate solution. The blood may then be taken to the laboratory and diluted as desired. One of the superficial veins at the bend of the elbow is usually selected as most convenient. The skin is thoroughly cleansed and sterilized. It is seldom necessary to cut through the skin. The needle is easily plunged into the vein which is made prominent by drawing a soft rubber catheter about the upper part of the arm and holding it with an artery clamp.

Of the 79 cases which I have examined, 37, or 46.8 per cent. were positive. These represent a variety of cases. The streptococcus was isolated 18 times, the staphylococcus pyogenes aureus 5 times and the bacillus typhosus 14 times. The pyogenic organisms were found in puerperal sepsis, septic arthritis, endocarditis, osteomyelitis and cellulitis.

Cultures for the diagnosis of typhoid fever were made in 29 instances, 5 of which proved later not to have typhoid fever. Of the remaining 24, 14, or 58.75 per cent. were positive. According to the period and result of Widal reaction the results were as follows:

---

* Since reading this paper 94 other blood cultures have been taken. 25 cases of typhoid fever gave 19 positive results. Of the 6 negative cases 3 were after the third week, and no absolute diagnosis was made on 2 others. Of 8 cases of pneumonia only 3 were positive. Of the remaining 61 where a bacteriemia was suspected for various causes, 39 were negative. Of these many were of endocarditis and acute arthritis, nearly all of which were negative. The positive cases showed 9 streptococcus, 7 staphylococcus aureus, 3 staphylococcus albus and 1 bacillus coli communis.

|           | Cases. | Widal.    | Cultures. |
|-----------|--------|-----------|-----------|
| 1st Week ............ | 7 | 28 P. C. | 71 P. C. |
| 2d Week ............. | 8 | 62 | 62 |
| 3d Week ............. | 6 | 83 | 50 |
| Later ............... | 3 | 66 | 33 |

*Conclusions.*—Bacteriemia is the rule in most acute infections and may be made a means of accurate diagnosis in a typical case, when cultures from the blood are properly taken and carefully cared for. The finding of positive results under such circumstances is of absolute value from a diagnostic standpoint, and in the case of pyogenic organisms is of therapeutic value in relation to vaccine treatment. The finding of negative results does not preclude a bacteriemia, but the methods now employed make the blood culture one of the most reliable means of laboratory diagnosis.

1249 Dean Street.

REFERENCES.

1. Spassokukotzky., Abs. in *Jour. A. M. A.*, Jan. 1, 1910, p. 88.
2. Cannon. Quoted by White. *Jour. Exp. Med.*, May, 1889, p. 425.
3. Van Eisenberg. Quoted by Rosenberger, *Am. Jour. Med. Sci.*, 1903, p. 246.
4. White. *Jour. Exp. Med.*, May, 1889, p. 425.
5. Kahn. *Med. Record*, 1903, Je. 17.
6. Evans. *Wis. Med. Jour.*, Mar., 1911, p. 591.
7. Libman. *Med. News*, 1903, p. 733.
8. Libman. *Johns Hopkins Hosp. Bul.*, Ju., 1906, p. 215
9. Straus and Clough. *Ibid.*, Aug., 1910.
10. Rosenow. *Jour. Inf. Dis.*, 1904, p. 280.
11. Kingsley. *Jour. A. M. A.*, 1905, p. 871.
12. Cole. *Johns Hopkins Hosp. Bul.*, 1902.
13. Prochaska. Quoted by Straus and Clough (9).
14. Wolf. *Jour. Inf. Dis.*, 1903, p. 446.
15. Epstein. *Am. Jour. Med. Sci.*, Sept., 1907.
16. Coleman and Buxton. *Ibid.*, Ju., 1907.
17. Epstein. *Ibid.*, 1908, p. 190.
18. Joslin and Overlander. *Boston Med. and Surg. Iour.*, 1908, p. 667.
19. Kayser. Quoted by above (18).
20. Peabody. *Arch. Int. Med.*, Feb., 1908, p. 149.
21. Peabody. *Jour. A. M. A.*, 1908, p. 979.
22. Todd. *Ibid.*, Mar. 5, 1910, p. 755.
23. Ruchland. *Wis. Med. Jour.*, Mar., 1911, p. 597.
24. Rosenberger. *Am. Jour. Med. Sci.*, 1903, p. 234.
25. Libman and Celler. *Ibid.*, Sept., 1909.
26. Libman and Celler. *Ibid.*, Oct., 1910.

# THE TOXEMIAS OF PREGNANCY.*

## By Victor A. Robertson, M.D.,

of Brooklyn, N. Y.

THERE can be no doubt that in most of the cases of pregnancy that come under our observation we have to consider a pathological condition in which many toxic symptoms may occur. We must discard our old ideas that many of the discomforts and unpleasant symptoms that may arise may be neglected or belittled because reproduction is a natural and essential function. The morning sickness, headache, nervous irritability, and later, traces of albumin in the urine and perhaps slight edemas, indicate toxic influences at work from which every pregnant woman must be guarded.

When we consider the additional strain laid upon the excretory functions, due not only to the maternal metabolism, but the fœtal as well, we can understand why it is that women who enjoy good health at other times suffer during pregnancy from an auto-intoxication or toxemia.

In no branch of medicine can an incompetent practitioner do more harm, yet obstetrics is not taken as seriously as it should be, and every physician should realize that alarming complications can arise at any time in patients apparently in a normal condition.

It was formerly very generally accepted that the fundamental and predominant lesion in the toxemias and eclamptic conditions in pregnancy was a nephritis with consequent failure of kidney function. Renal changes, it is true, as evidenced by albumin and casts during life and inflammatory conditions in the kidney at autopsy, have been found, but when compared to more marked changes in other organs they could only be considered not as the characteristic lesions, but secondary to those in the liver. Pathological alterations in the liver that were constant and characteristic have been identified by many observers so that we can consider the toxemia of pregnancy to be largely due to impaired hepatic function or hepato-toxemia. The main feature of this condition is an alteration or perversion of the normal functions of the liver, which fails to destroy or oxidize certain poisonous products of metabolism passing through it. Later, secondary renal changes occur, which in turn lead to further retention of toxic products, and thus a vicious circle is formed.

Although the etiology and pathogenesis of the toxemias of pregnancy are still to some degree in dispute, they may be divided into, *first,* toxic vomiting; *second,* acute yellow atrophy of the liver; *third,* nephritic toxemia; *fourth,* pre-eclamptic toxemia, and *fifth,* eclampsia.

## Toxic Vomiting.

The persistent vomiting of pregnancy, although occasionally reflex in character due to an incarcerated retroflexed uterus or some other abnormality, is in the vast majority of cases toxic in character. Examination of the urine should be carefully made. Basing our diagnosis on the presence of albumin and casts is not enough, as at times they may be absent. The urea output is of vastly more importance, and not merely the urea percentage, but the whole nitrogen partition should be determined, which should contain the proper proportion of the nitrogen compounds, especially urea nitrogen and ammonia nitro-

---

* Read before the *Brooklyn* Pathological Society, October 10, 1912.

gen, which are normally 75 per cent. and 5 per cent., respectively. Creatinin and the purin bodies are about 4 per cent., leaving the remainder of undetermined nitrogen.

In toxic states the ammonia nitrogen may rise to ten or even forty per cent. Williams considers the presence of 10 per cent. ammonia nitrogen an imperative indication for the induction of abortion. Still further morbid constituents of the urine to be looked for are indican, acetone and diacetic acid. This brings us to the consideration of another pathological state in the toxic vomiting of pregnancy of which several cases have recently come under my observation, and that is, the acidosis of pregnancy.

The urinary findings in this condition are misleading if only albumin and casts are looked for. There may be no evidences of renal irritation, but heavy reactions for acetone and diacetic acid are always present. In the process of normal metabolism a number of acid products are formed as intermediary substances that undergo further oxidation. Some of these acid bodies, as, for instance, carbonic acid, are eliminated by the lungs; others, such as phosphoric, sulphuric, hydrochloric and uric acids, through the kidneys, never as free acids, but always combined with alkalies. The alkali lost is replaced by the ingestion of food and in addition the body possesses a reserve supply of alkali in the blood. Acid intoxication ensues whenever there is increased production of acid products with reduced excretion from some retardation or perversion of normal oxidation. Following this as a natural sequence we find a reduced alkalinity of the blood and the appearance in the urine of acids and acid bodies not normally found or present only in small quantities.

The acids that may be considered are many, but more particularly oxybutyric acid and its oxidation products of acetone and diacetic acid. Oxybutyric acid has a large share in producing the intoxication that occurs in other disturbed metabolic conditions, notably diabetes. It is also found in starvation states in various poisonings, after anæsthesia in acute yellow atrophy of the liver and in puerperal eclampsia. Its occurrence in diabetes is dependent on two factors, the removal of carbohydrates from the dietary and the ingestion of too much proteid and excessive use of fats.

We can readily see the method of its production in pernicious vomiting, as there is failure of the stomach to retain food with consequent carbohydrate starvation and the organism is compelled to oxydize large amounts of the bodily fat. This suggests the rationale of the successful treatment of this condition by the use of carbohydrate feeding and some of the sugar yielding foods, and even sugar itself.

This pathological state of acidisis in pregnancy is well borne out in the history of a patient under my observation a year ago.

The patient comes of an ancestry showing marked metabolic defects. Her mother and two maternal aunts are diabetics and her father suffers from gout. She is the mother of five children, the writer having been the accoucheur in the last four deliveries. Last year she returned to town, pregnant one month.

In former pregnancies nausea and vomiting always began a few days after conception and persisted more or less through the whole period. These symptoms were, however, somewhat amenable to treatment and were never so uncontrollable as seriously to interfere with nutrition. However, in this pregnancy the vomiting was persistent and soon became pernicious in character and controlled by no form of medication.

No physical abnormality such as a misplacement of the uterus or other morbid condition of the genitalia was present.

The urine was examined but nothing suggestive was found as it was limited to an examination for albumin and casts which were absent and the urea output was normal in amount. As this vomiting was uncontrollable and had lasted several weeks the patient became much reduced in strength and as her condition became more critical the termination of the pregnancy by abortion was suggested and consent given.

At this juncture the writer returned from his vacation and another examination of the urine was made which showed the following urinary output for 24 hours: 36 ounces; spec. gravity, 1019; highly acid; 8.4 grains urea to the ounce; no sugar; faint trace of albumin; no casts; decided reaction for indican and an extremely heavy reaction for acetone. The next day the findings were practically the same with the additional presence of a marked trace of diacetic acid.

The therapeutic indications being plain, stomach lavage with large quantities of a soda bicarbonate solution was employed, accompanied with colonic flushings with the same solution. Large amounts of lactose by the mouth and enemata were also given. The vomiting quickly came under control, ceased entirely on the third day, and the patient's subsequent history was uneventful.

At times during the pregnancy when slight symptoms of nausea appeared, they always yielded to the alkaline treatment. The urine became alkaline within 24 hours after beginning treatment and was free from abnormal acid products in a few days. Delivery was normal at full term.

### Acute Yellow Atrophy of the Liver.

Acute yellow atrophy or malignant jaundice in pregnancy is a rare disease. It has never come under my personal observation. Jaundice with vomiting and diminished volume of the liver are characteristic symptoms. The urine is bile stained and contains albumin and casts. The urea is markedly decreased, with an increased nitrogen ammonia. Acetone in large amounts is also found. Leucin and tyrosin may be present.

Treatment is practically *nil.* Efforts should be made to eliminate toxins by purgatives and colonic flushing. Attempts to control the vomiting are usually futile.

### Nephritic Toxemia.

Nephritic toxemia is found in pregnancy, but in the writer's experience is in many cases secondary to the toxic liver states already described. In some cases it is associated with a pre-existing chronic renal lesion which becomes aggravated by the pregnant state. In this condition headache, visual disturbances, edema of face and ankles, high tension pulse, with increasing amounts of albumin and casts, are present. Toxic vomiting is not a prominent symptom. The nitrogen partition may be normal. Uremic poisoning occasionally develops and the fœtus dies and is expelled prematurely. A restricted diet with eliminative measures is usually followed by a lessening of the symptoms. If the albumin increases and the urea decreases in amount, with the appearance of eclamptic symptoms, the induction of premature labor is indicated.

### Pre-eclamptic Toxemia.

The pre-eclamptic toxemias occur generally in the latter months of pregnancy. The symptoms may be slight or there may be profound intoxication. The urinary output may be greatly diminished, with the appearance of albumin and casts. In milder cases the total nitrogen content may vary little from the normal, but in the severe types there may be a decrease of the urea nitrogen with an increase of the ammonia nitrogen. Under appropriate treatment the toxic condition may be controlled by eliminative measures as indicated in toxic vomiting states. Prophylactic treatment is not always successful and the condition may lead into the fifth division of toxemias, *viz.*:

## Eclampsia.

Eclamptic convulsions may appear without warning, but in the majority of cases premonitory symptoms of the pre-eclamptic state are present. The toxic symptoms of edema, headache, nausea, vomiting, nervous instability and visual disturbances precede the attack. The urine is diminished in quantity; albumin casts and decreased urea output are present. In some cases the urine may appear normal, casts and albumin being absent, but the disturbed nitrogen partition with a low urea nitrogen and a high ammonia nitrogen give warning of the toxic state. In addition, the acetone bodies are frequently found.

Still another condition bearing on the toxemia of pregnancy can be considered and that is, disturbed thyroid function. We know there is a physiological hypertrophy of the thyroid during the parturient state. It is due to the increased activity of the gland to influence the additional metabolism of the liver necessitated by pregnancy. When this normal enlargement fails toxic conditions are apt to develop. When, on the contrary, hyperthyroidism, such as is found in Graves disease, develops, metabolic disturbances also take place. We are as yet in ignorance as to the exact role this ductless gland plays in metabolism, but it has been suggested that the addition of thyroid material to the circulation stimulates glandular activity and also produces antibodies.

## Conclusions.

All these toxic states in pregnancy insensibly merge one into another and several of them may be operating at one time, and successful treatment should be largely prophylactic. Owing to the frequency of renal and hepatic lesions the urine should be frequently examined, not in a perfunctory manner, but to a degree of thoroughness that will determine not only the absence or presence of albumin and casts, but the urea ratio, the nitrogen partition, indican, acetone and diacetic acid.

Some criticism has been raised as to efficacy of laboratory methods of investigation. These should not be used to the *exclusion* of the physical examination, but as affording a valuable means of adding to our information in any given case, and should *always* be *co-related* with the bedside methods of diagnosis of the clinician.

We must not relax in physical methods of diagnosis or fail to remain acute observers of all the objective signs of disease, and give *all* the findings in every case due consideration.

Treatment in toxic vomiting is rest, lavage with large quantities of soda bicarbonate solution, dextrose or lactose by mouth and enemata, colonic flushing and a non-proteid diet. In pre-eclamptic states dietitic and eliminative measures may be used. When convulsions appear, the pregnancy should be terminated, the method of delivery being dependent on the period of pregnancy and the condition of the cervix, which determines whether it should be dilated by manual traction, incision, dilating bags or nature, supplemented by version or forceps. Cesarian section or vaginal hysterotomy may also be indicated.

# PATHOLOGICAL CONDITIONS WHICH ARISE DURING PREGNANCY AND WHICH JUSTIFY ABORTION.*

## By O. Paul Humpstone, M.D.,

### of Brooklyn, N. Y.

THE indications for therapeutic abortion are undergoing a revision these days in the light of the advances of the pathology of pregnancy. Alas, in the morally weak minds of many of the profession this revision has come to include sociologic and economic indications which are contrary to the laws of nature and the state, and contrary to the best interests of the home, the nation, and civilization.

Therapeutic abortion is the induction of abortion by a physician to save the life of the mother, and is only to be accomplished after consultation has carefully considered the dangers and determined its necessity. Conservative as we should be in meeting this problem, it is not to be forgotten that we may be too conservative, and wait too long until abortion will not save our patient, and this applies particularly to pathological conditions which are directly due to pregnancy.

These are some of the more serious manifestations of the toxemia of pregnancy, the exact cause of which we do not know but now fully believe to be either some toxin obtained from the fetal or placental metabolism affecting the normal maternal metabolism; or else some disturbance of the maternal metabolism, most probably in the ductless glands, which makes the maternal excretion of the normal fetal products of metabolism impossible. This toxin has a most marked effect on the liver, on the entire nervous system, the kidneys, the heart and the blood vessels. These pathological effects being manifest clinically by persistent vomiting, continued high blood pressure, loss of flesh, muscular weakness, various psychoses, diminished urine with its disturbed protein excretion. Any one of these symptoms may demand abortion.

Persistent vomiting, when associated with a pulse rising to 100 or over and a little fever, and rapid loss of flesh, is an absolute indication for abortion; and it is to be remembered that it is very easy to make the mistake of carrying these patients too far before relieving them. If the vomiting does not cease after ten days of suitable treatment and the pulse is 100 or over, no time is to be lost. These cases are to be carefully differentiated from the malingering hysterical cases of vomiting.

Continued high blood pressure, over 150, if associated with dyspnea and renal insufficiency and not responding in a few days to suitable treatment, is another absolute indication.

Muscular weakness increasing with the associated pains of a developing multiple neuritis, especially if there is present any psychosis, is an absolute indication; on the other hand, any increasing psychosis, even though there be absent any signs of the involvment of the peripheral nerves, is an indication.

Last of these toxic causes is the rare type of nerve affection, chorea gravidarum, which is an absolute indication.

Besides the toxic causes, we have two other causes directly attributable to the pregnancy itself which demand immediate abortion.

---

* Read before the Brooklyn Pathological Society, October 10, 1912.

The one, an incarcerated retrodisplaced pregnant uterus, caught beneath the sacrum, which cannot be reduced under anæsthesia. The other, an acute hydramnios in the early months of pregnancy, with its associated cardiac insufficiency.

The second class of cases demanding immediate abortion are those in whom exists some disease which would be aggravated to the point of endangering life if pregnancy continued, and in which we may hope to considerably prolong life by ending pregnancy. We include in this class heart disease, kidney disease, tuberculosis.

*Heart disease* complicating pregnancy always presents a problem demanding the closest of observation and the keenest of judgment. Views on this question vary, from abortion for every case of heart disease, to the opposite opinion that abortion is never indicated in heart disease. In dealing with this question we have always to consider not only whether it is possible to carry pregnancy to viability, but also how much invalidism and shortening of life will be caused by allowing this pregnancy to continue. It is undoubtedly a fact that life will be more or less shortened by pregnancy occurring in a patient suffering from endocarditis. The patient and her husband are entitled to an opinion in this matter. Two valvular lesions are, in my opinion, absolutely indicative of abortion; the one, aortic stenosis, the other, mitral stenosis with or without insufficiency.

In cases with simple insufficiency of the valves, the most favorable cases are mitral insufficiency, when compensative hypertrophy is sufficient. These cases regularly do well. The important point to remember is, has this heart compensation been broken without pregnancy, and how many times, and how badly? If the compensation has been sufficient for ordinary health, pregnancy may be tried with the understanding that should a break in compensation occur which is not easily controlled by proper medication and rest, the immediate termination of the pregnancy is indicated.

In *chronic diffuse nephritis,* with exudation of finely and coarsely granular casts, where chronic uremic symptoms have persisted, it is out of the question to expect such damaged kidneys to be sufficient for pregnancy. The same holds true for the chronic diffuse nephritis without exudation, with its associated arterial thickening, blood pressure and weakened heart muscle.

These cases are to be sharply differentiated from cases which have had one or more attacks of acute nephritis with or without pregnancy; such cases demand the most careful of observation but are not in themselves necessarily indicative of abortion.

*Tuberculosis* is very unfavorably influenced by pregnancy. In my opinion, in any case in which active pulmonary tuberculosis is manifest early in pregnancy, abortion should be performed. In the so-called arrested cases without systemic symptoms it is, I believe, justifiable to allow pregnancy to continue unless there are evidences of the disease lighting up. In the advanced case of tuberculosis it is well to remember that the emptying of the uterus is likely to be followed by a very rapid fatal termination of the malady.

The last condition for which therapeutic abortion is indicated is not an absolute one. I refer to a pelvis so contracted as to be an absolute indication for delivery by the abdominal route. I do not believe we are justified in saying to all such women that they must go to term and have a Cesarean. Such a patient still has the right to choose between abortion and Cesarean at term, but it is our duty to influence her, everything else being equal, to carry her child.

# AFTER-TREATMENT OF OPERATIONS UPON THE THYROID GLAND.

## By Russell S. Fowler, M.D.,

Chief Surgeon, First Division, German Hospital of Brooklyn; Surgeon, Methodist Episcopal Hospital of Brooklyn, Brooklyn, New York.

*THE Primary Dressing.*—The primary dressing should be applied as for all operations on the neck requiring extensive dissection. In addition a loosely rolled compress, four inches in length by one in thickness, should be placed to either side of the trachea on the skin, to exert slight lateral pressure. In case of scabbard trachea, the retaining bandage should be reinforced by a sufficient number of turns of a plaster-of-Paris or starch bandage to ensure the retention of the neck in a straight position, otherwise the turning of the head might interfere seriously with respiration. The fixation bandage should be so placed as to allow of ready access to the wound. In exophthalmic cases, the dressing should consist of an abundance of fluffed-out gauze loosely applied and loosely bandaged in place to provide ready absorption of the discharge.

*General Rules.*—The patient is placed in bed in the elevated head and trunk position to lessen the amount of oozing and the possibility of secondary hemorrhage. The degree of elevation will depend upon the amount of shock. Murphy proctoclysis is given in all cases. It is particularly indicated in cases which have lost considerable blood and in exophthalmic cases. In exophthalmic cases, it is imperative that the tissues get water to combat the effect of the hyperthyroidism set up by the operation. In these cases, it is well to give a hypodermoclysis of 500 to 750 c. c. immediately after the operation. In case, Murphy proctoclysis is not retained on account of intestinal relaxation, repeated hypodermoclysis should be used (250 to 500 c. c. every three hours). All cases are given fluids by mouth as soon as anæsthetic vomiting has ceased and a return made to normal diet as quickly as the stomach will tolerate it. As soon as the patient is strong enough, usually at the end of twenty-four hours, the head of the bed is lowered and the patient given a back rest. At the end of the second twenty-four hours the patient is allowed out of bed in a chair and at the end of the third twenty-four hours may walk about if so inclined. In exophthalmic cases, the course is not so rapid. There is usually some rise in temperature for the first three days and in the bad cases some acceleration of pulse. The patient also complains of headache, is restless, and the sleep is interfered with. Drugs have little, if any, influence unless the cause is neurotic when morphia will aid in controlling the restlessness. Usually the cause is not free enough drainage or absorption of thyroid secretion, in spite of free drainage. The treatment is first to see that free drainage exists and in addition to force the ingestion of water. The Murphy proctoclysis is given as fast as it can be absorbed and if the symptoms persist hypodermoclysis is added, 750 to 1000 c. c. being given at first and 250 to 500 c. c. at four hour intervals. In exophthalmic cases also all sources of irritation should be avoided. If symptoms of hyperthyroidism develop, the patient should be placed in a separate quiet room with special attendants. In these cases, the entire problem resolves itself into free drainage and dilution of the toxins.

*Care of the Wound.*—There is a rise of temperature for the first few days. This is due to traumatism to the remaining portion of the gland incidental to the operation, and absorption of wound secretion.

It need occasion no alarm in any save the exophthalmic cases. In other than exophthalmic cases, packing used to control oozing or drains are removed at the end of forty-eight hours and a small drainage strip introduced. This is renewed every forty-eight hours as long as drainage continues. The character of the drainage will be straw-colored serum, becoming somewhat gelatinous as the amount decreases. Sutures are removed on the fifth day. In exophthalmic cases the dressing, except the drains, should be removed as frequently as soiled and dry fluffed out gauze loosely applied. It is important that the gauze quickly absorbs the secretion and thus aids the drains. The drains themselves (glass spools with gauze and green silk protective strip) are removed on the fourth day or as soon thereafter as the lessening of the amount of drainage permits. As long as they drain, they are not disturbed. Upon their removal green silk protective strips are substituted. These are renewed every forty-eight hours until all drainage ceases. In removing the original drain, the glass spool is first removed and on the following day, the gauze and green silk protective drain. If any retention of secretion occurs, the drain is to be immediately removed and a tube drain inserted. If, in spite of this symptoms of hyperthyroidism persist, the wound is to be opened sufficiently to ensure free drainage.

*Secondary Hemorrhage.*—This should be a rare complication if the operation has been properly planned, *i. e.,* if the thyroid vessels have been ligated as the first step in the operation and if all minute bleeding points have been secured by ligature or circumsuture. Its occurrence necessitates tamponade of the wound for forty-eight hours. The tamponade should be carefully removed and renewed to avoid recurrence of the bleeding.

*Disturbances of Respiration.*—These may be due to tracheitis from pulling upon the trachea in the course of the operation; to edema of the trachea from sudden removal of the pressure in scabbard trachea; to collapse of the trachea following removal of pressure in scabbard trachea; to occlusion of the trachea from sudden turning of the neck in scabbard trachea; to injury to the recurrent laryngeal nerve, causing paralysis of the corresponding vocal cord, resulting in aphonia, weakened voice, or foreign body pneumonia; bilateral injury to the recurrent laryngeal resulting in asphyxia. These complications are almost always preventable; gentleness in manipulation, maintenance of the head in the position in which breathing is easiest in scabbard trachea, leaving the posterior portion of the capsule intact to avoid injury to the recurrent laryngeal. In regard to laryngeal paralysis, the nerve may have been pressed upon by the enlarged thyroid and hoarseness and possibly aphonia been present before the operation. If the pressure has not been too long continued, the symptoms will gradually disappear following relief of the pressure. Paralysis and collapse of the corresponding vocal cord will follow injury to the nerve, while if both nerves are injured bilateral paralysis will result and death from asphyxia follow unless the condition is promptly recognized and tracheotomy performed. The injury to the nerve may be by section, clamp, ligature or traction in dislocating the enlarged lower lobe.

If due to clamp, ligature or traction, the resulting hoarseness will gradually disappear as the nerve resumes its function. Months may elapse before this occurs. Even if the nerve has been completely sectioned with resulting weak and hoarse voice, the condition will improve very materially, for in time the opposite vocal cord encroaches on the paralyzed cord and so lessens the gap between the two. Suture of the cut nerve has been performed with resultant restoration of function.

Care in swallowing must be exercised as a foreign-body pneumonia is apt to ensue. If these patients temporarily cannot swallow as occasionally occurs nourishment is given by stomach tube. In scabbard trachea discomfort due to the distortion of the trachea will persist for some time.

*After Care of Enucleation of Thyroid Tumors* (*adenometa and cysts*).—The wound is drained and a copious dressing applied. In this and in similar operations involving more or less traumatism to the substance of the gland, in spite of most careful hemostasis during the operation oozing will follow. If more severe hemorrhage occurs, perhaps caused by post-anæsthetic vomiting, the blood will first fill the cavity in the gland from which the tumor has been removed, and, if drainage is not free, will then extend beneath the deep fascia. In the latter event, there will be danger of asphyxia. Treatment consists in the removal of a sufficient number of sutures to permit the free escape of the effused blood.

*Escape of gland secretion* may occur in cases in which there is much tearing of the gland tissue. The secretion escapes into the tissues of the neck and forms a soft swelling in and around the gland if drainage is sufficient. If rapidly absorbed, symptoms of acute thyroidism will appear. The treatment is to open the wound and provide efficient drainage.

*Complications due to Interference with the Function of the Thyroid and Parathyroid Bodies.*—*Tetany.*—Fortunately this complication is rarely seen at the present time; formerly it was a common complication, following thyroidectomy and was thought to be due to the removal of the entire gland; but now it is known to follow only, and not necessarily always, the removal of the entire gland; but now it is known to follow only, and not necessarily always, the removal of the parathyroid bodies.

When this fact became recognized, the technic of thyroidectomy was improved to safeguard the parathyroids by leaving the outer and posterior portion of the capsule. According to the latest statistics, the complication now occurs in less than one-half of one per cent. of cases; even this for a preventable complication would seem high.

Tetany first makes its appearance a few days following the operation. The first symptoms usually appear in the upper extremities; a tingling or twitching of the muscles may be first noted, convulsive seizures follow, the fingers are first flexed and then rigidly contracted; the wrist and elbow are flexed and the knee and hip extended. The feet are in plantar flexion and supinated. The muscular contractures are tonic, continue for a variable length of time, and recur at intervals. The muscles of the face and neck may become involved. Formerly in about 60 per cent. of the cases death followed in a few days. The diphragmatic muscles are at times involved. The onset of this complication sometimes occurs at the end of weeks or months following the operation. If the patient survives the first few days, the tetany may rapidly subside after a duration of eight to fifteen days; in some cases, it is prolonged for months and years with remissions. Finally death results from respiratory paralysis. Occasionally a case will recover.

*Treatment.*—As soon as the first symptoms appear, the patient should be given parathyroid gland extracts; the diet should be light and low in nitrogen. Elimination should be increased by active stimulation of excretion through the skin, bowel, and kidneys. Saline infusion is useful in diluting the toxemia and increasing the elimination.

Transfusion will temporarily check the symptoms. Intravenous saline infusion acts in the same manner. Feeding with parathyroid glands and injection of parathyroid emulsion temporarily and often rapidly stops the symptoms. Following any of these methods the symptoms may be held in abeyance for twenty-four hours. The use of these measures, however, will probably not prove of any permanent value, should all of the parathyroids have been removed, but if, as is conceivable, one or more of the parathyroids were removed and the remaining one traumatized during the operation, then, in the event of the development of tetany, the above mentioned measures would be of extreme value in tiding the patient over until the traumatized parathyroids resumed their function.

*Beebe's nucleo-proteid* is of value particularly when combined with parathyroid feeding; fresh ox parathyroids are used. The administration of soluble calcium salts will quickly stop severe tetanic symptoms. In a case of Halstead's in which the administration of parathyroid gland extracts had averted tetany for two years, the attacks were also averted during the third year by the use of calcium salts.

Experimental transplantation of parathyroids in animals has proved successful in about 60 per cent. of cases according to Halstead. In some of his experiments a beginning tetany was tided over by the administration of *calcium salts*. Eiselberg transplanted a parathyroid in a woman who had suffered for many years from severe tetany following parathyroid extirpation. In Kocher's experiments transplantations into the tibia are made in two stages; first the tibia is opened and a small cavity made by forcing a silver ball into the marrow; the wound is then closed. After several days, when granulations have formed the silver ball is removed and fresh gland tissue implanted in the resulting cavity. In this manner interference by hemorrhage is avoided. Kocher found that this method proved efficacious in dogs. One of his most interesting observations is that resection of the bone containing the implanted tissue quickly caused death from acute tetany.

*Myxedema* (cachexia strumipriva) develops slowly and for this reason seldom comes under the notice of the surgeon as the case has long since passed from under his observation. Only rarely does acute myxedema develop. Usually it is months before the disease is noticed. The most marked early symptom is increasing anemia. Gradually all parts of the body become affected. The skin is at first waxy and pale; later, owing to the almost complete inhibition of the sweat and sebaceous glands, the skin becomes dry and fissured. Following this, the skin becomes thick and brawny due to an edema which affects the entire body; this edema is general and does not pit upon pressure. It has no resemblance to nephritic edema and cannot be massaged away. The hair, particularly of the head and pubes, falls out. A curious fact in this connection is the growth of coarse hair in parts of the body which are normally free from hair. The body temperature is lowered, the skin is cool. In the majority of cases the pulse is slowed, though in rare instances, it may be increased. The amount of urine is diminished and its specific gravity is below normal. More marked even than the bodily changes is the change in mentality. Slowly but steadily the intelligence of these unfortunate patients disappears; the speech becomes slow and stuttering; movements become uncertain; memory is lost; the features are dull and apathetic.

The process is a slow one and may continue for years, the patient finally dying from gradually increasing cachexia.

Cases in which an accessory thyroid is present or in which a portion of the thyroid is left may present the early symptoms of myxedema, but upon the hypertrophy of the remaining thyroid tissue these symptoms will gradually disappear.

*Treatment.—Thyroid Therapy.*—Malignant disease constitutes the sole indication for the entire removal of the thyroid gland. Such cases, and in cases in which but a small portion of the gland has been left, are to be watched carefully. In the first instance, it is better to begin thyroid feeding at once; in the second as soon as it becomes apparent that the amount of thyroid tissue remaining will not be hypertrophied sufficiently to provide the secretion necessary for metabolism. By means of thyroid feeding, we may hope to avert indefinitely the changes which inevitably follow the removal of all thyroid tissue. In many cases, this treatment will prove successful. In cases in which symptoms of myxedema have already appeared, feeding will prevent an increase of the symptoms and cause their gradual disappearance. The secretions become normal, there is an increase in weight and the mentality is improved. The final condition of the patient becomes quite normal. Whether this is true in every case, it is impossible to state at the present time. The treatment must be continued indefinitely. At intervals of weeks or months, the treatment may be discontinued for a time, if there are no symptoms, in order to determine if hypertrophy of remaining thyroid tissue or accessory gland has occurred. Upon the occurrence of any symptoms treatment is to be immediately begun. Chloral hydrate is a useful adjunct to thyroid feeding. The implantation of normal thyroid tissue is the ideal treatment, but naturally presents great obstacles. The conditions necessary for success are, a fresh portion of active gland and a favorable implantation soil (Kocher). *Administration of thyroid preparation.* As the secretion of the thyroid gland in large doses is a powerful poison, care must be exercised in its administration. The dosage must be determined in the individual case. The fresh gland was formerly given twice a week, one-half a sheep thyroid at a dose, cut up raw and spread on bread. This was made more palatable by the addition of a little pepper and salt. At the present day a dried extract of the gland is prepared in tablet form. Each tablet represents five grains of the dried gland. The dose of this dried extract is one tablet given after a full meal once a day for several days; if no bad symptoms are noted a tablet may be given twice a day. The number may subsequently be increased to from three to five tablets a day. The actual strength of the extract varies according to its manufacture. A more staple preparation is thyroidin (three grains of iodin and one grain of the dried gland) or thyroid colloid, the active principle of the thyroid gland. The dose of the latter is one-half to one grain, but it is better to begin with the smaller dose and test the tolerance of the patient before giving larger doses. Should an overdose be given very alarming symptoms will arise. A single dose may prove too large or a series of moderate doses may prove cumulative. Acute thyroidism will develop. The temperature rises rapidly, the pulse becomes rapid, small and irregular; there is headache, vertigo, nausea, pains in the joints and muscular tremors. Upon the appearance of these symptoms, the drug is to be discontinued at once.

301 DeKalb Ave.

# NOTES ON TRACHEAL INSUFFLATION.*

## By William C. Woolsey, M.D.,

of Brooklyn, N. Y.

ALL apparatus so far devised for tracheal insufflation anesthesia has been costly, cumbersome and suitable for hospital use only. Elsberg's, Janeway's and Boothby's are the models generally employed and they represent patience and skill in their construction, they are perfectly efficient and solve perfectly the various mechanical problems of the anesthesia. Can we obtain satisfactory results from a simpler form of apparatus? The writer believes that we can. Tracheal insufflation anesthesia not only fulfills the demands of intrathoracic surgery, where elevated intrapulmonary pressure is a requisite factor, but is also being strongly advocated by those of experience, for general anesthesia in other fields of surgical work as well.

1. Tracheal insufflation narcosis has special virtues which recommend its selection as the anesthetic of choice in any prolonged hazardous operation where the added toxæmia of an anesthetic must be reduced to the utmost and every factor of safety conserved.

2. It is specially indicated in operations about the oral and nasal cavities where inspiration of blood and operative debris would not only hazard the patient's life but also interfere with the operator. The constant return flow of air current makes aspiration of foreign mouth contents practically impossible. See experiments of Meltzer & Githens (*J. A. M. A.*, LVII, Aug. 12, 1911) in which charcoal and purposely ejected stomach contents were made to fill the pharynx during insufflation and none entered the lung or bronchi.

Reports of five hundred cases of insufflation in man from the pen of Dr. Elsberg of Mt. Sinai Hospital, New York, and many smaller series from other hospitals in Boston and New York all go to prove the absence of harm from the introduction of the tube.

All of my hearers have recognized that the one disturbing element in a majority of narcoses has been some form of obstruction to respiration in that part of the airway between the teeth and the trachea. Collapsed alæ nasi, recedent tongue and jaw or paralyzed epiglottis are the obstructions which not only cause asphyxia but also interfere with the inspiration of sufficient ether into the lung to produce the desired anesthesia. Consequent upon this obstruction and the persistence of too superficial anesthesia the anesthetist increases the quantity of ether, raises its concentration to so high a degree that a vicious cycle of toxæmia of anesthetic and too superficial anesthesia is the result.

Tracheal insufflation anesthesia, by conveying the anesthetic vapor with an abundance of air for respiration, direct to the bronchi, does away with all obstruction to respiration and toxic dosage referred to above, and in addition to assurance of constant dosage of anesthetic independent of the respiratory act, it furnishes at all times that degree of perfect oxygenation necessary to smooth, harmless anesthesia.

Elevation of intrapulmonary pressure to forty millimeters of

---

* Read before the Brooklyn Surgical Society, March 7, 1912.

mercury is sufficient to produce relative apnœa in man, but such a degree of pressure is unnecessary and inadvisable. In ordinary intrathoracic surgery where acute pneumothorax is to be prevented, fifteen to twenty millimeters of mercury are all that is necessary. In other narcoses even as low a pressure as ten millimeters will insure proper ether dosage and proper oxygenation, the patient's own respiratory efforts being sufficiently active to prevent any carbon dioxode accumulation in the bronchi themselves or the other intrapulmonary dead space where the insufflation air current is but partially active as a means of ventilation.

Damage to lung tissue from such pressure is remote indeed if possible. The experiments of Quimby, of Boston (*Surg., Gyn. and Obst., xii,* Nov., 1910), have shown that pressure in a lung sufficient to fill the opposite plural cavity after a unilateral pneumectomy, has caused no damage to that lung. The very low pressure required in general anesthesia for other than interthoracic surgery cannot possibly cause damage.

Experiments by Prof. Yandel Henderson at the Yale physiological laboratories have demonstrated that "artifically induced hyperpnœa through a tracheal tube by means of a powerful apparatus which not only inflates but also deflates the lung at the rate of sixty to seventy respirations a minute, does not cause sufficient acapnia to induce fatal apnœa vera" (Henderson: *Amer. J. Physial.,* xxv. No. 6).

Therefore tracheal insufflation anesthesia is considered to furnish constant minimum dosage of anesthetic, insures perfect oxygenation of the blood, carries on respiration without obstruction from the dead space between the teeth and epiglottis and through its positive intrapulmonary pressure allows intrathoracic surgery, free from acute pneumothorax.

The apparatus here presented includes a nitrous oxid and oxygen attachment because the writer's experience has been directed along the line of using these gases by the tracheal insufflation route.

Nineteen cases have been thus anesthetized at Kings County and St. John's hospitals, none for actual intrathoracic surgery, but in brain cases, amputation of legs in infirm alcoholics, exsection of carotid for inoperable malignancy of mouth and neck and abdominal sections. Small amounts of ether have been used in some cases but less and less as experience proved the absolute efficiency of the nitrous and oxygen.

Details of these cases and confirmation of the actual value of the technic are held for future report and further experience.

The apparatus consists of two bottles, the first containing water, into which three delivery tubes convey the air from the foot pump, and the nitrous, and oxygen from their respective tanks. These tubes act as sight feeds, the gases bubbling through water at a rate always controlled by the valves on the tanks or the force of the pumping. In the center of the top in one bottle is the mercury manometer and safety valve which registers its twenty millimeters of mercury and then blows out, thus preventing any possible overdistention of the lung from spasm of the glottis or similar obstructive accident. After the manometer does blow out the mercury resumes its position and is ready to again register the pressure. It is one of the essential factors in a safe intracheal insufflation apparatus.

The second bottle contains the ether. A valve on its top is so arranged that the gas current can be directed all across the bottle to the tracheal tube, all through the ether or any part either way, thus allowing any desired percentage of ether to be carried into the tracheal tube or none.

The water in bottle one is hot, therefore heats, filters and moistens the insufflated gases before they reach the lung. When simple ether vapor is to be used, the foot pump supplies the pressure of air. When nitrous and oxygen are to be used the valve on the air tube is shut off and the gases flow direct from the tanks. On the nitrous tank is placed a pressure reducer, in order that freezing of valves and too great initial pressure. of gas stream may not interfere with constant flow of nitrous through the bottle.

Tracheal insufflation seems to offer an ideal field for nitrous oxid and oxygen, on account of, *first,* the elimination of all mechanical obstruction to respiration between the mouth and the trachea, *second,* the exhibition of nitrous under slight positive pressure direct to the pulmonary capillaries, *third,* the partial elimination of the diluting nitrogen of air in the lungs by the comparative apnœa present, and *fourth,* the absence of the cumbersome face mask of ordinary use.

# Announcement

## APPLICATIONS FOR MEMBERSHIP TO BE ACTED UPON AT THE JANUARY (1913) MEETING.

PROPOSED BY RUSSELL S. FOWLER.

HAROLD K. BELL, 825 President Street, Brooklyn P. & S., N. Y., 1910.

DAVID SHERMAN, 272 Ninth Street, Brooklyn, L. I. C. H., 1896.

CHRISTIAN W. JANSON, 949 Bushwick Avenue, Brooklyn, Cornell, 1902.

PROPOSED BY FRANK T. DE LANO.

CHARLES J. PFLUG, 53 Stuyvesant Avenue, Brooklyn, L. I. C. H., 1903.

PROPOSED BY JAMES COLE HANCOCK.

LE ROY P. VAN WINKLE, Amityville, L. I. C. H., 1903.

DAVID CORCORAN, Central Islip, P. & S. N. Y., 1905.

WALTER RAYMOND TERRY, 1085 Gates Avenue, Brooklyn P. & S. N. Y., 1905.

ALFRED SHIPMAN, 572 Halsey Street, Brooklyn, P. & S. Keokuk, Iowa.

WILLIAM WENDELL HALA, 763 Second Avenue, Astoria, Drake University, Maryland, 1905.

J. CARLISLE DEVRIES, 72 Van Siclen Avenue, Brooklyn, N. Y. Univ., 1905.

PAUL E. WESENBERG, Linden Avenue, Brooklyn, Vanderbilt University, 1908.

GEORGE W. HARGUT, St. James, L. I., L. I. C. H., 1887.

SAMUEL HENRY RABUCK, Huntington, L. I., Rush M. C., 1896.

# EDITORIAL

## VALEDICTORY.

F OR eight years, it has been the privilege of the writer to edit the transactions of tne Associated Physicians of Long Island, first in the form of a yearly volume and for the past six years as a monthly Medical Journal. The work has brought the writer into close association with many of the physicians of Long Island, whose co-operation was essential to the continuance of an independent medical association on Long Island. The Journal has been the means of attracting many new men to the association, and has increased its influence with the growth of the society. It now is the official depository for the transactions of the more important medical societies of Long Island and therefore will take its place among the medical histories of the State.

During the past year, the business management of the Journal has been taken charge of by the Publication Committee and under their guidance the business affairs of the Journal have been placed upon a firm basis. It has allowed us greater latitude in the editorial work, and has opened up the avenues for establishing permanently a medical journal of great usefulness.

Upon the editor has devolved the working out of most of the details of the publication, both editorial and executive.

The editor wishes to express his thanks to the publication committee which has stood by him so loyally, and through whose efforts the continuance and increased usefulness of the Journal has been made possible.

The writer finds it necessary to lay down his editorial pen, owing to the pressure of other professional and literary duties which make it impossible for him to longer devote the time required for the work involved in such a publication as the Long Island Medical Journal. In resigning as editor of the Journal, he does so with great regret.

To the new editor, Doctor Henry G. Webster, he expresses the wish that the duties he is about to take up will bring him much pleasure and profit. The recognized ability of the new editor ensures the successful development of the Journal.

PAUL MONROE PILCHER.

## THE ASSAY OF PROFESSIONAL TYPES.

THEORETICALLY, the thoroughly trained physician ought to be very versatile and efficient in action and very wise and inclusive in his varied counselings. But practically, it is interesting to note his shortcomings, not in any spirit of captious criticism, but merely as a part of the never-ending study of man and of mankind. The physician is one kind of man and cannot claim to be exempt from searching observation. It has become instinctive with him just now to resent examination, for most of the data bearing upon his activities that do not flatter him are not compiled in good faith. It is not good form to dwell upon the shortcomings of the doctor, unless one can do it with the tact and wholesomeness of Dr. Delatour. It must profit the doctors and must not put them too distinctly on the defensive. Much could be crudely said that is better left unsaid, a triumph in itself of good judgment, a vindication of discretion, and a proof of kindliness. So it is upon thin ice that we are venturing, but it is not in the spirit of rushing fools that we approach it.

Here we should like to preface our remarks with the explanation that what we have to say is conceived from the standpoint of him whom to malign has never been considered a grievous offense, but who by reason of his big heart and naive characteristics seldom points out the beams in his neighbors' eyes, but who nevertheless has observed and thought much and is without serious illusions—the general practitioner. What does he see that he does not audibly comment upon? One would suppose that one who has been indicted upon so many counts, who has been damned for uncountable sins of omission and cursed for innumerable faults of commission, should be tempted to retaliate more often. He is even alleged to be disappearing, like the Indian and the bison. Nowadays when we say "doctor" we don't necessarily mean this near-dodo. He is only taken into account when it is considered in order to pillory someone. What then can this pseudo-wraith say? We say for him that it is his sweetness of soul that accounts for his placid kindliness, but we fear that his habitual critics will find a more plausible explanation—to them—in stupidity and guilt. One can speak plainly in dealing with the general practitioner, it will be noted. Tact is not so essential here and the ice is never so thin as to be impassable.

Yet properly looked at, every surgeon or specialist is a general practitioner in a sense. When, however, he essays to play the rôle in anything like full measure he is apt to be as ridiculous as the general practitioner who essays to play surgeon. If the patience of the specialist or surgeon is frequently tried by the shortcomings of the general practitioner, it is equally true that the "placid kindliness" of the latter is just as often subjected to severe jolts. This is something not often divined or respectfully considered.

Perhaps the loss of the old-fashioned doctor will entail the disappearance of such great-hearted and broad-minded types as the authors of "Rab and His Friends," of "The Autocrat of the Breakfast Table," and of the *habitant* poems (Drummond). Literary attainments of high order are not often revealed nowadays by medical men, and we are seldom treated to such productions as that of our fellow townsman—"The Doctors of Samuel Johnson and His Court." Many doctors perform too much upon one string; let us hope that the time will never come when most of them will do so. The assay of the physician's value ought to necessitate the broadest measurements, else we stand convicted of intellectual provincialism and an attenuated type of professionalism. This should apply to every physician. All but the supercilious doctor—always an uninformed "shut-in"—find one man in the last analysis as good as another, nearly always. Many of us, by the way, have discovered the curious fact that it is possible for a man to be prominent in the profession and yet harbor the most snobblish and even vicious notions concerning men far outranking him in both human and divine value. Yet to judge even such a man sanely we must judge the whole man.

The dearth of brilliant literary efforts to-day on the part of medical men is doubtless explainable in part by reason of the fact that the best physicians find in sociological and other practical interests an outlet for their surplus energies. Abstractions and pen and ink idealizations have given place to service. All the professional types assay higher in value than ever before, except a certain class, the product of mercenary proprietary schools in recent years. But these are negligible bands in the professional spectrum. In the professional character picture the shortcomings common to us all should be viewed as the penumbra wherein the shadows serve the better to reveal the high lights. A. C. JACOBSON.

## THE MODERATE DRINKER.

THE presence of alcohol in some form from the beginning of recorded events has graced the table of hospitality and its use through custom has become a seeming requisite of honor to the welcomed guest. The fleeting exhilaration consequent upon its use undoubtedly creates a spirit of cordiality and fraternalism; artificial it is true, but charmingly delightful to the poor devil who free from the stressing importunities called forth by his struggle for existence, finds himself in an atmosphere of merry abandon, roseate with opportunities and bewilderingly pleasant. Verbiage as light and frothy as hillocks of sea foam nestling upon the beach falls upon his ear as scintillating wit, and to him "For He's a Jolly-Good-Fellow" possesses a melody sweeter by far than Verdi's classic "Holy Mother Guard His Footsteps." We who have participated in such inanities and insanities for which Oh, Bacchus! you were responsible and we the willing worshippers, must in the future quaff the sparkling fluid servant to Moses' rod, if we desire to preserve the highest standard of our natural endowments, according to Colonel Louis Mervin Maus, Medical Corps, U. S. A., Chief Surgeon, Eastern Division, who, in a paper, entitled "Should Total Abstinence Be Required of Officers in the Military Service," read at the meeting of the military surgeons of the United States held recently in Baltimore, forcibly advocated the adoption of the affirmative answer to his query. Colonel Louis Mervin Maus commenced his dissertation by humorously alluding to his past minor transgressions against the law of total abstinence, thus disarming any possible criticism, and "many who came to scoff remained to pray," listened with rapt attention to the doctor's words.

He conclusively proved by competent scientific authority that former opinions of alcohol had been revolutionized through laboratory and psychologic research. We all recognize the lamentable effects of hard drinking but that it is difficult to convince the moderate drinker—a man who drinks two or three times a day—that he exceeds the safety limit to body and mind. When warned he will reply, Why! whiskey in moderation is a stimulant and food. A traditional fallacy. Exhaustive experimentation has shown that it is a depressant after its primary stage of excitement. The influence of alcohol on the nervous system continues from twenty-four to seventy-two hours and affects thought and action during that period. It does not relieve fatigue through stimulation, but by deadening sensation. The typical effects observed in moderate drinkers are a weakening of the higher functions and a corresponding exaggeration of the lower ones; a loss of mental alertness and the finer conception of originality; a lowering of the moral standard and lessening of self-restraint; that it makes men less cautious and impairs judgment and ability to arrive at normal conclusions. The once brilliant mind fades away to be replaced by lowered moral tone. The health of cells depends upon the condition of the nuclei and proto-plasm. Alcohol is a protoplasmic poison inhibiting cell growth, restricting the production of anti-bodies and neutralizing the action of the bacterial toxins in the blood. Sir Benjamin Richardson showed that under the influence of alcohol temperature was lowered from three-quarters to three degrees. Nansen and all other explorers inveighed against alcohol in frigid climates.

In summarizing Doctor Maus said: "That after a careful study of alcohol as a beverage, he was unable to find one single beneficial or useful purpose it serves in the human economy, on the other hand, even in moderate quantities it reduces every one's efficiency and impairs mental and phisical conditions. Medical officers, the proper performance of whose duties involve the safety and lives of others, should especially be debarred from the use of alcoholic drinks so as to conserve their mental capacities to the fullest extent. In view, then, of our knowledge of the subject, has the Government the right to prohibit the use of alcohol amongst public servants. Every officer who accepts a commission in the Army and Navy, relinquishes in part his civil rights and personal liberty. In orders, commands and duty, the Government provides ample pay and allowance and obligates itself to pension officers on age and length of service, or for mental and physical disability contracted in the line of duty. For this reason, we hold that the Government has the right to require every officer and enlisted man to safeguard himself against disease and vicious habits inimical to health and efficiency. Sanitary orders are issued guarding by modern means against amoebic dysentery, cholera, typhoid fever, small pox and diphtheria. Why not enforce abstinence of alcohol which is the underlying cause of venereal diseases, impaired health and non-efficiency in public servants? In answer to interference with personal liberty, one's rights only invite activities that are not detrimental to others or communities."

Few will attempt to controvert Colonel Maus' deductions that alcohol is not necessary to the human economy, that man maintains a better correlation of bodily metabolism when totally abstemious, that even in moderate quantities alcohol is destructive to all life. Logically then we must agree with the Colonel, that when the lives of others, in fact, communities and counties are imperilled by reduced efficiency of those in charge, the cause of this inefficiency should be removed. Military officers and medical men are ever the subjects of emergency calls involving life and death. There is no gainsaying the proposition that they should be in full possession of their mental powers when such a demand is made upon them. The practice of moderate or occasional drinking is not so bad in itself, but the temptation at times to exceed moderation is very great. Therefore, a habit of total abstinence is a safeguard. To look for universal teetotallism is but a chimerical idle dream, but to hope for teetotallism amongst men of intellect entrusted with gravest responsibilities, possessing a conscientious regard for a divine duty is not a far fetched thought. It may be slow of growth, but conscience will ripen its fruition and the ideal be realized.

JOHN C. MAC EVITT.

## COMMISSIONS TO INVESTIGATE ANIMAL EXPERIMENTATION.

MANY practitioners in this country have considered it unnecessary to fight the various propositions made by the Anti-Vivisectionists to have committees appointed to investigate laboratories where medical research is being carried on. They can see no harm in allowing these investigations to be carried on. They do not realize, however, that the committees appointed for such investigations are generally made up of persons who are entirely ignorant of the true purpose of research work and incapable of judging the degree of suffering which the experiments cause. Even this objection has been overcome in England and commissions have been appointed, which are capable of judging such matters wisely.

The result of these investigations in England has twice been favorable to the continuance of animal experimentation, and yet, despite the fact that the verdict of the commissioners was overwhelmingly in favor of the experimenters, they supply the illogical and untruthful leaders of the Anti-Vivisection movement with much material for misrepresentation.

In 1875, Queen Victoria appointed the Royal Commission to investigate the medical laboratories of Great Britain, and that commission found no abuse of the privileges granted to the medical men. The report, however, was followed by the passage of a restricted law which has greatly hampered research work in England. All this, of course, seems illogical and yet it is a fact that, if these commissions are appointed, the result of their investigations, whether they are favorable or not to the research laboratories, still have acted harmfully to the profession.

P. M. P.

## WHAT IS PROGRESS?

"IT would be happier for a race to be free and diseased rather than healthy and enslaved." We do not know who the author of these words was. We recently encountered them in a book by Berry Hart, the eminent gynecologist and teacher, of Edinburgh. They excite thought.

There is an implication in the quotation that freedom entails disease and that health connotes slavery. If this were true what hope would humanity have?

Because love is blind—and free—people marry with little or no thought concerning heredity. Were they to follow the rules of Galton, the great student of eugenics, perhaps the race would be better, considered from certain points of view, but certainly it would be less free. There are those who would institute legislation in respect to marriage—

legislation along so-called scientific lines. In fact the thing has been done here and there. We fancy that we can regulate affection and control natural selection, but Nature seems to take no defects into account in the carrying out of her biologic programme. Our problem, the problem of a higher civilization, seems to be the thwarting of natural laws with no penalties in the way of lessened freedom, unhappiness and balked progress. This is "some" problem. The eugenic programme is supposed to make for a healthier race, yet according to the thinker whom we have quoted it will probably make for racial deterioration, in a sense, as well. Would this be progress? What is progress?

William Winter, the noted critic, in a recent speech before the Lotos Club, spoke of the vaunting of progress as a vain thing, so long as our prisons are overcrowded and our State Hospitals overflowing, and so long as discontented poverty is embattled against entrenched wealth, not to mention other counts. On the day following Winter's address the New York *Times* printed an article which purported to be the Church's view of progress. After recounting the facts indicating progress under the administration of a distinguished prelate about to be raised to very high office the *Times* article stated that "in addition, the number of reformatories, asylums and homes under his care have multiplied exceedingly."

Th progress of William Winter is clearly not the progress of the *Times* nor that of the distinguished prelate. Winter cannot think of an advanced and free race as greatly diseased, while the *Times* and the prelate are seemingly content to accept an unhealthy society as a progressive society. There is much confusion here, as everywhere in human thought and action. So we shall not attempt to define what progress is. We have no zeal for crystallizing and reducing to static order that which we would better think of after the manner of G. K. Chesterton. Such definitions must be left to the final eugenic product, that perfect being who shall combine all excellences—except, probably, humanness.

Arthur C. Jacobson.

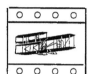
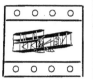
### THINGS THAT NEVER HAPPENED

On the first day of June the Court of Appeals affirmed the judgment of the Appellate Division, from which an appeal had been allowed and taken, in the case of Binks *vs.* the State and City of New York, for $5,000 damages sustained through an attack of typhoid fever. The full amount sued for was awarded.

\* \* \* \* \*

The May session of the State Legislature saw the final passage of the Eugenics bill. The governor will sign it. One provision of the bill makes the State liable for certain preventable defects in children. Thus a child contracting a disease through palpably bad housing conditions can recover damages, the alleged facts to be passed upon by a permanent State Hygiene Commission. Naturally, it is expected that the institution of this measure will radically affect the hygienic and sanitary activities of the State. This bill was introduced and passed at the behest of the profession, which is now not only unified and powerful in state affairs and alive to and informed upon the problems of sociological medicine, but has fully regained its erstwhile lowered caste.

\* \* \* \* \*

At the last monthly meeting of the Metropolitan Medical Association papers on the following subjects were read:
A Justification of Fee Splitting.
The Problem of Prostitution and its *Solution.*
Ethical Advertising: Means and Methods.
X-Ray Treatment of Locomotor Ataxia.
A Plea for the Recognition of the so-called Irregular Cults and a Plan for their Co-ordination and Regulation as Minor Phases of Legitimate Medical Practice (by the State Commissioner of Education; Discussion opened by a Regent of the University).

\* \* \* \* \*

It is authoritatively announced that representatives of all the "independent" medical journals in council assembled have agreed to excise all objectionable matter from their advertising columns, the reform to be instituted before the expiration of the current year and to be under the auspices of the Council of the American Medical Association. This is regarded as not only a triumph of good taste, but as a distinct professional advance. It will now be in order for certain journals to die as tastefully and utterly as possible.

\* \* \* \* \*

Hereafter, the visiting surgeons at the Perkins Memorial Hospital, according to a recent ruling of the Board of Governors, will rank according to the amount of private room business they send in. They will also receive a commission of 10 per cent. on the profits accruing therefrom.

\* \* \* \* \*

The beneficent bequests of the lately departed Snooks, the great philanthropist and multi-millionaire, to the *Kings* County Medical Society, are being applied to the purposes designated by the testator with all possible dispatch. The bowling alleys and swimming tank to be placed under 1313 are already contracted for and the squash and handball courts should be completed within a month. The moving picture equipment was installed last week. The grill room promises to be the coziest corner of the building. The great library endowment will easily place us ahead of the Library of the Surgeon-General's office, the Library of the New York Academy of Medicine and the Library of the College of Physicians of Philadelphia. Regarding the pension fund, a large number of physicians eligible for its benefits by reason of twenty-five years' practice have sent in the data required by the trustees of the pension fund. These data, which must be properly attested and authenticated, must show the applicant's average yearly income for the entire period of the applicant's professional life, the pension equalling half of said average income. It is extremely doubtful if even now the doctors will keep their accounts properly.

Many disaffected physicians of the metropolis went about in bands one night last month, smashing windows in the business section.  They worked under the leadership of Dr. George Pankhurst.   The doctors' grievance, it appears, is the fact that only a few of the profession are accorded the privilege of attending their own hospital patients, while the rank and file enjoy no institutional privileges or courtesies, nor are even conceded to possess elemental rights in this field of civil practice.  The anti-militant faction favors a test case in the courts.

* * * * *

All the medical schools of New York City closed their doors yesterday, not to reopen them for a period of ten years.  It is the mature conviction of their faculties that such a step will further the best economic interests of the profession, and, indeed, that it is imperative.

---

### WHEN GABRIEL BLOWS HIS TRUMP WILL WE STILL BE

—Devising new operations for the repair of the female perineum?

—Attempting to abort pneumonia?

—Dealing futilely with charity abuses?

—Removing alleged adenoids when the site of obstruction is in the anterior nares?

—Treating medical colitis as surgical appendicitis?

—Giving iron and arsenic to overworked, underpaid and underfed industrial slaves?

—Overtreating gonorrhea?

—"Instructing" children in sexual matters so far as anatomical and physiological facts are concerned and expecting that in some mysterious way this instruction will safeguard them as they grow older against the lure of the erotic? (after being given a course in Hamlet with Hamlet left out the discovery of the complete play will not fascinate them).

—Doing a vast amount of hospital and other work for nothing?

—Witnessing the chloroforming of public medical servants of the Wiley type by beaurocratic tools of the interests?

—Multiplying the registration area statistics by two in order to arrive at approximate ideas as to the country's morbidity and mortality?

—Treating victims of tuberculosis under ridiculous economic conditions and cooly watching, like an association of ghouls, the destruction of our brothers?

—Dispensing roof paint in journalistic containers and labeling the stuff wine of science—in violation of the as yet unwritten Pure Truth and Wisdom Act?

—Making shift without a National Department of Health?

A. C. J.

---

### SUGGESTIONS FOR A MEDICAL PARADE IN BOHEMIA, PLANNED TO SYMBOLIZE THE PROFESSION'S ECONOMIC CONCERNS.

Battalion of able-to-pay hospital and dispensary patients, under command of feeble-minded staff physicians.

Corps of ten cent medical company doctors in charge of trained keepers.

Automobiles containing comatose medical group uninterested in present-day economic problems.

Float carrying lecturers upon naively conceived economic remedies; also "extemporaneous thinkers."

Semi-secret proprietary detail man, in gilded chariot, attended by medical postilions.

Corps of bill collectors.

Dead beat, suspended by the thumbs.

Display of scalps belonging to members of the League for Medical Freedom. Only truthful expert witness now living in captivity.

Float carrying heroic figure, surrounded by worshipping physicians, typifying the Triumph of the Semi-Secret Proprietary.

SQUAD OF LODGE DOCTORS.

Nine tons of ethically doubtful proprietary advertising matter, dragged by harried looking editors.

Perpetrators of long-winded, rehashed papers, in chains.

Catafalques bearing nearly moribund faculties of proprietary medical schools.

Authors and manufacturers of useless text-books, bearing heavy crosses.

Heroic figure, "The Thinker," after Rodin, representing the awakening of the profession.

A. C. J.

## TO-MORROW'S MEDICAL NEWS.

Several thousand people able to pay moderate fees will be treated free in the dispensaries of the city.

Every ten seconds a baby under one year of age will die somewhere in the civilized world.

Several hundred prescriptions for semi-secret nostrums will be written by indolent and incapable physicians.

Several debilitated young women who work ten hours a day in factories, at ten cents an hour, will apply to their physicians to be "built up."

An absolutely normal appendix will be found upon opening the abdomen of a patient suffering from "acute appendicitis."

An incipient cancer of the cervix and several cases of "closed" tuberculosis will pass unrecognized through the hands of physicians.

Ten per cent. of sugar will be found in the urine of a surgical patient who has failed to heal.

The Wassermann reaction will be found still positive in a patient in the early stages of syphilis after most intensive courses of salvarsan and mercury.

A physician will receive a check from a surgeon for having acted as "first assistant" at an operation on a referred patient who has paid the operator what he supposes to be the operator's bill and the physician what he supposes to be the physician's bill, but who has no knowledge of the aforesaid transaction.

Several score physicians will be consulted by young matrons by reason of delayed menses and fear on the part of the latters' friends and relatives that they are "not strong enough" to bear children.

In a young woman lithographer, who has inhaled bronze dust regularly for ten years in the course of her work and who is the sole support of her mother and young sister, will be found the signs of incipient tuberculosis.

A hundred or more young men will have their prostates massaged and their urethras irrigated for the fortieth time, with no apparent diminution in shreds or bacteria.

The consummation of many "combined vaccine" successes will be noted.

A. C. J.

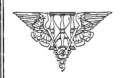 **Society**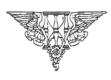

**Transactions**

## TRANSACTIONS OF THE BROOKLYN PATHOLOGICAL SOCIETY.

*Stated Meeting, October* 10, 1912.

The President, PAUL M. PILCHER, M.D., in the Chair.

### The Pathology of Pregnancy.

DR. ELI MOSCHCOWITZ, of New York City, presented a paper with the foregoing title, illustrated by a lantern slide demonstration of the various pathological lesions which occur during pregnancy. Sections of endometrium were shown by Dr. Moschcowitz, demonstrated by lantern slides, showing the fallacy of our former judgment calling for currettement; the pathologist has shown the gynecologist that currettement is not so frequently indicated.

### Pathological Conditions which Contraindicate and Prevent Pregnancy.

DR. GEORGE McNAUGHTON read a paper with the foregoing title.

### Pathological Conditions which Arise During Pregnancy and which Justify Abortion.

DR. O. PAUL HUMPSTONE read a paper with the foregoing title, which is published in full on page ——.

### The Toxemias of Pregnancy.

DR. VICTOR A. ROBERTSON read a paper with the foregoing title which is published in full on page ——.

*Discussion.*

DR. WILLIAM P. POOL, in opening the discussion, said:

The doctor always prefers to prevent rather than cure, and one thing which struck me during Dr. McNaughton's remarks was that it often comes within our power to prevent pregnancy in patients who are so afflicted that they cannot well bear that condition. It not infrequently is possible for the gynecologist, for instance, in operating upon a patient whom he knows to be afflicted with a dangerous heart disease, or nephritis, or other condition contraindicating pregnancy, to exsect the tubes. It is a simple thing to do. This might be done either in the course of an operation for some other cause, or we might even go further in some cases and advocate such an operation as preferable to pregnancy.

It is all very well to give instructions not to become pregnant but such instructions are often wittingly or unwittingly disregarded.

The conditions as mentioned by Dr. McNaughton seem to me a positive contra-indication to the condition of pregnancy, tuberculosis in particular. While it is perfectly true that very few infants, indeed, are born with active tuberculosis, it cannot be denied that they very quickly acquire it if the mother have the disease in any active form, to say nothing of the effect which parturition inevitably has upon the patient. I think that we have sometimes been deceived by the appearance of health which occurs in many of these cases of tuberculous women during the period of pregnancy. This readily gives way to a swift decline, during lactation, if that be permitted, or, in any case, during the period of the puerperium.

The insane or feeble-minded certainly should not be allowed to become pregnant. An eminent criminologist has advised vascetomy in males and salpingectomy in females to prevent the continuance of species among these people. He even advocates allowing them to marry. They are entitled to life and liberty and the pursuit of happiness, within reasonable limitations, as well as any one. This would certainly be an ideal method of preventing the propagation of feeble-minded children and reducing the number of those unfortunates from whom the criminal class is largely recruited.

36

Another class of cases in which we might easily guard against the ill-effects of pregnancy is in the women who apply to us after previous confinements, from which they have suffered extensive injury to the pelvic floor, and to the supports of the uterus, and present a sagging of the pelvic viscera, amounting in some cases to a complete procidentia. By proper plastic operation such cases may be cured and will remain cured permanently if further child-bearing be avoided. But if there be a subsequent parturition, the surgeon's work is likely to be entirely undone, and the last state of the patient may be worse than the first. This is a matter of frequent experience. And after a woman has been invalided by child-bearing and restored to health by operation, it does not seem fair or right that she should be deliberately exposed to the same danger again. In repairing these torn and overstretched structures, what is easier than to pull forward the fundus of the uterus through an incision in the anterior vaginal wall and exsect the tubes from the horns of the uterus. Of course, such a sterilizing operation must first be consented to by the patient.

The absolute and relative indications for abortion as mentioned by Dr. Humpstone seem to me extremely well set forth. I would only emphasize what he has already said—the necessity for early action in cases where we become convinced our treatment is not gaining ground, in the toxemias particularly. The continuance of high tension, of vomiting, loss of weight, etc., in spite of active treatment, calls for early interference. In this connection, I think it should be emphasized that we cannot depend too much upon laboratory diagnosis in these cases. We can learn after a certain amount of experience, more by frequent clinical observation of the patient than from the test tube, and I think that such observation should be insisted upon always.

One thing in particular of which I would speak is the tendency to heart failure in cases of persistent vomiting. We do not know the poison, the physiological chemistry of this process is very vague, but we can easily determine the force and frequency of the heart and general condition of the circulatory system by the use of the finger on the pulse, the manometer, and the stethoscope: clinical means of observation. A continuous failure in this line should be met with immediate abortion because it is difficult to say how long such a heart may hold out, and sometimes such cases get away from us before we know it.

Dr. A. A. Hussey, in discussion, said:

One great advantage, I think, of going over this subject at this time, is to emphasize the fact that pregnancy has a pathological side. The general public does not realize this fact. Personally, I believe that is one of the great factors that leads up to midwives confining 50 per cent. of the population in New York to-day. If the people in general realized that pregnancy was a condition associated with danger, they would undoubtedly employ physicians rather than women without medical training, and it is by discussing these things and bringing the matter to their attention that we can prevent a great deal of suffering and loss of human life.

In discussing the points that occurred to me in the papers, I would emphasize first that the prevention of many of these conditions is possible, I think, by careful watch of the patient during pregnancy. For instance, one of the complications given to-night for the induction of abortion is incarceration of the uterus. This is preventable and there should be no occasion for having to induce abortion in such cases if the physician has seen his patient regularly. When a pregnant patient has a retroverted uterus, unless the uterus is firmly adherent, it should be lifted up before it becomes incarcerated, but if this does occur, it should be freed by a laparotomy, and not by induction of abortion.

In regard to syphilis as a cause for the prevention of pregnancy, of course we would all say that active syphilis is a true cause for the prevention of impregnation. It usually causes of itself sterility, abortion or premature labor, or syphilitic babies that die soon after birth. But syphilis is a curable disease. There was the case that I saw about three years ago of a woman who aborted at the seventh month at Low Maternity and who gave a distinct Wassermann reaction. She was sent back to her physician for anti-syphilitic treatment and was delivered by me later of a full-term, perfectly normal child. Syphilis was there not an indication for the prevention of impregnation, but an indication for treatment which afterwards gave a healthy living child. I think we can accomplish somewhat along this line, and not condemn a woman because she has syphilis, to a childless life, but encourage her to take treatment so as to have healthy children later.

The toxemias of pregnancy of which we see so many in the hospital are either pernicious vomiting in the early or eclampsia in the later months. These conditions are very trying, as we all know, and are very difficult to treat. The vomiting of pregnancy is one in which I am free to admit I have occasionally fallen down. My tendency, perhaps, has been to wait too long before causing abortion. I think that may be the tendency of the general practitioner. Therefore, I think that instead of holding back on the therapeutic abortion in bad cases of toxic vomiting, we should be perhaps rather more ready to induce abortion in this class of severe cases and do it early. In my opinion, eclampsia is always an indication for emptying of the uterus, and emptying it at once.

Another cause that occurs to me, which I think was not mentioned, is antipartum hemorrhage or placenta previa.

In reference to the toxemias of pregnancy, I think that with careful study we can differentiate the nephritic from the hepatic type. In my experience eclampsia comes most frequently from hepatic intoxication. We occasionally see uremic poisoning which may simulate true eclampsia, but in the great majority of cases of acute eclampsia the lesion originates in the liver, and the clinical course of the case bears this out. Some serious cases I have seen have had no albumin in the urine before attacks, but they always have albumin after the onset of convulsions, and that is to us a warning not to pay quite as much attention as we have heretofore to the routine examinations of the urine, but depend more upon the general examination of the patient. Every time we see the patient we should not only examine the urine, but we should also examine her blood-tension and examine the general condition of her digestive apparatus, and question her carefully in regard to her general physical condition. In other words, make a picture of the case, not from the laboratory, but clinically. We can do a great deal for patients if we watch them.

I do not agree with one of the speakers in the question of abortion in contracted pelvis. I do not think that with the results that this speaker is getting in Caesarean sections for that conditions that he has any grounds to claim that abortion is indicated in a contracted pelvis.

DR. F. C. HOLDEN, in discussion, said:

DR. TREMBLY, of Saranac Lake, who has had a very extensive experience with tuberculosis associated with pregnancy, some three years ago read a paper before the Section of Obstetrics and Gynecology in the New York Academy of Medicine, at which time he took up in detail the subject of tuberculosis in pregnancy. The summary of what he had to say was somewhat as follows: That no woman with tuberculosis should be allowed to become pregnant, but in event of that unfortunate occurrence taking place, it was the duty of the physician immediately to empty the uterus. In cases where pregnancy had advanced to later months of pregnancy and was doing fairly well, it is well to let such cases continue to near term, and in the event of the woman being a primipara, or the baby being large, to induce labor one or two weeks before term to insure less difficult labor; also that these cases should never be allowed to have a long second stage of labor. As soon as the cervix is fully dilated under ether-oxygen anaesthesia, forceps should be applied and delivery done so that there should be as little wear and tear as possible incident to this stage of labor.

As regards heart conditions: I would say that every heart is a heart unto itself. Where there has been broken compensation on any previous occasion, it is very safe to say that it will recur with greater severity and more danger to the patient on each succeeding pregnancy. Therefore, I believe that in cases of broken compensation there should be an immediate emptying of the uterus. The same ruling applies to the management of the second stage of labor in heart cases which has already been spoken of in tuberculosis.

I had the opportunity during the last year of having under my care a woman, 34 years of age, who had previously had been emptied by a very eminent New York gynecologist, after consultation with two equally eminent men, because she had what is said to be a very bad heart. She became pregnant again and took the matter up with me, and after taking counsel with an obstetrician and a general medicine man I told her that if she cared to share the responsibility with me we would try to carry her along and see how the heart behaved. Her nine months of pregnancy were absolutely uneventful with no broken compensation, or other cardiac disturbance. She went into labor spontaneously at the expected time, unfortunately had a premature rupture of the membranes, but nevertheless went on and after a period of five hours had nearly full dilation of the cervix. Up to this time, the heart showed no signs of fatigue. Under ether-oxygen anesthesia, I did a medium forceps operation and delivered without difficulty an eight and a half pound live child. The woman's convalescence was absolutely uninterrupted and uneventful. She is nursing her child very satisfactorily.

In reference to syphilis: I think as Dr. Hussey does, that we have all seen syphilitic woman who have been cured and have subsequently been delivered of perfectly healthy children. I have in mind at the present time a case of a woman whom I confined three times who had some three years before her marriage a chancre on her lip with secondary lesions.

In reference to Dr. Pool's remarks regarding the advisability of affording a woman who has been operated on and cured for procidentia the use of sterilization operation, I cannot say that at the present time I am entirely in accord with his views in the matter, as I have seen women so cured and subsequently delivered without a recurrence of the original disastrous results.

On the other hand I think that any woman with an absolute contraction of the pelvis has a right to be sterilized and that we are not justified in telling her that she should submit to the Cesarean operation if she again becomes pregnant. To my mind there is quite a difference between a case of procidentia which may have been produced by faulty obstetrics and the case of an absolutely bony pelvis.

DR. RALPH H. POMEROY, continuing the discussion, said:

I desire to set up a new propaganda. I am proposing that we initiate a movement to educate ourselves and the public to look upon pregnancy in the individual woman as a pathological process throughout.

Dr. Moschcowitz has pointed out to us the definite fact that the impregnated ovum attacks the maternal structures by a process of cell invasion exactly simulating the progress of a localized malignant growth. It is in no light vein that I urge you to note that a woman is subjected throughout each pregnancy to grave burdens of toxic metabolism affecting her general organic health; that for nine months she carries in her body a neoplastic parasite; and that at any stage of her "hostessship" a riddance of the parasite involves a varying degree of surgical disaster.

The mortality of childbirth is certainly as high as one mother and five infants in every two hundred deliveries. The primary and secondary morbidity is certainly high enough seriously to detract from the physical efficiency of womankind, collectively and individually, yet neither State, public nor medical profession looks upon pregnancy as coming properly under the necessity of medical supervision.

It has been related this evening that more than fifty per cent. of the births in New York City are conducted without such medical supervision. The law allows it, the public prefers it, and the profession weakly concurs. Until it is acknowledged by all three that the pregnant woman is individually a pathological subject, we cannot expect the practice of obstetrics to keep any pace with its status as a science and an art.

DR. J. D. SULLIVAN, in discussion, said:

This discussion to-night has been very interesting from a scientific point of view, but, like the last speaker, my feelings have been jarred by the principles enunciated here.

I think from a sociological, moral and patriotic standpoint that we are away below par, very inferior to what the human race should demand of the medical profession. Human life deserves more consideration than seems to have been accorded to it. The human embryo is so sacred that it should not be destroyed on account of some curable ailment or imperfection on the part of the mother: and I suppose a good many of you know that race suicide is depopulating the country at a very rapid pace. Were it not for the immigrant population of this country we would be in a sorry plight in propagation as compared with other nations. We would be dwindling. The advocates of race suicide say that when a patient is sick and incidentally becomes pregnant, then we must kill the child to save the mother. We have often heard, "Thou shalt not kill!" It appears to me to be more scientific and more humane to put the patient under rational scientific treatment and cure the toxemia, or whatever the disturbance may be, and give the prospective infant a chance to live. I believe it is a point that should be developed before the society. I am sure I have seen many patients with tuberculosis who fared better by letting their pregnancy continue than by interrupting it. The same is true of syphilitic patients. Syphilis is a curable disease. Why not treat the disease according to approved standards and leave the mother and child to thrive the best they can with the aid of nature.

DR. J. S. WIGHT, in discussion, said:

Some of the questions brought out here this evening were very interesting, particularly that case of Dr. McNaughton's of early tuberculosis. While it is perhaps not borne out, it is suggested in the investigations of Dr. Saleeby where he found that the placenta is a natural filter and shuts out organisms and poisons from the fetus, but in the presence of alcoholic addiction, where his investigations have been largely carried on, he finds that this filter has been broken down so as to allow of the passage of these organisms.

A topic which is interesting to every one of us is that of heredity, and while a great deal has been brought out that is new, we are perhaps not conservative enough in passing laws and enforcing laws for sterilizing human beings. Nature has the tendency to drag back to the normal. The only thing we really know about heredity is the effect of the dominant determinants and the results where two feeble-minded people or two people who have what might be termed the presence or the absence of something are married; then their children are all feeble-minded or they have, with very rare exceptions, the presence or the absence of something. So it seems to me that the question of sterilization might wait for further investigations. There are, of course, cases where it would be right to stop a line of feeble-minded people and criminals, as, for instance, such families as the Kallikak family, which has been written about, and the Jukes family, but it seems to me that we are rushing into this problem with solutions without due consideration.

DR. S. R. BLATTEIS, in discussion said:
A plea has been made in behalf of the unborn infant. May I make a similar plea for the lining membrane of the uterus?

The first operative work given a hospital interne is a curettage; the first thing an ex-interne does when he gets into practice is a curettage.

The endometrium has been the scapegoat for a great many things. I do not believe, and there are others who think the same way, that the endometrium is there for the purpose of indiscriminate interference, and that its removal is a cure-all for metrorrhagia, menorrhagia, and dysmenorrhoea. To think so is a fallacy. Whatever pathological changes are produced in the endometrium are the results and not the causes of any of the former conditions, and it is admittedly illogical to encourage a surgical or medical proceedure which attempts to remove the effect and not the cause of a condition.

You have seen slides and have been told, that the pathological changes (excepting tumors, benign or malignant), observed in the endometrium are very slight, and one is at a loss to adopt a classification useful for clinical purposes.

In an examination of hundreds of curettings, one sees (besides the changes incident to menstruation) either a simple diminution in the number and atrophy of the glands, and a corresponding increase in the interglandular tissue or an increase in the number of glands with the interstitial tissue less in evidence. Curettage for diagnostic purposes is a different subject.

So the idea that denuding the uterus of its lining membrane as a panacea should be generally and vigorously discouraged.

## TRANSACTIONS OF THE BROOKLYN SURGICAL SOCIETY.

### Stated Meeting, June 6, 1912.

### The President, JOHN A. LEE, M.D., in the Chair.

#### Ulcer of the Stomach with Recurrence of Symptoms after Operation.

DR. W. B. BRINSMADE reported the following case:

About a year ago he operated on a woman for gastric ulcer. All of the characteristic symptoms were present. She had on the anterior wall of the stomach a thin ulcer about the size of a half dollar, and the doctor simply infolded the ulcer, sewing over the peritoneum and making a fold in the stomach, and leaving the stomach in apparently very good condition as regards the function. The ulcer was far enough from the pylorus, so that it did not interfere with its function. He then discovered a chronic appendicitis and removed the appendix.

The patient gained thirty pounds during the summer and came back to her work as a school teacher.

Last Christmas she began to have a return of symptoms, with vomiting, and the characteristic symptoms of gastric ulcer with gastric hemorrhage, which she did not have before. Blood finally appeared in the stools and she was unable to do her work, but did not wish to take a vacation if it could be avoided.

She was operated on last Monday and the seat of the old ulcer was occupied by a larger area of induration than was present the first time. The indurated area was easily removed entire, and the stomach was repaired, but the fold caused by the former operation was so extensive as to make the operation of gastro-enterostomy extremely difficult.

The doctor stated that in future, he would either excise the ulcer in such cases or would perform a gastro-enterostomy at the time of the first operation.

## Compound Fracture of the Skull.

Dr. J. H. Long reported the following cases:

Case I.—This patient, H. S., 26 years of age, dentist's assistant, was admitted to the Brooklyn Hospital on Dr. J. E. Jennings' service on August 19th, 1911. A steam tank over which he was working exploded, causing the following injury:

A deep stellate laceration over the left frontal region from which blood was flowing freely and brain was protruding. The cavity of the left frontal sinus was visible. His pupils were unequal; he had vomited blood and was wildly delirious.

The patient was immediately anesthetized with chloroform and the wound slightly enlarged and the soft parts retracted. This disclosed an opening in the skull about the size of a twenty-five cent piece from which one fissure extended across the median line, another into the temporal region and two more upward and backward, including between them a depressed area about the size of a twenty-five cent piece. Through the opening, the fragments of inner and outer table and underlying dura, which had been driven into the brain were removed, also the posterior wall of the left frontal sinus which was detached and imbedded in the frontal lobe. The brain was retracted away from the median line to see if there was hemorrhage from the longitudinal sinus where the inner fissure crossed it. There was none. The brain was then retracted toward the median line to see if the fissure which extended toward the temporal region was causing hemorrhage from the meningeal artery. None was found. The depressed upper fragment was elevated and left in place. A zinc oxide gauze pack was placed against the lacerated and bleeding brain tissue which was protruding at the opening in the skull and dura and the soft parts closed around the packing.

There was a copious discharge of bloody cerebro-spinal fluid for a few days. Delirium lasted seven days. Following the removal of the packing, there was a protrusion of the brain tissue. This was kept in with packing until granulations formed and the edema subsided. The scar filled in the bony and dural defect and there is no brain hernia. In spite of the fact that this was a compound comminuted fracture and that the opening of the frontal sinus gave communication between the brain cavity and the nose, there was no infection. His present condition is excellent; so far there has been no cerebral disturbance.

Case II. Patient, a school boy five years old, brought in on the ambulance and admitted to Dr. Jennings' service, at the Brooklyn Hospital. He fell down a flight of stairs, striking his head, sustaining a punctured wound of the right vertex, and out of that was oozing blood and brain tissue. When pressure was applied, the skull could be seen to give and crepitus was evident over quite an area on the right side. He suffered from shock but was conscious. With chloroform, a small incision was made and then enlarged and a fracture was found with two triangular separated depressed fragments. From the apex of the anterior one a linear fracture extended forward beyond the hair line without laceration of the dura. From the apex of the posterior one, fracture and laceration of the dura, with one-eighth inch separation, extended down under the occiput. The injury was so extensive that the edges from forehead to occiput could be separated by pressure. The dura anteriorly was intact, the posterior portion being torn. The brain was protruding between the edges of the wound in this portion, i. e., from the crown to the occiput. It was possible to raise the anterior fragment without detaching the dura. The posterior fragment had become detached from the lacerated underlying dura but was replaced. An attempt was made to get the dura together at the point where it was torn, but this was not possible, so it was packed with zinc oxide strips from the apex of the posterior fragment to the torn portion of the occiput to hold the brain in place, and it was thus partially closed.

The patient had a temperature for about a week ranging from normal to 102 degrees, the pulse was 100 to 150 for three weeks. He cried freely for two days and was miserable generally, but after that he was fairly comfortable and was a good patient. The first dressing was done on the fifth day.

At the end of the seventh day, the packing was removed. The seventh day the left hand and arm and the side of the face began to twitch, once in three seconds. Patient was dressed again and considerable edema and protrusion and some discharge were found. The posterior fragment was raised away up, so it was removed and the twitching improved for a little while. The next day he was twitching again just the same. He was dressed again with a wet dressing and all pressure was removed and the twitching stopped for a few hours and then began again. The wounds healed nicely after that. The twitching lasted three days. On the twenty-sixth day, there was considerable protrusion of the brain. This was treated with pressure and adhesive straps which kept it pressed in, and it healed over in spite of the infection. During one of the late dressings another piece of bone, the anterior fragment loosened and came away.

On the twenty-seventh day, after the operation, there was a discharge from the left ear and pain in the right ear, and the day after that he had a typical measles rash. During the measles, the skin which had been holding well, broke down again, and there was considerable discharge. Then he got over his measles and went home. It was a genuine case of measles in an epidemic of measles. He was home four days and came back with a temperature of 104 degrees, with pain and tenderness over the left ear. This was thought to be a mastoid case, but the ear drum was punctured and a little serum appeared and the trouble subsided. Later, while attending the dispensary, another little spicule of bone was removed. The patient has had no paralysis. His only sign of trouble was that when he first got out of bed, his right leg was thrown out when walking. He seemed to have some difficulty with his balance, but he had no paralysis and no atrophy, and now walks perfectly.

### Stricture of Common Bile Duct.

DR. WILLIAM LINDER reported the following case:

Patient, S. B., aged fifty-one, admitted to hospital November 16, 1911. Was operated upon for right inguinal hernia four years ago.

Eight months ago patient for the first time was suddenly attacked with moderately severe epigastric cramps occurring two hours after his meals. The pain lasted three hours, was not accompanied by chills or fever, nor was it followed by jaundice. Two months later had a similar attack. Patient was then well for six months. Three weeks before admission, patient suffered a third and more severe attack. This time vomited a few times, the vomitus consisting of food taken, no blood. During week before admission, the patient noticed that his face became yellow, stools clay-colored, bowels constipated, no chills or fever, no appetite. Lost forty pounds during last eight months.

A diagnosis of a stone in the hepatic or common duct was made. Nothing was palpable in the abdomen.

Dr. Linder made a Miculicz incision, starting from the ensiform cartilage one inch from the median line going down one inch from the umbilicus, and cutting across the rectus muscle so as to have a good exposure. The gallbladder was found contracted and a stone was found in the hepatic duct. There were considerable adhesions of the gall-bladder. The gall-bladder was excised and the cystic duct clamped and slit down and the stone was milked out of the duct. A probe was passed down to the duodenum and a free flow of bile occurred, the usual rubber tube was sutured in position and a drainage tube was passed along side of it, to provide for leakage.

The patient gained five pounds after the first operation and was perfectly well for four months.

The gall-bladder showed chronic suppurative cholecystitis and streptococcus pyogenes breves.

Four months later patient came back, having become gradually completely jaundiced. Nothing palpable in the abdomen.

Dr. Linder made a diagnosis of obstruction of the common duct at the point of drainage. He reopened the patient one inch to one side of the former incision, making the same incision, and after freeing the omentum, which was adherent to the abdominal scar, he began to look for the sharp border of the gastro-hepatic omentum. Raising the duodenum, he began to dissect blindly the duodenum in order to expose the common duct. The common duct was followed up and a mass of adhesions were found around the hepatic duct, consisting of complete cicitrisation. A longitudinal incision was made in the long axis of the hepatic duct and it was found that the proximal end of the duct was very much dilated where the common duct was normal in size.

A small rubber tube was inserted in the hepatic duct, and the other end was inserted in the common duct. The tube was covered with peritoneum and on top of this the duodenum was grafted. The point of incision of the duct was drained with a split rubber tube, containing a piece of gauze. However, for twenty-four hours, there was no leakage and the drainage tube was removed and the patient made an uninterrupted recovery, bile being present in the first bowel movement. The urine has lost the bile and the patient has gained 25 pounds.

The present position of the tube is uncertain. It is not known whether it has been passed or not, but it gives him no trouble.

This brings up an important point in duct surgery. While direct anastomosis was done by Kocher and William Mayo, when the stricture was lower down, yet in this case it was impossible to bring the proximal end of the hepatic duct to the duodenum, although it was mobilized, and this case proves that such a procedure is feasible.

In spite of these two incisions, the patient has an absolutely firm abdomen. In closing up such wounds, if the posterior sheath of the rectus is carefully stitched and the anterior sheath is stitched to the aponeurotic layer, there is no weakening of the abdominal wall.

### Intestinal Obstruction Due to a Perforating Tubercular Ulcer of Small Intestine.

DR. WILLIAM LINDER reported the following case:

Patient, N. B., aged forty-three, admitted February 22, 1912. Has had a bilateral inguinal hernia for the past ten years. Obstinate constipation for years.

Four days before admission, patient was suddenly taken with severe abdominal cramps located about the umbilicus, which persisted up to the time of admission. Vomited persistently greenish material of fecal character and odor. Bowels did not move in four days and no result by enemas; no gas passed. No fever, no chills or sweats. On examination, patient appears acutely ill. Abdomen distended, tympanitic and rigid, diffuse abdominal tenderness. Bilateral inguinal hernia larger on left side. Dr. Linder put his finger into both inguinal canals, which were very much dilated, and, as far as he could determine he could not feel a knuckle of intestine in either canal, nor did the patient feel any pain.

An incision was made to the left of the median line, below the level of the umbilicus. A knuckle of ileum was found strangulated at the internal ring. A piece of gut the size of a ten cent piece, was found so much pinched that the circulation did not return with hot irrigations. The intestine was invaginated and a circular suture was made, after making sure that gas could be passed. The right internal inguinal ring containing sac was inverted, cut off and sutured. An ordinary Bassini was done, bloody fluid was found in the peritoneal cavity. The abdomen was closed in layers with no drainage. The patient made an uninterrupted recovery and left the hospital with no trouble on March 19, 1912.

Patient felt very well for seven weeks, when he was taken with sudden severe pain in the upper abdomen, radiating to the lower abdomen. He soon vomited the stomach contents, and had eructations of gas. Next day, after the enemas, patient passed a small fleshy blood tinged mass along with fecal masses, flatus and mucus.

On examination, patient had tenderness over the old scar and an indefinite mass could be felt there.

A lower right rectus incision was made and the intestine was found kinked upon itself several times and adherent, some coils being firmly united to the scar on abdominal wall. The gut was thickened, markedly congested and freely bleeding, with plastic exudate about the loops of intestine. Part of omentum was markedly thickened and inflamed. It was necessary to remove about eighteen inches of small intestine and the pathologist reported the presence of tubercular ulceration and perforation of the small intestine. A lateral anastomosis was performed with broad implantation. The patient made a good recovery.

### Resection of the Tongue.

DR. WILLIAM LINDER reported the following case:

About four months ago, a patient was admitted to the Jewish Hospital suffering with ulceration of the tongue. The clinical picture was that of carcinoma of the tongue. He had some glandular involvement on the right side of the neck. A section was taken which the pathologist reported to be carcinoma.

Operation was proposed and accepted, the Whitehead being performed. It was a very extensive operation, going down to the base of the tongue, entire floor of the mouth, the left half being involved. The cervical glands were removed by a curved incision. The lingual artery was ligated at the usual point and then the tongue was removed by mouth. The ease with which such an extensive operation can be done on the tongue in the mouth, is surprising. The patient is a laborer, works daily, eats anything and everything, and it is remarkable how well he speaks.

These cases are frequently lost through aspiration pneumonia. This case showed the value of introducing the anesthetic through a catheter. There was no difficulty at all in passing the catheter very nicely. It was clamped on the side of the mouth. The patient was in a sitting posture where the operator could see well, and the operation was bloodless. The lingual artery was tied on one side and the other side was clamped in the mouth when it was reached. There is a little hardness of scar tissue in the mouth at present, which is not a nodule.

### Discussion.

Dr. M. Figueira, in discussing this case, said that he had done an operation in cases of this kind that he considered better than the usual operation which is done. Some years ago, Dr. Dawbarn advised the removal of the external carotid artery in inoperable carcinomata of the neck. In a case such as Dr. Linder's, in which the tongue and glands are involved, the external carotid artery can be ligated and divided just above the origin of the superior thyroid artery and then the different branches can be ligated. A long incision can then be made along the lower jaw and all of the diseased tissue and glands can be removed. The mouth can then be opened and the tongue operated upon without hemorrhage. It is a perfectly dry operation.

It is a noted fact that the malignancy and rapidity of growth of malignant tumors is connected with an increased blood supply and that when perchance they stop growing or show a tendency to disappear, this is connected with a decreased blood supply. This is the theory on which this operation is based. By cutting off the supply of blood to the parts, the return of disease may to a certain extent be prevented. The operation may be done in two stages. The artery can be ligated on one side and one-half the tongue removed and then in a week or so, the other side may be removed and in that way the operation is completed. The results are better and recurrence is less likely to take place, because the supply of blood is cut off.

### Two Cases of Gall Bladder Disease.

Dr. C. E. Lack reported the following cases:

Case I. Patient, 50 years of age, had repeated attacks of gall-stone colic during January and February. There had also been symptoms of severe disturbance in the upper abdomen, following these attacks. An operation, in April, revealed an empyema of the gall-bladder which had ruptured. The gall-bladder was bound down by adhesions and the liver was so displaced that the gall-bladder had become encysted. In order to drain it, the ribs had to be resected. The patient is now recovering.

Case II. Patient who also had repeated attacks of gall-stone colic. The patient was removed to the hospital and was operated upon by Dr. Delatour, who found a gall-bladder containing 750 stones. The appendix was also chronically inflamed and was removed.

### Carcinoma of the Cecum.

Dr. W. A. Gildersleeve reported the following case:

A woman, 35 years of age, had suffered two hemorrhages from the stomach six years ago. Two years ago, there was a third hemorrhage. Latterly there had been a steady loss of weight and considerable flatulence, but no severe pain. Examination revealed a mass low down in the right iliac fossa about the size of a fist. Uterus freely movable. Operation revealed a large carcinoma of the cecum with some involvement of the ileum. Four inches of the cecum and two inches of the ileum were removed and a lateral anastomosis was done. A colon infection followed. Patient died October 7th.

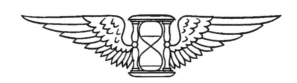

# LONG ISLAND MEDICAL JOURNAL

VOL. VII.    FEBRUARY, 1913    NO. 2

## Original Articles.

### THE PREVENTION AND TREATMENT OF URETERAL FISTULA, WITH REPORT OF A RECENT CASE.*

By Walter A. Sherwood, M.D.,

of Brooklyn, N. Y.

A N ureteral fistula may be defined as an abnormal opening through which urine is discharged from the lumen of the ureter either into the cavity of the uterus, some part of the alimentary canal, the vault of the vagina or upon the surface of the body. These fistulæ are in very rare instances of congenital origin; occasionally they are the result of ulceration such as is caused by the incarceration of an impassable renal calculus, or, as is most common, they owe their origin to accidental traumatism.. The last named variety is invariably the result of operative efforts in the domain of pelvic and lower abdominal surgery and is the principal concern of this paper.

As an outcome of an increasingly better appreciation of the anatomy and pathology of the pelvis and its contained viscera, together with continued advances in operative technique, accidental injuries of the ureter have grown to be of comparative infrequence.

*Frequency.*—In 1904, there were collected from the records of the Gynecological Clinic of Johns Hopkins Hospital, 30 cases of ureteral injury; 19 of these were the result of 156 operations for cancer of the cervix uteri, the remaining 11 cases being gathered from the records of 4,513 patients representing all other pathological conditions of the lower abdomen and pelvis. Of the 30 cases of injury to the ureter 10 resulted in persistent ureteral fistulæ.

It seems reasonable to assume that even under the most ideal conditions of knowledge, experience and improved technique, and in the hands of the most skilful and dextrous operators, this unfortunate accident, although theoretically avoidable, will continue to happen in a varying small proportion of our pelvic cases.

In order that we may be reminded of the safeguards at our disposal for the prevention of this accident and that we may be prepared to meet its effects when it does occur, it seems proper to review some of the most essential features of the subject and to present in connection therewith the report of a recent illustrative case which well typifies the remote results of ureteral injury, the problem of its diagnosis and one satisfactory method of its surgical treatment.

---

* Read before the Greater New York Medical Association, December, 1911.

*Anatomy.*—Although unnecessary to recall the anatomical structure, course, and relations of the ureter, it may be said that a knowledge of its normal blood supply and especially the arrangement of the periureteral plexus will explain why this duct may be stripped up from its retroperitoneal bed for its entire length without injury and at the same time why a comparatively slight traumatism of a small area of the ureteral wall may result in localized necrosis and the subsequent formation of a fistula. (See Figure 1.)

*Etiology.*—Among the conditions in which operative treatment may result in injury of the ureter and the permanent establishment of a fistula may be mentioned the following:

1. Cancer of the cervix, extensive operation for which is by far the most frequent condition resulting in ureteral traumatism.

2. Any abnormality which produces a lateral displacement of the cervix, thus distorting the normal relation and position of the ureter. This is particularly true of cervical and intra-ligamentous fibroids, as well as intra-ligamentous cysts and inflammatory exudates at the base of the broad ligaments.

3. Masses adherent to the posterior parietal peritoneum covering the ureter.

4. New growths and cysts of retroperitoneal origin.

5. Deep and extensive pelvic dissections in such conditions as carcinoma of the sigmoid, rectum and prostate.

6. Almost any other pelvic condition in proximity with the ureter.

Concerning the cases of injury to the ureter which are recognized at the time of operation, it need simply be mentioned that proper steps should be taken for their immediate repair by one of the accepted methods of uretero-ureteral anastomosis or uretero-vesical implantation, as seems indicated according to the conditions of the individual case.

With these we are not especially concerned; nor is this paper intended to include those cases which result in spontaneous closure within a few days or weeks, but only those in which there is a persistence of the fistula as shown by a continued discharge of urine through the abnormal opening for months or years after operation and in which, perhaps, attempts have been made to effect a closure without success.

The infliction of an injury which may result in a permanent ureteral fistula is produced in one of the following ways:

a. By the application of a clamp or ligature.

b. By the use of the cautery.

c. By complete or partial severance with knife or scissors.

d. By tearing the ureteral wall or interfering with its blood supply in the digital enucleation of adherent masses and the separation of dense adhesions.

*Classification.*—Ureteral fistulæ may be complete or partial, the former term being applied to those cases in which all of the urine from the wounded duct is discharged through the abnormal opening, the partial variety being one in which part of the urine escapes by way of the abnormal opening, the remainder finding its way into the bladder through the distal end of the wounded ureter, which may not be completely occluded.

The lesion is almost always unilateral, though a few cases have been reported in which the patient survived injury to both ureters through the prompt establishment of a bilateral fistula.

*Symptoms.*—The symptoms of ureteral fistula depend upon the location of the abnormal opening, the vault of the vagina being the most common and natural site for its occurrence. From the false opening there is a more or less constant discharge of urine, mixed with debris, epithelial cells and in most cases pus and bacteria. This is often ascribed by the patient to a lack of bladder control. This constant leakage of urine with its subsequent local irritation and excoriation of the skin or mucous membrane is a most distressing symptom and as a result of it there ensue mental depression, a desire to avoid people and a gradual general physical deterioration. There is a more or less constant sense of local discomfort and in most of the cases periodic attacks of pain and fever caused by imperfect drainage and the absorption of infected urine. There may be also an accompanying cystitis which adds much to the pitiable condition of the patient. The more remote effects are the symptoms of ascending infection and the development of pyelitis and pyelonephrosis. When sepsis becomes established, the mental and physical suffering is such as to cause these patients to spend most of their time in bed.

*Course.*—The course of such a fistula, if unoperated, is one of persistent physical impairment with constant likelihood of ascending infection and all of its accompanying dangers.

A few cases have been reported in which spontaneous closure with a return to health has occurred after persistence for a period of months or years.

This can only be explained by absence of infection, occlusion, urinary absorption and a final cessation of function of the kidney on the affected side.

*Diagnosis.*—The diagnosis of the existence of a ureteral fistula is usually simple and depends upon the history of a previous operation and the discharge of urine from one of the abnormal openings before mentioned.

It must be differentiated from vesico-vaginal, vesico-rectal and vesico-uterine fistulæ as well as abnormal communications between the bladder and the surface of the abdomen. This differentiation can easily be made by over-distension of the bladder with a colored fluid and noting the presence or absence of this fluid in the fistulous tract.

If operative treatment is to be considered, it is a matter of first importance to determine which ureter is the one involved and this can only be accomplished with the aid of the cystoscope and the ureteral catheter, the use of which will also determine the presence or absence of renal infection and the functional ability of the kidney; important considerations in the choice of a proper method of treatment. An X-ray picture in conjunction with the ureteral catheter may also be of service in distinguishing between the normal ureter and its diseased mate.

*Prophylaxis.*—Much can be done to lessen the number of cases of ureteral fistula by a fundamental familiarity with the anatomy and pathology of the pelvic viscera, especially in their relation to the ureter; by the discreet use of ligatures, clamps and cautery; by the old and well-known rule of keeping close to the uterine wall and cervix in the removal of new growths, cysts and inflammatory exudates; by the avoidance of mass ligatures in the tissues lateral to the cervix; by an immediate recognition and successful primary repair when the ureter has been divided or torn and finally by the routine practice of ureteral catherization as a preliminary to operation in all cases involving deep and extensive pelvic dissection and where, as the result of a laterally displaced cervix, the normal position and relation of the ureter is disturbed. This procedure in the hands of a skilful cystoscopist takes but a few minutes of time and serves during the operation as a sure and constant guide in safe-guarding a duct which, if injured, may result in prompt death or the establishment of a condition which means chronic invalidism; a condition which, no matter how unavoidable it may seem to have been, reflects no credit on the surgeon. I can, therefore, see no objection to the more general recommendation of preliminary ureteral catheterization as a routine practice in a larger number of our pelvic cases.

*Treatment.*—The surgical treatment of a persistent ureteral fistula must be decided on the merits of the individual case. These patients, although highly neurotic and worn out by years of suffering are willing to accept any plan of treatment which offers them a hope of ameliorating their mental and physical suffering.

One of three courses may be pursued:

*First. Uretero-vesical implantation.* This is the ideal operation and the method of natural selection in the absence of renal infection and other contra-indications, and if successful, gives promise of a most satisfactory result. It is contra-indicated when a severe ascending infection is present and when the fistulous opening is high up in the ureter.

*Second. Nephrectomy.* This plan of treatment may be adopted in the cases in which an operation for implantation has failed, where the kidney is the seat of a bad infection and where the fistulous opening is too high to permit of an anastomosis with the bladder. It is needless to add that it should never be undertaken without a positive assurance of a normal kidney on the other side.

*Third. Maintenance of the fistula.* By this is meant the continuous provision for free drainage. This plan is indicated in those cases in which for any reason one of the other methods cannot be employed.

In reference to the proper method of effecting a uretero-vesical implantation, it seems to the writer that the intra- or transperitoneal route for exposing the ureter is preferable to the extra-peritoneal method in that it gives much freer access and exposure for the necessary manipulation, an advantage of sufficient importance to overweigh the slight danger of infection which with proper precaution and provision for drainage is not of much moment.

For the statistics and many of the more important data contained in the foregoing remarks, I am indebted to an excellent monograph on the subject of Ureteral Fistula by J. A. Sampson of Albany, which was published in the May number of *Surgery, Gynecology and Obstetrics,* 1909. I am also indebted to this author for the use of the first drawing which has been utilized in the preparation of this paper for the purpose of illustration.

### REPORT OF CASE.

In conjunction with these observations, I herewith submit the report of the case of Mrs. B. S., aged 36, married, who was referred to the writer by Dr. J. C. Graham and admitted to the Methodist Hospital on September 4, 1911, with the following history:

Eight years previously, while in the British West Indies, she had been subjected to an abdominal hysterectomy for a uterine fibroid. She stated that ever since this operation, there has been a constant leakage of urine from the vagina, which she thought was due to a lack of bladder control. Urine was also passed at regular intervals in the normal way. There had been a gradual deterioration in her general health with much despondency and during the last two years, she has been confined to the house or bed. Three attempts had been made through the vagina to control the leakage, none of which were successful. She has had frequent attacks of abdominal pain with fever and prostration. One month before admission to the hospital urination became painful and difficult with much burning. The urine was dark in color and had a foul odor. After each attempt at urination a few drops of bright red blood were passed. During the last two weeks, she has complained of dull aching pain in both kidney regions. She has lost considerable weight.

At the time of entering the hospital, her chief complaints were the constant leakage of urine from the vagina, with local discomfort, difficult urination, fever and prostration.

Physical examination reveals the scar of former operation; abdomen otherwise negative except for slight tenderness on deep pressure over the left kidney which is not palpably enlarged.

Vaginal examination reveals evidence of a former complete hysterectomy. At the vault of the vagina, there is a circular area of ulceration about 1½ inches in diameter. Near the centre of this area are two small fistulous openings through which a probe can be passed in a tortuous direction upwards and backwards for a distance of an inch. From both openings cloudy urine is being discharged a few drops at a time. All attempts at examination caused so much discomfort that further examination was not attempted until September 7, at which time a cystoscopic examination was made under general anæsthesia by my colleague, Dr. Roger Durham, with the following result:

Bladder capacity 6 ounces. More than this causes leakage from the urethra, but no increase in the discharge from the fistulous openings. The urine in the bladder is clear and does not contain blood. The bladder mucous membrane appears normal, but the organ seems rotated on its axis as if pulled by adhesions. There are no areas of intravesical ulceration and there is no fistulous opening. The left ureteral orifice is lower than that of the right side. A ureteral catheter can be freely passed on the right side for the entire length of the ureter and from this orifice jets of urine were seen to be ejected in the normal way.

On the left side the catheter met an obstruction one inch from the ureteral orifice and could be passed no further. No urine passed through this orifice into the bladder.

A second confirmatory cystoscopic examination was made a few days later at which time an X-ray picture was taken, showing the ureteral catheter following the normal course of the right ureter.

The urine from the right kidney was normal except for a slight trace of albumin and a moderate number of leucocytes. No urine could be obtained from the left kidney except through the fistulous opening and as this was contaminated, examination of it was of no value in determining the condition of the renal function on the affected side.

With the evidence furnished by the examination of Dr. Durham, it was demonstrated that the fistulous opening was situated on the left side about one inch above the ureteral orifice.

In view of the fact that there was no marked evidence of a renal

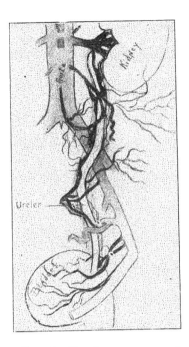

Fig. I.—Showing arrangement and source of ureteral blood supply—(after Sampson).

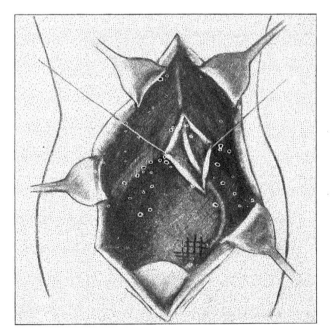

Fig. II.—First step in operation of utero-vesical implantation. Exposing ureter at pelvic brim. Posterior parietal peritoneum incised and retracted. Fistulous tract indicated by crosses.

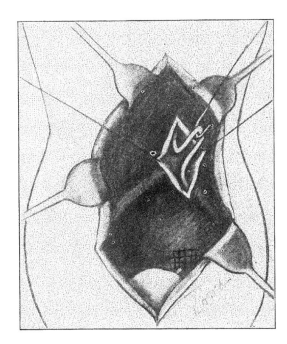

Fig. III.—Second step. Ureter drawn up from below previous to severing it just above fistulous opening.

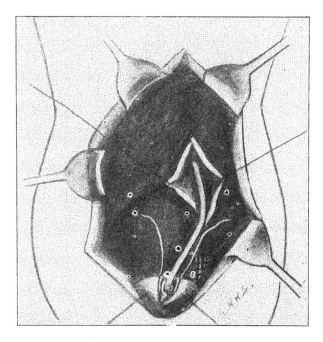

Fig. IV.—Third step. Divided ureter being implanted into posterior wall of bladder.

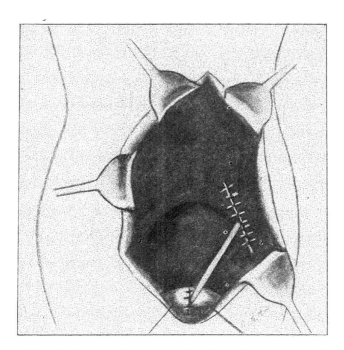

Fig. V.—Implantation completed. Note changed course of ureter, part of which is no longer retroperitoneal.

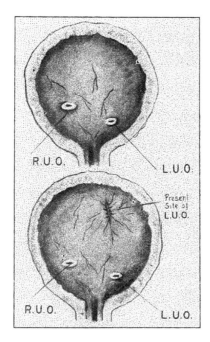

Fig. VI.—Cystoscopic appearance of inside of bladder before and after operation. U. O. = ureter opening.

infection, it was deemed advisable to attempt a uretero-vesical implantation, an operation which seemed best adapted to the conditions as found with the choice of a secondary nephrectomy in the event of failure. The conditions were explained to the patient and accepted.

On September 27, after the preliminary passage of a catheter into the right ureter, the abdomen was opened through a five inch left rectus incision. The intestines were pushed upwards and to the right side and retained there by gauze pads and the Trendelenburg position. (See Figure II). An opening was made in the posterior peritoneum and with the catheter in the right ureter as a guide, the left ureter was identified as it passed over the brim of the pelvis. With an aneurism needle the ureter was stripped up for a distance of five inches from its retroperitoneal bed, care being taken to preserve the loose areolar tissue surrounding the duct in which the ascending and descending branches of the various arteries could be plainly seen. (See Figure III).

The ureter was ligated at the lowest point which could be reached which was estimated to be 1½ or 2 inches above its orifice into the bladder and just above the fistulous opening. It was severed at this point and brought out in front of the incision in the posterior peritoneum. The duct was not dilated and appeared normal in size and consistence. The stump was cauterized with carbolic acid.

With two sutures in the bladder wall as anchors, a slit one inch in length was now made through the bladder wall on the posterior surface a little below and to the left of the fundus. Two sutures were introduced through the wall of the severed ureter about ¼ of an inch from its end which was now inserted into the bladder opening and secured at its posterior extremity by passing the above mentioned sutures through the bladder wall and tying them. (See Figure IV). A curved probe which was introduced showed the lumen of the ureter to be patent. The wound of the bladder was next repaired with a double layer of chromic gut sutures which also included the wall of the ureter.

The posterior peritoneum was sutured, allowing the ureter to pass out near the lower angle. (See Figure V). A wicking drain was inserted down to the site of the anastomosis and brought out at the lower angle of the wound which was closed by the usual layer method. A permanent catheter was introduced through the urethra and retained by a suture to the edge of the meatus.

The patient suffered considerable post operative nausea which continued for several days. The wound was first inspected on the fifth day at which time some omentum was found to have been extruded between the skin sutures. The patient was taken to the operating room and on removing the skin sutures it was found that there was a complete separation of muscles, fascia and peritoneum, an unfortunate accident which could only be explained by the quality of the catgut, no trace of which could be found in any part of the wound. At this time, the wicking drain was removed and the finger passed down to the site of anastomosis revealed evidence of satisfactory progress in the process of repair.

The wound was carefully resutured and from this time on the patient's convalescence was uninterrupted. There was never any further leakage of urine. The wound healed by primary union. The catheter was removed on the twelfth day after which no difficulty was experienced in holding the urine for six hours and voiding it without pain. She was up and around at the end of three weeks, gaining rapidly in health and strength and much improved in mental attitude.

She was discharged from the hospital on October 29th at which time a cystoscopic examination by Dr. Durham revealed the following:

Bladder capacity, 7 ounces under moderate dilatation. Bladder wall normal and not twisted on its axis. The newly made left ureteral orifice now appears in a retracted portion of the posterior wall of the bladder above and median to the old orifice. From the new orifice which is slit-like, urine is seen to drop into the bladder at regular intervals. (See Figure VI.) The passage of a ureteral catheter was not deemed advisable. The ulceration at the vault of the vagina is entirely healed and there is no discharge.

A personal communication received by the writer from the patient together with a report from her physician, Dr. Graham, shows a continued improvement in general health with entire freedom from all local symptoms.

For the satisfactory outcome in this case, I am much indebted to the valuable suggestions and services of Dr. Durham in the establishment of an accurate diagnosis, which made possible the choice of a proper method of treatment.

REFERENCES.

J. A. Sampson, *Surgery, Gynecology and Obstetrics,* May, 1909.
Kelly, Operative Gynecology.
Bovée, The Practice of Gynecology.
Kelly and Noble, Gynecology and Abdominal Surgery.

## ANOTHER ASPECT OF THE HOSPITAL PROBLEM.
### By "Medicus."

THERE are occasions, when, having read something which especially stirs my emotions, an impulse bids me take pen in hand. This occasion has come: I have just finished reading Dr. Pilcher's splendid article in the December JOURNAL, on "Professional Responsibility for Faulty Hospital Organization." We all know him and love him. His is the life we all would emulate. I would not take issue with him on these questions for his position has been such that it would take a larger experience than mine to successfully question his conclusions. The question, however, which has arisen in my mind is, has he stated the whole case? Perhaps some of the points which I shall take the liberty of bringing up he did not present for lack of space or time, but they are points which the medical profession as a whole must consider, and I have failed to see them fully and frankly discussed elsewhere.

Lest any one in reading the following should exclaim, "he is a *destructionist* and a *pessimist!* out with him!" I shall take the liberty of forestalling the criticism by saying, "quite the contrary; I am not, as my friends will tell you." But in this instance, some *destruction* is necessary before *construction* can take place. I hope, if the editor will permit me, to take up the constructive side before finishing.

In the first place, honesty is always the best policy, whether honesty with the public in such a fight as that which clusters around the question of vivisection and public hygiene, or honesty with ourselves. We should be as honest and just in judging ourselves, as we are in judging those matters which are without the pale of our profession. Where does the ultimate responsibility lie that such a state of things exists as Dr. Pilcher mentions in the first paragraph of his article and which we all know about?

I judge it must have been with the system and not with the individual. Being granted, how comes it that such a system exists? It has been stated that it exists because of lack of co-operation among physicians themselves. Quite true. Why do they not co-operate? I'll answer this question by saying because a system has grown up which makes it highly undesirable from any point of view for them to co-operate with each other, and the leaders in medicine, particularly in the large centers, have unwittingly fostered the growth of this system. The very nature of our profession as a business proposition makes ultra-competition destructive and friendly co-operation constructive. In the second place, the profession as a whole has not yet shown itself capable of rising above the personal point of view and acting for the best interests of the community and its own best interests. Mr. Fagan is calling our attention to the dangers of unionism in the management of railroads, and his view is taking a firm hold on the thinking public. The same principle holds good in the medical profession. Like railroad unionism the stand it takes toward itself has the disadvantage of trying to level all before it. Because a man is licensed to practice medicine, that is all sufficient and the medical profession has never allowed the least interference, and rightly so, with its prerogative of judging itself. On the contrary by a policy of *laisser-faire,* it has never, except in extreme instances, sought to govern itself.

Now this brings up two sides of a very important question, and I will discuss the last point first. Perhaps it can be best done by pointing to some concrete examples. It has been said with some show of authority that ten per cent. of the medical profession is addicted to the use of morphine. Personally, I doubt it. Having been thrown with large numbers of the profession in years past, I can count on the fingers of my hand the men known as morphine users. Has any one heard of an expulsion from a Medical Society or revocation of license, because of mental and moral irresponsibility following the use of morphine? If there have been such, they have not come to my notice. What protection has the public, whose confidence as a class we so much desire, if the medical profession does not act in such cases?

This brings up the still more tender point of the use of alcoholic beverages. I doubt if there is a man who reads this article who does not know of several who are mentally and morally unfit to practice medicine from this cause. I have in mind a hospital not two hundred miles from New York, where that question is now being considered. Shall a surgeon be expelled from the staff of that hospital for doing irreparable damage, time after time, while under the influence of liquor? The appointing power is in the hands of a very sensible Board of Trustees. One of the members said to me within a month, "We have the power to appoint the Staff and we don't want it. We were obliged to take it some years ago, because of the perpetual bickerings and medical politics which cropped up at every point when these questions were considered and we found as a matter of practice that if the Board did not settle these questions, they either were not settled or they were settled purely on grounds traceable to personal animosities or attractions. We have rarely if ever been able to get a disinterested opinion on an abstract basis of right and wrong on any question which involved the relationship of the physician to the hospital. We do not assume to judge the professional capability of any practitioner of medi-

cine; we are not in a position to do so, but those who are in the position to judge, will not judge for us."

I have known of several instances of this question of the use of
alcohol on the part of hospital practitioners, but I have never yet known
of an instance where such a man was dropped. Their "influence" was
too great or a halo had been placed about their heads as the result of
long service, and allowed to continue, they have in every instance died
in harness, ultimately because of their habits. Recently, in England,
several thousand railway operatives struck because an engine driver,
a member of the union, was discharged for entering and drinking at a
public bar, and as travelers we say that it was a dangerous precedent
for the railway authorities to yield and ignore even such appearance
of evil. How much more scrupulous should the physician be in this
respect!

Where is the courage which bids a Lazear to die of yellow fever
that mankind might be saved? Where is that courage which every
member of the medical profession uses daily in such ways as protecting
a "grasping" life insurance company from extortion and thereby loosing
a source of income? When it comes to dealing vigorously with situations like those given above, that courage seems to be supine. About
the only proposition it seems willing to attack at present is the abor-
tionist.

This leads up to the point of co-operation, first mentioned. To be
honest, I must reason out why it is not advantageous for physicians to
co-operate. To do that I must be again honest, and above all things
fearless, even at the risk of causing pain. The "captain of industry"
who is behind the breastworks is anxious to have himself protected by
the laborer in the ranks of medical industry and he wonders why the
laborer doesn't do it. He talks of many things such as benefits to the
community, best service to the largest number, conditions under which
the finest scientific work can be done, and other equally abstract and
beautiful platitudes, and he is undoubtedly correct. Then why doesn't
the laborer respond as he always does in every other altruistic thought
that is put to him? I think I can answer the question, at least partially.

In the first place, the average practitioner who watches the game,
is not at all sure that picking out the best men for the use of the hospitals is done on a merit basis. He has seen money, nepotism and too
many other sinister influences at work. He has also seen men take and
try to carry hospital positions, who though admittedly competent, carried too much, so much that their work was not done properly. Some
years ago the *New York Herald* published a list of the attending staffs
of the largest Manhattan hospitals; the motive for such a publication
being known to many of us. The duplication of positions clearly indicated where the major medical and surgical influences lay in that
field. After a certain point of efficiency is reached, these men are practically self-appointed in their various positions. Do they pretend to tell
the rest of the profession that *they* are the only ones who are competent from the standpoint of highest scientific attainment to hold them,
and is that the reason why they consent to remain there? Is the motive
altruistic? If it is, why do the "captains" consent to allow such a state
of things to exist that only the unfit inhabitants of the public ward
and the multi-millionaire can afford to have the best the profession can
give, while the man who can afford two dollars an office call is allowed
to employ a relatively unfit laborer in the vineyard of medicine, or at

least one who is considered as incompetent for hospital work, because of lack of opportunity or desire or ability to make himself better? These observations open up many other questions which would be themes for profitable discussion.

In the second place, the average non-hospital practitioner will not assist the "captain" in pulling the latter's chestnuts out of the fire, because he sees in the hospital a growing menace to his livelihood. As a rule, he has no other desire than to earn such an income for himself and family, as will return to him who has spent money, time and effort to attain a scientific and professional training, a fair compensation. In the face of all the forces combining to crush him, he gives 25 per cent. of his effort to bad debtors and the poor, where there is no glory nor legitimate advertisement for consultation work; and still the number who will do abortions for hire is extremely small. Yet, he sees constantly patients leaving him and going to the hospital dispensary and to the hospital ward because they can get their needs supplied, "without money and without price." Even when that harm has been done him, the best taken away from him and the skimmed milk left, is he always sure of getting the skimmed milk? By no means. Wouldn't it be an odd thing to have a gastro-enterostomy case referred back to the original physician by the hospital surgeon on leaving the hospital, the former being called by name, unless the two stood in direct friendly relationship? Where is the dispensary or hospital which makes it a practice of diligently protecting the interests of the non-hospital practitioner, or ever asks the slightest question as to the previous medical attendance? This brings up another question, that of the "specialist," who is so often a hospital attaché. Some two years ago, a professional friend of mine who is an especially competent gastro-intestinal specialist made this statement. "The mass of practitioners do not send me cases because they want to. They send them because they are obliged to. Even the major portion of my practice walks into my office without reference at all, because the individuals have heard of me." I asked him to consider for a moment and tell me why. He said he couldn't, that he knew he was competent in his line, and yet he was unable to command the respect of his fellow practitioners sufficiently to draw practice through the profession and it was a source of great disappointment to him. I asked him to follow this invariable rule in the future: in every non-referred case to enquire the previous medical attendance, whether the patient had had attendance in the present difficulty or not. Then he was to adopt one of two procedures, to act through the previous attending whether the case had been referred or not, or to send the patient to one in the locality in which he lived. He has done so, and he tells me that his reference practice has increased five-fold since, and that he has made personal friends with many physicians who in return have repaid him many times. Shall specialists be pirates in the profession, or shall they be the helpful ones? Some day some specialist will discover how to act toward his brother practitioners and he will make a fortune, and make it in the easiest way imaginable by little work and high pay for what he does.

I might take up several points along this line but lack of space forbids. I have abundantly destroyed in the hope to adequately reconstruct. That shall be my task now. In doing so, I ask your attention to the contrast presented by the following two statements, both taken from Dr. Pilcher's article:

Dr. Farrar Cobb: "Allow me to emphasize again that the work

of a large number of men operating intermittently with relatively small
material and experience cannot be compared fairly with the work of
one highly-trained man with abundant material." I hardly think any
one will quarrel with that. It's the truth if anything was ever the truth
but it isn't the whole truth. . Here is what Dr. Neuman of Vienna says:

"As the head of Gremial Hospital, a state institution, I receive $1,-
600 a year salary. Every patient in my department has my personal
attention. My assistants have to work. If they do not study and work,
they must leave." Here again is the truth but not the whole truth
and wherein will the two indicate the proper direction along which
evolution shall go?

Shall I take the liberty of outlining? In the first place on leaving
the hospital, every young physician should have abundant opportunity
to connect himself with some institution in some capacity, and in such
a way that by hard work and attention to study, he may advance
along some chosen line. If he does reasonably good work, say for instance in the out-patient department, he should have a small salary, and
be encouraged by opportunity to study individual bed cases under the
direction of the assistant attending. He should *not* be permitted to go
into a room with fifty patients and told that he *must* get through in one
hour to make room for some one else. In other words, the quality of
his work and not the number of patients cared for should be the criterion. By the time he is 35 years of age, as an average, he should by
virtue of his work be promoted to the position of assistant attending
at an advance in salary. In this position, he should have immediate
charge of the patients in the wards, but only a few of
them at one time, and under the direction of the regular
attending. Here again the quality of the work on the individual patient should be the criterion, not the number of
patients he may be able to send into the private rooms of that particular institution nor the number of operating rooms he can keep busy
during the morning by fleeing from one to another while the different
patients are being prepared for operation. There is a whole lot to
surgery besides what is done in the operating room. The number of
different things an attending can find out the matter with one patient is
of a good deal more importance than the number of different patients
who have one thing. It is right in this point that Dr. Cobb "falls down"
in his generalization. How many surgeons are there of the type he
mentions who can make a dependable microscopic diagnosis? How
many, I venture to add, have a working knowledge of dietetics? A
surgeon of reputation recently told me that he recommended albumin-
water as a post-operative diet. When I remarked that a patient must
take a lot of it to meet caloric needs, he promptly replied that it would
not take much, and then "it was so easily digested!"

At this period of his career, the young surgeon should
be doing the minor-major operations, the hernias, the appendectomies, etc. He should have few enough patients to make original
observations and do some clinical research work, and *study his cases,*
under the supervision of the attending. The full attending, reaching
this stage at the forty-fifth year, should then be in the full fruition of
his powers. He should confine himself to the real major operating,
such as goitre removal, gastro-enterostomies, brain surgery, etc. An
appendectomy at this stage should be to him very much as a boil is to
the present-day attending, except as it presents unusual difficulties or
complications, and be left to his assistants. After a man has done 250

appendectomies, further experience with that operation is gained at the expense of other fields of surgery where he should be proficient, such as scientific preparation for operating, the technique of recovery, better facility in medical diagnosis, and other numerous questions which arise and which, mayhap, now receive but scant attention. An attending can find plenty to do, under circumstances such as these, where by educating his assistants, giving direction to their work, and, master of the situation as regards his department, so control and manage things as to gain the greatest return for the smallest amount of work, *i. e.,* enormously increased efficiency. Finally comes the consultant, the graduated attending, who still preserves his interest in medical things, who desires special cases for original work. It should be his part to give advice and disinterested counsel in the management of the medical and surgical affairs of the hospital.

In closing, I am sure most have recognized the train of thought which runs through this whole article. I desire to stimulate co-operation among physicians by making it to their interest to do so. Increase the number of men who are connected with our institutions and put them under strict graded service, thereby giving greater opportunity to the profession at large to gain the advantage to be gotten from association with the best. Vigorous action, not only in protecting the interests of the "family doctor" against pirating, but in weeding out the unfit not only among the hospital practitioners, but the profession at large, thus further protecting the public against low standards of practice and incompetence, *is needed.*

To sum up, the problem must be solved not by increasing the amount of work already done by the few, but by educating the many to do each less but better work. To that end the hospital should not be regarded, in its last analysis, as primarily a place for the sick to be healed, but as a place for the sick to be healed *and for the real education of the profession.*

## EDITORIAL NOTE.

The unsigned contribution printed above was submitted with the understanding that the responsibility for proof of the facts stated should not be assumed by the JOURNAL. The publication of articles submitted anonymously or under a fictitious name is contrary to the policy of the JOURNAL, but in view of the discussion in regard to Medical Economics which is now so prevalent and as this contribution takes up a phase of the subject that the Editor does not recall having seen presented from just this view-point, he feels that it should be presented to the readers of the Journal, inasmuch as it calls attention to a condition which may seem very real to others in the profession beside the writer of the article.

The Editor may reasonably express some doubt as to the wisdom of too much public discussion about the short-comings of our profession. The devil can quote scripture for his use, and the public and lay-press are only too prone to acclaim apparent faults. Whether we do not present the appearance of disunion by our present attitude is a grave question. On the other hand the frank discussion of real short-comings can, in the end, produce nothing but good, and, as this particular article discusses its point of view temperately and in the spirit of earnestness, its appearance in these pages seems justified. H. G. W.

# BLOOD CULTURES; SIMPLIFIED BY NEW APPARATUS; DEMONSTRATION.*

## By William Lintz, M.D.,

of Brooklyn, N. Y.

*(From the Bacteriological Department of the Long Island College Hospital.)*

OF all clinical methods as yet devised for the purpose of diagnosis, prognosis and treatment of disease there is no method which finds so wide a range of usefulness and importance as that of culturing the blood for bacteria. True, blood cultures find their greatest usefulness only in infectious diseases and the complications they lead to. But then it is just these types of cases that form the major part of the work of the general practitioner, surgeon, and not infrequently of the obstetrician; and they are often cases that are extremely difficult and occasionally impossible to diagnose by other means. Positive blood cultures absolutely clinch the diagnosis as but very few other single procedures do; negative blood cultures are not so conclusive, although even they have significant values from a negative point of view, as we shall see later.

In no other disease has blood culture proven its usefulness as much as in typhoid. It has established a method of making the earliest possible diagnosis; it has revolutionized its pathogenesis; it has scientifically explained its relapses; for it is an established fact that typhoid bacilli occur in the blood so early, while the temperature is still rising, and so regularly, that bacteriologic examination of the blood may be regarded as the best means of diagnosis in the early stages of the fever, the period when definite diagnosis is most difficult yet most desirable. I have been able to cultivate the bacilli from the blood as early as the first and second days of the fever, long before the appearance of specific agglutinins, for it is not at all infrequent for the Widal reaction to be negative until the temperature has already reached normal.

During the first week of the disease the bacilli can be found in the blood in from 93% to 100% of the cases; during the second week in about 76% of the cases; during the third in about 56% to 60%, and in the majority of the cases the bacillus disappears from the blood about the end of the third week.

As to the pathogenesis of typhoid: in view of the early occurrence of the bacillemia, its persistence during the height of the attack, its relation to relapse and recrudescence indicate perhaps that the intestinal lesions of typhoid are not primary, but secondary from hematogenous invasion, and there is experimental proof that the bacilli enter the circulation by means of the tonsils.

As to prognosis: I have not found that the number of bacteria in the blood, as determined by plate cultures, stands in any relationship to the height of the fever or the general severity of the attack.

Whatever has been said of typhoid holds good for paratyphoid and paracolon bacillemia.

In the blood of pneumonia patients Prochaska, Philosofeff-Weber and Rosenow find the pneumococcus in 100% of the cases examined before the crisis. Blood cultures from hospital patients during all stages

---

* Read before the Medical Society of the County of *Kings*, December 17, 1912.

of pneumonia have yielded to me about 45% to 50% of positive results. Some of these cases developed physical signs of pneumonia twenty-four to thirty-six hours after the culture was taken.

In malignant endocarditis blood cultures are not infrequently the only means of making a positive diagnosis before the occurrence of emboli. The micro-organisms I found in the order of frequency are the streptococcus, pneumococcus and staphylococcus pyogenes aureus.

In blood cultures taken in numerous cases of rheumatism of all types I have been able to obtain the diplococcus rheumaticus in but four cases. The reason why the positive findings are so few is perhaps due to the fact that the micro-organism is but very infrequently present in the circulation, as it is encapsulated within the rheumatic nodules so characteristic of that disease.

In septicemias and bacteremias due to the pyogenic cocci, streptococci and staphylococci in particular, such as follow local abscesses, general infections, puerperal sepsis, pelvic cellulitis and cryptic infections of all sorts, blood cultures are of the greatest help.

In osteomyelitis of children I have obtained the staphylococcus pyogenes aureus with such constancy and so early in the disease, in some cases the positive blood culture preceding any focal osseous symptoms, that I wonder whether in children suppurative osteomyelitis is not always a primary staphylococcus bacteremia with secondary hematogenous infection of the bone.

A mastoid infection associated with a positive blood culture nearly always points in addition to a sinus involvement, although there may be no other symptoms pointing to that condition.

As to the importance of negative blood cultures: repeated blood cultures during all stages of tuberculosis have yielded but negative results, not only as regards finding the tubercle bacilli, but also the finding of any other micro-organisms of secondary infection, so frequently reported to be present.

Contrary to the accepted opinion that prior to death there invariably occurs an agonal invasion of bacteria into the circulation, blood cultures taken in vivo and post mortem from well preserved bodies show that the post mortem findings compare favorably with those taken ante mortem. Of special importance in this connection are the *sterile blood cultures* obtained post mortem in cases that have died from purulent peritonitis as a result of ruptured appendix, intestinal ulcer, gall-bladder, etc. If agonal invasion were so frequent, one has a right to expect positive blood cultures in these types of cases where the peritoneal pus is swarming with all kinds of bacteria. Therefore, post mortem blood cultures have a decided diagnostic importance and no autopsy is complete without them.

Examination of the blood in cases of measles, scarlet fever, diphtheria, poliomyelitis, tetanus, malaria, purpura hemorrhagica, syphilis and most cases of erysipelas have proven sterile.

A negative result may mean:

(1) That the bacteria sought are actually absent.

(2) That the disease may be an infection that is not due to bacteria demonstrable by present methods of blood culture, as syphilis; or

(3) That the bacteria are so few in number that they are absent in the quantity of blood examined; or

(4) It may be due to bacteria that either do not escape at all into

the circulation or that reach the circulation in small numbers or inconstantly so that they do not appear in the cultures.

(5) The bacteria may be present during chills and fever when they are swept into the circulation from the infecting focus, but the bactericidal power of the blood is still preserved and unless the blood is taken at a suitable time, the cultures are sterile.

(6) And finally, negative results are obtained when infected emboli and thrombi and not free bacteria, are circulating in the blood and produce metastases.

Repeated blood cultures will obviate most of the above-named difficulties.

The prognosis when bacteria are cultivated from the blood is not by any means always fatal. Contrary to the opinion of text-books, my experience has shown that the streptococcus is more fatal than the staphylococcus pyogenus aureus. The hemolytic power of the streptococcus is not in direct proportion to its virulence.

In spite of the great usefulness of blood culture, the general practitioner seldom avails himself of culturing bacteria in the blood, its use being restricted mainly to hospital practice. This is due to the *difficulty of procuring* the blood. By the methods at present in use the process of obtaining blood is exceedingly *cumbersome* and *contaminations are frequent,* so that one has to have special training in this line of work, for otherwise the results are not only unreliable but even misleading.

By the use of the method devised one can avail himself of blood cultures as readily as of the Widal reaction in typhoid.

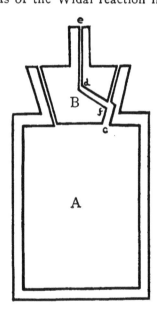

*Description of apparatus.*—The apparatus is composed of a glass bottle (a), containing *a ground air-tight* stopper (b); along the lower half of the inner surface of the neck of the flask, there is a longitudinal groove (c); the stopper contains a longitudinal canal (d), which opens above at (e), and below the canal is continuous obliquely downward and outward, opening at the ground side of the stopper at (f), which lies below the upper level of groove (c). It is evident that if the stopper is placed in the bottle so that the lower opening of the canal (f) opens into the groove (c) on the inner surface of the neck, the inside of the flask will be in direct communication with the outside by means of the groove (c) and the canal (d). It is also evident that by rotating the stopper sideways so that the lower opening of the canal (f) no longer opens to the groove (c), the inside of the flask is shut off from all communication with the outside of the flask (to facilitate rotation of the stopper a lubricant, such as graphite, is recommended). Place in bottle 0.5 gm. of finely powdered sodium chlorid, or 10 c.c. of 1% solution of ammonium oxalate in normal saline, or sterile $H_2O$. Replace stopper (f) so that there is communication between the lower opening of the canal in the stopper (f) and the groove (c) on the inner surface of the neck of the bottle. This will afford direct communication between the inside of the flask and the outside air. *Produce next a vacuum in the flask.* This can be accomplished in several ways, either by a water pump, vacuum pump, or by the simple aspiration of the air with an ordinary syringe. I found that the simplest way of producing a vacuum and at the same time sterilizing the contents of the flask, is by placing the flask in water (or brine) with its neck above the level of the fluid, and then boil the water. The heat will rarify the air in the flask and thus a partial vacuum, sufficient for all practical purposes, will be produced. The same result can be obtained with dry heat. Also aspiration of air with the mouth, as suggested by Mr. Layton is excellent. As soon as you have obtained the vacuum, irrespective of the method employed, break the communication between the inside of the flask and the outside air by turning the stopper sideways so that the lower opening of the canal in the stopper (f) will no longer be in communication with the groove (c) on the inner surface of the neck of the flask. Attach a needle (g) to the stopper directly or by means of a connecting piece of rubber, cover the needle with test tube (h) and sterilize the entire apparatus by boiling dry or steam heat. The apparatus is immediately ready for use at *any date in the future.* (The vacuum keeps).

*Use of apparatus.*—To use the apparatus one paints the bend of the elbow with tincture of iodin (or sterilize the part by any other method), plunges the needle in the median basilic or cephalic vein, and then rotates the stopper so that the lower opening of the canal (f) communicates with the groove (c) on the inner surface of the neck of the flask. The vacuum in the flask will rapidly suck in the blood from the vein.

Having obtained the desired quantity of blood, 10 c.c. being quite sufficient for all practical purposes, you break the communication between the inside and outside of the flask by rotating the stopper sideways, and then remove the needle from the vein. Cover with collodion the opening in the skin caused by the entrance of the needle.

The flask containing the blood is now thoroughly shaken. The sodium chlorid or ammonium oxalate or sterile $H_2O$ used prevents the blood from coagulating, but is not bactericidal. In fact, the bacteria commonly found readily multiply in it.

The blood thus obtained can now be taken or sent to the laboratory and subjected to the usual process.

Where one suspects the typhoid bacillus to be the infective organism instead of placing ammonium oxalate solution or salt, you put 10 c.c. of bile in the flask and after obtaining the blood in the manner described, incubate the mixture in the flask without further manipulation. Likewise, when suspecting the pneumococcus to be the cause of the bacteremia, one places in the flask a slightly alkaline solution of 10% peptone and 1% dextrose, as recommended by Wiens, and after obtaining the blood, one incubates the flask. Experience has convinced me that practically all micro-organisms found in blood grow readily on bouillon or glucose bouillon, so that if the blood is obtained in a bottle containing the latter media and the mixture is incubated, no further manipulation of the blood is necessary.

*The advantages of the method are*: 1. Contaminations are absolutely excluded.

2. (a) The general practitioner of the city *or country* can avail himself by this method of blood cultures, for the attending physician can procure the blood when he visits the patient and the flask can be brought to any laboratory for further examination. All one has to determine from now on is the micro-organism present; and it means no more than the determination of any micro-organism when pus is inoculated on an agar culture tube; hence the expense to the patient is but trivial. The cost of blood cultures by the present method makes it prohibitive for most patients.

(b) Furthermore, by the present method, the country practitioner could not avail himself of blood cultures. By this method he can send the flask containing the procured blood to the nearest laboratory by mail, for further examination. The flask can be placed and shipped in a thermos bottle or in the center of a roll of cotton wool which would prevent the lowered temperature from destroying the bacteria in the blood.

3. The sight of syringes, needles, test tubes, flasks, media, etc., frightens the patient, who in most instances anticipates a major operation. With this method he anticipates at the most no more pain than is caused by a hypodermic needle.

4. One has at all times a sterile apparatus which he can use at once as the occasion arises.

5. As the entire apparatus can be easily carried in the vest pocket, it is very convenient for obtaining blood outside of the laboratory.

6. The procurance of blood with this apparatus is so simple that anybody can undertake it.

7. By the use of this apparatus one obtains a nice, clear serum without hemolysis of the red cells, which is a particular advantage when the blood is obtained for Wasserman, Widal, meiastigmin or cancer reactions. Of course, this apparatus can be used for obtaining blood for any serological purpose.

8. The apparatus saves the outlay of expensive syringes, and, furthermore, will last a lifetime.

(*For discussion, see page* 80.)

---

# THE EYES OF OUR SCHOOL CHILDREN.

By James Cole Hancock, M.D.,

of Brooklyn, N. Y.

WHEN we consider the undoubted importance, both economic and physical, of the care of the eyes of our school children possibly the system in vogue at the present time for this purpose seems inadequate to meet the necessary requirements. Upon the other hand it is unquestionably true that much good has been done by the school physicians and that great benefit has been rendered the community at large through their efforts in connection with the care of pupils who suffer from errors of refraction or diseased eyes.

The physicians who make the school examinations for physical defects such as adenoids, enlarged tonsils, skin affections and eye troubles are medical inspectors of the Board of Health and beyond maintaining a card index relating to the physical conditions of the pupils to be kept in the schools as a record and referring those found mentally defective to the Board of Education physicians have no direct responsibility to, or direct connection with, the Board of Education. In other words, the Board of Education lays out school work to be done and it then becomes the school physician's duty to ascertain by examination who are unfit physically to perform the duties so laid out.

Although this paper shall have to do only with the *eye* disorders met with in the schools the rules relating to these apply to all other physical defects ascertained. Should a pupil be found upon examination by the school physician to have vision falling below the standard known as "normal vision," or to be suffering from any eye inflammation accompanied by a discharge, or an eye inflammation having the characteristics of trachoma, phlyctenular conjunctivitis or keratitis, a formal statement is sent to the pupil's parents giving the name of the affection and advising that the eyes need attention and that a physician be consulted. Provided no attention is paid this advice, after a few days, the school nurse calls at the home of the pupil and recommends to the parents that the suggestion be immediately carried into effect. If this visit of the nurse proves unavailing others are made by her and finally one or more by the school physician himself. These visits are made at intervals of not less than ten days in order to give the parents opportunity for complying. In addition to home visits consultations are held where doubting mothers may be instructed and defects demonstrated to them by actual tests. In cases where the parents are unable to take the child to the dispensary, the nurse will take the child herself. In certain selected cases, with the permission of the parents, the eyes are examined with atropine at the Health Department clinics. Trachoma is also operated upon at the Health Department eye hospitals. If the physician and nurse find that it is impossible for the parents to pay for proper glasses attempts are made through philanthropic sources to obtain free glasses for the pupil. Should the school physician become convinced that no argument or further effort will prevail he marks upon the pupil's card "treatment and advice have been refused," and this ends the matter until the pupil is re-examined when the school is again gone over. Where the eye disorder is of an inflammatory nature, possibly, probably or certainly contagious, and where it is accompanied by a discharge the pupil is immediately sent home and not allowed to return to school until under treatment and bringing a note from the physician in charge stating that there is no danger to others. When the parents of such a child refuse to consult a physician in the matter the pupil is not re-admitted to the school. If there is an attempt to return the case is reported by the class teacher to the school nurse who has power to exclude the pupil if in her judgment necessary. In all cases, where pupils have been examined for glasses or treated for inflammatory eye conditions, they are re-examined by the school physician and a record is kept as to whether the child is cured, improved, or not improved, and the case is then terminated.

In many cases parents do not appreciate the importance of the disordered conditions of the eyes and so pay them little attention, even after having received proper advice, while in others they cause the children to conceal the symptoms through the dread of most parents to have their children wear glasses. These are both decided obstacles in the way of getting results.

The physical examinations are supposed to be made at the beginning of the school year and continued until all the pupils in all the schools have been examined for physical defects. All who are found by the class teacher giving symptoms of eye disturbance in any form are supposed to be reported to the school nurse and by her to the school physician if in her judgment necessary.

We have mentioned the importance of the work, the methods employed and some of the obstacles encountered, now let us consider the results obtained. These, without a doubt, are decidedly beneficial, but existing circumstances make them less far-reaching and effective than they should be. First: All pupils with defective vision are sent home with a statement to the parents advising that a physician be consulted for examination and correcting glasses. This is a great step in the proper direction for much relief for distressing symptoms is obtained and the pupil enabled to continue the school work that would be impossible to be continued otherwise. Second: Contagious eye disorders have been practically eliminated from our schools and the milder forms remaining are in the majority of cases under treatment. Trachoma, which had a greater hold upon our school community three or four years ago than was generally believed, has been practically driven out and the comparatively few mild cases remaining are mostly under treatment and therefore less dangerous.

While the cases of myopia and marked astigmatism, because of the resulting defective vision, are easily found, the cases of hypermetropia are almost all overlooked, for with these the vision is usually normal and so comes up to the standard required. The reason the vision is normal here is because of the ability to strain the eyes and this "eye strain" is responsible for a very great number of reflex symptoms and disturbances, such as headache, nervous indigestion, dizziness and many other neurotic phenomena. "The nine o'clock headache" is not unknown in many households, but it is not generally thought that, beyond the disinclination for school, there is any real reason for it. The real reason many pupils dislike school, however, is that it makes their heads ache to go there and gives them many other unpleasant symptoms. Generally speaking all children before beginning school should have the eyes tested with atropine or an equivalent as this is the only sure way to bring to light hypermetropia, and by far the best way to determine the full amount of other forms of refractive error.

A paper of this kind should give proper credit to the school physicians. While it is impossible for them to give a great deal of time to this work in that time they really accomplish much good and could accomplish much more were there more active co-operation upon the part of the parents. It seems, however, that the present system could be greatly improved and this most important work rendered much more productive of good results.

To my mind, these physicians should be under the direction of the Board of Education and should receive salaries sufficient to enable them to give to the schools the time and attention really necessary to obtain truly satisfactory results. The small staff of school physicians at present seems quite inadequate to do the work justice and should be greatly augmented. Our smallest schools carry fifteen hundred pupils on the roll and the larger ones over four thousand. It is not physically possible for one physician to attend two or more of these schools and do his work better than in a superficial way, and the work is far too important to be so done. He does the best he can and much better than one in any other walk of life or profession would do for a salary so small.

While much if not practically all of this work might well be put under the head of "special" it seems to me that physicians who are called upon to perform the duties exacted should have previously received some special instruction and experience. By this it is not meant that specialists are necessary for this work, but that those who do it should be better informed concerning the physical defects most likely to come under observation.

There has been for a long time, and probably will be for some time to come, a decided difference of opinion between physicians in general and those having in charge the laying out of school work. Physicians are firmly of the opinion that there is by far too much home work, but this is stoutly denied by the school authorities. It seems to the medical profession that schooling should be largely confined to the school and school hours and that our young people should have more opportunity for out-of-door exercise and recreation. Three or four hours devoted to study outside the school building seems to us too much. The solution of the subject appears, however, to be for the future as sufficient interest cannot be aroused among the laity at present, and physicians, unfortunately, are but little consulted when matters of public importance are to be decided. Because of the, often excessive, use of the eyes required, at a time of life when all excesses are most influential for evil, it is my practise to order weak resting glasses for such of my patients as complain of their eyes tiring after, or while doing the necessary school work and this even when their eyes are proven to be perfectly normal. In this way many a pupil goes through school without real damage to the eyes. During vacations the glasses are not used and when the school work is finally finished, they are usually entirely discarded. Many a pupil comes to the end of the schooling with impaired eyes and the necessity for glasses who could as well have been spared the resulting annoyance and worse by this simple procedure. It is difficult to make parents see the importance of this simple relief because of the almost universal disfavor in which the putting on of glasses is held.

The number of schools assigned to each inspector depends upon registration. Each school physician has under his care about nine thousand children and it is impossible to examine the whole school even once a year. The children are examined in the following order: First, new admissions; second, graduating classes; third, children the doctor finds on going through each class having defective vision or other eye disorders who need immediate treatment; fourth, regular examinations by grades. Visual defects are not sought in grades below the so-called 2A grade. This practically means that no child is examined before learning to read letters. It presumably excludes from such examinations all who attend the kindergarten and this is important as children often are under considerable "eye strain" while in the kindergarten, though this is generally not supposed to be the case.

# EDITORIAL

## VALE ET SALVE.

WITH the current number of the JOURNAL, the editorial management changes. Dr. Paul Monroe Pilcher, who has piloted the destinies of the JOURNAL from its infancy, retires after six years of arduous service in its behalf. The result of his work is familiar to every reader of the JOURNAL. The Associated Physicians are to be congratulated, not only upon the results, but also upon the nature of Dr. Pilcher's services, for during his editorial management the JOURNAL has grown from a feeble infant of somewhat rachitic tendencies to a robust adolescence. That Dr. Pilcher merits the hearty appreciation of the Associated Physicians goes without saying.

His successor enters upon his duties with a standard already set so high as to occasion misgivings. It seems to him an appropriate time to point out to the Associated Physicians of Long Island that the LONG ISLAND MEDICAL JOURNAL is their journal and its editor their steward; that while upon him rests the duty of conducting the JOURNAL according to their wishes, the duty devolves on every one to help build up the JOURNAL to its highest efficiency by his hearty co-operation. Suggestions will be welcome, criticisms equally so. The interest of each member is besought, his active co-operation urged.

In order that the JOURNAL may represent the interests of all Long Island, it is necessary that every member should constitute himself a contributing editor. Items of personal interest from each town on the Island, contributions from all members, will help to stimulate a general interest in the JOURNAL that must needs make it an active influence in uniting the profession of Long Island in a common bond. The editor pledges his best efforts to this end. He looks to every member of the Society for practical help. H. G. W.

## THE AMERICAN SOCIETY OF MEDICAL ECONOMICS.

WITH the birth of the American Society of Medical Economics, the profession of medicine entered upon a new era. Incorporated December 18th, 1912, under the laws of the State of New York, that society is already engaged in the consideration of plans for the construction and establishment of a national organization which will devote its energies solely and exclusively to the systematic study of medical economics. For this reason, the society has the earnest support and co-operation of representative members of the profession, irrespective of schools of practice. This unification of the medical profession is unprecedented in its history. It has been the one thing needed for effective work. Realizing this, the incorporators of the American Society of Medical Economics, at their initial meeting, eliminated the word "school" from their deliberations. It is this unifying element in its foundation which promises the success of the present undertaking.

The objection may be raised that the movement is radical; the answer to this possible criticism would be that it is radical only in appearance, that it is, in fact, the culmination of a natural, steady growth; it is new only as the plant which breaks the ground is new; underneath is the germinated seed, the root drawing nourishment from a fertile soil. Progress is ever growth, adaptation, not revolution. It is not a sudden springing into being, it is a gradual development. But here the word gradual must be taken in a relative sense; for in the course of evolutionary processes, there occur, from time to time, upheavals which resemble destruction, but which in reality are the separation of elements for the purpose of crystalization. The Italian Renaissance was not, as its name suggests, a sudden bursting forth, it was a gradual ripening. The upheaval in France which history has named the French Revolution, crushed and scattered to the four winds the crumbling atoms of an unjust and despotic monarchy. This was an evolutionary upheaval, whose heated, whitened, scattered elements fell upon the site of the cruel and bloody Bastile, and, crystalizing, formed there an enduring monument dedicated to human liberty. The first gun fired in defense of the Union must not, in the light of evolution, be interpreted as a beginning. It bespoke an end. It sounded a death knell, the death knell of human slavery.

Birth is never creation. Back of every normal birth are all the natural, the evolutionary processes of coming into being—germination, nutrition, growth, development, fructification and ripening. The birth of the American Society of Medical Economics was a normal birth; back of it are all the natural, the evolutionary processes. The society is the natural result of the changed conditions confronting us, a knowledge of which has been thrust upon every member of the profession. For example; nothwithstanding the constant increase in population, the death rate in our own crowded community, in one generation, has been cut almost in two, and this is fairly representative of what is happening in other similar communities. When we come to look back of this fact for its explanation, we find that it lies in the wonderful achievements of medical and surgical science and that the work which accomplished these achievements has occupied the time and taxed the utmost energies of our profession, to the exclusion of every other thought, certainly to the exclusion of the study and consideration of any measure which would make for the betterment of its own condition. We find that in its splendid, its unvarying altruism, its zeal for the acquisition of knowledge, its magnificent self-abnegation, our profession has almost entirely forgotten itself. It has never paused long enough to care for its own comfort or to calculate its own advantage. It has been too closely attentive to its actual work to consider its own rewards or even its own just recompense. With these facts in mind are we not forced to conclude that it is indeed time to attempt the development of a science of medical economics?

Such a project should interest our patients as well, because, if it be true that our household affairs are unsatisfactory to us, our methods of management antiquated and inadequate, it follows that our working efficiency is thereby impaired. Moreover, the efficient servant is the contented servant, and it is here the patient has his obligation to that profession which has ever been foremost in the service of humanity. When we reflect upon some of the economic conditions which may be said to affect the general public; charlatanism and quackery, medical legislation, lodge and contract practice, medical charities, eugenics, the adulteration of food stuffs, milk supply, the substituting of drugs in the dispensing of physicians' prescriptions, abuses of quarantine, the effects on the health of children of school curricula, and the like, we cannot fail to realize that they have grown to such proportions as to require for their intelligent consideration and control the best efforts of a united profession.

What we need, then, is an organization which will welcome to its membership every practitioner of medicine. The American Society of Medical Economics offers itself as a nucleus for such an organization. The details of this or that question which the society hopes to solve, need not at present concern us. These are to be left, as they should be, until their disposition can represent the best thought of the medical world. What is needed now, what is absolutely essential, is the strength of numbers. Let us but make the membership of the society universal in the profession and its future achievements are assured. It will then be in a position to stand squarely and authoritatively before the general public, a representative body selected by the great profession of medicine, a body chosen for the exercise of delegated powers which for lack of time can not be exercised by our scientific organizations. The following are the names of the officers of the Society:

President, Dr. E. Eliot Harris; vice-presidents, Dr. Algernon Bristow, Dr. William Francis Campbell, Dr. Smith Ely Jelliffe, Dr. T. K. Tuthill, and Dr. Thomas F. Reilly; secretary, Dr. Dana Hubbard; treasurer, Dr. Royal S. Copeland, and historian, Dr. W. J. Cruikshank. Among the committees and the men selected to head them are: General Economics, Dr. L. Pierce Clark; Professional Conduct, Dr. J. R. Kevin; Medical Charity, Dr. W. S. Thomas; Education and Statistics, Dr. Alfred S. Taylor; Legislation, Dr. J. E. Wilson; Foods, Drugs and Sanitation, Dr. E. J. Kopetzky; Ways and Means and Inspection, Dr. Russell S. Fowler; Special Business, Dr. Irving Wilson Voorhees.

The American Society of Medical Economics enters upon its work with no lack of appreciation of its obligations, its duties and its responsibilities. It realizes that the problems which, in the course of time, it hopes to solve, present many new and involved questions requiring full discussion and the most intelligent and careful reflection. It is, therefore, convinced that in seeking the support and co-operation of every practicing physician and surgeon it is conserving the best interests of the medical profession and of the general public.

WILLIAM J. CRUIKSHANK.

## THE CRUSADE AGAINST VENEREAL DISEASE.

THE International Committee of Young Men's Christian Associations has recently sent out a card which carries the following declaration:

"In view of the individual and social dangers which spring from the widespread belief that continence may be detrimental to health, and of the fact that municipal toleration of prostitution is sometimes defended on the ground that sexual indulgence is necessary, we, the undersigned, members of the medical profession, testify to our belief that continence has not been shown to be detrimental to health or virility; that there is no evidence of its being inconsistent with the highest physical, mental and moral efficiency; and that it offers the only sure reliance for sexual health outside marriage."

The circular letter which accompanies it carries the approval of such men as Abraham Jacobi, William M. Polk, Walter B. Cannon, William S. Thayer and others, and the intention is to secure the signatures of a sufficient number of physicians of prominence to add to this declaration the assurance of ex cathedra authority. The ultimate plan is to make use of this with other material by placing it in the hands of such organizations as the Society for Sanitary and Moral Prophylaxis; the American Federation for Sex Hygiene; Public Health Departments; Young Men's Christian Associations, etc., for use in the campaign that they are waging against the spread of venereal disease.

To one who has watched with interest the growth of this organized effort to curb a plague which is fast becoming a national curse, this latest exposure of a public error seems a long step in the right direction, for it has been an argument that has been difficult to meet because of its widespread popular acceptation.

It may not be amiss to trace briefly the milestones in the campaign which has now assumed widespread significance. Although for years the medical profession has realized the inroad that the venereal diseases have made upon the health of the community; although they have appreciated the sufferings which have, according to the statement of the late Gaillard Thomas, been the forerunners of 60 per cent. of all operations upon women; and have shuddered over the pitiful array of blind babies who are, perhaps, the most heartrending victims of these accursed troubles, they have failed in concerted action, they have been only too prone to join the ranks of those who have let well-enough alone and have satisfied themselves with an effort to remedy what they should have striven to prevent. It is to the credit of Dr. Prince A. Morrow that, following his plea for the organization of the Society of Sanitary and Moral Prophylaxis in 1904, this organization sprang into existence a year later and has since spread to cover almost the whole country. It has drawn together not only physicians whose work has lain more particularly along these lines, but a very large number from all the walks of public usefulness—lawyers, clergymen, educators, social workers and men of business. Even with the weight of such influence behind it, the work has had to overcome no small obstacles, of which public inertia and prudery have been and are still the worst.

The American Federation for Sex Hygiene was next to take up the organized work, and since then the Young Men's Christian Association has conducted an orderly campaign through its various branches. In furtherance of the same work the New York State Legislature two years ago passed the Page Law which placed in the hands of the Health Department the power to determine the presence of venereal disease among women of the streets, a faulty step, but one in the right direction.

Efforts such as these, directed as they are against a vice ingrained in human nature, fostered by passion and ignorance, and working in secret, can make but slow progress. They should appeal to every thoughtful physician, not only upon the professional, but upon the paternal side, for the curbing of this insidious plague is of vast importance, threatening as it does the very grain and marrow of our national health. We have enthusiastically taken up the prophylaxis of typhoid, small-pox, of bubonic plague; we should heartily unite in this far-reaching step that seeks not only the physical but the moral uplift of our country.

H. G. W.

## TENEMENTS AND PHILANTHROPY.

THE sanitary tenement house, built for the poor, has not been a success, if some of its critics are to be believed. Not only that, it has tended directly to make the living conditions of the very poor worse, for the model tenement's presence raises the rents of the poorer structures 'round about it. Here again private philanthropy is confronted by the spectre which meets it at every turn—the Frankenstein who relentlessly points out the futility of tinkering with pitiable end-results, instead of playing the game of life fairly at all points. The truth is that more consumptives are made in the course of the earning of our great philanthropists' fortunes than the model tenements can ever prevent or cure—supposing that the very poor could afford to live in them. That human beings should have to live in tenements at all is a deplorable fact. So long as goodness and simplicity, commonly known as ignorance and feeble-mindedness, shall be exploited by craftiness, selfishness and legalized violence, commonly known as efficiency, fitness and power of organization and administration, so long will there be tenements. What is most needed to set right the ills of society is not direct action in any of the foolish and harmful forms adopted by so-called philanthropists or radical social agitators—equally vicious figures—so much as a certain negative attitude towards one's fellows, expressed for physicians by Hippocrates when he said: "Above all things, let the physician see to it that he do no harm," and for all men by Confucius in the words: "What ye would not that others should do unto you, do ye not unto them."

The "improvement of the condition of the poor" is a ghastly phrase and a necessarily ineffective programme, so long as economic and industrial exploitation goes on and our social ethics are shaped and financed by the Tartuffish vultures of the master class and their parasitic and sycophantic retainers of the press, the pulpit, the bench, the colleges and the political arena.

A. C. JACOBSON.

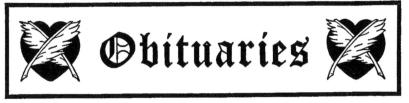

# Obituaries

DEPARTMENT UNDER THE CHARGE OF WILLIAM SCHROEDER, M.D.

## JOSEPH J. JACHES, M.D.

DR. JACHES was born in Russia in 1860 and died in Brooklyn, New York, October 20, 1912. He was graduated in Medicine from University of Moscow in 1886. He leaves a widow and three children—Julia, Helen and John.　　　　　　W. S., Sr.

---

## WILLIAM FREDERICK DUDLEY, A.B., M.D.

DR. DUDLEY was born in Brooklyn, New York, June 30, 1862, and died, after several months of invalidism, of infectious endocarditis, on October 22, 1912. He was the son of William H. Dudley, M.D., who was a native of Ireland, and of Charlotte Duckwitz, of New York.

His early education was received at the Polytechnic Institute, from which he received the degree of A.B. in the Class of 1883. He received the degree of M.D. from Long Island College Hospital three years later. His entire professional life was spent in Brooklyn. He was at different times physician to St. John's, Brooklyn, St. Christopher's and Long Island College Hospitals, to the Brooklyn Seaside Home for Children, and was Laryngologist to the Swedish and Norwegian Hospitals, as well as Instructor in Diseases of the Nose and Throat in the Long Island College Hospital and Brooklyn Post Graduate Medical Schools. Dr. Dudley was a member of the Medical Society of the County of Kings since 1890, serving five terms as Censor. In addition to the State and American Medical Associations he was a member of the Associated Physicians of Long Island, New York Academy of Medicine, The Brooklyn Pathological Society, and the American Rhinological, Laryngological and Otological Society. On November 19, 1890, he married Laura L. Bee, who, with four children— Frances H., Laura L., William and Gordon, survives him.

W. S., Sr.

---

## ALBERT NOCHIM MEHRENLENDER, M.D.

DR. MEHRENLENDER died at the Kings County Hospital on October 31, 1912. He was graduated from the New York University in 1893. He leaves a widow, Eva, and one child.

W. S., Sr.

---

## WILLIAM FREDERICK REX, PH.G., M.D.

DR. REX was born in New York City August 30, 1881, and died in Brooklyn, New York, November 1, 1912. His early education was received in the public and high schools of this City. He entered the New York College of Pharmacy, receiving the degree of Ph.G. in 1901, and that of M.D. from the Long Island College Hospital in 1905.　　　　　　W. S., Sr.

## HENRY GEORGE SMALL, M.D.

DR. SMALL was born at Exeter, Maine, May 25, 1852, and died in Brooklyn, New York, November 8, 1912. He was the son of John M. Small, M.D., of Maine. His medical education was received at the College of Physicians and Surgeons, New York, where he was graduated in the Class of 1875; he practiced medicine in this city during his professional life. From 1879 to 1890 he was a member of the Medical Society of the County of Kings and a member of Cornerstone Lodge F. & A. M. His widow, Araminta Small, survives him.                                     W. S., Sr.

## CLARENCE ALBERT BAKER, M.D.

DR. BAKER was born in 1863 and died at Yaphank, Long Island, November 9, 1912. He was the son of the late James J. Baker, M.D., who died in 1886. His early education was received at Cornell University and his medical education at the College of Physicians and Surgeons, New York, graduating M.D. in the Class of 1886. During his professional life he was at times Health Officer of Brookhaven, Physician to the County Almshouse and Childrens' Home at Yaphank and a member of the Suffolk County Medical Society and Associated Physicians of Long Island, South Side Lodge No. 493, Survassett Chapter No. 195, R. A. M., and Patchogue Commandery, No. 195, K. T. A widow and one daughter survive him.                                     W. S., Sr.

## CHARLES E. WELLS, M.D.

DR. WELLS was born in 1851 at Baiting Hollow, Long Island, and died at Sag Harbor, Long Island, November 14, 1912. He was graduated from Bellevue Hospital Medical College in the Class of 1889. Dr. Wells practiced at Sag Harbor during his professional life. He was at different times postmaster and justice of the peace, a member of the Suffolk County Medical Society and the Associated Physicians of Long Island from 1900, and Wampona Lodge, F. & A. M. He is survived by a widow, a son—Charles E. Wells, Jr.—and four daughters—Olive, Elizabeth, Isabelle and Alar Lynn Wells.                                     W. S., Sr.

## REV. ALBERT CARRIER BUNN, A.M., M.D.

DR. BUNN was born at Cape Vincent, N. Y., November 24, 1845, and died at Asheville, N. C., December 24, 1912. He was educated at Hobart College where he received his degree of A.M. His medical education was conducted at the University of Buffalo where he was graduated with the degree of M.D. in the Class of 1867. He practiced medicine at Westford and Morris, New York, until 1874, when he was appointed Medical Missionary at Wuchang, China, at which place he established St. Peters and The Elizabeth Bunn Memorial Hospitals. He was rector of the Episcopal Church of the Atonement 1881-1891, Church Charity Foundation 1891-1901, St. Matthew's Church 1901-1911. Dr. Bunn is survived by two sons, Captain Henry W. Bunn, U. S. A., and Albert C. Bunn, Jr. He was a member of the Medical Society of the County of Kings from 1893-1911.                                     W. S., Sr.

## EDWARD LEROY OATMAN, M.D.

DR. OATMAN died at his home in Brooklyn, New York, on December 26, 1912. His medical education was received at Bellevue Hospital Medical College, graduating M.D. in 1879. He practiced medicine at Nyack, New York; Southford, Connecticut; Brooklyn and New York City, New York. During his professional life he was Surgeon to the Manhattan Eye and Ear Hospital, Brooklyn Eye and Ear Hospital, Consulting Surgeon to the Nyack, N. Y., Hospital, and St. Mary's Hospital at Waterbury, Conn. A member of the Medical Society of the County of Kings 1899-1912, American Medical Association, and the New York Academy of Medicine. He was also a member of the Rembrandt, Brooklyn and Hamilton Clubs. He leaves a widow, Jean F. Hinman, and a daughter, Marjorie Jean, wife of Charles S. Munson. The funeral services were conducted by the Rev. John H. Melish, rector of the Holy Trinity Church.

His contributions to medical literature are as follows: 1903—Plastic Artificial Vitreous in Mule's Operation. 1904—Epithelial Cystoma of the Conjunctiva. 1904—Etiology and Pathology of Corneal Cysts. 1905—Cysts of the Pars Iridica Retinæ.

W. S., Sr.

## KERAN O'BRIEN, M.D.

DR. O'BRIEN was born in Brooklyn, New York, January 18, 1870, where he died January 6, 1913. He was the son of Keran O'Brien, of Ireland, and Flounda Stefani, of Switzerland. Dr. O'Brien married Mary J. Connelly, of Yonkers, N. Y. His early education was received in the public schools, St. Peter's Academy and St. Francis College. His medical education was under the direction of Dr. John Kepke, graduating M.D. from the Long Island College Hospital in the Class of 1901. He was a member of the Medical Society of the County of Kings from 1901, and the Associated Physicians of Long Island from 1901.

W. S., Sr.

## ROBERT BRADLEE WELTON, M.D.

DR. WELTON died in Brooklyn, New York, January 8, 1913, aged 70 years. He was educated at Harvard University and graduated from its medical department in 1868. In 1874 he began the practice of medicine in Brooklyn, New York, where he remained during his professional life. In 1879 he connected himself with the Medical Society of the County of Kings. He leaves a widow, Henrietta L., and three sons—Wendell P., Waldorf B., and Thurston S. Welton, M.D. Dr. Welton was a member of the Alumni Society of Harvard University and the Long Island Harvard Club.

W. S., Sr.

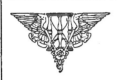
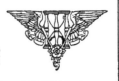

# Society Transactions

## TRANSACTIONS OF THE BROOKLYN PATHOLOGICAL SOCIETY.

*Stated Meeting, December 12, 1912.*

The President, PAUL M. PILCHER, M.D., in the Chair.

### The Experimental Pathology of Cancer.

*By William H. Woglom, M.D.*

DR. WOGLOM said:—"One is rather loath to present a full paper before the Society because the practical results thus far obtained in the laboratory have been so meagre. Much of the time has been spent in going over ground which has been already traversed theoretically in the past, and in confirming certain suggestions previously advanced on a basis of pure speculation, and discarding others.

"The question of the infectivity of cancer which periodically comes up for discussion in the medical press and in society meetings, is an example of a question which has been settled beyond reasonable doubt. There have been reported innumerable cases of transmission of the disease to a husband, a wife or to other people living in the same house, and the narration of many of them is like this: A man died of cancer of the stomach and three years afterward his wife died of cancer of the liver. When the study of mouse cancer was begun several instances were described where the disease attacked mice living in the same cage, and some observers were persuaded that mouse cancer must be contagious. But upon looking into the matter a little more closely it was found that most of these cancers appeared in the mammæ of old female mice.

"Now, the different species of animals are affected by cancer in different organs. The cow, for instance, suffers from cancer of the liver; the dog from cancer of the mammæ, while the human female suffers very frequently from cancer of the uterus and of the mammæ, and the latter organ is the one which is affected in the mouse. This is a perfectly valid explanation for the occurrence of these cases of cancers in one breeding establishment or in one cage. They were spontaneous almost without doubt, first, because they occurred in old female mice; second, they were found in the organ which is almost invariably affected in the mouse. It would have been a most remarkable coincidence if a cancer-bearing mouse in any of these cages had succeeded in infecting only old female mice and these at the point where spontaneous cancer occurs with the greatest frequency. The fact that cancer can be artificially transmitted from one mouse to another has been seized upon as proof that cancer is contagious, but this observation cannot be adduced as a proof because cancer fragments introduced under the skin of mice and rats have been carefully followed from day to day in the laboratory, so that one knows now just exactly what occurs.

"If a fragment of say, tubercular tissue were to be transplanted under the skin, the surrounding healthy tissues at the edge of that graft would gradually become tubercular. This is not the case, however, with cancer, for when it is inoculated under the skin of mice it is known that the surrounding cells never become cancerous. The parenchyma of this graft will proliferate, and the stroma will die, to be replaced by a new connective tissue scaffolding from the host; but not one cell of the host will take on the characteristics of cancer. This is not, therefore, an instance of infection in any wise; it is an example of transplantation, and cannot be used to uphold a theory of the infective nature of cancer.

"It has been found that animals can be immunized against the transplantation of cancer by preliminary inoculation with the tissues of the same species and, as Dr. Lintz has correctly said, the tissues must be alive and uninjured, and it may be that they must actually live for a few days in order that the immune condition may be evolved. In an immune animal there is no new supply of blood vessels; there is no provision stroma, and the graft lies in a cystic cavity and finally dies, the cells on the extreme periphery being the last to perish. The fact that the outlying cells are the last to succumb, although they would be the first exposed to antibodies in the tissues or fluids of the host, suggest very strongly that in mice resistant to transplanted cancer there do not exist any protective substances analogous to those discovered as a result of investigations in the domains of bacteriology and immunity. The peripheral cells do not seem to be actively injured, and remain alive longer than those in the center of the graft because they are able to obtain by imbition a supply of food-stuff sufficient for a short period at least.

"Surgeons have been aware for a long time that recurrences take place after the ablation of a cancer, from fragments which have escaped into the tissues. Laboratory investigation affords unqualified support of what Dr. Bristow has said of the unwarrantable practice of cutting into a cancer to excise a fragment for diagnosis. If a cancer be removed from a mouse and transplanted into other mice, it will grow in a certain number of them. But a graft of that cancer, introduced into the mouse in which it arose, will almost invariably grow because the cells are still in the soil to which they are accustomed, and are not forced to battle for their existance as they would be if they were introduced. Such experiments show the great danger to be apprehended from the introduction of the cells of a cancer into the patient in whom it arose spontaneously, and, on the other hand, the minimal danger to other persons.

"There has been going on for years a spirited discussion on the hereditary nature of cancer, and it has been possible in the past decade to approach this question from the experimental standpoint. In Dr. Bashford's laboratory in London, Dr. Murray has been breeding mice of cancerous ancestry, by which he means that cancer had occurred either in the mother, or in one or both of the grandmothers, or in all three. He finds that mice of cancerous stock are almost twice as likely to develop spontaneous cancer as those in which there has been no cancer in the mother or grandmother. These observations cannot be transferred in their entirety to man, because cancerous mice having been deliberately selected for breeding purposes, the taint was much stronger than it could ever be in man except by some unusually unfortunate chance.

"In the treatment of cancer there is nothing to offer. Wassermann, about a year ago, published some suggestive experiments in which he treated cancer with metals in the colloidal form, but Wassermann himself recognized all of the fallacies to which his experiments were liable and has continually emphasized his view that his results were to be taken merely as an interesting biological finding—nothing more. Fichera's treatment is founded upon certain fallacious premises. In the first place, normal tissue, whether embryonal or adult, can only prevent the development of a transplanted graft; it has no effect upon an established tumor. In the second, even though it were possible to cure transplanted tumors, there is no warrant for assuming that the effective agent would be efficacious against a spontaneous tumor, in which an animal's own cells are proliferating lawlessly. Such a tumor must be sharply distinguished from a transplanted growth, in which the proliferating cells are those of another animal—the one in which they first became malignant. Thirdly, the favorable results observed by Fichera in the rat, where his experiments were first undertaken, may not have been due to the treatment at all. Transplanted tumors not infrequently undergo spontaneous retrogression, which supervenes irrespective of any treatment whatsoever, and from causes about which we are still entirely ignorant.

"No advice regarding treatment has ever come from an experienced investigator of cancer either at the bedside or in the laboratory, except that which would urge any one who has the slightest suspicion of the presence of a malignant growth to put himself immediately and without reserve in the hands of the most competent surgeon that he can find. Early diagnosis and thorough excision offer the only hope of cure so far known."

## The Clinical Diagnosis of Cancer and Its Gross Pathology.

### *By Algernon T. Bristow, M.D.*

"With respect to the function of the surgeon in the macroscopic diagnosis of these tumors presented to us from time to time: As a matter of fact, the surgeon, to be a real surgeon, ought to be a pathologist and a bacteriologist as well, a pathologist for the purpose of being able to distinguish the true character of growths which present themselves at operation, such as in the case the other day mentioned by the chairman, and a bacterioligist because an accurate bacteriology is not only necessary to a correct surgical technic, in my judgment, but also because it is most illuminating with respect to treatment.

"There are a great many tumors which, macroscopically, I think it is impossible for a surgeon to more than guess at, but I think that many times the pathologist can do no more, and I sympathize with Dr. Murray when he speaks of the necessity of the pathologist having the entire tumor, and perhaps an experience which I had with him may illustrate very well the necessity of what he has insisted on and at the same time emphasizes the truth of what I have said in regard to the difficulties of making a diagnosis macroscopically.

"Five years ago a lady came to see me with a very small tumor in the breast, about the size of a chestnut. None of the familiar signs were present, no orange appearance of the skin, no evidences of adhesions of those processes of connective tissue which result in dimpling. I told her that I was unable to make a diagnosis without an exploratory incision. To this she demurred. We managed to get her to go to New York and I sent her to a New York surgeon, at her request, but he would not make a diagnosis and sent her back to me. Finally she accepted my original proposition to make an exploration and I took out the whole tumor, which I think is always very much better surgery than to make an incision in the tumor, as recommended by some English authors. The tumor was not very much larger than a good-sized chestnut. Dr. Murray took it to the laboratory. After about fifteen or twenty minutes, Dr. Murray sent over word that the tumor was benign and I might sew up the wound. I was just tying the last suture in the incision which I had made when Dr. Murray came rushing over in hot haste to tell me than he had found in another area distinct evidences of carcinoma. I was under the disagreeable necessity of allowing the patient to 'come to' again and telling her that a subsequent report of the pathologist had been received and that she had a carcinoma and that it would be necessary to remove the breast, which was done. She remained perfectly well for a year when I heard from her family physician that she had a moderate edema of the arm. She was in rosy health. I hoped that it was possibly one of those cases of edema that are sometimes due to a complete removal of the lymphatics. The edema subsequently disappeared, but later she came to me with a recurring edema of the arm. There was no evidence of recurrence in the scar. It was absolutely perfect. I cut down on the subclavian triangle and exposed the tissues, but I was unable to find any evidence of carcinoma at that time, so I closed the wound; it promptly healed and the edema disappeared. She went on for two years and then came back to me last spring when it was perfectly evident that she had a recurrence. She died about two months ago of recurring carcinoma.

"This teaches us that the small tumors are not the least malignant; the smaller the more malignant, and the more careful should be their removal. This emphasizes what Dr. Murray has said to us with regard to the necessity of having the whole tumor, because here was a case in which he had the whole tumor and yet it was only after persistent cutting up that he finally discovered the malignant portion.

"Another case which struck me somewhat similarly was a case in which I had made a diagnosis of fibro-adenoma of the breast. Now, when you have a series of tumors in the breast they are usually fibro-adenomata, but when you have one tumor it is usually cancer. In this case I took out these tumors, the report being that they were all fibro-adenomata. In five or six months the patient came back with another tumor and I took this out and sent it to Dr. Murray and I was astonished to get back from him a report that I was dealing with an adenocarcinoma, so I swept off the whole breast. That illustrates that even with the utmost care we still may miss a small carcinoma.

"The most difficult class of cases to diagnose clinically are certain tumors of the breast which simulate malignant disease, and the contrary. For instance, chronic mastitis very frequently simulates malignant disease and there is a nodular infiltrating carcinoma which simulates a chronic mastitis. I don't think, however, that the differential diagnosis here is of such importance for this reason: In those cases of chronic mastitis with sinuses and hard infiltration of the breast the woman is better off without the breast, first, because it is hopelessly crippled as to function, and, second, because such a condition as that affords a very excellent culture medium for the carcinoma to grow upon subsequently. There are however, a few cases where a carcinoma has engrafted itself (I say 'engrafted' because I think it best illustrates my point) on a chronic inflammatory process. I had at the County Hospital one of those cases of infiltrating carcinoma which resembled a blastomycosis of the breast. In that case I cut out one of the nodules in the skin for microscopic examination before I decided to do the Halstead-Meyer operation, and a report came back that it was a carcinoma—a duct carcinoma in that case.

"One of the peculiarities of duct carcinoma is the bloody fluid that may be expressed from the nipple by pressure on the breast. Of course it is also possible to have bloody fluid coming from an ordinary cyst, but there is nothing to me more suspicious than bloody fluid from a nipple in connection with a tumor near the nipple. They do not produce what the French call *peau de cochon*.

"A variety of carcinoma that is almost impossible of diagnosis until you have cut down upon it is the small carcinoma at the base of a very fat breast. There is rarely dimpling in those cases and it is necessary to expose the mass before you can come to any definite conclusions, at least in the cases I have seen.

"Another variety is the sub-pectoral carcinomas, which are probably due mostly to aberrant glandules from the breast which do not produce any pigskin appearance of the skin and produce no dimpling and no retraction of the nipple.

"I would like to say with respect to carcinoma of the male breast that this isn't very common, but is far more malignant than carcinoma of the female breast. Every case of carcinoma of the male breast which I have seen has ultimately terminated fatally in my experience. I had one case until quite recently under my care which illustrates this very well. A strong, healthy man three years ago was operated upon at Los Angeles for a growth in the breast and the report was that it was carcinoma. Evidently, a very partial operation was done in that case under the impression that a carcinoma in the male breast does not amount to as much as in the female breast. He came to me six or seven months after with a carcinoma. I promptly did a complete Halsted and made a very wide excision of skin. Dr. Murray made the examination and reported the disease as endothelioma. This man was in the habit of spending every summer in Paris and when he went back there last spring I gave him a letter to a French surgeon, because while I had done an extensive operation, I felt he would get a recurrence. In September I received a letter from the Paris surgeon advising me that a recurrence had taken place and that he had cut down on the original incision, which was entirely free from any appearance of malignant disease, but he found 5 or 6 centimeters of vein involved and thereupon he had abandoned any attempt at doing anything further. I saw the man on his return and he was then having edema of the arm with a good deal of pain and had nodules in his scalp. He had been treated by what is called in Paris cuprase. This is a colloid form of copper which comes in ampoules and he brought me a supply of these ampoules and I continued to use them so as not to discourage him, until he went back west. That is, I may say, a fatal case.

"In October I saw a lawyer who was brought to me by his family physician with an evident malignant disease of the breast and in that case I gave the family physician a very bad prognosis; I have no doubt that the subsequent history will show conclusively the extreme malignancy of cancer in the male breast.

"Now, take the malignant growths of the tongue. There is one thing which I have seen mistaken quite commonly for epithelioma of the tongue and that is gumma. Gummata, however, are usually one-sided or they are alone, in my experience, and do not involve the border of the tongue, and in almost all cancers of the tongue I have found a decayed or ragged tooth which has irritated the edge of the tongue and the epithelioma starts from the edge and grows inward. A very short course of iodid of potassium will clear up the diagnosis in those cases. Not seldom, but half a dozen times in the last few years I have had gummas of the tongue sent to me as epitheliomas, and in every instance the administration of iodid of potash has cleared them up, so that I was not dealing with an epithelioma but gumma.

"Tumors of the larynx are not easy of diagnosis. I doubt very much whether anybody is justified in making a diagnosis of epithelioma of the larynx by ocular inspection, because in two cases in which I have done complete laryngectomies for two years they were wandering around from clinic to clinic in New York, always with a diagnosis of benign tumor. In both of these cases I finally took out the entire larynx and microscopic examination subsequently made, one by Wright, of New York, and the other by Dr. Murray, showed the presence of malignant disease. The last that I heard from the first case was that the patient was still living and free from recurrence, and that was eight years. The second case lived a year, but the esophagus was involved and the most I could hope for was to postpone the evil issue.

# TRANSACTIONS OF THE MEDICAL SOCIETY OF THE COUNTY OF KINGS.

*Stated Meeting, November 19, 1912.*

The President, ELIAS H. BARTLEY, M.D., in the Chair.

As the Program for this meeting was provided by the Pathological Society, the transactions will be found under that heading. The coincidence of the meeting of the Clinical Congress of Surgeons of North America, under the auspices of the Kings County Society, and the regular meeting of the Pathological Society, made this arrangement desirable.

*Stated Meeting, December 17, 1912.*

The President, ELIAS H. BARTLEY, M.D., in the Chair.

Paper:

**Blood Cultures Simplified by New Apparatus; with Demonstration.**

*(From the Bacteriological Laboratory of the L. I. College Hospital.)*
*(See page 60.)*

*By William Lintz, M.D.*

DR. JOSHUA M. VAN COTT, in discussion, said:—"It certainly is a pleasure to have listened to a paper of the scientific type which the doctor has given to us.

"While he was reading I was reminded of the fact that probably the first of all secretions to be examined was the urine in the time of Hippocrates and with the first two periods of historic medicine there were scientists who examined urine by the sun and a flask for the purpose of determining the nature of disease, independent of the color and clarity of the urine. Then after that the feces and stomach contents, much more recently the contents of the stomach, then the sputum, and finally the blood has been utilized as a means of determining the facts of disease.

"Now, as the doctor has said, the reason why blood has lagged behind, the reason why so few men have utilized so important a fluid in the body for diagnostic purposes, lies in the fact of the difficulty of performing the operation and getting a sufficient quantity for the purposes of examination.

"This apparatus seems to have brought us a new era in the examination of the blood and, as Dr. Lintz has said, a child who has the nerve to do it can make a culture or gather the blood for examination.

"Now, it would be useless to go into any discussion of the technical part of the paper. There is no debate on it. The laboratory is teeming with the facts he has mentioned and which he brings to us in a new light of being entirely practicable, so that all I want to do is to cite a few cases of my own experience, cases where we obtained the blood at a moment's notice.

"The first case was that of a nurse at the Kings County Hospital who developed a high temperature and in whom there were some evidences of cardiac complication, and although typhoid had been suspected, the Widal was negative, but the blood culture showed the bacillus typhosus in large numbers.

"The second case, also at the Kings County Hospital, was that of a man who had a high temperature with some pain in the neighborhood of the gall-bladder. He was unable to answer any questions. The above symptoms pointed toward the gall-bladder. A culture from that man's blood yielded the very remarkable result of a pure culture of the bacillus of Fraenkel.

"The third case was one of a cystic goitre. The cyst was removed by one of our best surgeons in this town and the patient afterwards developed a secondary hemorrhage. The bleeding was so rapid and so great as to make it necessary to go into the wound immediately and she became infected. She had a curve which resembled somewhat the curve of typhoid fever. A suggestion was made, as she had given a history of malaria, that it was a case of complicated malaria. A blood culture was made in this case and streptococcus obtained without any difficulty.

"Personally, I feel greatly indebted to our colleague for having devised a method such as this and it seems to me it is a disgrace if any of us men fail to use this method in obtaining a culture of the blood for any diagnostic purpose."

Dr. Jacob Fuhs, in discussion, said:—"I have seen the apparatus used at the Long Island College Hospital and was surprised at the simplicity of the method of obtaining blood for cultures.

"A member of the house staff, who had had no experience with the apparatus, required only a few simple directions to apply it successfully.

"Its sphere of usefulness will be large, as it requires no complicated technic and also because it can be utilized not only for blood culture work, but also for making cultures of other fluids, such as exudates, etc. In the past, blood cultures were only taken in a limited number of cases, owing to the necessity of calling in a trained bacteriologist, entailing considerable expense. Even in hospital work I found that there were difficulties owing to the complicated methods and the possibility of contaminations.

"These disadvantages are overcome by this simple apparatus, which does not require much technic and only a moderate outlay.

"The great diagnostic value of blood cultures cannot be over-estimated. Almost every case of typhoid fever gave a positive result even in the early stage and before other diagnostic means determined the nature of the disease. About 50 per cent. of the cases of pneumonia showed a positive blood culture. Most of the latter were of a severe type of infection. In chronic infectious endocarditis blood cultures are of prognostic and diagnostic value. It is true that the diseases just mentioned can often be recognized without resorting to blood cultures, still in some cases it affords the only means of arriving at a correct understanding of the case.

"This is well illustrated in the early stages of typhoid fever, when it is difficult to differentiate between that and Brill's disease, meningitis, paratyphoid, and even appendicitis.

"The everyday use of blood cultures, made possible by the simple apparatus, will mark a decided advance in the methods of diagnosis available to the general practitioner."

Dr. John O. Polak, in discussion, said:—"What Dr. Van Cott and Dr. Fuhs have said covers the question as to the value of blood culture, but I cannot let this admirable paper of Dr. Lintz go by without congratulating him and the profession at large on his perfection of such a simple apparatus.

"Perhaps it has been my privilege to have as many blood cultures made in our work in sepsis as almost any one in Brooklyn, and I can see particularly the value of this simple apparatus for this purpose.

"There was one point which the doctor brought out which I think should be impressed particularly—and that is, that we do not get, in a very large number of cases, positive blood cultures in infections; the facts that he brought out as to the reasons for this are the points that we must remember. Most of our infections, particularly those infections post-partem, are local infections, and we do not get blood cultures in local infections in a large number of instances. Again, thrombophlebitis is a very common infection following abortions and labors, and, again, we find in these cases that unless we are so unfortunate as to get portions of emboli in the blood we will not get a positive blood culture.

"In regard to the bacteremias, the streptococcic and staphylococcic, the blood cultures are fairly constant, although we have found that we may frequently make three, four or five blood cultures before getting a positive one. That is accounted for, as the doctor has said, by the small number of bacteria to the cubic centimeter, and, again, there are periods in which the bacteria are not in circulation in the blood.

"I want to say this one thing and that is, the value of blood cultures cannot be over-estimated in the management of these cases. It is only by knowing what is in the blood or what is not in the blood that we are in a positive position to pursue the proper treatment of these conditions.

"Again I want to congratulate him on the simplicity of this apparatus and the admirable presentation of the subject."

Dr. Luther F. Warren, in discussion, said:—"It seems that there can be little to add to this quite comprehensive presentation, but there are one or two points possibly that cannot be too well emphasized, and that is the importance of early diagnosis in a great many cases. We see this particularly in typhoid, when we remember Coleman's work across the river, where he had six hundred cases and of those six hundred cases 10 per cent. of them never gave a Widal, while 90 per cent. gave very positive blood cultures. Now, this 10 per cent. that never gave a Widal, I think, speaks of the self-evidence of the importance of blood cultures. Then, again, in paratyphoid and paracolon infections it is usually our first light in a great many cases.

"I am glad the doctor brought out the failure to get positive blood cultures in tuberculosis. After the work of Rosenberger we thought that possibly the tubercule bacillus could be cultivated in a great many of those cases of tuberculosis, and this work has stimulated a great deal of work. I think it is definitely decided by those doing the most good work at present that cases of tuberculosis do not show a positive blood culture of the tubercle organism, with the exception of possibly one or two instances, one of them purely of the miliary type and another one of occasional occurrence in very advanced forms of the chronic ulcerative type.

"In regard to pneumonia: it is very interesting to see certain workers get a large percentage of cases, and Rosenow reports 90 per cent. more than any other worker. Cole of Johns Hopkins reported 30 per cent. in severe cases only. This may be due to several things, as has already been said, and one of them is that not enough blood is taken. If this be true, then it seems to me that possibly our little apparatus is a little too small in a certain number of cases. Another thing which seems to me to be a potent thing is that our cases of septic chronic endocarditis are very frequently negative and we get them positive more often when we use large amounts of blood, and possibly this apparatus is too small to give a higher percentage of cases unless we get another apparatus, which can be very easily designed, but then that would mean that, as Dr. Lintz has said, it could not be put in our vest pockets.

"There is another thing also which seems important to me and that is that when we have blood, as soon as it is diluted with some culture medium, very frequently it will have bactericidal properties which destroy the organism. This, however, is well taken care of by a larger bottle. Ewing says he does not believe that over 2 or 3 c.c. of blood should be placed in 100 c.c. of bouillon, for instance, and Webster says that not over 3 c.c. to 100 c.c. of bouillon. This will have to be taken care of by a larger bottle. I know these are rather exceptional and not the usual run of cases. That must be taken into consideration."

Dr. William Lintz, in closing the discussion, said:—"I have nothing to add except to say that bottles can be obtained and do come in all sizes. There is one that is much larger, filled with bile. In case we have typhoid the bacteria grow very well on this and experience has shown that the presence of gram-negative motile bacilli is pretty sure to be typhoid; so that the blood does not have to be manipulated at all. Blood obtained even in a small bottle is by far larger in quantity than is ordinarily obtained for the purposes of blood cultures with a syringe. Most syringes are not over 10 c.c., so that even a small bottle contains more than 50 per cent. of the blood usually taken. As to the bactericidal power of the blood: If one uses, however, a certain medium, like bile, for typhoid, and for pneumococcus, if one uses a 1 per cent. peptone solution plus a 10 per cent. glucose media, not only do the pneumococci grow very well on that, but the bactericidal power of the serum is also obviated; or if one uses ammonium oxylate, or salt, or sterile water, all bactericidal effects of the serum will be obviated. Of course, if, as has been suggested, the bottle is too small, one can make bottles limited only by the four walls of the room if necessary, but it isn't necessary."

---

# TRANSACTIONS OF THE BROOKLYN SURGICAL SOCIETY.

*Stated Meeting, October 3, 1912.*

The President, Richard W. Westbrook, M.D., in the Chair.

### Cancer of Breast With Foreign Body in New Growth.

Dr. Burr B. Mosher reported the following case:

"The case is that of a woman with a tumor in the breast. She consulted me about a year and a half ago. The growth was not large. An operation was advised and accepted, and on removing the tumor I discovered a needle which was within the growth. The microscopist reported the growth as carcinoma.

"In inquiring about the needle I learned that it had been in the breast 27 years."

## Unusually Large Uterine Fibroma.

Dr. Burr B. Mosher reported the case as follows:
"The second case is interesting to me because the text-books state, and I think the usual history we get is that of menstrual disturbance with a large uterine myofibroma.

"This patient, 36 years old, had absolutely no disturbance of the menstrual function; she menstruated regularly, had never borne children and only presented herself for treatment because of the size of the tumor.

"She made a good recovery from hysterectomy and I present this case simply to emphasize *that all cases* of uterine fibroids do not necessarily have a disturbed menstrual function."

### Discussion.

Dr. J. C. Kennedy, in discussing Dr. Mosher's case, said:
"It is strange how those needles travel. A clergyman a few months ago asked me to see him in reference to a pain in his back. On running my fingers over the back muscles I came across a sharp instrument which proved to be a needle, and he told me that twelve years before it had entered his foot. It was removed."

Dr. H. B. Delatour, in discussing Dr. Mosher's cases, said:
"The tumor presented is interesting on account of the size and ease with which Dr. Mosher said it was removed. It is curious that these large tumors so frequently are free of adhesions. I believe tumors that are smaller, that are confined to the pelvis, more frequently set up inflammatory trouble and so become adherent more frequently than the larger ones.

"That there was no disturbance of menstruation is well explained by the fact that it was a subperitoneal and not a mural or submucous fibroid.

"I have never seen a foreign body in a new growth of the breast. It is certainly interesting to have this case presented.

"I was quite interested the other day to see the recall of the Mayor's permits for playing balls in the street. As I read it it made me think of two cases operated last spring where carcinoma of the breast was directly traceable to the reception of a blow from a ball in the street."

Dr. J. C. Kennedy, in discussing Dr. Mosher's case of uterine fibroid, said:
"I have a lady now in the hospital on whom I did a hysterectomy for a small uterine fibroid. She complained of marked bladder trouble and to make sure that her bladder symptoms were not entirely due to the fibroid, I had her cystoscoped. Through the cystoscope we thought we had discovered a tumor on the posterior wall of the bladder, or perhaps an encysted stone. Dr. Williams, the X-ray expert, gave a negative report as to the stone. It was found at operation that adhesions had drawn the fibroid uterus back in certain positions of the body, and placed the cervix snugly against the posterior wall of the bladder, producing the elevation which we had seen and which resembled in every way a tumor. In contrast to this very large fibroid without symptoms, we have here a very small fibroid producing marked bladder symptoms."

## A Report of Three Cases of Acute Knee-Joint Infection.

Dr. John B. Sullivan reported the following cases:
Case I. On March 19, 1898, I was called to see Mrs. G., aged about 25 years, and found her afflicted with an acute septic fever and her left knee very much swollen and painful. About two months previous to that time she had an abortion and in the meantime her uterus was curretted three times. My diagnosis was acute suppurative infection of the knee-joint, secondary to an infected uterus. She was sent to St. Mary's Hospital and an incision made on each side of the patella into the joint, and a considerable quantity of pus evacuated. The knee was covered with a wet antiseptic dressing and a Buck's extension applied. After this the pain was relieved, the swelling subsided and her temperature soon became nearly normal. No farther local treatment was required. The convalesence was rapid and at the end of three weeks she left the hospital in very good condition. Soon after her arrival home passive motion of the knee-joint was instituted and gradually increased until the joint was completely restored to a normal condition. Fourteen years have elapsed since this patient was treated for that affliction and the joint has remained perfectly sound and normal up to the present time.
Case II. In July, 1903, Mr. J. H. P., a young man who was under treatment for gonorrhœa, was seized with pain and swelling in his right knee, which increased daily in severity until he was unable to leave his bed. The capsule of the joint became greatly distended and fluctuation was quite dis-

tinct. The leg was flexed to about 45 degrees and any attempt to extend it caused intense pain. He had only a moderate degree of fever and his general health was good. As the usual treatment was of no avail I aspirated the joint and withdrew about four ounces of serous fluid. This gave him great relief from the pain and he remained comparatively comfortable for about two days; but as the fluid began to accumulate the pain returned and increased in proportion to the distension of the joint capsule. Four days after the first operation I reaspirated the joint and drew off about three ounces of a straw-colored fluid. Again the pain was relieved and the inflammatory symptoms gradually subsided. A wet dressing combined with moderate compression was the only local treatment thereafter required. No other complication ensued and the patient made a rapid and complete recovery. This was plainly a case of Neisserian infection, commonly called "gonorrhœal rheumatism." Judging from my experience with other cases of this type, the patient's suffering was very much mitigated and his recovery hastened by the withdrawing of the effusion.

CASE III. This presents a rare and very interesting pathological condition. On October 13, 1905, I was called to Stamford, Conn., to consult with a physician of that town. The patient was a gentleman about 40 years of age who had always enjoyed good health up to about two months previous to that time, when he was taken ill with typhoid fever. In the fourth week of his illness, when the fever was abating, he began to have pain in his right knee which was continuous day and night, gradually increasing in severity until it became intense. About one week after the onset of the pain the knee began to swell. He was informed that it was a rheumatic affection and would soon disappear. He endured this condition for another week and as his distress was becoming intolerable, a consultation was requested. On examination I found the knee greatly swollen, the skin tense and glossy, the subcutaneous cellular tissue infiltrated and firm, with deep fluctuation very distinct. It appealed to me as a case demanding immediate intervention and I suggested that we aspirate the joint then and there. His attending physician objected and said that he could not approve of any such procedure and would give his consent only on condition that I would assume all the responsibility for any damage resulting from the operation. An aspirating needle was immediately sterilized and introduced into the joint and about six ounces of a sero-purulent fluid withdrawn. This fluid was subsequently examined and found to contain the bacillus typhosus. No other micro-organism was identified. The patient experienced great relief by the aspiration and remained comparatively comfortable thereafter except that any motion of the joint was attended with pain. I did not see him again until November 4th, three weeks after the date of my first visit, when he came to his home in Brooklyn. Then I found the limb encased in a plaster of Paris cast which was applied to immobilize the joint during his journey home. The cast was removed and the limb found to be swollen very much from the ankle to the middle of the thigh. There was quite a firm fixation of the knee joint, apparently a fibrous ankylosis. Any attempt to flex it would cause great pain. His general health was fairly good. An alum-acetate solution was applied to the limb. The swelling gradually subsided and he was soon able to move about on crutches. Several attempts were made to produce passive motion in the knee-joint, but each effort was followed by such a degree of inflammation that we were obliged to desist.

By the latter part of December, about six weeks after his arrival home, he was able to come to my office on crutches. But in January following, an inflammatory focus developed on the tibia of his left leg which remained hard for a considerable length of time—then suppurated and was opened. During the next year several other foci of infection appeared on the right leg above and below the knee. These all suppurated and delayed our efforts in making passive motion to restore the function of the joint. Still, during the second year of his ailment he attended to his ordinary business and was encouraged to move the joint as much as possible. The patella had become quite firmly fixed and strong fibrous adhesions surrounded the joint and motion was limited to about ten degrees from a straight line. During the third year strenuous efforts in the way of massage, superheating and forced flexion and extension were practiced and continued until the function of the joint was restored to nearly its normal condition.

Comments: When a joint becomes infected the damage comes primarily from the virulence of the infecting micro-organism and the accumulation and pressure of the products of infection held under tension by its capsule. If this condition persists for any considerable length of time the endothelial cells lining the synovial membrane are destroyed. A contraction of the muscles above and below the joint occurs as a result of the inflammation pressing the articular surfaces together and conducing to ankylosis. Besides, as the inflammatory effusion into the joint increases in amount, the ligaments become stretched and conditions favoring an easy deformity or dislocation obtain. Viewing a knee in such a pathological condition, the indications for treatment are manifestly to relieve the interarticular pressure either by aspiration or incision without drain and the application of a Buck's extension to overcome the contractions of the muscles involved. To epitomize, the cardinal points in the treatment are: Aspiration or incision without drainage, and Buck's extension.

## Discussion.

Dr. Lewis S. Pilcher, in discussing Dr. Sullivan's cases, said:

"In regard to the treatment and the results in cases of acute knee-joint infection, I can recall many experiences in dealing with that condition in the past. I remember most clearly, because I see him quite frequently, a gentleman of about the age and general physical conformation of the patient that Dr. Sullivan has presented here tonight. He developed an acute suppurative infection of his knee-joint, did this gentleman, which we aspirated, and then opened and drained the joint, and were fortunate in securing in due time a favorable outcome.

"This young man at the time was engaged to be married and the day had been set for his marriage, and after he was up and about the main thing which troubled him was whether he would be able to kneel at the altar at the time of the ceremony, and he set himself at work to loosen up that knee so that when the time for the ceremony should come he would be able to perform his part properly, *and he did!*

"There is at the present moment a great deal of interest over certain questions of the management of these knee-joint infections, involving the point especially as to whether it is proper to introduce a drainage tube into the joint at these times or whether we should content ourselves with simply opening the joint and washing it out and then protecting it. I infer from Dr. Sullivan's case histories that the latter is practically his method of proceeding, adding to it the Buck's extension so as to overcome, as it does admirably, the tendency to muscular contraction or all fixation results which might be produced if that were omitted. Some of our greatest authorities tell us that that is the way to do and condemn in unmeasured terms the introduction of a drainage tube within a cavity of the joint. I'm not sure but that they're right.

"Practically in all the cases which I have had to deal with in the past I have, however, felt that it was my duty to introduce the drainage tube into the joint. In many cases I have passed a drainage tube through the subquadriceps bursa, through and through for a time. From the good effects which have been accomplished in the cases which have been under my care I have naturally been strengthened in the impression that such a course was the best thing to do. I have, however, been very much impressed with the positiveness and the reasonableness of the statements which are now being made as to the possible damage which can come to the delicate endothelial lining of the knee-joint from the presence within of such a foreign body as a drainage tube, and I should be inclined if another case present itself to treat it upon the more conservative method, which at the present time seems to be gaining general approval.

"I would be very much interested in the further discussion if my colleagues would take up this point and give their experiences in the use or non-use of drainage tube reaching the cavity of the knee-joint in dealing with these septic infections of the joint."

Dr. Algernon T. Bristow, discussing Dr. Sullivan's cases, said:

"The surgery of septic knee-joints has long been one of the terrors of the profession. In the old days, before our time, an infected knee-joint was the signal for an amputation. Then we adopted the method of free drainage by passing drainage tubes through and through the joint, or by separate drains on each side. Too frequently we were obliged to amputate to save the patient's life. We went a step further to secure complete drainage and making a U-shaped incision, flexed the joint, laid back the patella and retained the joint in the semi-flexed position, but I confess that the results which I got from this heroic treatment still left much to be desired.

"In these cases of knee-joint infection much depends on the resistance of the patient and the virulence of the infecting organism."

Here Dr. Bristow went on to speak of the character of the different infections, and said:

"A pneumococcus infection is always a very serious affair; so is the streptococcus and the staphylococcus aureus. When these infections occur in conjunction with a diminished resistance on the part of the patient, the results are apt to be bad.

"The Bier congestive treatment is distinctly advantageous and should not be neglected. If to this method we adopt the line of treatment laid down by Dr. Murphy of Chicago, which practically is the treatment which Dr. Sullivan has outlined here for us, first, the Buck's extension in order to keep the articular surfaces apart; second, aspiration of the joint, so as to relieve the pressure on the endothelial cells, and third, the injection into the joint of a 2 per cent. glycerin-formalin solution, we shall in the majority of cases get better results than with the older methods. Finally, I believe that vaccine therapy has an important place in the treatment of these serious conditions."

Dr. H. B. DELATOUR, in discussion of Dr. Sullivan's cases, said:

"I quite agree with all Dr. Bristow has said and what Dr. Sullivan's cases certainly illustrate, but I have had quite an extensive experience with injuries in the knee-joint that were suppurative and I must say that I cannot feel with Dr. Murphy that the drainage tube is such a sure producer of an immobilized or ankylosed joint. I would not introduce a drainage tube in a joint if I did not feel it was absolutely necessary to do so. In many cases I have simply aspirated and washed out, some cases with a weak bichlorid solution, and have gotten splendid results; but I have seen many cases in which the drainage tube has been passed through the joint in which drainage has been kept up for a fairly long period without destruction of the joint, and I cannot feel with Dr. Murphy, who is so very positive in his statement that never must we introduce a drainage tube in a joint if we expect to have a mobile joint afterwards. I feel very positive that that statement should not go unchallenged."

Dr. WALTER TRUSLOW, discussing Dr. Sullivan's cases, said:

"I would like to lay a little emphasis on the last point Dr. Bristow made—the question of Dr. Murphy's use of injection of some material into the joint.

"A comparatively extensive experience at the County Hospital with these joints, many of them, however, being cases of tubercular origin, leads me to believe that the conservative methods are often faulty.

"I have not used the drainage tube, but I believe that we must do everything that we can to insure the separation of the bony parts involved, so that in time they may heal and adhesions be prevented. Dr. Tunstall Taylor of Baltimore is now working on a paste, composed largely of paraffin and glycerin, making a semi-solid mass, which is injected into the joints—injected almost to distension, perhaps to temporary discomfort of the individual. He finds as a result that the mass he thus injects takes about six weeks to be absorbed, during which time—not neglecting the extension that has been mentioned and not neglecting the previous aspiration—the parts have a better chance to heal, adhesions rarely occur, and good motion is usually obtained."

Dr. ALEXANDER RAE, in discussing Dr. Sullivan's cases, said:

"One of the principle advantages in the use of the extension seems not to have been mentioned. It has been found in cases of ankylosis that in cutting through the tissues there was no material which really interfered with the flexion of the knee-joint until the capsule itself had been reached; so that it is not so much the contraction of the muscles of the extremity bringing together the articular surfaces, but rather the approximation of the surfaces which permits the undue shortening of the inflamed capsule, that causes the fixation. So that here is an added element for the recommendation of the use of the extension."

Dr. JOHN D. SULLIVAN, in closing the discussion, said:

"Dr. Rae's remarks, I think, are very true. The arthritis is generally followed by a considerable amount of contraction of the capsule and ligaments of the joint, sometimes to such a degree that a cutting operation is required to release them. Buck's extension tends to prevent, or at least diminish, these contractions and adhesions.

"In regard to Dr. Truslow's remarks about the injection, of course, that is something new; it has not been practised yet. I should think such an injection would tend to stretch the ligaments of the joint and also the capsule and thereby tend, as I claim in my paper, to favor an easy deformity or dislocation. One of the results of having a joint filled with fluid for a long time is that the ligaments become stretched, the bones sag, in the knee-joint the tibia falls backward as a rule. I have seen a good many cases in which there was a backward subluxation of the tibia, simply from distension. I should imagine that would be an objection to it unless it is quickly absorbed.

"In regard to the injection of a 2 per cent. solution of formaldehyd in glycerin, that is Dr. Murphy's treatment, and it is very good. I know that Dr. Lee did it in one case he had at the hospital. He aspirated the joint and injected a 2 per cent. solution of formalin in glycerin, and he aspirated two or three times and got very good results. In cases where the micro-organism is in the joint, I think that would be a good thing, but we must remember that this is not a surface infection; the infection does not take place on the surface of the endothelial side; the infection takes place in the membrane, in the dense synovial membrane, then sets up a synovitis, and the fluid in the joint is the result of the inflammatory process.

"Dr. Murphy says that in a large number of experiments which he made—cases he examined—in 7 per cent. of them the germ was found within a week, and only in 7 per cent., and it was several weeks before 80 per cent. of the cases showed a micro-organism in the fluid which was drawn. This 2 per cent. solution is not an antiseptic; it is not a germicide; he does not claim that for it; he claims it makes the fluid in the joint a poor culture-medium for the germ; not only that, but it produces a phagocytosis in the joint. That treatment wasn't known when I had these cases.

"In regard to drainage, I think a good many surgeons admit that the contact of any hard substance with a synovial membrane, or any serous membrane, like the pleura and peritoneum, destroys the endothelial cells of the membrane. Now, destroying the endothelial cells does not produce ankylosis, but favors it. But it is a fact that the presence of any foreign body and air in contact with the endothelial cells irritates them—does damage to them, and finally destroys them.

"I am very much opposed to drainage wherever I can safely omit it, even in the peritoneal or pleural cavities. I think it sets up a good deal more inflammation and consequent adhesions than would occur without it.

"I think it is a good thing to avoid opening a joint if it is possible, and in future I would aspirate and introduce this 2 per cent. solution of glycerin-formalin. Dr. Murphy insists that this solution should be prepared at least twenty-four hours before it is used, as it takes that length of time for it to dissolve. He injects only about 10-15 c. c. into the joint. That is only a small quantity and cannot do much harm; in fact, cannot do any harm. I would aspirate, inject, and, if necessary, re-aspirate and re-inject, and keep on as long as the patient's joint is safe and the patient in good health, rather than incise, as opening incurs a greater risk than aspiration, although my friend in Connecticut had a holy horror even of aspirating the joint."

## Dislocation of Scapula.

DR. STEPHEN L. TAYLOR presented the case history and photographs of the patient. The photographs show an unusual deformity of the right scapula, the lower angle and inner border projecting abnormally. The patient, a man about 60 years of age, a bayman by occupation, while attempting to lift a heavy weight experienced severe pain in the region of the right shoulder and noticed he could not use his arm. He consulted a physician, but no deformity of the shoulder was observed. The disability has continued. Eight months after the accident he was examined by me and these photographs were taken. The patient is emaciated. This is on account of a chronic illness, probably cancer of the stomach. There is no deformity of the structures about the shoulder other than that shown of the scapula. No muscular atrophy apparent. The muscles are wasted, but no more so on the right side than on the left. Motions of the hand, wrist, elbow and shoulder are normal, except that they are weak and awkward. Loss of power is especially noticed in attempting to lift or carry objects.

Dislocation of the scapula, I find, receives little attention in surgical works. Congenital elevation of the scapula or Sprengel's deformity, a displacement upward of one or both scapulæ in varying degrees, often associated with lateral curvature or torti collis, is frequently reported, about 90 cases having been reported since 1891, when the condition was first described. I have been able to find little mention of displacement of the scapula due to muscular exertion. In the Wharton and Curtis text-book of surgery, under the heading of dislocation of the scapula, a deformity similar to the one shown in these pictures is described and is said to be the result of the slipping of the angle of the scapula from its normal position beneath the latissimus dorsi muscle. It also states that this is not an infrequent accident with children and is brought about by attempting to lift the child by one arm. Fowler's Surgery refers to dislocation of the scapula and states that it is no longer considered due to displacement of the inferior angle from beneath the latissimus dorsi muscle, but is probably caused by an injury to the posterior thoracic nerve, resulting in paralysis of the serratus magnus muscle. In an article on injury to nerves by Dr. George Woolsey in *Keen's Surgery* is this statement: "The long or posterior thoracic nerve is not uncommonly compressed or contused by heavy weights on the shoulder or by contraction of the scaleni in excessive muscular strain." This seems to be the most satisfactory explanation of this condition. For treatment of this condition there is little recommended. The wearing of a tight bandage over the lower part of the scapula to help hold it in position is the only suggestion made which would seem to be applicable to this case.

*(Concluded from meeting of June 6, 1912.)*

### Perforating Ulcer of the Duodenum.

Dr. W. A. Gildersleeve reported the following case:

A woman, 34 years of age, gives a history of stomach trouble for six years. Fourteen months ago, she began to have severe colicy pains in the upper abdomen. This attack lasted four weeks. Two weeks ago, she began to have sharp pain in the upper abdomen after taking food. No vomiting, but nausea. Has had black stools. March 6th was awakened at midnight with very sharp pain in upper abdomen; four hours later, examination showed the abdomen greatly distended, rigid, and a general tenderness, especially marked in upper right quadratus. Abdomen was opened revealing gas and intestinal contents free in peritoneal cavity. A perforating duodemal ulcer was located in the two portions of the duodeum. Sutures could not be used on account of the infiltration. The opening was covered in by suturing the colon over it. The peritoneal cavity was sponged dry and a drain passed down to the perforation under the kidney fossa. The patient made an uneventful recovery and left the hospital in good condition.

Dr. John Horni reported the following three cases:

### Empyema of the Gall-Bladder and Gangrenous Appendicitis.

Patient admitted to German Hospital having been sick three days, complaining of sharp pain in the right iliac fossa, temperature 101 degrees, pulse rapid, no vomiting. Appendicitis was diagnosed. Operation revealed a gangrenous appendix and distended gall-bladder which was found to contain pus.

### A Case of Oxyuris Vermicularis Simulating Appendicitis.

Patient a girl, eight years old, admitted to German Hospital, sick and ailing for some time, pain over the region of the appendix. No temperature and no rapid pulse on admission. Appendicitis was diagnosed.

Operation revealed an appendix very much distended, but not much injected. On removing appendix, it was found filled with a tiny worm, which, on examination proved to be the oxyuris vermicularis, which are looked upon as harmless, still in this case it produced a sick and ailing youngster for some months, showing that these pin worms should be attacked as soon as discovered in a youngster and proper medication applied.

### Rupture of the Gall Bladder.

Patient, Mrs. H., referred to hospital for an appendectomy. Forty-eight hours before admission, had a fall and complained of pain in the right iliac fossa. No vomiting, slight jaundice. Abdomen distended. Appendicitis was diagnosed. On opening the abdomen, bile flowed freely, from abdominal incision. The peritoneal cavity was filled with bile, appendix was normal. A perforation was found in the base of gall-bladder admitting tip of little finger, no gall-stones. Gall-bladder was apparently in a healthy condition. The gall-bladder was drained and patient is now making an uneventful recovery.

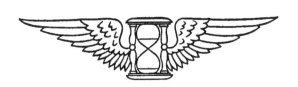

# LONG ISLAND MEDICAL JOURNAL

| VOL. VII. | MARCH; 1913 | NO. 3 |

## Original Articles.

### VESICAL CALCULUS.

#### By Edward L. Keyes, Jr., M.D.,

of New York City.

THE limits of this paper prohibit any intimate discussion of the more unusual features of vesical calculus, and grant opportunity for only a swift survey of the symptoms, diagnosis, and treatment of this condition. Yet, such a survey, founded upon a personal clinical experience, rather than upon text-book rules, may, we trust, prove not entirely valueless.

The symptoms of stone in the bladder begin with the history. This may, or may not, include attacks of renal colic, as the stone slips from the kidney into the bladder. In our experience a minority of bladder stone cases give such a history, for curiously enough a colic seems more likely to transmit a stone that will pass from the bladder without our assistance.

If the patient's history begins with such a colic, a greater or less interval of time intervenes, during which the stone remains "silent" in the patient's bladder. This interval may extend to a number of months, or even years, while the patient suffers, to all intents and purposes, no discomfort from his visitor. But when the stone begins to irritate the bladder and to cause frequent and painful urination, or even cystitis, the course of the disease becomes characteristically remittent, i. e., the symptoms of irritation never entirely disappear, and more or less frequent exacerbations occur, which our forefathers aptly termed "a fit of the stone."

The frequent and painful urination is characteristically more severe by day than by night; more severe when the patient goes about than when he sits still. Yet this rule is broken by innumerable exceptions, upon which we shall dwell in a moment.

Analysis of the urine of a patient suffering from stone in the bladder is likely to reveal a few blood cells, though the presence of even microscopical blood is not constant. On the other hand, occasional slight hemorrhage of prostatic origin, occurring at the termination of urination and accompanied by a good deal of pain, may be due to stone; but is so much more suggestive of tuberculosis as to have no diagnostic value. Pus may or may not be found in the urine.

On the other hand, the symptoms of stone in the bladder, like those of stone in the ureter or kidney pelvis, are often simulated by other maladies. Thus the most characteristic traditional symptom of bladder stone is sudden stoppage of the urinary stream, due to obstruction of the urethral outlet by the stone. Now not only is this symptom a rather unusual one when stone is present, but the stoppage is far from uncommon when the patient has a tumor in his bladder, a hypertrophied prostate, or simply one of those many functional derangements of urination, which so frequently follow gonorrhea or accompany sexual neurasthenia. Moreover the typical picture of stone in the bladder may be precisely mimicked by renal, or reno-vesical, or prostatic tuberculosis, so that for diagnostic purposes the clinical picture of stone is worth almost nothing at all.

Furthermore, some patients can carry a stone in the bladder for many years without symptoms. This may be due to various causes. Thus, the infant that urinates frequently, and cries and is fretful, may be said, clinically, to have no symptoms of stone, for its parents and physician pay no attention to this stone, and the child is finally brought to us with a stone the size of a walnut, and with the statement that its symptoms have existed for only a few months. At the other end of life the old man does not suffer from stone in the bladder because this stone, lying in a pouch behind the prostate, or in a saccule, does not irritate the bladder neck, and does not add materially to the symptoms of urinary retention from which the patient already suffers. On the other hand, one occasionally meets patients in middle age with no recognizable prostatic hypertrophy, yet with a surprising absence of symptoms of stone in the bladder.

Such a patient came to me in 1904, with the history that he had been refused life insurance on account of albumin. His only symptom was that horseback riding made him pass blood, though it did not increase his urinary frequency in any way. I saw a great deal of this patient from 1904 to 1908, during which time he never had any urinary frequency and only rarely bled. I then asked Dr. Cauldwell to X-ray him, thinking that he might find a stone in the ureter, and to my great surprise this operation disclosed two stones in the bladder, almost spherical, and each measuring about 3 cm. in diameter. Litholapaxy was performed upon this patient, and when last seen, a few months ago, he had no return of his stone.

Having thus endeavored to shake your confidence in the so-called clinical picture of vesical calculus, let me present to you one symptom upon which some dependence can be placed as being strongly suggestive of this condition. This is stinking urine without grave kidney lesion and without retention of urine in the bladder. This stinking urine without renal or vesical retention is but rarely seen. Rather more frequently a patient comes with vesical retention, submits to the irrigations and catheterizations calculated to relieve this condition, and yet the urine continues to stink. This is very suggestive of stone.

By the same token, a purulent urine that becomes absolutely clear and free from pus under treatment suggests that no stone is present.

## DIAGNOSIS.

Let us pass, however, to the definite surgical measures for ascertaining the presence of calculus in the urinary tract. First among these stands the radiograph, and when vesical calculus is suspected one should always have a radiograph taken—not, curiously enough, for the purpose of diagnosing the presence or absence of stone in the bladder, but for the purpose of ascertaining the presence of stone in the ureter or kidney pelvis, which may simulate stone in the bladder or may be associated with it. (Though let it be said, parenthetically, such association is not the rule.)

The radiograph, however, is singularly negative in the detection of vesical calculus. The late Dr. Tilden Brown reported a case cystoscoped by him and sent to a radiographer, with the statement that stone had been seen in the bladder. Yet repeated radiographs failed to show this stone. I have had an experience precisely similar; though the stone in Dr. Brown's case was a large one, while mine was small. This simply means that certain vesical calculi are singularly bereft of lime salts in their construction.

An older diagnostic implement is the stone searcher. This, especially in the hands of the expert manipulator, is a very delicate diagnostic instrument, and one that may do service in persuading irritable patients that they have stones by the briefest possible manipulation. Yet the inexperienced manipulator can do little with the searcher, and even the most expert cannot expect to disclose by its use the presence or absence of prostatic hypertrophy, or bladder sacculation, nor can he discern by its use the presence of renal deficiency or infection on one or both sides, all of which complications enter into the case when operation is contemplated—all of which may be disclosed by cystoscopy. The cystoscope, therefore, like the X-ray, is the essential instrument for the diagnosis of vesical calculus. Even the cystoscope is by no means infallible in the diagnosis of stone. Apart from the fact that the examination may fail to reveal a stone in a saccule, it is liable to two grave misinterpretations. An old clot often looks exactly like an acid stone, while a stone covered with fibrin often looks exactly like a sloughy, malignant tumor. But the mere knowledge of these possible errors, and a little poking with the ureter catheter almost invariably suffices for a diagnosis.

## TREATMENT.

Small vesical calculi, like small ureteral calculi, may pass spontaneously. Yet there is not the same incentive to wait for such passage, since vesical calculi may be crushed in a few moments. If the patient is not over-sensitive this operation may be performed in the physician's office under local anesthesia.

At the other extreme, large stones, or stones complicated by bladder tumor, or sacculation, or by prostatic hypertrophy, obviously require suprapubic cystotomy for their removal, for the management of the complications, and for drainage, though in some instances this last may be dispensed with and the bladder sewed up tight, if we remember the cardinal rule, that free drainage must always be supplied through the suprapubic tissues down to the sutured viscus.

But between the wee stone, almost small enough to pass, and the huge or complicated one, there are many calculi not more than four or five cm. in their greatest diameter and uncomplicated by anything worse than cystitis and perhaps a slight pyelonephritis. What shall be the operation of choice in these cases? Shall we perform litholapaxy or lithotomy? The older generation succeeded very well with the former operation. My father, for instance, performed almost two hundred litholapaxies and never lost a patient under sixty years of age. But stones in the bladder are relatively infrequent in this part of the globe, while ambitious general surgeons are far more common than the teeth of a hen. Consequently these patients are thinned out, as it were—distributed in small number to a very large number of operators, who have little especial interest in this particular class of patients and less experience in the various delicate features which they present. Such men do not perform litholapaxy, and it is much better that they should not, for one has only to hear of the distinguished surgeon who dragged forth a piece of small intestine in the jaws of his lithotrite, to realize that unskilled fingers have difficulty in recognizing the position of the lithotrite within the bladder.

Litholapaxy is one of those operations whose first ten victims should include all the mortality that an operator is ever to have. But for uncomplicated stones the specialist will continue to prefer litholapaxy to lithotomy on account of the lesser mortality and the greater rapidity of convalescence. After a litholapaxy the patient may perhaps not be detained in the hospital at all, and many usually leave as early as the fourth or fifth day; while lithotomy, under the best of circumstances, detains him in bed a week, and may lay him up for three or four weeks. But the selection of operation in any given case must lie with the operator. None of us can consider the performance of repeated litholapaxies, year after year, in almost infinite sequence, on old prostatics, as an ideal condition, though we still occasionally meet patients who insist upon this form of treatment. On the other hand, few of us would deem it wise to perform all of our litholapaxies in the office, urging the patient to return for repeated partial crushings and washings almost after the manner of the ancient lithritist. Yet the late Dr. Chismore, of San Francisco, founded an enviable reputation upon his method of operation.

But let us not try to be more specific where we should inevitably fail either to interest or to persuade you. Let us hope that the dispute between litholapaxy and lithotomy may continue vigorous and interminable. Yet let us also hope that the rival camps will occasionally call a truce and urge subscription to one thesis for the edification of the young. When in doubt, cut.

# THE NORMAL CEREBRO-SPINAL FLUID: ITS PHYSIOLOGY AND CHEMISTRY.*

By Phebe L. DuBois, M.D.,

of Brooklyn, N. Y.

THERE is very little written in English about the cerebro-spinal fluid. My sources of knowledge have been three French books written by Anglada, Milan, and Cathelin, respectively, two Oliver Sharpey lectures by Mott and an article by Cushing.

Cotugno discovered the cerebro-spinal fluid in 1764. He observed it only in the cadaver and thought it present only after death. He found it in fish and turtles, but not in birds and dogs. He always remained in doubt of its reality. He thought the arachnoid space was filled by serous vapor, but reasoned that its condensation would not give as much fluid as was present at death and so thought there must be water there during life.

* Read before the Medical Society of the County of Kings, November 19, 1912.

Haller found fluid in the cord, but did not realize that it circulated. He compared it to the fluid in the pericardium and peritoneum and thought it was a transudate that collected all along the way, there being no relation between that in the ventricles and in the spinal canal. He said that a serous vapor was continually exhaled from the free surface of the pia mater and the ventricles.

After Cotugno and Haller no one mentions cerebro-spinal fluid until Magendie redescribed it and thought he was the first to discover it. It should be remembered in connection with him rather than Cotugno, because he pointed it out during vivisection and discovered the connection between the ventricles and sub-arachnoid spaces by means of the foramen that bears his name.

The presence of fluid in the ventricles had been known a long time, but numerous controversies had always existed about it. Galen, Willis, Vieussens, Litre, and Schneider believed in the existence of water in the ventricles. Coiter, Hilden, Bohn, Verdue, Lieutaud, Haller, and Cotugno believed in a serous vapor capable of condensing under the influence of pathological causes. Magendie demonstrated absolutely that it was a liquid and not a vapor during life.

The study of the cerebro-spinal fluid may be divided into three periods. The first or anatomical period extended from the 18th century to the first part of the 19th. The physiological began in 1840, with Magendie and has extended up to the present time with Bourguignon, Longet, Claude Bernard, Paulet, Mosso, Salathe, Francois Franck, Talkenheim, Nanyn, Richet, etc. They studied the role and chemical constitution, the communications of the ventricular spaces and the sub-arachnoid, the pressure of the liquid, and the relation of the circulation in the brain and cord with the cerebro-spinal fluid and Richet and Franck established their laws of the synchronism of the flux and reflux of the cerebro-spinal fluid depending on the movements of inspiration and expiration. With Quincke, who inaugurated lumbar puncture in 1891 began a new period—the clinical period which gave to physicians a way of investigation and study. Since this time, the discoveries have been more and more numerous and one may truly say that the three methods, anatomical, physiological and clinical, receive help from each other. Thanks to the work of many investigators the origin and destination of the cerebro-spinal fluid is at least partially understood.

Its composition is against its being a transudation from the blood or a lymphatic secretion. Mott gives the following facts to prove this conclusion. (1) It contains .02% of protein against 7% in blood plasma and 4.5% in body lymph. (2) There is an absence of lipochrome. (3) There are no leucocytes in normal fluid. (4) In typhoid, there is an absence of agglutinins. (5) It has no hæmolytic action on the blood corpuscles of other animals. (6) It contains no alexins. With few exceptions experimental observations on men and animals have shown that drugs or bacterial toxins administered by mouth or subcutaneously do not pass into the cerebro-spinal fluid. The cerebro-spinal fluid and brain are not stained with bile in the great majority of cases of jaundice. Cavazzini found that the injection of lymphagogues in some cases increased it. The facts speak against its being either a transudation or a lymph secretion, although it is generally admitted that the perivascular lymphatics open into the sub-arachnoid space.

Willis in 1664 called attention to the glandular nature of the choroid plexus. Petit and Girard published a monograph on the secretory function and morphology of the choroid plexus of the central nervous system taking up the systematic study of the plexuses in different animals belonging to different classes of vertebrates in 1902. They state that Faivre in 1854 affirmed the intimate relation of the choroid plexus with the spinal fluid.

The work since has progressively tended to support this view of its source. Microscopic sections of the choroid plexus show tufts of vessels surrounded by a loose connective tissue covered by a single layer of cubical-spheroidal or polyhedral cells lying on a basement membrane. Around the arteries and arterioles numerous nerve fibres are seen in the form of a plexus. Comparison with the lachrymal gland shows that the epithelial cells of the choroid plexus present a very similar appearance. The histological evidence is all in favor of the choroid plexus being a gland with an external secretion, but with an internal destination. It thus constitutes a mixed type of gland intermediate between a ductless gland and a gland with a duct. Its mode of formation is effected in an inverse manner, epithelial invagination for a gland with an excretory duct, ependymal invagination for the choroid plexus. In the former case, the vascularization is peripheral, in the later it is central.

If we accept these observations as conclusive proof that the choroid plexus is the source of the cerebro-spinal fluid and that it is continually secreting this fluid then we can understand its unique chemical composition and its freedom under normal conditions from corpuscular elements. We know that it is reproduced very rapidly. Patients after fracture of the skull or removal of nasal polyps have been known to lose more than a litre in 24 hours. Matthieu reports having seen after vertebral traumatism the loss of 2-4 litres per day. The normal amount in a man of ordinary height is 62 grams according to Magendie and 125-155 grams, according to Cotugno—probably the latter estimation is more nearly correct. The quantity is greater in proportion to the size in adults than in infants because of the development of the brain—deeper convolutions. The amount also varies with the height of the individual and the time that elapses between death and the autopsy.

The fluid secreted in the ventricles escapes from the 4th ventricle into the sub-arachnoid space by the foramen of Magendie and the foramina of Luschka. Mott describes these openings thus—"When the cerebellum is raised posteriorly so as to expose the tela choroidea one sees at the level of the calamus scriptorius a round or oval opening with irregular borders as if torn. This orifice connecting the 4th ventricle with the sub-arachnoid space was first pointed out by Magendie and has since been called after its discoverer. It is situated in the mid-line and measures 7-8 mm. in length by 5-6 mm. in breadth. The foramina of Luschka are a pair of lateral orifices connecting the 4th ventricle with the sub-arachnoid space. They occupy the external extremity of the lateral recess which the cavity of the fourth ventricle forms and from which emerge the origin of the mixed nerves. Through the foramina of Luschka the choroid plexus of the 4th ventricle passes."

Mott goes on to say that the existence of the foramen of Magendie has been doubted by Cruiveilhier, Reichert and Kolliker who regarded it as an artifact. The foramina of Luschka have been described by Marc Sie and Hess. Hess met with them in 51 out of 54 subjects examined so that they must be fairly constant.

The fluid escaping into the sub-arachnoid space fills up all the cracks and crevices and by its mechanical action as a water pad protects the brain and cord. The blood vessels of the cerebro-spinal axis have comparatively thin walls and the arteries relatively few muscular fibers and vasomotor nerves. The uniform pressure of the fluid sleeve which surrounds the blood vessels serves to support their column of blood. The whole central nervous system being contained in a closed space, the cerebro-spinal fluid fills up all the space which is not occupied by tissue or blood, serving thus to equalize the pressure throughout the whole cranio-spinal cavity. It also serves as a self adjusting mechanism by maintaining a uniform equalization of the blood supply to the nerve elements during the rhythmical variations of the respiration and circulation. The headache, vertigo and vomiting that sometimes follow lumbar puncture have never been satisfactorily accounted for. They may be due to a disturbance of the equilibrium of osmotic pressure—i. e., there may be a secondary hypertension following increased irritative secretion, or perhaps the brain deprived of its water mattress suffers contusions against the walls of the cranium.

There is good reason to suppose that the cerebro-spinal fluid is constantly being secreted, but it cannot be constantly secreted and not flow away. According to Cathelin it escapes along the lymphatics of the cranial and spinal nerves passing through the paravertebral lymphatic glands and eventually arriving in the venous circulation through the receptaculum chyli and thoracic duct.

Flatau demonstrated by injecting into a rabbit's olfactory nerve that the fluid follows the course of the perineural sheath, then passes directly into the lymphatic net work of the nasal mucosa arriving at the glands of the neck and the naso-pharyngeal cavity.

Hill and Cushing from their observations believed that the cerebro-spinal fluid made its escape from the cranium by means of the veins opening into the longitudinal sinus. Cushing agrees with Adamkiewicz that there exists a free communication between the sub-arachnoid space and the longitudinal sinus. He questions the correctness of Key's and Retzius's hypothesis that the Pacchionian bodies act as filters for they do not exist in very young children nor in some of the lower animals.

The nature of these openings of the sub-arachnoid space is not known, but they probably run obliquely forward like the veins into the sinus and probably have a valvular action so that the fluid can flow into the sinus, but blood cannot flow back. Mercury injected into the sub-arachnoid was found in the sinuses, jugular veins and right heart. A non-absorbable gas introduced into the sub-arachnoid space produced death by cardiac air embolism and if the jugulars were exposed bubbles of it could be seen pouring down toward the heart. Exposure of the cervical lymphatics and of the thoracic duct on the other hand showed in all instances a complete freedom from gas.

Mott suggest that cerebro-spinal fluid may reach the venous blood by way of the capillaries. He says that the lymphatic sheaths of the vessels of the central nervous system are intracerebral and intraspinal prolongations of the sub-arachnoid space. Also he says that probably a canalicular system surrounds the cells and vessels which is in direct communication with the sub-arachnoid space. This system contains a fluid of non-proteid nature, probably, therefore, the cerebro-spinal fluid, which may serve as the ambient fluid of the neurons and play the part of lymph in the central nervous system.

From all this it would seem that while the origin of the cerebro-spinal fluid is pretty generally agreed upon, its destination and means of exit are not.

As I have stated before, with few exceptions experimental observations on men and animals have shown that drugs and bacterial toxins administered by the mouth and subcutaneously do not pass into the cerebro-spinal fluid. Yet much smaller quantities of these same substances injected into the sub-arachnoid space produce much more marked and more rapid onset of symptoms. Lewandowsky observed that a few centigrams of sodium ferrocyanide injected into the sub-arachnoid space produced toxic symptoms rapidly while the injection of from 4-6 grams into the jugular veins of rabbits of the same weight produced no specific symptoms. Behring found that hens injected subcutaneously or intravenously with tetanus toxin suffered no effects, but when it was injected into the cerebro-spinal fluid they died from typical tetanus.

Jacob introduced methylene blue and iodine into the cerebro-spinal fluid and was able to demonstrate their presence in the brain several days later, although they were gone from the cerebro-spinal fluid.

Aside from its mechanical role the function of the cerebro-spinal fluid is not very well known. It is not even definitely known whether or not there is an exchange of substances en route between its secretion by the choroid plexus and its removal by lumbar puncture.

Normal cerebro-spinal fluid is a clear colorless liquid looking exactly like water, but it does not wet the sides of a test tube so much. The specific gravity is 1003-1004. Quincke found the pressure to be from 40-150 mm. of water normally. We approximate the pressure by the number of drops per minute. The normal reaction is alkaline, but it becomes acid soon after death. The cryoscopic point is .55°C. Normally cerebro-spinal fluid when heated gives a faint opalescence. It contains a small quantity of serum globulin, mineral matters, in particular sodium chloride, traces of fat, cholestrin, glucose and urea. There has been some question as to what the reducing substance is, whether it is glucose or pyrocatechin. Halliburton says it is glucose and that it is increased after successive punctures. Normal cerebro-spinal fluid does not contain fibrin or fibrinogen. It should be classed with the aqueous humor and the amniotic fluid. It is totally different from the liquids of the serous cavities and the lymph. It is poor in cellular elements, must be centrifuged a long time, and then only a few lymphocytes and desquamated endothelial cells will be found.

In examining 465 spinal fluids at the Research Laboratory, we have found a number of normal fluids. We depend upon the stained sediment, Noguchi's globulin reaction and the albumin reaction in judging whether or not a fluid is normal.

# VENEREAL PROPHYLAXIS IN THE NAVY.*

## By T. A. Berryhill, M.D.,

Medical Inspector, U. S. Navy.

WHEN I first entered the Navy, twenty-seven years ago, an old Medical Director said to me, "Doctor, the Navy would be a nice place in which to practice medicine if the men had neither tonsils nor testicles," and I have found his statement true, as these two sets of organs indirectly produce more sickness and more sick days in the Navy than all other causes.

The question of venereal diseases in the Navy is one of great importance, as they produce more morbidity than any other disease.

For the year 1909 there were 11,064 admissions, giving 139,396 sick days, with a rate of 199.17 per 1000. In 1908 the admission rate was 127.76 per 1000. This sudden jump was caused by having every case of venereal disease admitted to the sick list by orders from the Bureau of Medicine and Surgery. Prior to 1909 probably less than half the cases of venereal disease was entered on the books for record.

These figures show that about 200 men in every thousand, 20 in a hundred, or one man in five, in the Navy, is infected with some venereal disease. It would be interesting to be able to compare the rate in the Navy with the rate in civil life, but unfortunately there are no statistics of any value for the civil population. As some of the states, notably California, have passed laws making it obligatory to report all venereal diseases, we may soon have some figures with which to make a comparison. I have little faith in the accuracy of statistics of this kind, for only a small proportion of men having gonorrhœa go to a physician for treatment, for every "rounder" has a number of prescriptions for this disease and is always willing to prescribe for other unfortunates. I venture to believe that the rate of venereal disease among the young unmarried civil population is equal to that in the Navy.

One-third of the patients seeking free treatment at the free dispensaries do so for venereal disease. Morrow estimates the number of syphilitics in the United States at 2,000,000. If the proportion between syphilis and gonorrhœa found in the statistics of the Committee of Seven in 1901 in New York City of nearly one to ten obtains for the whole country, the number of people having venereal disease would reach nearly 20,000,000. Of 30,000 prostitutes in New York City in 1897 (35,000, according to Mrs. Goode), one-half were or had been infected with syphilis. Venereal diseases always increase after a foreign war with occupation by the troops. Many young married men become infected and spread the diseases on returning home.

Under the present method of admitting to the sick list all venereal cases, we now approximate the admission rate of the U. S. Army for primary venereal disease, viz.: Navy 160.40, Army 174.84 per thousand. This admission rate is much higher than in the navies of some other nations, viz.: German 66, French 75, Italian 83, British 120 per thousand. How much of this difference is due to methods of recording cases I am unable to state, but in all these countries there is some control of prostitution, with the exception of England, where they

* Read before the Medical Society of the County of Kings, January 21, 1913.

treat the condition as we do in this country, by shutting the eyes to it. While the navies of all the European countries show a lower rate than ours, the armies of these countries show a much lower rate than their navies, probably because the soldiers stay at home and many marry and thus do not run the risk the sailors do by stopping in different countries.

Germany, France, Spain, Hungary, Portugal and Russia all have some method of supervision over prostitution and, although this supervision may be enforced in a lax manner, as it usually is, there can be no doubt but that it exercises a beneficial influence.

There is another reason for the higher rate of venereal disease in our Navy than that of European navies and that is that our men receive higher wages than the sailors of foreign navies and therefore have more money to spend in the gratification of their desires.

The average age of our ship's company, officers and men, is 25½ years. Most of the sailors are recruited from the young men of the middle West and have never seen salt water till they are sent to a training station on the coast. It seems that something should be done to protect them from the dangers of the big cities, especially from the curse of venereal infection. We are trying to do this in the Navy, but are receiving no assistance from the cities where our men spend their liberty and money, except for the Naval Y. M. C. A. branches. A sailor in a strange town has three places where he may go and be welcome; a church, a bar-room or a brothel. As there is no segregation of prostitutes in any of our coast towns, the streets are full of street-walkers who find an easy mark in our unsophisticated young seamen and the natural result follows. The New York city law which allows the physical examination of women arrested for certain causes and their treatment in hospital, if found suffering from venereal diseases, is one that might be of great benefit if it could be strictly enforced. Its weakness is that the arresting officer must have absolute evidence or he will not be upheld. Such evidence is hard to procure. In some of our smaller coast cities efforts to control these diseases could be carried out with more success than in a city of the size of New York. Take the cases of the cities where three of our training stations are located: Newport, R. I., San Francisco, Cal., and Norfolk, Va. The admission rates for all venereal diseases in 1909 were: at Newport, R. I., 75.6; at San Francisco, Cal., 124.4, and at Norfolk, Va., 331.6 per thousand. These cases occurred amongst boys from 17 to 20 years of age. Certainly in a small city like Norfolk effective work could be done by the authorities, as it would not be difficult to spot all the prostitutes and make them keep healthy or stop their trade. Unfortunately we are confronted with the irrational attitude of the Anglo-Saxon race that this question should not be recognized as existing, although prostitution is probably the oldest profession in the world and will continue with us as long as man's passion persists. When that passion ceases the race will end. I recognize the difficulties of control of this question, but even if only one diseased prostitute is cured it will prevent many men from contracting disease.

That the medical officers of the Navy have been aware of the importance of venereal diseases as a cause of great loss of efficiency is demonstrated by the many reports and papers sent in to the Department. In fact there has been so much written and said about it that it has become a common belief that all sailors are diseased, just as all sailors are supposed to be drunkards, when, as a matter of fact, alcoholism in the Navy is very small, being only 5.9 per thousand during 1910, while in 1900 it was 10.8 +.

Since the discovery of the cause' of gonorrhœa and its mode of attack in the urethra, it has been the belief that could a germicide be introduced soon enough, the disease could be aborted.

Metchnikoff had demonstrated that in experimental syphilis the hard chancre could be prevented by calomel.

These two facts form the basis of the prophylaxis in these two diseases.

We are indebted to the Germans for the practical application of this knowledge.

In 1904, a year before Schaudinn discovered the treponema pallidum, I was on a naval vessel in the West Indies. We ran across a German man-o'-war having about the same number of men as our ship. In comparing notes with the medical officer I found he had only two cases of gonorrhœa on his ship, while I had twenty. He told me the men on his ship used the contents of a prophylactic package which they purchased from the canteen, whenever they were exposed to venereal infection. This package contained an antiseptic ointment and an injection of a silver salt. I reported the matter to the Department but heard nothing from it at that time.

In 1907 an energetic medical officer on the Asiatic Station became so interested in the German method of prophylaxis that he tried it on his ship, with such success that he interested the Fleet Surgeon and the Commander-in-Chief. Reports were made to the Bureau of Medicine and Surgery and attracted instant attention. The reports were published in the *Naval Medical Bulletin* and soon many ships were using the method. It was soon found that without the co-operation of the commanding officers but little could be accomplished, as many men refused to take the treatment and many denied having been exposed. Gradually the line officers began to see the benefit of the work and they issued orders that all men who had been exposed to venereal infection should appear for treatment. Should he deny exposure and subsequently show a venereal disease, he would be punished for lying and concealing a disease. Thus armed with authority we can now go ahead with the work. The men are given lectures at stated periods, which become drill periods, and are now no more remitted than the drills at the guns. The Bureau of Medicine and Surgery has issued circulars of a confidential nature describing the venereal diseases and giving advice to those having these diseases. The lectures are given by a medical officer and consist of general subjects of hygiene of ship's life and of the venereal diseases.

The manner in which the prophylaxis is carried on in most ships is as follows, with slight variations in different ships: A duplicate of the liberty list is given to the medical officer every day. Upon the return of the men from liberty, they are each asked if they had been exposed during their liberty. If they answer "yes" they are given the treatment. If "no" they are checked off the list. These lists are filed for reference. A place is provided in the sick bay where treatment is administered. This is equipped with wash basins, cotton and syringes. It is under the supervision of one of the nurses.

The man is required to wash his privates with a solution of bichloride of mercury 1-2000. He then washes in pure water and takes an injection of about two drams of a solution of argyrol, 10 per cent., or protargol, 2 per cent., which he retains three minutes by the clock. He then smears the penis with a 50 per cent. ointment of calomel and lanoline. This ointment is to be thoroughly rubbed into all folds of skin around the glans and prepuce and also cover the body of the penis. This is left on.

The success of this treatment is not yet apparent in the general statistics of the Navy, but every medical officer with whom I have spoken about it believes in its efficacy. It is certainly true that it is reducing the amount of primary syphilis.

In this connection I desire to give my experience of the results obtained on the U. S. S. Nebraska. The ship had been on the southern drill grounds at target practice for several weeks. We came into Hampton Roads and, on September 16, 1909, gave liberty to one hundred men. Most of these men went to Norfolk. I decided I would start the prophylactic treatment on this liberty party. On their return after twenty hours liberty, they were asked if they had been exposed to venereal infection. Ninety answered in the affirmative. They were given the treatment. Upon following up these men for a number of weeks, none were found to have contracted venereal disease. From September 16 to December 31, 1909, there were given to the ship's crew 14,000 liberties. Of this number 1,134 admitted exposure and took the treatment. During this time there was no chancroid, no syphilis and only two cases of gonorrhœa among those taking the treatment. I attribute this result to the great care exercised by the nurses in charge of the treatment and to the fact that we used argyrol instead of protargol, which is very painful, and will not be retained a sufficient length of time in the urethra to be efficacious.

At the Training Station at Norfolk the prophylactic treatment was begun late in 1909 and continued during 1910. As before stated, the venereal rate during 1909 was 331.6, while for 1910 the rate had been reduced to 281.7 per thousand. While this was not as great a reduction as was expected it shows progress.

Almost all the reports from ships show a decreased percentage of disease among those taking the treatment and particularly in the rate for syphilis, which is very much reduced. There are various reasons why the results are not better. Some men who deny exposure on return from liberty find themselves with a venereal disease later on. They then go on liberty, return and take the treatment and then claim the treatment was not efficacious. Then there is a large class who get extended liberty and others who overstay their liberty. These men usually get the treatment too late to be of use.

It has been thought that if men took with them on liberty a prophylactic package and used it immediately after exposure we could reach this class of men, but many men are exposed in places where there are no facilities for washing and then there are others who would be ashamed to use the treatment in the presence of the woman, fearing to cast reflections on her cleanliness, and again there are others who are exposed while under the influence of alcohol and who do not care.

The Surgeon General has recommended that the pay of a man with venereal disease be forfeited during his disability and that all persons in the naval service, especially those afloat, be examined physically once a quarter and that such examination be required by regulation.

If these regulations were enforced it would cause all men to be more careful in taking the treatment and would prevent the concealment of disease.

From the decrease in the number of cases of syphilis it is believed that the treatment is more potent in this disease, when given late, than in gonorrhœa or chancroid. If this is so it is worthy of continuance, although the expense is very great.

It is the hope of my corps that when we can make every exposed man take the treatment we can reduce the primary infection of these diseases to less than 30 per thousand.

I have recently received the reports of the Surgeon General of the Army and the Surgeon General of the Navy for the year 1912. It appears that the War Department has become interested in the question of venereal prophylaxis and has issued a general order, which has the force of a regulation, that all men who have been exposed to venereal disease will upon their return to camp or garrison report to the hospital for the application of the prophylactic treatment, and that twice a month all enlisted men will be examined physically, and should a man be found suffering from a venereal disease after failing to take the prophylactic treatment, he is to be brought to trial before a court martial. During the last session of Congress a bill was passed providing that no money should be paid any man in the Army who was on the sick list for any disease contracted on account of his own misconduct. This gives the Army medical officers all the authority they need to cope with these diseases. The venereal rate in the Army for 1911 was 163.85 per thousand, as compared with a rate of 155.51 in 1910. Upon analysis it is found that there was a decrease of 8.92 per thousand for gonorrhœa and a decrease of 1.38 per thousand for chancroid, while the increase was due to syphilis alone, it being 17.65 per thousand. The increase of syphilis from 26.65 per thousand in 1910 to 44.30 per thousand in 1911 was due to the use of the Wasserman reaction, which has been extensively used in all of the commands.

The report of the Surgeon General of the Navy shows some improvement in the rate of venereal diseases for the year 1911. In 1909 the rate was 199.17, while for 1911 it is 183.56, a decrease of 15.61 per thousand. While this is not as good as was to be expected, it must be noted that we are working under difficulties, as only on certain ships is the taking of the prophylaxis compulsory. The best criterion as to the efficacy of the treatment would be statistics giving the number of infections after taking the prophylaxis. In every report from a ship where this treatment was used it is shown that the number of infections taking place subsequently was exceedingly small and leads us to believe that should all the exposures be given the prophylaxis, inside of eighteen hours, we could reduce the rate, as I have before stated, to less than 30 per thousand.

*(For discussion see page 117.)*

# THE VALUE OF THE GONORRHEAL COMPLEMENT FIXATION TEST AND THE WASSERMANN REACTION IN DETERMINING THE FITNESS OF A PERSON TO MARRY.*

By Max Lederer, M.D.,

Brooklyn, N. Y.

THE observations herewith recorded are based upon the personal examination of about 1,000 cases by the syphilitic complement fixation test and a small number of cases tested by the gonorrheal complement fixation properties, the work having been done in the laboratory of the Jewish Hospital.

The syphilitic cases giving a positive reaction during any stage of the disease can be dismissed with the statement, that the reaction is always a definite contra-indication to marriage. The question of syphilis is here considered mainly from the standpoint of the male, as it is the male who usually seeks for advice on this point. I might here state that during the last two years of this work at the hospital, which covers a series of from 300 to 350 reactions, we have not obtained a positive reaction in any case which was definitely non-syphilitic.

The negative reactions must be divided into several classes. Given a case with a history of recent infection, and as a result of that recent infection a positive reaction, the case receiving a sufficient amount of treatment, and as a result of this treatment a reaction that becomes negative and staying negative for a reasonable length of time, we can safely assume, theoretically, I think, that such an individual is not capable of transmitting syphilic infection, having a syphilitic offspring, or developing parasyphilis. Of course, the Wassermann reaction has not been in use long enough for us to definitely state that a series of negative reactions means that a patient is absolutely free from syphilitic taint. The only interpretation that we can put upon such a state of affairs to-day is, that the disease is under control, and thus we must still adhere to the old idea in advising a person whether to marry or not; that is to say, that the old idea of treatment for a reasonable length of time must be adhered to, in order to be absolutely sure that there will be no syphilitic sequelæ of any nature. I have had several individuals come to the office for that advice, and have advised them that if their reactions remain negative without anti-specific treatment for two years after the cessation of such treatment, that they may safely marry. This rule, of course, is arbitrary and has been adopted as the result of experience.

It goes without saying, that the presence of clinical symptoms of syphilis, even with a negative reaction, means interdiction of marriage. There is also a class of cases in which the individuals have a moral fear of syphilitic infection, in whom it is impossible to get a history, or to find any definite signs of the disease. We might even call this a form of syphilophobia. As an example of this type, there comes to mind a manager of one of the large cabarets of New York, who thought he had come in contact with several questionable people, and for that reason was afraid to marry on account of the fear of syphilis. His physician, whom he went to, finding no evidences of disease,

---

* Read before the Brooklyn Pathological Society, January 9, 1913.

advised a blood examination and sent him to me. The result of the reaction was negative, the individual's mind was relieved and he married with a clear conscience. The uncommon reaction is the negative one with the presence of syphilitic symptoms following syphilitic history. This type of reaction is extremely uncommon, but must be borne in mind.

In those cases which are under treatment, and give a negative reaction, the serologist might report freedom from disease because of insufficient history. To report such an individual with a negative reaction as safe to marry, would be wrong, for as mentioned above, a patient under treatment does give a negative reaction and yet may have uncured syphilis. I might here mention that another class of uncured syphilis in which a negative reaction occurs without treatment, is during the chancre stage before the fourth to the sixth week of the appearance of the initial lesion. In our experience, it has been rather uncommon to obtain a positive reaction before that time.

Another class of cases is that on which light has recently been thrown, cases of infection many years before, that develop cerebrospinal symptoms such as tabes, general paresis, etc. In these individuals, one may get a negative or only a faint reaction in the blood, whereas the cerebrospinal fluid uniformly gives a strongly positive test. I remember one case which later developed into typical tabes, in which the blood gave an absolutely negative reaction and yet the fluid by lumbar puncture gave a strongly positive reaction.

It must be borne in mind, that in all of the cases in which one obtains a negative reaction, that it is very, very unsafe to venture an opinion, unless one gets in addition a history of the case, as there may be facts or conditions which will give negative reaction, and yet there may be present a syphilitic taint in the system. It is unjust to the serologist and to the patient also, to confine the former simply to the result of the examination of a specimen without saying anything about the history. Furthermore, in this connection, quantitative estimation of the amount of syphilitic antibody must be necessary in order to arrive at a definite conclusion.

The question of transmission of infection during the stage when the reaction is negative, either when the patient is under treatment, or perhaps even after the patient has been pronounced cured, is a question open to argument. Theoretically, I believe we can assume that as long as the treatment is sufficient to control infection, and so cause the blood to give a negative reaction, the disease ought not to be transmissible. As I mentioned before, though, the work in this line has been of too short a duration to enable us to arrive at definite conclusions from facts or statistics. We have been working with the Wassermann reaction but six or seven years. and the question whether in an individual who has had syphilitic treatment for syphilitic infection, the reaction will remain negative for the rest of his life, is still open.

In gonorrhea our experience has been rather limited on account of the difficulty of obtaining antigen. The technic of the Wassermann reaction and the gonorrheal complement fixation test is identical, except that the specific antibodies sought for in gonorrhea are bound by a different antigen. That used in gonorrheal complement fixation test is a watery extract of the gonococcus. The point of practical value is that both tests can be done on one specimen of serum. It is not necessary to puncture the patient's vein twice. The technic of the gonorrheal complement fixation test is rather more difficult because of the instability of the antigen, and the results as yet are probably not so reliable as those obtained with the Wassermann reaction. The latter has become very practical in our hands, the laboratory results, as a rule, agreeing with the clinical findings.

The importance of determining whether an individual, and this affects the female as well as the male, is cured of gonorrhea, is apparent when we consider that most authorities regard this disease as being incurable in from 75 to 90 per cent. of cases. The test is reliable from the negative standpoint insofar that one never obtains a positive reaction in a negative case. McNeil and Schwartz, whose work covered a fairly large number of cases, arrived at this conclusion.

A point to be borne in mind regarding the gonorrheal complement fixation test is that in those cases where the disease is in its early stage a diagnosis is easily made; where the pathological process is limited to the anterior urethra in men and to the vagina in women, the reaction is always negative. In these cases we have other evidence, the symptoms—and smears. Where the complement fixation test is a necessity, is in those cases of latent gonorrhea without clinical symptoms such as in gonorrheal prostatitis, gonorrheal salpingitis, gonorrheal rheumatism, etc. We had this brought to our minds in a rather forcible manner in a case that occurred at the hospital in our early work with the fixation test. In this case, the attending physician made a diagnosis of gonorrheal rheumatism, but the man absolutely denied any history of infection. A gonorrheal fixation test done on his blood proved strongly positive. In view of the history, I was a little bit doubtful, and sent a specimen of the serum to Dr. McNeil, who confirmed the positive reaction. Dr. Louria, attending on the case, then had one of the internes vigorously massage the prostate. The secretion obtained was sent to the laboratory, and examination revealed the presence of numerous pus cells containing Gram negative diplococci, which, on culture, proved to be Neisser organisms. The evidence was laid before the patient, and he finally confessed that he had had specific urethritis six years before.

In going over the last article by McNeil and Schwartz, one is struck by the figures relating to latent gonorrhea: 31.4 per cent. of a large number of cases of prostatitis which had been regarded clinically as cured, gave positive reactions. In a large number of cases giving a history of infection three years before and considered cured, 54.8 per cent. give positive gonorrheal complement fixation tests.

If we consider, then, the unreliability of our present methods for the detection of latent gonorrhea, such as examination of smears and cultures, any added facilities that we can make use of should certainly receive a thorough trial. This is especially true for gonorrhea, and a positive test may prevent much unhappiness and invalidism. It is true that in the face of a negative reaction we must still rely upon our doubtful and difficult cultural methods.

Therefore, the serologist to-day is competent in many instances to decide whether from the standpoint of syphilis or gonorrhea or both, a man or woman may or may not safely marry. There is no maybe or perhaps. The family physician must answer yes or no, and if he works hand in hand with the serologist, it is certain that a more definite decision can be arrived at than in former times.

THE Fifteenth Annual Meeting of the Associated Physicians of Long Island (Forty-fifth Stated Meeting) was held January 25, 1913, at the Library Building of the Medical Society of the County of Kings, Brooklyn. The meeting was called to order at three o'clock by President William B. Brinsmade, there being more than a quorum present.

As the minutes of the previous meeting had been published in the JOURNAL it was decided to omit them at this meeting.

The Membership Committee reported favorably upon the following applications:

Christian W. Janson, 949 Bushwick Ave., Brooklyn.
David Sherman, 272 Ninth St., Brooklyn.
Harold K. Bell, 825 President St., Brooklyn.
Charles J. Pflug, 53 Stuyvesant Ave., Brooklyn.
Louis Ashley Van Kleeck, Manhasset, Long Island, N. Y.
Paul E. Wessenberg, 7 Linden Ave., Brooklyn.
Walter Raymond Terry, 1085 Gates Ave., Brooklyn.
Samuel H. Rabuck, Huntington, Long Island, N. Y.
Alfred Shipman, 572 Halsey St., Brooklyn, N. Y.
David Corcoran, Central Islip, Long Island, N. Y.
LeRoy P. Van Winkle, Amityville, Long Island, N. Y.
Richard P. Williams, Farmingdale, Long Island, N. Y.
William W. Hala, Astoria, Long Island, N. Y.

These names being voted upon, the Secretary was instructed to cast one ballot electing these gentlemen to membership.

Dr. William H. Ross, Chairman, read the following report of the Publication Committee: "We believe that the JOURNAL shows the result of hard work. We hope that it merits your commendation. It is now started toward the goal that it is expected to reach. It is not yet all that it should be; but a continuation of the same kind of effort and support already shown will make it so. Remember that it is yours—the only journal in a territory of three million people and more than three thousand physicians.

The advertising is a subject of discussion and criticism. To us it resolves itself into this: the income from the advertising makes the JOURNAL possible. Without it it could not be published.

The Committee from time to time have rejected or discontinued some advertising offered.

We have not thought it advisable to set an ideal standard because we have to have the money. The standard, however, compares favorably with that of other journals.

The Committee feels that should we eliminate more, it would seriously interfere with paying our bills.

We believe also that if it was finally reduced to only one advertisement there would be some one to criticise that; and so, feeling that it is not possible to satisfy every one, have used good judgment in following the present plan.

A year ago the affairs of the JOURNAL apparently touched low-water mark. Since then there has been a gradual improvement. It is expected that this upward tendency, gathering momentum as it moves onward, will finally land this publication in the front rank of current medical literature.

Dr. Paul M. Pilcher, who has ably edited the JOURNAL for six years, or since its foundation, has felt it necessary to resign the work because of other increasing responsibilities.

The Committee have recommended to the Board of Directors the election of Dr. Henry G. Webster. The Board has elected him.

The publication committee wish to record their appreciation of the services rendered the JOURNAL by Mr. Albert T. Huntington. His advice has been invaluable. The excellent typographical appearance of the JOURNAL is due to his painstaking interest. Many of the changes in the editorial make-up are also due to his knowledge of men and what is needed to make a Twentieth Century journal. It is the hope of the retiring publication committee that his services can be called upon at any time that the necessity may arise.

The JOURNAL is now printed by the *Brooklyn Eagle.*

The large amount of work has made it necessary to employ a clerk to do stenographic work and typewriting, to assist generally in making up the JOURNAL, to attend to getting new advertising and collecting money, to follow up delinquent members and to assist in the clerical management of the affairs of the Association. This is a charge against the JOURNAL.

The JOURNAL cost, for the year 1912, including salaries, $4,359. The advertising yielded $2,579. The net cost to the Association is, therefore, $1,780.

The income from advertising is now $350 per month. There has been a steady increase during the year. It is reasonable to expect that there will be a continued increase in this source of income because the JOURNAL is more attractive to advertisers than it was last year.

The present amount per month, you will notice, will give $4,200, almost enough to pay the cost independent of the funds of the Association.

The Committee begs your indulgence for its shortcomings; and yet a good deal has been accomplished. With a continuation of good, hard, loyal work, the JOURNAL will become a publication of which you will all be proud, and will finally completely demonstrate one of the reasons for the existence of the Associated Physicians of Long Island." The report was accepted.

The report prepared by the Historical Committee was then read and follows: "A feeling that is human within us directs that our first duty at our annual meeting is to record the names of those of our members who have completed their life work among us, and to note their devotion to the practice of the healing art. They each in turn were an honor to the profession and a benefit to the community in which they lived. The Association has been made stronger by their connection with it, and as members were active in all things that tended toward its prosperity.

And in respect to their memory—their names and date of membership are herewith recorded.

| *Membership.* | *Date of Death.* |
|---|---|
| 1899-1912—John Henry Baker Denton, M.D. | February 26, 1912 |
| 1906-1912—Frederick Henry Colton, A.M., M.D. | March 6, 1912 |
| 1905-1912—Harold Flagg Jewett, M.D. | April 12, 1912 |
| 1900-1912—Herbert Cooper Rogers, M.D. | April 29, 1912 |
| 1912-1912—William Vincent Dee, M.D. | March 18, 1912 |

1899-1912—William Frederick Dudley, M.D........October 22, 1912
1900-1912—Clarence Albert Baker, M.D..........November 9, 1912
1900-1912—Charles E. Wells, M.D..............November 14, 1912

The various Universities and Colleges represented in the new members are as follows:

| | | | |
|---|---|---|---|
| University Cornell ....... | 7 | Long Island College Hosp.. | 37 |
| University Kentucky ...... | 1 | College Phy's & Surg, N.Y. | 20 |
| University and Bellevue... | 7 | Bellevue Hosp. Med. Coll.. | 8 |
| University Naples ........ | 3 | Albany Med. College...... | 1 |
| University Christiania .... | 1 | Baltimore Med. College.... | 4 |
| University North Western . | 2 | Pulto Med. College ....... | 1 |
| University Johns Hopkins. | 1 | Jefferson Med. College .... | 1 |
| University Penn. ........ | 1 | Hahnemann Med. College, | |
| University Harvard ...... | 1 | Phila, Pa. ............. | 1 |
| University New York ..... | 6 | N. Y. Homo. Med. College. | 21 |
| University Berlin ........ | 2 | N. Y. Ecl. Med. College... | 4 |
| University Michigan ...... | 1 | Unknown ............... | 1 |
| University Dorpat ........ | 1 | | |
| University Yale .....:.... | 1 | Total ................ | 135 |
| University Vermont ...... | 1 | | |

The work of the Historical Committee during the year has progressed with good results, the blanks have been bound in three large volumes and are in the library of the Medical Society County of Kings, that Society having set aside a place for their keeping.

The LONG ISLAND MEDICAL JOURNAL has published obituary notices of our deceased members during the year and as we all look for a little praise, when we feel that we have done the right thing, it is justly due the Editor of the above named JOURNAL for the manner in which he presented the last number of obituaries of our deceased members.

Again I must thank the Secretary of our Association for assistance during the year and with the hope that during the coming year, each member who has not done so will give a little attention to the memorandum blank sent him."

WILLIAM SCHROEDER, SR., M.D.

The report was accepted and ordered placed on file.

The report of the Secretary was then read and accepted. The Secretary reported that the usual meetings were held and well attended. That during the year 66 new members have been added to the roster, 13 of whom are from Queens, Nassau and Suffolk Counties and 53 from Kings. That there have been during the year 10 deaths and 5 resignations and that the total membership at the present time is 851, 8 being honorary members. Of the active members 217 are from Queens, Nassau and Suffolk Counties and 626 from Kings County.

The Treasurer's report was then read and having been audited by Dr. George F. Little, was accepted and ordered filed. The Treasurer reported a balance of $61.68. Dr. Delatour's motion for a vote of thanks for Dr. Charles B. Bacon upon his retirement from the Treasurership was carried.

Under the head of Unfinished Business H. B. Delatour presented the report of the committee appointed to further consider the proposal in the President's address concerning autopsies.

"The report of your committee at the October meeting met with enthusiastic support. Since that time a quiet campaign has been carried on. The public press took the matter up and commented favorably on it, from one end of the country to the other. Many communications have been received from medical societies, inquiring as to our plans. Several letters have been received from individuals requesting us to arrange that autopsies be performed. The fact that an autopsy may be performed in the bedroom of the deceased and without mutilation has attracted much comment. Several instances have occurred in which the agitation of this subject was the determining factor in getting permission for autopsy. Altogether your committee feels that the matter is of great importance; and that it has received such general support that we are prepared to make the following recommendations:

1. Establishment of a Bureau of the Association to be known as the Humanic Bureau.

2. The object of the Bureau shall be to promote a campaign of publicity in the profession and the laity in regard to the necessity and desirability of autopsies.

3. To communicate and arrange with the pathologists of the hospitals located in different localities to the end that autopsies, when desired, may be properly and promptly performed.

4. To prepare and send to every physician on Long Island, with the request that he sign it, a card to read as follows:

"I appreciate the necessity of autopsies and the benefits to be derived therefrom. It is my desire that at my demise my body be autopsied, if the physician in charge so request. I will endeavor to remove the prejudice against autopsies which seems to exist in the minds of the laity."

It was moved, seconded and carried that the report be received and that the recommendations be acted upon one by one. After discussion by Drs. Bartley, Brush and Onuf the recommendations were approved by the vote of the Society. Dr. James M. Winfield's motion that the incoming president be empowered to appoint a committee to continue this work was seconded and carried.

The following resignations were received and accepted: Harold Bryn, John L. Moffatt and E. Charles Rose.

The Nominating Committee, through the Chairman William H. Ross, presented the following names to fill the various offices for the year 1913 and there being no other nominations the Secretary was instructed to cast one ballot for their election:

President, Samuel Hendrickson, Jamaica.
First Vice-President, James P. Warbasse, Brooklyn.
Second Vice-President, Guy H. Turrell, Smithtown Branch.
Third Vice-President, Dudley D. Roberts, Brooklyn.
Secretary, James Cole Hancock, Brooklyn.
Treasurer, Edwin S. Moore, Bay Shore.

After the new President was introduced the President turned the meeting over to the Chairman of the Scientific Committee who introduced Dr. John E. McWhorter, who gave a most interesting demonstration of the application of the Cinematograph for the study of development in vitro, and the growth of tissues both normal and neoplastic. Dr. William H. Woglam followed with an interesting discourse on "Some Recent Aspects of Cancer Research."

The Scientific Session was attended by about two hundred members and guests who showed by their enthusiasm that they fully appreciated the excellence of the program.

Dr. Lewis M. Pilcher proposed a vote of thanks for the gentlemen who had furnished the scientific session and this was carried with a will.

The dinner was served at the Hamilton Club and although only attended by seventy members and guests was a most enjoyable affair and to be regretted by those who missed it. Addresses were made by Drs. Brinsmade, Webster, Moore and Hendrickson and these were followed by a "mighty good" moving picture show.

JAMES COLE HANCOCK, *Secretary.*

---

# Editorial Review

## ARTHRITIS DEFORMANS.

### By Jaques C. Rushmore, M.D.,

of Brooklyn, N. Y.

THE term arthritis deformans includes all forms of deforming arthritis save those of known etiology. As our knowledge of etiology increases, the general class of deformities included under this term becomes less. The two great classes now remaining under this division are trophic in character and are known as rheumatoid arthritis and osteo-arthritis.

The former is an atrophic condition and usually polyarticular. The latter is a hypertrophic condition and usually monarticular, in which increase of bone structure is coincident with bone destruction, but exceeds it.

The polyarthritis of childhood, known as Still's disease, belongs under this heading, but in the general acceptance of the term, arthritis deformans is not so considered and is probably infectious in character.

The toxic joint conditions common to all ages and usually monarticular, form a distinct class with a definite symptomatology and pathological and radiographic findings.

The joint condition exhibited in rheumatic fever is distinct in its clinical course and differs markedly from arthritis deformans in that it never results in permanent joint injury and shows no bone change. As to its etiology, it is generally accepted as due to the streptococcus rheumaticus and is amendable to vaccine therapy and the salicylates.

The neurotrophic joint change, known as Charcot's joint, occurring in tabes dorsalis, properly belongs to this class as a trophic joint disturbance but differs from rheumatoid and osteo arthritis in that the condition is of known etiology.

The purely bacterial joint conditions are not of this classification. Periarthritis is associated with many joint changes and conditions and should not be described as a distinct class of arthritis deformans.

Spondylitis deformans should not be considered under this head, as there is a periosteitis of the vertebra and ossification of the vertebral cartilages and not cartilage disorganization. Whereas, in both osteo and rheumatoid arthritis, there is true joint disorganization.

Villous arthritis is an entity in which there is a redundance of synovial tissue without other involvement of the joint.

Coxa vara senilis is a softening of bone structure producing a flattening of the head of the femur with a lessening of the angle of the neck. There is no hypertrophy of bone structure.

Rheumatoid arthritis seldom occurs before the latter part of the second decade, more commonly in the third decade, rarely after the fourth. Women are more subject to it than men. There is often a history of a long enteric disturbance, as typhoid fever or a severe nervous strain.

The mode of onset suggests two distinct types, although they are similar as to joint changes and treatment. In one, the onset is vivid with a rise in temperature, increase in pulse rate and prostration. Many joints are involved simultaneously or in rapid succession. The temperature drops by lysis, the joint changes persist. This type certainly suggests a bacterial invasion in its reaction.

In the other, the onset is slow. There is no general reaction, many joints are involved simultaneously but gradually. There is commonly a history of stiffness of the muscles of the neck and of a rubbing sound of the temporomaxillary joint. These patients often wear glasses for muscle strain of the eye without any definite eye change. The entire muscle tonus is low and often relief is first sought for painful feet.

In rheumatoid arthritis the pulse is persistently high, ninety to one hundred. The blood pressure is not altered.

The vasomotor disturbance suggests a relation to Raynaud's disease, the fingers and toes blanching and turning gray. The extremities are usually cold. In the very early stages the joints cause moderate pain and become stiffened and slightly enlarged. The hips and shoulders are seldom, if ever, involved. In the upper extremity, the fingers, carpus and elbow are involved in frequency in the order named.

In the lower extremity the knees are involved as commonly as the tarsus and toes. The character of the knee joint and the constant strain is probably an element.

Interosseous muscular atrophy is early and conspicuous.

Ulnar deflection of the hand and fingers with abduction of the toes and eversion of the feet is usual. The anterior metatarsal arch is often flat with resultant callosities. The interosseous muscular atrophy makes more conspicuous the joint enlargement, and the hands present a gnarled appearance.

At first the joint enlargement is restricted to the soft parts and periarticular tissues without deformity. An indurative myositis is usually associated and is a large factor in the pain.

Later the bones rarify, flatten out on their articular surfaces and become roughened. The cartilages become absorbed and ankylosis results.

The whole picture suggests a systemic condition of which the articular changes are an expression rather than a causative factor and the treatment belongs properly to the internists.

Osteo arthritis belongs more properly to the latter decades of life.

It seldom begins before the fifth decade and more commonly in the sixth. It affects both sexes equally.

It is usually insidious in its onset and has a predilection for the greater joints, as the knee, hip and shoulder. It is generally monarticular when affecting the hip or shoulder, but not uncommonly attacks both knee joints.

The involvement of both knee joints is successive and not simultaneous. The second involvement tending to be dependent on the first in that greater strain is put on the sound knee with resultant disturbance.

The joint condition does not affect the general physical condition, save indirectly through loss of functions.

Pain is not conspicuous in the early stages; stiffness, grating and inability to go about as formerly is first complained of. A high chair is preferred because of the difficulty in rising from a low seat. Later, pain becomes conspicuous on use, due to involvement of the joint cartilages, but while at rest there is little discomfort.

The joint enlargement is general with slight excess of synovial fluid. Later irregular bony exostoses appear, giving the joint a roughened appearance. Muscular atrophy is secondary and dependent upon disuse, for in the early stages the limbs are well rounded. Motion is moderately limited and not due to muscle spasm but to bony mechanical destruction. The joint change is primarily in the bone and destruction and proliferation take place at the same time, the proliferation being in excess.

The bone proliferates irregularly and the osseous spurs penetrate the joint cartilages and destruction results through pressure. The articular surfaces become more irregular and the ends of the shafts broaden, with exostoses developing.

The ligaments of the joint are subject to great strain and become relaxed. Ankylosis may result through ossification of the exostoses of the opposing articular surfaces. There is a traumatic osteo arthritis in which exostoses appear shortly after the injury that is purely proliferative in character and which might be described as a reactive bony hyperemia with excessive bone production.

Heberden's nodosities, a proliferative osteo arthritis of the phalangeal joints, occur both with the typical monarticular osteo arthritis and rheumatoid arthritis and present a clinical appearance that is distinct.

Rheumatoid arthritis is more amenable to treatment than osteo arthritis, and if sufficient work and attention can be given to this condition much can be done. It is, however, a condition that cannot be entirely relieved, as true joint changes take place.

There is no specific. Vaccine therapy, save in the type with acute onset, is of little value. Thymus gland as a therapeutic agent is still in the experimental stage and is not entirely free from disagreeable, if not dangerous, effects. Thyroid gland is of no value. These patients as a class are poorly nourished, with low hæmoglobin percentage and low elimination.

They should be placed upon a generous diet rich in fats and the coarser vegetables. Sugar and alcohol must be eliminated from the diet. It is my custom to put these patients on five meals a day.

Daily they should be given lactic acid bacilli in some form, preferably in milk. As an intestinal eliminative, half grain doses each of blue mass and powdered ipecac at night, followed by thirty grains of magnesium sulphate in the morning, act well. It is my custom to continue this for three weeks, intermit for a week, and repeat. Colonic irrigations three times a week are used when conditions permit.

To increase the elimination of the kidneys such a diuretic as Basham's mixture in one or two drachm doses well diluted three times a day with increased intake of water is excellent. The iron in this preparation also raises the hæmoglobin percentage.

Sedatives in some form are usually required. Aspirin is useful for pain. Jones, of Bath, greatly favors guiacol carbonate in five grain doses.

Locally, deep massage is of the greatest importance and should be given daily. General massage should not be given at the same time as it counteracts the local effect.

A valuable adjunct to the massage is a hyperemia of the joints as produced by the Bier hot air box. Massage not only washes out the joint but relieves the accompanying indurative myositis. Passive hyperemia as produced by the Bier bandage is not successful.

Fixation of the joints by splints and plaster of paris dressing is to be avoided as far as possible, and if used, should not be allowed to remain for more than ten days because of the possible resultant ankylosis. Shoes, strapping and weak foot plates aid greatly in getting the patient about if the lower extremities are involved.

Little can be done in the treatment of osteo arthritis. These patients if heavy with involvement of the knees are relieved by reducing the weight and using proper shoes and plates. Heat and light massage of the joints gives some relief. The actual cautery used lightly is often of value.

Internally the extract of thyroid gland in doses of one or two grains daily often is of great value and should be continued over a long period with intermissions.

# EDITORIAL

## NEW ACTIVITIES OF THE DEPARTMENT OF HEALTH.

THE Health Commissioner of the city of New York has announced the establishment of a clinic for the diagnosis of venereal diseases, as well as one for the treatment of the same, and is, it is understood, planning the erection of a hospital for venereal disease in addition to the contagious hospitals it already operates.

The reasons for this action on the part of the Health Department are not stated in the circular, nor is it quite clear why this somewhat radical departure has been taken. Considered in connection with the Department's action in discontinuing the free administration of antitoxin and its contemplated action in removing to contagious hospitals all such cases as cannot receive prompt injections at home, it would seem that the Department had decided to take upon itself a variety of functions that cannot be strictly regarded as included in our understanding of the accepted functions of a Department of Health. There can be little question that the present attitude of all our government departments is just now more than suggestive of paternalism, a distinctly un-American attitude. There are excellent reasons why the Government should direct organized efforts to prevent the spread of disease and to protect the health of the citizen whether he cares to be protected or not. The economics of this position are clear and require no discussion. In so far as enforced treatment can be counted on to eradicate disease and thus tend to increase the safety of the citizen, the organized efforts of a Department of Health seems justified, and this may be conceded as the only reasonable argument for the present activity of the Health Board.

The Department of Health, constituted as it is, should represent the concrete idea of co-operation between the body of trained physicians who constitute the medical profession and the public spirited citizens who represent the idea of public safety. The moment that the Health Department oversteps the idea of preventive measures, the moment that it usurps the function of the physician as laid down in the various legislative acts relating to medical education and license to practice, the moment it places in the hands of untrained and unqualified persons the function of diagnosis, it arouses the strongest antagonism on the part of the very profession from whose ranks it must draw its essential material.

In the circular already referred to the Health Commissioner lays down certain restrictions as to what patients may be examined at the venereal clinic. In order to carry assurance to physicians that their interests will be safeguarded, he first declares that only those applicants shall be received who come armed with a physician's certificate. So far so good. In the next breath he states that those who have no doctors need not bring a certificate. No mention is made of the means to be employed to ascertain whether a physician is in attendance or not. If past experience be any guide the profession of the city of New York will view with some misgiving this latest incursion into the realm of medical practice by the Department of Health, for it is distinctly a step toward practical Socialism and another signboard pointing to the time when physicians in America will be compelled to take up and face the situation that now envelops the profession in England and in some of the continental countries, where as a concrete reward for years of study, for enthusiastic self-sacrifice and for the real altruism which practically every doctor exhibits, he may look forward to a pension at the end of an underpaid and overworked professional life in the service of the government such as practically levels him to the lot of the bullock that monotonously turns the water wheel.                                                     H. G. W.

## MIRACLES FROM THE LAY-PRESS.

FROM time to time the news columns of the daily press announce, with every appearance of sincerity and often with details of time, place and circumstance enough to insure credence, such wonders of modern surgery as to stupefy, bewilder and benumb the most imaginative. Now it is the human heart that has been removed by two surgeons, repaired, purified and replaced. Again, the eye of a sheep is reported as successfully implanted in a human orbit. The crowning achievement seems to be the replacing of a portion of a human brain by that of a dog, an epoch making event recently reported in an otherwise trustworthy and respected New York daily. Whether some men might not be permanently benefited by the substitution of a good canine brain for a questionable human one is a thought worthy of consideration.

The glow of pride that warms the doctor's heart when he reads of such an achievement, the eager joy with which he welcomes the news of such a wonderful step in advance is only equaled in human experience by those keen delights that have come to us in childhood when we have rapturously absorbed the stirring adventures of Jack the Giant Killer, or possibly have read for the first time the fascinating, if apocryphal, narrative of the chances that befell Sindbad the Sailor. What if today's edition does deny yesterday's report? What if we are assured that it was not the whole brain, but only the dura that was inserted? We have had the thrill, and a credulous public has learned of another gifted surgeon whom it may patronize in case of need. Without going into further detail one might readily enumerate a number of newspaper accounts, some of them illustrated and provided with display head-lines in Sunday editions, that should make the slow plodders of the medical profession blush with shame to think they have fallen so far behind in accomplishment.

The point in all this is the harm that comes to the medical profession and the public alike from the publication of such uncensored reports. Consider the gorgeous possibilities of that operation on the wounded heart—think for one minute of the bitter disappointment of the credulous sufferer from heart disease who rushes to his family counselor with this cheering bit of medical progress only to learn that his heart disease cannot be cured in any such spectacular way; and so on through all the list of discoveries whereby the blind are made to see and the dumb to speak by miracles of surgery vouched for on the authority of reputable newspapers. Such passing notoriety as accrues to the doctor whose performance is heralded in the public press is more than offset by the false light in which he is displayed to his fellows, while the harm done to a reputable physician by a garbled account of what may be a really creditable performance may cling to him for years.

And the moral of this, as the Duchess said to Alice in Wonderland, is, that corn, and not pearls, is the proper porcine diet and the lay-press should censor its medical news. H. G. W.

## AN ABUSE OF PUBLIC CHARITY.

THERE has recently been brought to the writer's notice an arrangement connected with the city hospitals that raises a question as to how far the purely charitable institutions of the city are available for destitute patients and whether certain privileges that are now granted in connection with them are not detrimental to the hospital, to the medical staff and to the patients. If our information is correct, the Department of Public Charities of New York City, in certain of the hospitals under its charge, permits patients who are not strictly charity patients to pay for board and lodgings at a fixed per diem rate, the explanation given being that this charge is intended to act to deter those who can afford to pay something for their care from entering a free hospital. It is, of course, recognized that emergent cases such as are not infrequently brought in by the ambulance must receive such treatment as the urgency of their condition demands, irrespective of their ability to pay, and that some of this class of patients are abundantly able to pay well for their care while in the hospital. It is argued that the city should be paid for the care of such patients provided their condition is such as to prohibit their removal to a private hospital. It seems fair that the attending staff in such a case should not be expected to render gratuitous service, but should be entitled to a fee proportioned to the financial standing of the patient.

Now, if provision is made whereby patients who can pay a hospital charge are admitted side by side with those who actually cannot pay, an anomalous condition is created. Let it be understood that the reputation for surgical and medical work of a high grade attaches to all our city hospitals and that many of the attending staff are men pre-eminent in the profession whose reputation is likely to attract patients. It is evident that under present economic conditions a man who is not particular as to his personal comforts and who places economy above fairness may without difficulty obtain admittance upon the payment of a small fee and enjoy the benefits of excellent professional attendance to the detriment of staff and hospital alike. It is even conceivable that a member of the staff might be tempted to obtain admittance for a patient of his own under similar circumstances and thus work injury to the rest of the staff as well as to the reputation of the hospital. The problem that the city is to solve is not an easy one from the standpoint of the medical staff. It may seem a little hard that association with a charitable institution, while enhancing their professional capacity and reputation, precludes them from enjoying an income such as may be expected from association with a private hospital. To meet this condition the plan has been tried in some localities, notably in Massachusetts, of setting aside a pavilion to which members of the attending staff may admit their private patients, the hospital charges being graded according to accommodations. While this plan has much to commend it, it is intrinsically opposed to the idea of city care of the sick. It must not be forgotten that the ward charges of the average private hospital are practically identical with the amount charged by the city hospital for some of their accommodations, the charity hospital thus entering into direct competition with the private hospital. Thus it will be seen the charge which is made ostensibly to deter those who are able to pay from entering the charity hospital is actually an invitation for them to avail themselves of the advantages which are found in the modern construction and complete equipment of a hospital backed by the city's budget.

If an editorial suggestion may be permitted, it seems wise to adopt in the conduct of the charity hospitals, whether under the care of the Department of Charities or Health, the same arrangement now in force for the state hospitals for the insane, that is, a paid staff, whose work may be graded according to length of service but strictly limited to the service of the hospital. Men thus attached will sooner or later obtain a standing such that their abilities will create a demand for their services sufficient to insure them a competence upon retiring from the paid staff. The hospital might well have in addition a staff of active consultants to supervise the work of each department chosen for peculiar ability in their particular line of work. These men should have the privilege of active participation in operative or other work in return for the demand on their time which the position involves.

While there may be objections to such a plan thus roughly sketched, it has advantages that make it worthy of consideration.

H. G. W.

## THE TREND OF MEDICAL ECONOMICS.

EVERYONE has noted the great increase of professional interest in economic problems. The medical press shows it markedly and not only are medical societies giving such problems considerable space in their deliberations, but new societies are in process of formation which will make them the chief topics for discussion. What is the meaning of it all, and what will it lead to? Will there be witnessed any change of heart on the part of the eminent gentlemen who are now serving institutions notorious for the abuse of medical charity? Will it be found too late a day to reform practices as deeply rooted as it is possible for them to be, and to repair the souls of men who, though at the top of the profession, possess the moral outlook of an Archbold? Can grave evils be eradicated and habitual offenders be born again? Does this medico-economic movement represent a mere aspiration of idealists who are not "practical men," and will it achieve nothing great, or more worth while than the establishment of bill collecting bureaus, political auxiliaries, and sordid alliances of unfit practitioners for whom economic death would be a logical destiny? What is it we are hearing, yelps of richly deserved pain or the voices of prophets and saints and splendid, efficient souls? Is there a flowering of the spirit of good men, or a jaundice of little souls? The tangible results of the movement will answer our questions.

A. C. JACOBSON.

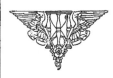 **Society** 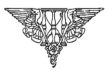 **Transactions**

## TRANSACTIONS OF THE MEDICAL SOCIETY OF THE COUNTY OF KINGS.

*Stated Meeting, January 21, 1913.*

The President, JAMES M. WINFIELD, M.D., in the Chair.

### Venereal Prophylaxis in the Navy.

THOMAS A. BERRYHILL, M.D., Medical Inspector, U. S. Navy, read a paper with this title (published on page 97).

DR. HENRY H. MORTON, in opening the discussion, said:—"I have, of course, been very much interested in listening to the Doctor's paper in which the first thing that strikes me is the very large rate of venereal disease which the Navy men have; 170 per thousand I believe he stated was the normal rate before prophylactic measures were introduced. Compare these figures with the present rate—1,134 men exposed, with only two cases of gonorrhea,—and you can see what prophylaxis accomplishes.

"The question of prophylaxis in gonorrhea was begun to be worked on some six or seven years ago. When I was in Germany six or seven years ago Dr. Frank had just been trying his experiments with patients in his clinic and he saw that prophylaxis really does protect. He experimented as follows:—

"He chose six men, telling them beforehand what he was going to do and paying them to allow themselves to be experimented with. He inoculated them with gonorrheal pus. Three of the men used the prophylactic installation of one of the silver salts (protargol), and the three men who received the instillation did not develop gonorrhea, while the other three did. Then he reversed the experiment and the fellows who escaped the first time were inoculated and did not develop gonorrhea while the others did.

"These experiments were not carried on by Frank alone, but were also worked out by Kopp of Munich and, I think, Neisser.

"Now, several years ago, acting on Frank's suggestion, I had a druggist make up some little tubes of prophylactic consisting of albargin in solution and containing a proper dose suspended in glycerin. The tube orifice is covered with paraffin, which is broken off and then the injection is delivered and held in the urethra for about five minutes. Frank in his prophylactic tubes used protargol at first and afterwards albargin, because it is found to be less irritating and can be used in weaker doses.

"At the time the druggist made these up for me we wanted to try it out thoroughly so as to be sure we were really going to have something that would destroy the gonococci. Dr. J. Sturdivant Read took some cultures of gonococci in test tubes and he tried these, adding the 5 per cent. albargin to the cultures and found that they destroyed them to some extent; then he tried the 10 per cent. strength and finding that that was much more efficacious, he finally increased it to 15 per cent. albargin in glycerin, destroying nearly all the cultures in the test tube, so we decided that the 15 per cent. was the proper strength to use for the suspension in glycerin. It is not irritating, although it is a much stronger solution and can be used by way of irrigation. The glycerin also protects the mucous membranes somewhat: it is only necessary to use a few drops, and it is only held there a short time.

"Dr. Berryhill spoke of the experience on the German ships. That was borne out by a statement of a friend of mine, Surgeon-Major Roscher, now of Berlin, who was with the German troops at the time of the invasion of China during the Boxer rebellion. The German sailors and soldiers going ashore were provided with a package of the solution of protargol. Now, the Germans when in service are very obedient and do as they are told, and when they were told to use this protargol instillation they used it and Roscher told me that in every case where the men used the instillation (and they used it in nearly all cases) gonorrhea was prevented. In dealing with large numbers of men in the navy, however, in order to make prophylaxis really useful it must be compulsory.

"In reading over the statistics I think it is necessary that we analyze them a little and I believe it will be found that the general total of venereal disease has not been so materially reduced as we might suppose, but that instead it is only in certain particular ships where prophylaxis has been properly carried out that this great cutting down in the amount of venereal disease has been accomplished, for on listening to Dr. Berryhill's paper I am led to suppose that on many of the ships prophylaxis is imperfectly carried out and that it is only where it is carred out with care that such wonderful results as 1,134 exposures with two cases of gonorrhea, are found. Dr. Pugh, who is the surgeon on one of the vessels of the United States Navy, told me of his experience when his ship was at Goldfields, Nicaragua, and the men had been ashore a good deal. Those hot countries are very full of venereal diseases, but the Doctor told me that of 700 exposures, which were regulated by prophylactic treatment, it was found that on returning to the Brooklyn Navy Yard there were only about three men sick with venereal disease. Now, that is certainly a very remarkable result and simply shows that prophylaxis does protect the sailors and other people as well.

"The question of houses of prostitution must also be considered, while we are talking on this subject. What is to be done with them? This thing has been talked of and written about in the medical and lay journals. In *McClure's Magazine* and even in the *Ladies' Home Journal* of Philadelphia, there were articles about the 'black peril' in the South as distinguished from the 'white peril' (consumption) in the North. The subject of venereal diseases is one which interests every physician whether he be doing genito-urinary work or not. It is unquestionably a most important subject, particularly when it comes to the question as to what can be done to lessen the amount of venereal disease and thereby lessen the ravages and harm which gonorrhea and syphilis are responsible for in the community. I think as physicians we all feel the correct thing to do is to license prostitution, to segregate prostitutes and to have regular inspection by the Board of Health or some other department of the city that should be delegated to look out for that particular question.

"Of course, by inspection of these houses you would not stop all venereal diseases, but women would be found before they could have an opportunity to infect a number of men and these women could then be isolated in the hospital where they would be taken care of until the lesions had been healed. But such a system of segregation, of inspection, would be entirely incomplete without proper hospital system attached to it, where the women would be taken care of while being cured, because it is their trade, their means of livelihood, and if their way of living were cut off they would starve or become a burden on the community, so, therefore, it will be seen that any system of that sort must take into consideration the question of what should be done with the diseased women while they are being looked after and under treatment.

"A system of licensing and inspection would also do a great many other things; for instance, it would stop police graft, because these houses are breaking the law and are only allowed to go on because they pay, and by paying hush money they are enabled to break the law. Licensing the houses would stop the graft.

Another thing it would do is this: if women are detained in these houses against their will and we had regular inspection, the proper authorities would become cognizant of the fact that they are being held against their will and they could be removed and put in proper places and have an opportunity of changing their way of living if they choose to.

"I think that this policy of shutting our eyes to this thing has done a great deal of harm. The gynecologists see it in the sterility in women who have married men who have had gonorrhea; the general practitioner sees it in the cases of late syphilis, locomotor ataxia and infantile syphilis and inherited syphilis, and every one practising medicine sees the effects of syphilis and gonorrhea, and, therefore, we must look not only at the more immediate results of cases of gonorrhea or chancre, but also at the far-reaching effects on the whole human race, and I think it is our duty as physicians to do all we can to bring about a sensible method of regulating this question of prostitution by a plan where it can be properly taken care of and looked after because we cannot stop it."

DR. HOMER E. FRASER, in discussion said:—"It has been a great pleasure to listen to this paper on venereal prophylaxis in the Navy.

"My remarks will be brief because I have had no practical experience in the matter. The Doctor states that they have considerable difficulty in the Navy, where the men are under more or less discipline, in getting them to submit to prophylactic treatment. In dispensary and private practice the individual you see is already infected and the disease active before he comes under your observation.

"I do not think that there can be any question as to the albuminates of silver being a gonorrhœal prophylactic if used at the proper time and strength. Cases in which infection has taken place but a short time, the first twenty-four hours of urethral discharge, have in a certain number of my cases been aborted and the urine rendered clear in one week by the energetic use of albuminate of silver.

"No doubt, if prophylaxis was universally carried out it would be the means of protecting the public from venereal disease. The public does not seem to be much interested in prophylaxis. I cannot recall, in my office or dispensary practice, of having over two or three men ask me if there were not some means of preventing infection. After explaining that there was such a preventive treatment they did not even take the trouble to ask the name of the drug of for the prescription.

"As the Doctor has said many of the young enlisted men are from the middle West and without much worldly experience and early contract venereal disease. The same is more or less true in civic life. It is the inexperienced youth that is most prone to venereal infection. It is this class that in a large part support the street-walkers who are almost invariably diseased.

"One infection does not mean that prophylaxis will in the future be employed because the individual does not expect to expose himself again and if he does he is so certain that his partner is free from disease that it is hard to convince him that he is mistaken even after he has been infected.

"I do not believe if the medical officer in the Navy directed the sailors going ashore to step up and take prophylactic drugs along with them that one in five would avail himself of the opportunity, because he does not expect to become exposed to disease, but because of drink or temptation their good resolves fail.

"Venereal prophylaxis has been known and more or less employed by the medical profession for the past five or six years, but it does not seem to have interested the public to any great degree, and unless the profession can impress the public with the importance and value of it in the future, it will be little employed. It is not peculiar that the public shows no great zeal in this matter. It is known that vaccination is a sure preventive of smallpox yet general vaccination is not the rule but has to be made more or less compulsory by school laws and health board scares. The same is true in regard to the vaccination for typhoid. People know that they can have treatment that will prevent them from having typhoid but there is no great rush to be vaccinated. They are willing to take a chance and the same is true in venereal disease. I do not look for any great lessening of the disease through prophylaxis.

Dr. THOMAS A. BERRYHILL, in closing the discussion, said:—"It is true that a great many people refuse to take prophylaxis, although they are pretty certain they are going to be exposed and may get diseased.

"Now, in the Navy, we cannot expect to accomplish much unless we get the authority of the Navy Department itself making it obligatory on the men exposed to take this treatment. We have not got this authority, but the Army has. We usually follow the Army; that is: They get a good thing and we try to get it also. We hope to have prophylaxis made obligatory.

"I think that all statistics will be rather disappointing unless only the cases taking the prophylaxis are considered. The great increase in the Army, you can see, occurs because they are taking a Wassermann reaction of nearly everybody in their commands and that brings out the latent cases and does not mean that the initial disease has increased at all.

"In the Navy, as Dr. Morton says, there is only a part that gets this treatment. The part that gets it are those people who are on the receiving ships and those afloat and not those ashore. There is a large number of men ashore that never get this treatment. They could go to the hospitals, or get treatment at the dispensaries if they wished, but probably one-third of the men will never have prophylactic treatment if they do not take it themselves."

# TRANSACTIONS OF THE BROOKLYN SOCIETY FOR INTERNAL MEDICINE.

*Stated Meeting, December 27, 1912.*

The President, EDWARD E. CORNWALL, M.D., in the Chair.

### Report of a Case of Acid Auto-Intoxication.

*By Dr. C. Eugene Lack.*

DR. C. E. LACK, in closing the discussion, said:—"As far as the ammonium salts are concerned the urea was apparently not broken up inasmuch as the patient was passing the normal percentage of urea; whether she should have passed the normal daily quantity we have no method of finding out.

"Regarding the patient's diet we know, of course, that patients under many conditions may have acetone and that it is a normal constituent of urine, and these diabetics from whose diet the carbohydrates are excluded and given fats frequently pass acetone and fats are broken up, producing acidosis; the same holds good as to exclusive proteid diet, and it is a disputed question whether the proteids are more responsible for the acetone or the fats. Van Norden, of course, claims that the absence of carbohydrates is responsible for the acetone.

"This patient admitted that she ate considerable meat, although with her meat she ate carbohydrates and had starches, but her meat diet was not sufficient in itself apparently to account for her condition. Then, the remarkable part of the diminution of acetone lies in one's ability to quickly free the patient from it. They react quickly to the carbohydrate addition. In twenty-four hours your patient may be free from acidosis by a carbohydrate diet. We can have large quantities of acetone in the urine without apparently any symptoms. It is a question whether this patient was suffering from acetonemia and whether her symptoms were the symptoms of acetonemia or just those of a sick girl and with this illness acetone in her urine was discovered, or whether she had a chronic eclamptic state without having large amounts of urea in her urine, or could it be an hysterical condition? Her pain at the present time is severe and she gets just exactly into the state that those patients do who are in the acute pain of kidney stone and immediately the pain subsides she is just as happy as anybody can possibly be. To my mind, she is not hysterical. Was her condition due to anaphylaxis? Did the ether anesthesia have anything to do with it? Was the anaphylaxis due to the blood of the infant being anaphylactic to the blood of the mother, which it frequently is, being a foreign proteid? Those are the questions which I say are still unanswered and I dislike very much to report a case which is unfinished, in which the findings haven't been completely studied. Then arises a question as to her sugar. Was it due to reactive or intestinal putrefaction? Was it a symptom from the intestine reacting through the pancreatic duct causing pancreatic disturbance, and does it make any difference regarding the percentage of sugar as far as the symptoms are concerned? She only had one-quarter of one per cent."

DR. TASKER HOWARD, in discussion, said:—"I think it would be rather interesting to know what the ammonia was doing all that time. Was the ammonia estimated in the urine? Often in the acid intoxications the urea is diminished because it is diverted in the ammonia stage to neutralize the acid. I think that that is sometimes the case in pregnancy (but as to this I would like to find out from those who know more about it), in that type of intoxication where there is a good deal of involvement of the liver. We know that with acetonuria we find a large amount of ammonia present in order to neutralize the acid."

DR. EDWARD E. CORNWALL, in discussion, said, that it is well known that acetone is found in a number of conditions besides diabetes mellitus. It occurs in cases where there is carbohydrate starvation, which may happen in certain cases of gastro-intestinal conditions, where there is great loss of appetite, vomiting or diarrhœa. It may happen if the diet is badly arranged so that there is too much meat and fat and too little carbohydrate. It has been observed after operations, plainly due to the deprivation of food.

Apropos of oliguria without evidences of kidney disease, Dr. Cornwall reported a case of a boy of fifteen, whose excretion of urine was not more than five or six ounces daily for five days: the urine was apparently normal. There was nothing of significance in the previous history of this case except the taking of a considerable dose of belladonna shortly before the appearance of the oliguria. No drugs were given to this case, and his recovery was complete after five days in bed on a modified milk diet.

## General Discussion of the Treatment of Thyroid Disease.

DR. H. B. DELATOUR, in opening the discussion, said:—"The treatment of the thyroid I will consider simply as we see it in the form of goitre. We must remember when cases of goitre present themselves to us, as Dr. Longmore has already told us, that a great many of them respond very nicely and permanently to medical treatment. They are not all surgical cases and there are certain classes of them that are not suitable for surgical intervention.

"We must recognize, first of all, the enlargements that occur at puberty and during the menstrual periods. These cases, if properly handled, seldom require operative interference and it is considered a mistake to operate in the young for goitre unless there are symptoms of pressure or a very decided enlargement, or the general symptoms become rather acute, for it is generally recognized that the young stand the goitre operation very much less satisfactorily than the adult. We know, also, that in pregnancy the thyroid enlarges and will stay enlarged possibly during the entire term of pregnancy and even without any treatment, it will disappear until another pregnancy takes place. In these cases the goitre, except for its appearance, seldom gives any symptoms. Some cases appear to be worse after surgical interference, but those cases are exceptional. Unfortunately certain cases do not come to the surgeon until it is too late for a satisfactory operation. These are the cases of hyperthyroidism that have been allowed to go on. These cases are not benefitted and seem to be worse after operation and it is in this class of cases that Mayo has used the X-ray treatment as a preliminary to operative interference. He claims in a certain number of cases that, after prolonged treatment by numerous exposures to the X-ray, the gland undergoes some change, and then operative interference is more successfully carried out. I had one case in which that seems to have been true.

"We must bear in mind, that it is not always necessary that the gland should be enlarged, to insure benefit from surgical intervention. This is not generally understood. In cases of hyperthyroidism where the gland is apparently not enlarged a decided benefit is frequently derived from a removal of a portion of the gland. In certain cases the operation is indicated, not because of any general symptoms, but because of the pressure of the enlarged gland on the trachea or esophagus, or on the vessels of the neck, and in certain other cases from the tumor being a positive annoyance to the patient. In these cases frequently the gland is the seat of a cyst and simple enucleation of the cyst without any removal of the gland tissue will effect a complete cure. These are the simplest of all the cases we have to operate.

"In the very severe cases of hyperthyroidism, operative interference must be preceded by very careful medical treatment, rest in bed and a general preparation of the patient for operation. Some of these patients seem to be very easily frightened. Gerster cites a case of a patient who was suffering from extreme hyperthyroidism on whom he proposed to operate. The day and hour for the operation had been set, a few days only intervening, and before the time for the operation came the patient suddenly died. He ascribes this to the fright. In a similar case he followed the teaching of Crile, of preparing the patient for the operation by slowly bringing her to the point without knowing that operation is to take place. In his second case Gerster had administered ether to the patient at intervals—I don't know how short or long the intervals were— but in increasing quantities, the patient considering it a simple therapeutic measure applied for the cure of the goitre. The ether was given for a short time one day and at the next sitting for a longer time, until finally the patient was completely anesthetized and allowed to come out again and a certain period of time allowed to elapse again when the operation was set and the patient was completely anesthetized and operation carried out. In that way the patient was brought to the operating table without knowing beforehand that the operation was actually to take place. That patient made an excellent recovery. He cites these two cases as being almost identical in their clinical symptoms.

"In some of the severe cases ligation of the arteries, the superior thyroid, sometimes of both the superior and inferior thyroids, is indicated and the results are quite satisfactory. In some cases it seems to have little or no effect, or only a very temporary effect. The best results of removal are obtained in patients in middle life in whom the goitre has existed for some time and the symptoms of thyroidism have come on slowly.

"After the thyroid has been removed and pregnancy takes place, the greatest care must be taken in the watching of such patients, for these people tend to develop most severe toxemias and eclamptic seizures. It is well to bear in mind when having to do with women who have been operated for goitre and in whom pregnancy develops that you have a serious condition to watch out for, for these patients are very likely to get into serious trouble. The loss of the gland seems to have a decided effect on the general health of the patient.

"Another thing that I wish to speak of is carcinoma of the thyroid. Carcinoma of the thyroid gland is not exceedingly rare, but we must not be discouraged when the pathologist reports carcinomatous disease as his finding after the gland has been removed, for if it is true carcinoma it is a very slow-growing carcinoma and has but very little tendency to recur. I recall two cases in which two of our best pathologists in town and one other, making three in all, unknown to each other, made a positive diagnosis of carcinoma of the removed gland and one patient is now living seven years and the other five years, without any sign of recurrence and, of course, in each case the entire gland was not removed. One of the most marked cases of hyperthyroidism I ever saw was in a young man. I removed half his gland and the improvement was immediate. His pulse came down from 160. His severe nervous symptoms rapidly disappeared. He went back to his work and went along very comfortably for about three years, when he had a shock which upset him and his symptoms re-appeared. At the first operation I removed the left half of the gland. After the recurrence of his symptoms two years ago, I removed the right half of the gland, simply leaving the isthmus, and from then to now, after two years, he has had no recurrence of the symptoms.

"Whether we are getting more goitres in this neighborhood now than we used to have, I cannot say, but I know we are getting more cases for operation. Only today I had seven cases in my office. Four had been operated; three had not; two of them were cases of young women who came to me two years ago with decided enlargement of the thyroid, both of them under 20 years of age, and today the glands are apparently no larger than normal. Three of the cases were cases that I operated recently and the symptoms immediately disappeared after the operation, and the fourth was an old lady, 67 years of age, who had an immense goitre. An attempt had been made to remove it a year before coming to me and the gentleman who had cut into the goitre got severe hemorrhage and was afraid to proceed with it and he packed the wound and she left the hospital with an open wound which continued to bleed for a year off and on. The first time that I saw her she was covered with blood. She had nearly a whole roll of absorbent cotton on her chest and it was more or less saturated with blood. It looked like a most hopeless condition. I sent her to the hospital simply to have her where she would be well taken care of and because I didn't want to tackle the job at once. She was given X-ray treatment every three or four days for about six weeks, and at the end of this time the wound had completely closed and the woman's general condition had improved very materially. I then proceeded to operate and without any great difficulty removed three-quarters of her thyroid gland. It is now a little over a year since that was done. She came back to me today very much worried, fearing she had the same trouble recurring on account of some difficulty in breathing, but she has an asthmatic condition and she had merely taken a fresh cold and this had disturbed her breathing and for that reason she was afraid she had a recurrence of the growth."

DR. EDWARD E. CORNWALL, in discussion, said that he endorsed Dr. Longmore's high estimate of the value of rest and diet in the treatment of hyperthyroidism and his low estimate of the value of any particular kind of drug treatment in that condition. He further said that in hyperthyroidism, as in any condition where a particular toxemia existed, it was rational treatment to diminish the work of the body as much as possible by lessening any other toxemias that might be present, and he spoke of the toxins from intestinal putrefaction which could be lessened with ease and advantage in this condition. He also alluded to recent investigations which seem to show a dependence of various organic functions on the stimulus of internal secretions: how the glycogenic function of the liver seemed to depend on an internal secretion from the pancreas, the secretion of gastric juice on an internal secretion from the pyloric end of the stomach, the secretion of the pancreatic juice on an internal secretion from the duodenum, and intestinal peristalsis on an internal secretion from the spleen. The internal secretion of the thyroid, he said, had been studied longer than most of them, and it seemed, broadly, to have some kind of control over oxidation in the body, so that hyperthyroidism might be understood in a way as bringing about excessive oxidation, and hypothyroidism as resulting in suboxidation.

Dr. C. E. Lack, in closing the discussion, said:—"I would like to report a case along with Dr. Longmore's where Beebe's serum was used, a case of goitre in which there was no question about the hyperthyroidism. The patient had numerous attacks of thyrotoxicosis. The diagnosis was positive.

"In the case which I refer to Beebe's serum was administered with Beebe's help and under his supervision. This patient had more than 200 injections of serum and made a perfect recovery. The only symptom, if there is any symptom, is that at times the patient is fearful lest may be he has not recovered. It was a long treatment, over a long period of time, and the only reason he was held to it was because of the relief he received through administration of the serum. Dr. Beebe has reported more than 1,500 cases in which his serum has been administered and by now the number must have increased to nearly 2,000, and while he is, of course, very optimistic regarding his serum, I cannot help but believe that his reports are truthful.

"This case was taken early. He had no medical treatment before the administration of Beebe's serum.

"The rest treatment in this case was not very positive. During his treatment the man went into business deals and was successful at times, so that he had all the elements that would preclude the possibility of recovery from the medical treatment, but Beebe's serum seemed to hold him and cure him. To my mind, it is a valuable adjunct to any treatment, but it takes a long time and the patient must be well conserved."

---

# TRANSACTIONS OF THE BROOKLYN GYNECOLOGICAL SOCIETY.

*Stated Meeting, November 1, 1912.*

The President, ALBERT M. JUDD, M.D., in the Chair.

### Report of a Case in Which Adrenalin Solution was Used to Control Bleeding in Repair of a Recto-Vaginal Fistula.

*Dr. S. J. McNamara.*

Discussion by Dr. A. A. Hussey.

Paper:

### Amputation vs. Repair of the Cervix Uteri.

*Dr. S. J. McNamara.*

Discussion by Drs. Gordon Gibson, J. O. Polak, George McNaughton, F. J. Schoop, W. B. Chase, O. P. Humpstone, Horowitz, Carroll Chase, W. H. Cary, A. R. Matheson, V. L. Zimmerman, A. M. Judd and F. C. Holden.

As the transactions for this meeting have not reached the JOURNAL, the Program only is printed.

*Stated Meeting, December 6, 1912.*

The President, CARROLL CHASE, M.D., in the Chair.

### Malignant Endocarditis in Infants.

Dr. L. J. J. COMMISKEY presented two specimens of hearts from newborn infants showing vegetations on the valves, hemorrhagic vegetative endocarditis, with the following notes:

No. 5. M. F., normal spontaneous labor; normal baby for first 24 hours, then had bleeding from the rectum; this continued despite treatment and the child died on the fourth day. Symptoms those of external hemorrhage and the loss of blood. Temperature never above 98⅓ F.

Mother's history negative, including negative Wassermann reaction.

Post-mortem. Gastro-intestinal tract filled with fluid blood and small clots. Hemorrhage into the myocardium, especially along the coronary arteries and the auriculo-ventricular junction; vegetations on the tricuspid valves.

No. 31. L. McK., rapid spontaneous breech labor; weight 5 lbs. 9 oz.; normal baby until fourth day, when it commenced to bleed from the skin at the junction with the cord, which was still attached and dry. The bleeding continued and the baby died on the fifth day; seemingly there was not enough blood lost to cause death from hemorrhage. Temperature varied between 97.4 and 99.2 F.

Mother's history. Positive Wassermann reaction, tubercle bacilli in sputum with physical signs of disease in both lungs. Urine contained a moderate amount of albumin but no casts.

Post-mortem. Congenital syphilis of the liver and vegetation on mitral and tricuspid valves of heart.

### Discussion.

Dr. A. M. Judd said:—"They are beautiful specimens. I wish to say that they show the excellent work that the pathologists of the Kings County Hospital are doing under the present *régime.* We have a man from Manhattan, Dr. Haller, who is doing magnificent work. These specimens also call to our attention the remarkable work that is being done by Dr. Commiskey in the treatment of bleeding babies. In former years the great majority of babies with hemorrhage died, unless it was of a slight character from the vagina, which, I think, can hardly be classed with those of the severe type. In the years I have been connected with the hospital I have seen at least thirty babies die from hemorrhage. The only babies we lose now are those where the hemorrhage is so severe that they die from the primary condition, or those which are septic. Dr. Commiskey classifies these cases as septic, syphilitic, and those in which there is an absence of or diminution of fibrinogen or other elements of the blood. During the time he has been treating these cases by means of the injection of whole blood. He has had fourteen cases and has lost a very small number."

Report of cases:

Dr. Cary:—"I will take a moment to call the attention of the members to a case which I briefly reported to the Society some time ago and presented a specimen of tumor of the placenta. The woman had been delivered that day. I subsequently sent the specimen to the Johns Hopkins Hospital for examination by Dr. Williams. I have received a letter from Dr. Williams in which he states that the specimen is a sarcoma of the placenta. I have not had a chance to look up the literature but will report the specimen in detail later."

### Current Opinion of the Toxemias of Pregnancy.

Dr. William Pfeiffer read a paper with the above title.

### Discussion.

Dr. A. A. Hussey said:—"I want to compliment Dr. Pfeiffer on the excellence of his paper. The subject is very complex and one on which few of us have any very definite ideas, but are apt to change our ideas about eclampsia, depending upon our last experience. I shall not attempt to discuss this paper in detail, but simply speak of a few points occurring in my own service. The etiology of eclampsia is entirely indefinite and undetermined and the best we can do, as the author has said, is to consider it as disturbed metabolism, whatever that may be. Probably the predisposing cause has a great deal to do with it. I have seen cases where the previous condition of the liver, stomach, and duodenum might have had something to do with the onset, and we have all seen cases where pathological conditions in the kidneys had undoubtedly a great influence, especially in pernicious vomiting, where there has been previous trouble in the stomach and duodenum, and perhaps an ulcer, which has set up trouble at the commencement of or during pregnancy, and the vomiting is continued by the ulcer. Or the trouble may have its seat in the gall-bladder. I believe that if we knew more about the pathology from actual pathological work, we would be able to eliminate many that we used to regard as reflex. I have never seen a case of pernicious vomiting of pregnancy which I believed to be due to malposition of the uterus, nor have I seen any effect from treatment of the uterus or from reposition. The doctor struck the keynote when he said that the care of the patient during pregnancy was the principal thought. I have never seen a case where the patient was sufficiently intelligent to follow the advice regarding diet, hygiene and exercise. The women who come to my hospital service are those who sit around and take no exercise, and most of the gentlemen here who are doing hospital work will bear me out in that statement. In regard to treatment I have settled on one plan, and that is to empty the uterus as soon as I can get the patient on the operating table. By that method I save more patients than when I used temporizing treatment. If any one thinks the Strogonof method is easy I want him to sit beside a patient for twenty-four hours and then tell me about it. I tried it and lost three out of four

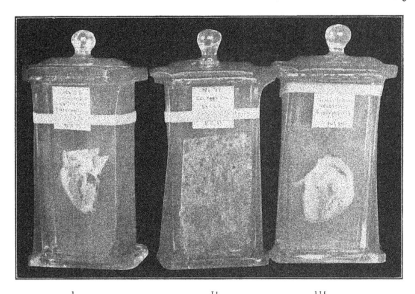

I., III. Hemorrhagic Vegetative Endocarditis.
II. Eclamptic Liver.
Illustrating Dr. L. J. J. Commiskey's contribution,

cases, and then began to empty the uterus, provided the patient was not moribund. Other doctors try the conservative methods and their patients are sent to the hospital in a moribund condition, too late to help them. In the cases in which I have operated early I have saved four out of five. I deliver cases in the easiest manner that presents itself. Where the cervix is open and the parts soft I use instruments, and if the parts are rigid I prefer vaginal hysterectomy. If the delivery is rapid the loss of blood is not great. I want to emphasize one thing, and that is, the use of a pack in the cervix to stop excessive hemorrhage. In regard to treatment by drugs, I must express my preference for chloral, morphine, and bromides, by rectum or otherwise. Dr. Stewart, with whom I was associated formerly, was very fond of veratrum, and I saw many cases die of edema of the lungs from its use. I think it is a dangerous remedy and can do harm."

Dr. H. A. Wade said:—"The etiology of the toxæmia of pregnancy has never been at all clear. The explanation is advanced by Dr. Cornwall that the toxæmia is a mixed one, produced by the toxins which come by way of the placental circulation from the fœtus as a result of the fœtal metabolism; and those toxins which belong to the mother and have no necessary relation to pregnancy; and that these toxins are always present in every pregnancy; and that the toxæmia becomes pathological only when the toxins overwhelm the maternal organism either because the liver cannot destroy or the kidneys cannot eliminate these poisons in sufficient quantities.

"Whether this be the true explanation or not, my experience has taught me that if we empty the colon of putrifiable material by proper attention to diet, it will be rarely necessary to empty the uterus for the relief of this condition.

"What effect the thyroid secretion has upon pregnancy is at present not thoroughly understood; but it is a significant fact that in severe toxæmia occurring in the later months of pregnancy, we do not find the usual slightly hypertrophied, actively functionating thyroid gland normally found in pregnancy.

"When necessity arises for emptying the uterus, the choice of method is dependent upon the condition of the cervix, the condition of the fœtus, the skill of the obstetrician, and the environment of the patient. Women ill with toxæmias of pregnancy should always have the benefit of hospital care. In the presence of a rigid cervix, after the twenty-eighth week of pregnancy with the vaginal tract fairly free from the suspicion of microbic infection, through unclean handling, the best interests of the mother and of the child demand an abdominal Cesarean section."

Dr. J. O. Polak said:—"We have to thank Dr. Pfeiffer for the presentation of a very able paper; one of the best, I believe, I have heard on this subject. Of the theories that have been discussed on toxemia of pregnancy I think the most important are practically summed up under two heads—faulty fœtal metabolism and its consequences, and the entrance of the poisoning elements into the placental blood, and the disturbance of maternal metabolism. The more I read of the etiology of eclampsia the more indefinite is my knowledge of the condition. We stand where we stood several years ago. We know that it occurs in a pregnant woman, and that it is because she is carrying a child, and whether it is the fœtal or maternal condition, or both, that is at fault is not for us to settle now. It is sufficient for us to know that we have a toxemia, and that it differs in its effects in the early months from that which we have to deal with in the later months of pregnancy. In the early months there is a change in the liver, beginning in the center of the lobule, and in the later months the effect is upon the perilobular tissue, the lesion being a perilobular thrombosis and extending from the periphery inward. This, I believe, is generally admitted. In the early months it is exceptional to find blood pressure increased, even in excessive vomiting; it may not reach over 100 to 110, and may be as low as 90. In the later months the blood pressure is the earliest and most constant index of the toxemia; it is more pronounced in the nephritic type. Another point is the leucocyte count. It has so much to do in pregnancy for or against the individual. Where the leucocyte count is low the condition is more serious. I must take exception to the suggestion of the Russian method that has been used by Davis—I do not believe in it. Chloroform should not be used under any circumstances to control the convulsions of eclampsia. Its effect upon the liver cells is very much like that of the disease itself, and some of the patients who have died under its administration have died from its destructive effects upon the liver structures, not from the toxemia. We are now using oxygen and ether. It controls the convulsions equally as well as chloroform. There are four or five points that I should like to speak of in treatment. 1st, we must minimize the amount of metabolic products by limiting the nitrogenous food; 2d, aid in the elimination of the poisonous elements, and 3d, reduce blood pressure. If these do not reduce the toxemia, as will be shown by relieving the danger signals, then with the first convulsion the uterus must be emptied. The records of the last six years show that we have lost just one single case in our service from eclampsia, and that was a case brought in, as Dr. Hussey has said, where the physician had procrastinated for a long time. When once the uterus is emptied the reaction is usually prompt, and the convulsions cease at once in over 60 per cent. of the cases. How shall we empty the uterus? The uterus must be emptied in such a way that the patient is not traumatized, and shocked. Understand that the patient is a poor operative risk. We have been too free with our *accouchement forcé*. In the early months, that is, up to the seven and a half or eighth month, if we have a rigid cervix, I prefer vaginal hysterotomy. I do not think the hemorrhage is to be feared. I have felt that it is very much like a phlebotomy and the patient may be benefitted by it. I can conceive of only a few conditions in which abdominal section may be necessary. If the patient is toxemic and has had several convulsions, the child is usually toxemic and its viability impaired. So, in the interest of the child, it may be necessary. In such cases the condition stands as it does for the consideration of Cesarean section without toxemia; the size of the child; the condition of the parts; and the necessity for rapid action. On the other hand, in the majority of cases at or near term spontaneous labor is possible, and it may be terminated by forceps, or often simple rupture of the membranes will control the convulsions. Veratrum is an excellent drug, but unfortunately it is not always used in sufficient dosage. Five or ten drops given occasionally will do no good. We have to sit by the patient and inject fifteen, ten or five drops, as necessary, and repeat, watching the pulse and blood pressure, keeping the pulse at 60 and blood pressure below 120 mm. If we do this, in 99 out of 100 cases we can look for good results. It is good in near term eclampsias, and in women in labor."

Dr. V. A. Robertson said:—"I would like to speak of a case which I brought to the attention of the Pathological Society some time ago—a case of the acidosis of pregnancy, not always recognized, and the recognition of which depends upon a rather elaborate examination of the urine, as mentioned by Dr. Pfeiffer. The ordinary examination of the urine is not always a fair criterion of the condition of our patients, as I have seen cases of eclampsia where the urine examined the day before did not show any abnormal signs. The case I refer to showed absolutely no abnormal elements, such as albumen and casts, during the period of the woman's greatest toxemic symptoms. This is the case mentioned by Dr. Pfeiffer. She was the mother of five children and the family history showed marked metabolic defects, as the father was gouty and the mother diabetic, as were two maternal aunts. This woman enjoyed good health during the non-pregnant state, but toxemic symptoms always developed as soon as she became pregnant, and especially hyperemesis. About eighteen months ago this patient returned from the South while I was out of town, and was treated for this condition. When she came under my care the vomiting was pernicious in character and had been for several weeks. None of the ordinary remedies seemed to be of any use. Examination of the urine showed none of the usual signs of toxemia, no albumen or casts, and urea output normal. A nitrogen partition was not made as it is a very difficult and elaborate method of analysis. I found the woman almost in extremis from the persistent vomiting. Further examination of the urine showed indican acidosis, and marked traces of acetone. The treatment instituted was stomach lavage, bicarbonate of soda by mouth and rectum, lactose and cereal gruels. Within twenty-four hours the symptoms were under control, and at the termination of pregnancy she had a normal delivery. In these cases bicarbonate of soda can be given *ad libitum,* and with its use the urine becomes alkaline. It has been said that we can divide these toxic cases into hepatic and nephritic, and unquestionably this will include a vast majority of them. I think, however, cholelithiasis is sometimes a cause of toxic conditions. One patient I had a few years ago had made several attempts to carry a child but had been compelled to give up the trial and submit to emptying the uterus to relieve the toxemia. I tried various forms of treatment but without effect and finally had to terminate the pregnancy. When pregnant she had been troubled with discomfort and flatulence after eating, and most of the time had constipation. Physical examination elicited no symptoms of gall stones. She went for a trip in the South and was taken ill in Florida and when she came home showed the classical symptoms of gall stone colic. A diagnosis of cholelithiasis was made and an enlarged and thickened gall bladder with several calculi was removed. The patient has had uninterrupted health since the operation."

DR. A. M. JUDD said:—"I feel that we all owe to Dr. Pfeiffer a just tribute for the great amount of work he must have given to the preparation of the excellent paper he has read this evening. It gives evidence that he has spent in its composition many hours that should have been devoted to rest. I have brought to-night a specimen right in line with the subject of the evening's paper—a section of the liver taken from a patient whom I lost in an eclamptic seizure. This patient was in coma when I saw her; delivery did not stop the convulsions and she died before any further measures could be taken. The specimen shows the necrosis found in such cases. I feel that this was a case of the hepatic type of eclampsia. Reference to the photo will show you the areas of necrosis present all through the liver. I call my eclampsias all toxic. but what the toxic substances are none of us know at the present time. In the early stages of pregnancy there are undoubtedly many cases of reflex vomiting, due to mal-position of uterus or old inflammatory conditions. I have seen many such cases relieved by proper measures. Increased blood pressure to me, as it is to Dr. Polak, is one of the first symptoms I look for where there is any suspicion of trouble. In the maternity wards of the *K*ings County Hospital we carry this out by having the blood pressure taken once a week or oftener if necessary, and if the pressure goes above 150 we start treatment. We use thyroid extract in these cases. I am a strong believer in veratrum but have seen it used where it was not well used, too much veratrum being given. As Dr. Polak states the pulse must be watched and you must go according to that. The idea to be observed in the administration of veratrum is that whatever the dose may be, you must secure the therapeutic effect, that is, a diminution of blood pressure to 130 or 140 and a reduction of the pulse to 60. The cases that have gone into collapse after veratrum are cases where too much was given or its use was not guarded by means of a blood pressure apparatus. Dr. Hussey says that the cases that have come under his care in the hospital are under exercised and over fed. That is contrary to my experience, which has been the opposite, for mine are over exercised and under fed. Cases from the tenement districts are not apt to be well cared for. The eating they do is more apt to be of the kind that leads to toxemia. Regarding the use of the cervical pack for hemorrhage in hysterotomy, it is, in my opinion, contraindicated. I like to bleed them and have never seen a dangerous hemorrhage. I feel that most of the men taking part in the discussion, although they may advise conservative measures, are too apt when put up against a case to adopt extremely radical measures."

Dr. W. B. Chase said :—"Just one or two simple points. In this day with our better knowledge there is very little venesection, but when it was more frequently used they must have had beneficial results or it would not have been used in these cases. What was its mode of effect? Was it from a lowering of blood pressure, or by getting rid of blood already contaminated? I am inclined to believe it was from its effect upon the blood pressure. Is there any risk from the use of veratrum? It is a powerful drug. Yet one of my colleagues, a physician of large experience, told me that he had looked over the literature but could not find any cases of poisoning from that drug, or cases where it had produced edema of the lungs. It is said that we have a perfect antidote for veratrum in morphia. I do not believe that you can give veratrum in unlimited amounts and then use morphia as an antidote, but it will overcome the effects in moderate amounts."

Dr. F. W. Shoop said :—"I should like to speak of the effect of the toxemia on the milk of the mother, and what effect it has on the baby when it is nursed. I had one case where the baby died forty-eight hours after birth. The nurse said it had been smothered by the mother. I believed death to be due to the toxemic poison in the milk."

Dr. Holden said :—"One reference to the use of chloral as to whether it has any degenerative effect upon the liver. Dr. Corrigan had made a number of experiments with this drug and decided that it had no degenerative action on the liver."

Dr. Pfeiffer, in closing the discussion, said :—'I wish to thank the members for their cordial reception of my paper. It is my maiden effort before the Society. There will always be differences of opinion in societies of this kind but these differences are apt to come from differences in view point. In answer to Dr. Shoop's question I think the death of the baby was due to the toxic effect of the milk. The entire theory of the condition points to the breast as one of the excretory outlets for the poison."

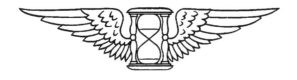

# LONG ISLAND MEDICAL JOURNAL

VOL. VII.            APRIL, 1913            NO. 4

## ⚙️riginal 🅐rticles.

### THE BROOKLYN EYE AND EAR HOSPITAL.

#### By James W. Ingalls, M.D.,

Brooklyn, N. Y.

*But it is worth while to study yesterday in order to learn wisdom for to-morrow.*—LYMAN ABBOTT.

D URING the early part of the last century, a number of the larger cities of the country established hospitals, or infirmaries, for the special treatment of diseases of the eye and the ear. For instance, the New York Eye and Ear Infirmary began its work in 1820, when the population of New York was approximately 120,000. The Massachusetts Charitable Eye and Ear Infirmary was established in 1824, when Boston had a population of 40,000 or 50,000. The Wills Eye Hospital in Philadelphia was opened in 1834. But Brooklyn had a population of more than 350,000 before any special provision was made for the destitute who were suffering from affections of the eye or ear. However, in the spring of 1867, Dr. Arthur Mathewson suggested to his friend, Dr. Homer G. Newton, that they endeavor to interest influential people in behalf of an institution for eye and ear patients. Soon Dr. Cornelius R. Agnew, of New York, became deeply interested in this work of charity. Dr. Agnew's extensive influence and high professional attainments contributed much to the success of the undertaking. The good people of Brooklyn quickly responded, and in this response Mr. Simeon B. Chittenden took a leading part.

On the evening of March 2, 1868, a number of charitably disposed gentlemen met, at the residence of Mr. Simeon B. Chittenden, to consider the advisability of establishing an eye and ear hospital, in the city of Brooklyn. Subsequent conferences were held, and it is evident that not much time was wasted in deliberation, for the minutes show that, in about six weeks from the date of the first meeting, a house, on the northeast corner of Washington and Johnson Streets (a site now occupied by the Post Office) was fitted up for a temporary dispensary and hospital. The Brooklyn Eye and Ear Hospital was opened April 15, 1868, for the treatment of indigent persons, suffering from diseases of the eye or ear.

The Charter for the Hospital was granted by the State Legislature May 4, 1868. The list of names of the Incorporators and the Board of Directors is essentially a muster roll of the leading citizens of Brooklyn forty years ago. The Incorporators were: Horace B.

Claflin, Benjamin D. Silliman, William C. Rushmore, Archibald Baxter, Cornelius D. Wood, Josiah O. Low, Reuben W. Ropes, Nathan D. Morgan, Alexander M. White, Samuel McLean, Edward ·Carey, Charles L. Benedict, Jacob Campbell, John A. Prentice, Jonathan Ogden, Frank Woodruff, Coe Adams, Henry Sanger, Henry G. Reeve, Augustus E. Masters, Simeon B. Chittenden, Henry E. Pierrepont, Francis Vinton, Cornelius R. Agnew, M.D., Edward G. Loring, M.D., Arthur Mathewson, M.D., Homer G. Newton, M.D.

During the first year the Directors were: Horace B. Claflin, William C. Rushmore, Cornelius D. Wood, Archibald Baxter, Reuben W. Ropes, Rev. Richard S. Storrs, D.D., Nathan D. Morgan, Frank Woodruff, Josiah O. Low, Edward Carey, Simeon B. Chittenden, Rev. Francis Vinton, D.D.

The Medical Officers for the first year were: Cornelius R. Agnew, M.D., Edward G. Loring, M.D., Daniel B. St. John Roosa, M.D., Arthur Mathewson, M.D., Homer G. Newton, M.D.

That such an institution was sadly needed in Brooklyn, is evidenced by the fact that nearly 1,500 patients were treated the first year. Therefore the Directors were soon obliged to consider the question of more commodious quarters. And at the January meeting in 1869, an agreement was made to purchase the property at 208 Washington Street for the sum of $17,000. This building was remodeled and used for a hospital until 1882.

In 1871, aid was granted by the State of New York. However, the Hospital records show that when the check was received, "Dr. Agnew moved that the Treasurer be instructed to return the check, already received from the state, with the resolve of this institution not to receive 'state aid.' Motion was seconded and carried."

Although this hospital was originally intended for the reception of patients suffering from diseases of the eye or ear, yet, later.it was deemed advisable to supplement this work by establishing a clinic for diseases of the throat and skin. In 1872, this department was opened by Dr. Samuel Sherwell, who continued in active service more than forty years. In spite of the fact that the intimate relation between the throat and the ear had been recognized for a long time, yet, so far as can be learned, this hospital was the first eye and ear institution in the world to establish a throat clinic in connection with the other work of the hospital. The wisdom of this innovation has been shown by the fact that many other similar institutions subsequently adopted this plan. The following figures amply justify the statement that the development of the throat clinic has been truly remarkable. The Annual Report for 1874 shows that, during that year, 152 patients were treated for diseases of the throat. Last year, 1912, the clinic for diseases of the throat and nose treated more than 4,000 cases.

In 1877, the department for the treatment of diseases of the nervous system was established by Dr. John C. Shaw, who had formerly served as house surgeon at this hospital. He continued as chief of the clinic until the time of his death in 1900.

In the course of a few years, it became evident that a larger building would be necessary to accommodate the ever-increasing number of patients. In 1881, the construction of the Brooklyn Bridge and its approaches compelled the hospital to find a new location. The Directors met the crisis with characteristic promptness and liberality. A special meeting was held, November 7, 1881, to consider the advisability of purchasing the Juvenile High School building, on Livingston Street.

"This three-story structure, 45x78 feet, was open on all sides to the light and air. The property also included two adjoining lots on Schermerhorn Street. This all could be bought for $47,500."

The acquisition of this property was, in a large measure, due to the activity of the Rev. Richard S. Storrs, D.D., who used his influence in securing funds, and also to the generosity of Mr. George I. Seney, who gave $25,000.

However, extensive alterations and repairs were needed in order to transform an antiquated school building into a suitable hospital. The solution of this problem was assigned to Dr. Edward R. Squibb, who served as chairman of the building committee. It is unnecessary to add that the work was done carefully and conscientiously.

Late in the fall of 1882 everything was completed and the hospital entered upon a wider sphere of usefulness. The annual report for that year, in alluding to the new location, said: "The Board can confidently present it to its supporters as a large and well appointed hospital, entirely sufficient for many years to come." When this statement was made the hospital was treating annually about 5,000 patients. But in a few years the number ran up to 7,000, and again it became evident that more room was needed. In 1891 additions to the building were made, so that the capacity in some respects was nearly doubled. Even this improvement sufficed for a short time only.

In 1906 the widening of Livingston Street necessitated the destruction of about one-quarter of the hospital building. In order to make up for this loss and also to provide more extensive facilities, the board of directors purchased an adjacent structure, which had formerly been occupied by the Commercial High School, on Schermerhorn Street. The solution of the difficulties confronting the hospital at that time was described by the chairman of the building committee, Dr. William Simmons, in the November number of the *Brooklyn Medical Journal*, 1906. The following is an extract:

"For several years the Board of Directors had been considering the erection of a new hospital. Although the hospital property comprised five lots, the shape of this plot was unsatisfactory for the kind of building needed for the work of the institution, unless a very large sum were to be spent in its construction; but no other site which could be obtained seemed so desirable. With these problems, as well as with the financial one, the Board of Directors was struggling, and no new building was in sight, when the calamity came of the destruction of a large part of the working space of the hospital.

"Most fortunately, just at this time the Board of Directors was able to secure three lots on Schermerhorn Street, adjoining the two already owned by the hospital and directly in the rear of the Livingston Street building. This plot had a building with a frontage on Schermerhorn Street covering its entire length, with a depth of forty-two feet; on the rear of the plot was a building of slightly smaller dimensions, and the two were joined by a wing on the west. These buildings came in direct contact with the hospital building on Livingston Street. They were originally built for factory purposes, but were remodeled several years ago at considerable expense by the Board of Education for school work, and had been occupied suc-

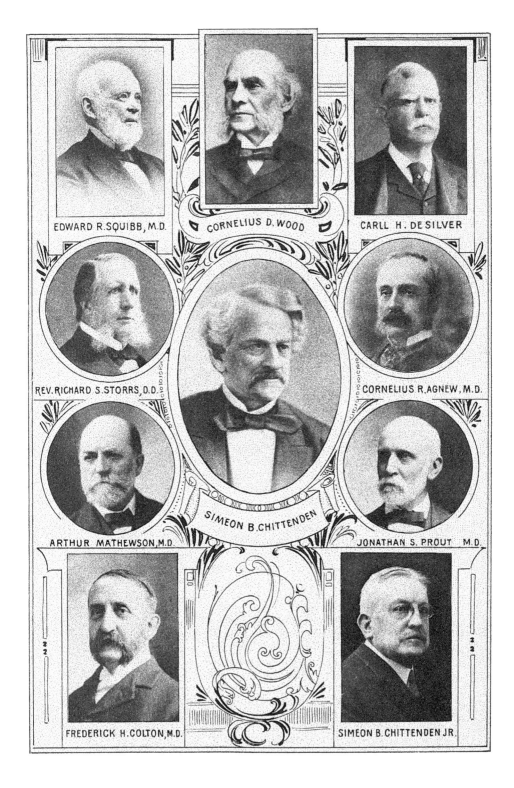

EDWARD R. SQUIBB, M.D.

CORNELIUS D. WOOD

CARLL H. DE SILVER

REV. RICHARD S. STORRS, D.D.

CORNELIUS R. AGNEW, M.D.

ARTHUR MATHEWSON, M.D.

SIMEON B. CHITTENDEN

JONATHAN S. PROUT M.D.

FREDERICK H. COLTON, M.D.

SIMEON B. CHITTENDEN JR.

cessively by the Manual Training School and the Commercial High School.

"The lease held by the city was just expiring, and the Commercial High School was about to move into its new home, when the Board of Directors purchased the property.

"The Building Committee had for several months been working on the problem of a new building and had developed plans for a building which should have a street frontage of one hundred feet and a depth of eighty feet, with four stories, basement and sub-cellar. This was to be of iron and brick construction, thoroughly equipped in the most modern manner for the large work which the needs of this great city demand in the care of the poor suffering from diseases of the eye and ear. The estimated cost of this building was $200,000.

"But the final hurried condemnation for the widening of Livingston Street and the demands by the city to vacate immediately the condemned premises threatened to throw the hospital out of a home. The Building Committee saw, in the acquisition of the adjoining property on Schermerhorn Street, the possibility of a temporary home and at once set about to make a virtue of necessity."

The work of reconstruction was begun in July, 1906, and completed the following spring. The old building had about forty beds for indoor patients. The enlarged premises provided eighty beds. Space for treatment of dispensary cases was more than doubled. Two operating rooms were furnished with modern equipments. Yet, in spite of these increased accommodations, only a few years passed before the hospital was again overcrowded.

The Brooklyn Eye and Ear Hospital has been very fortunate in having as presidents of the board of directors men of exceptional qualifications. Mr. Simeon B. Chittenden,* one of the founders, was chosen as the first president, which position he held for fifteen years. He was succeeded in 1883 by Dr. Edward R. Squibb,* who served one year. Dr. Squibb's successor was Mr. Cornelius D. Wood,* who continued in office sixteen years. He was followed by Mr. Carll H. De Silver,* who continued as president from 1900 to 1909. The next president was Dr. Frederick H. Colton,* who had served as secretary of the board for thirty-one years. Dr. Colton was elected president in 1909, and remained in office until the time of his death, March 16, 1912. The vacancy was filled by the election of Mr. Simeon B. Chittenden, son of the first president of the board of directors.

The following gentlemen constitute the present Board of Directors:—Mr. Simeon B. Chittenden, President; Mr. Howard O. Wood, Vice-President; Frederick D. Bailey, M.D., Secretary; Mr. Daniel V. B. Hegeman, Treasurer. Mr. Alexander E. Orr, Mr. Henry D. Atwater, Mr. Crowell Hadden; Mr. Isaac H. Cary, Mr. Edgar McDonald, Mr. Robert B. Woodward, Mr. Martin Joost, Arthur Mathewson, M.D.; Charles Schondelmeier, M.D.; Mr. R. Ross Appleton, Mr. Frank D. Tuttle, Mr. James N. Wallace, Rev. Edward F. Sanderson.

Dr. Arthur Mathewson, after thirty-three years of active service, resigned in 1901 and was appointed consulting surgeon. Dr. Jonathan S. Prout began service in 1869; he resigned in 1902, and was appointed consulting surgeon. Dr. Samuel Sherwell, after forty years of service, resigned in 1912 and was subsequently appointed

---

* Deceased.

consulting laryngologist. Dr. John C. Rushmore was appointed a member of the surgical staff in 1872. He is still in active service at the hospital. Of the founders of the hospital, only two survive, Dr. Arthur Mathewson and Dr. Homer G. Newton.

The following medical officers died while they were connected with the hospital: Dr. Orestes M. Pray, attending surgeon, died April 23, 1869; Dr. Cornelius R. Agnew, consulting surgeon, died April 19, 1888; Dr. Edward G. Loring, consulting surgeon, died April 23, 1888; Dr. Richmond Lennox, attending surgeon, died November 14, 1895; Dr. John C. Shaw, physician to the department of neurology, died January 23, 1900; Dr. William H. Haynes, physician to the department of neurology, died November 15, 1902; Dr. William Waterworth, attending surgeon, died May 11, 1904; Dr. Daniel B. St. John Roosa, consulting surgeon, died March 8, 1908; Dr. Edward L. Oatman, pathologist, died December 26, 1912.

The annual report for 1912 shows that since the hospital opened its doors, in the spring of 1868, more than 450,000 patients have received treatment. These figures need but little comment, since they speak for themselves. These figures signify that thousands of deaf persons have had their hearing restored; that thousands of men and women have regained their sight; that thousands of poor children have been helped who otherwise would have been sadly handicapped in the struggle for existence.

Of course, it is not claimed that all these would have become blind, even if they had not applied for relief. Also it is not claimed that medical or surgical skill has been able in all cases to restore sight that had been destroyed by accident or disease. But it is emphatically asserted that many have regained their sight who without treatment would have become hopelessly blind and dependent upon public charity. Very few persons ever stop to consider the economic value of hospitals when regarded as repair shops for disabled human machines. Suppose a baby suffering from ophthalmia neonatorum is brought to an eye clinic. With skillful care it is reasonably sure that the little one will have good sight. However, without such care, it is reasonably sure that the child will be blind for life. In attempting to treat a case of this sort the doctor is confronted with a serious responsibility.

For there is at stake a greater monetary value than the infant's weight in gold. Of course, this seems like a very wild statement. But let us get down to facts in the case. The little patient weighs ten pounds. An avoirdupois pound of gold is worth approximately $300. Ten pounds would be worth $3,000; hence the baby's weight in gold is equal to $3,000. Now, how much does it cost the state to maintain a blind person for life? Competent authorities* estimate that the approximate cost is $10,000. This sum, it will be noted, is more than three times the baby's weight in gold. And this does not take into account the diminished earning capacity of the individual. Therefore it follows that the statement which seemed wild was extremely conservative.

---

*New York State Jour. of Med.*, June, 1912. The Prevention of Blindness and the Instruction of the Blind Child. By G. E. de Schweinitz, M.D., Philadelphia, Pa. Read at the annual meeting of the Medical Society of the State of New York, at Albany, April 16, 1912. Dr. de Schweinitz referred to paper on Prevention of Infantile Blindness, by C. F. F. Campbell, Annals Amer. Acad. Polit. and Social Science, March, 1911.

The Christian charity which prompts good people to care for blind children is very highly commendable. But is it not also the part of common sense, as well as of charity, to aid in the attempts to *prevent* blindness?

During the year 1912 the hospital treated 21,993 patients. This large number shows that the demands upon the institution have increased more rapidly than the population. The causes for this condition are numerous. Years ago, little or no attention was paid to the defects of sight or hearing among school children. But now many of these defectives are sent to the Brooklyn Eye and Ear Hospital. Also parents and teachers are beginning to appreciate the beneficial effects of the treatment of adenoids and other diseases affecting the nose or throat. Thirty years ago comparatively little was known regarding eye-strain as a cause of headaches. At the present time, the fitting of glasses forms a large part of the work of the dispensary. All these causes, and many more that might be mentioned, have made this and similar institutions far more effective than in former years.

So much for the past, but what of the future? "A condition and not a theory" confronts the hospital. At the recent rate of growth, the hospital in 1914 or 1915 will be required to treat 25,000 cases. During the past year many patients needing operations have been turned away on account of lack of room. If the present accommodations are insufficient, what will be the condition when thousands more apply for relief?

---

## THE LIGAMENTS OF THE PATELLA.*

### By James P. Warbasse, M.D.,

Brooklyn, N. Y.

THERE is great discrepancy among anatomists in their descriptions of the aponeurotic and ligamentous attachments of the patella. Some assert that the quadriceps tendon is inserted in the upper margin of the bone and that the patellar ligament springs from the lower margin of the bone, inferentially leaving the patella a connecting link, as it were, between the quadriceps muscle and the patellar ligament.

Meckel says that when the tendon of the rectus femoris approaches the patella it becomes broader, and is attached to the upper edge of the bone, and is ultimately united with the tendons of the other extensors. He says the vasti tendons are attached to the upper and lateral margins of the patella.

Luschka says that the rectus femoris tendon blends with the tendons of the cruralis and vasti, and this common tendon sends a superficial layer in front of the patella, which is closely adherent to the front of the bone.

Quain describes the rectus femoris tendon as forming a flat band which is attached to the upper border of the patella, being joined with the tendons of the deeper portions of the quadriceps and forming with them the common tendon of insertion. The vasti, he says, are inserted into the upper part of the lateral borders and into the sides of the rectus tendon. "The common tendon, in which the four por-

---

* Read before the Brooklyn Surgical Society, December 5, 1912.

tions of the quadriceps muscle terminate below, is broad and flat, and is inserted into the fore part of the upper border of the patella, a few fibres being prolonged over the anterior surface of the bone into the superficial portion of the ligamentum patella."

Gray has it that the rectus femoris is inserted into the patella in common with the vasti and crureus, and that the vasti are inserted into the lateral borders of the patella and blend with the great extensor tendon. The superficial fibres of the ligamentum patellæ, he says, are continuous across the front of the patella with the superficial fibres of the quadriceps extensor tendon.

Cunningham does not describe any of the fibres of insertion of the quadriceps as passing in front of the patella, but finds the rectus femoris tendon inserted into the upper border of the patella, and receiving laterally parts of the insertion of the vasti. Neither of the vasti does Cunningham describe as sending fibres of insertion in front of the patella. The fascia lata of the thigh, he says, forms the lateral ligament and is attached to the borders of the patella.

Piersol does not trace the fibres of insertion but states that the rectus femoris is inserted by the ligamentum patellæ into the tubercle of the tibia.

Sobotta says that the conjoined tendon embraces the entire upper and lateral margins of the patella, which serves as a sesamoid bone, and continues to the tuberosity of the tibia as the patellar ligament, the actual insertion of the quadriceps being the tibia.

To increase the number of references would be to increase the confusion of description.

For the surgeon the important point is that all of these fail to describe the ligamentous continuations of the quadriceps insertions which pass not only in front of the patella but also on either side of the bone. Observations on the living patient and dissections upon the dead have impressed me with the strength of the ligamentous tissue through which the pull of the quadriceps muscles is transmitted to the tibia.

It is neither true that the patella is wholly a sesamoid bone developed in the tendon nor that the tendon of the quadriceps is wholly inserted into the bone. A portion of the tendon is inserted into the upper part of the patella, and ends there, as is shown in the dissections herewith presented; but the most important part of the tendinous terminations of the muscles pass in front and to the sides of the patella to find attachment below the knee joint.

After removing the skin and superficial fascia from the front of the knee, the strong enveloping fascia lata is exposed. This lies closely adherent to a second layer of tendon in front of the patella. The two may easily be dissected apart. The deeper prepatellar tendon is directly continuous with the terminal tendon of the rectus femoris, into which is inserted also fibres from the vasti. These three muscles are so closely adherent by their terminal tendon and muscular substance to the fascia lata that it also serves as a part of their insertion.

The strong fascia lata embraces the patellar ligament below the patella and virtually becomes a part of that ligament. It is attached to the tibia on either side of the ligament in the form of a V, the apex of which embraces the tubercle of the tibia, the arms running upward upon the lateral ligaments of the knee joint. (Fig. 1.)

That portion of the quadriceps tendon lying in front of the patella carries fibres directly from the rectus femoris and the vasti. (Fig. 2.) It is dense, glistening, and in the common transverse fracture pulls out into a fringe as it is torn across. It is inseparably united with

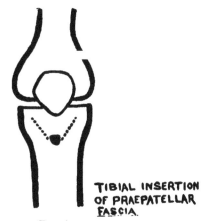

TIBIAL INSERTION OF PRAEPATELLAR FASCIA.

FIG. 1.

the periosteum. In origin and texture it is clearly tendinous As it passes below, the ligamentum patellæ takes its rise from it. It continues its fibres into the ligament. Laterally it is closely adherent to

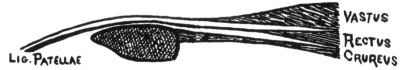

VASTUS
RECTUS
CRUREUS

LIG. PATELLAE

FIG. 2.

the fascia lata as it passes from the sides of the patella (Fig. 3) and becomes incorporated into the lateral ligaments of the knee joint while the fascia lata lies over it and is attached to the bony prominences about the knee.

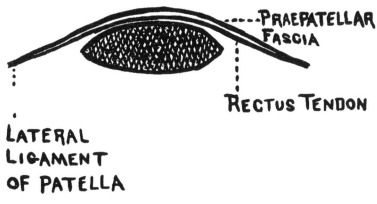

PRAEPATELLAR FASCIA

RECTUS TENDON

LATERAL LIGAMENT OF PATELLA

TRANSVERSE SCHEME

FIG. 3.

Thus this double ligament connects the sides of the patella with the head of the tibia, with the head of the fibula, the tubercle of the tibia, and the tibial surfaces above it. It transmits the pull of the three great extensors around and independent of the intervention of the patella—in front and to the sides of that small bone.

That part of the extensor tendon which is inserted into the upper end of the patella arises largely from the crureus muscle.

The ligaments of insertion of the vasti are represented in all three structures—prepatellar fascia, prepatellar tendon, and the suprapatellar tendon. The rectus insertion passes directly in front of the patella to the ligamentum patellæ. The crureus is inserted by a strong, thick ligament into the upper border of the bone.

This ligament of the crureus is the structure which is commonly identified as the quadriceps tendon—which it obviously is not.

It is of surgical interest that the strong rectus tendon not only passes in front of the patella but blends laterally with the prepatellar fascia to form the lateral patellar ligament, which ligament represents an important part of the insertion of the vastus externus and internus. The action of the quadriceps extensor muscles is transmitted to the leg through the patella slightly, but mainly through the ligaments in front of and at the sides of the bone. In repairing the transverse fractures of the patella the suturing of these ligaments is the main feature of the operation. This not only means suturing the conjoined prepatellar ligament but also the lateral ligament, the transverse tear of which shows that it sustains a similar traumatism to that which causes the patella to be rent in two.

*(For discussion see page* 164.)

---

## ECONOMIC FACTORS IN THE DOCTOR'S FUTURE.*

### By William Francis Campbell, M.D.,

Brooklyn, N. Y.

THE three great professions, law, theology, and medicine, have had a unique position in the life history of the race. They have loomed large in human experience because they have ministered to a very personal and individual need.

In the dim dawn of civilization we hear naught of music, of painting, of sculpture, of engineering, of architecture, of journalism; but what savage tribe without a chief to maintain law and order; without its priest to propitiate a higher power; without its medicine man to assuage pain and alleviate disease?

The three great professions are great because they are fundamental. Because they have built bridges over which every son of man must travel in his journey from the cradle to the grave.

Law bridges the gap from disorder to order; theology from the material to the spiritual; medicine from disease to health. The traveler cares little whether the bridge is ornate, who were the engineers who planned, or the workmen who wrought; one paramount question concerns the individual who crosses: is it safe, is it serviceable, is it efficient?

---

* Read before the Caledonian Medical Society, February 17, 1913.

The law of progress is the law of change. To cease to change is to cease to live; only the inorganic is stable. The problem of this generation is different from the problem of the last generation just as the problem of the next generation will differ from ours. The practise of medicine is not what it used to be because the human need is not what it used to be. In the memory of those of us who began the practise of medicine but two decades ago the change is most striking. We recall the epidemics of diphtheria, scarlet fever, measles, la grippe, and the summer diarrhœa of infancy. We recall practitioners who made thirty and forty calls a day. The writer, after he was graduated, was called upon to relieve an established physician, and made from twenty-five to thirty calls and saw from fifteen to twenty patients in the office daily. This was twenty-five years ago. How has the problem changed? The old economic law of supply and demand is inexorable and the equilibrium is maintained irrespective of individual protests. What are the facts?

Let us contemplate this important law as applied to the practise of medicine as it presents its problem to this generation. First, as to the demand. Let me reiterate some important and well known facts in order to clearly spread before you the evidence. During the last twenty years the death rate in New York City has been materially reduced, while the population, on the other hand, has notably increased. In other words, the demand for the services of the doctor has decreased while the population has increased, and this decrease in the demand for the doctor is due to the efforts of the doctor himself. For the highest function of the doctor is to be a teacher, and a teacher is one who is showing his disciples how to get along without him. From this high position the physician can never descend without violating the traditions of the centuries and forfeiting his honored place in the scheme of civilization. The doctor has been teaching the public how to get along without him.

Take a concrete example within the life experience of most of us. Note what the doctor has done as a teacher in the problem of tuberculosis. The public have been taught by the doctor how tuberculosis is communicated; that sunshine and fresh air are its most potent enemies; that vitiated air is its friend; that the most potent vehicle for the spread of the disease is the expectoration of the patient, and in no instance must it be deposited where it may become dried and be disseminated through the atmosphere, and thus endanger the lives of others. These facts the public have not been slow to appropriate and apply, with the result that consumption is fast decreasing, its curability is unquestioned, and its ultimate extermination is not an impossible dream. The doctor has been teaching the public how to get along without him.

Now, this campaign of education is not going to stop. It is only in its infancy. One of its most important phases is the present system of school inspection, which is producing far-reaching results. The handicaps of life early recognized are ofttimes ameliorated and sometimes cured; the final product must be more efficient men and women physically and mentally. We have not been content to teach the public ordinary cleanliness; we have taught them extraordinary cleanliness. The public begin to appreciate that it is not the dirt that is seen, but the dirt that is unseen by the naked eye, wherein lurks the deadly foe. They begin to understand that there are forms of life so small that the eye cannot detect them, so small that they are revealed only by a powerful microscope; that a particle of dust is not mere inert, inorganic matter, but that it is pulsating with life, and that the same laws which govern the infinitely great also operate in the life of the infinitely small. The public recognize that the micro-organisms are their deadliest foe, and thus armed they possess the secret of disease. The doctor is teaching the public how to get along without him. But not only this,—the doctor is providing the means never before so scientific and efficacious in ameliorating and eliminating disease. The beneficent accidental discovery of Jenner is the foundation stone for modern scientific therapeusis. The vaccines and serums are multiplying and daily demonstrating their efficiency in curing the diseases which twenty years ago we fought with the haphazardry of empiricism. The shotgun prescription is replaced by the glandular extracts and the immunizing and protective sera. Tetanus, diphtheria, pneumonia, typhoid, meningitis, the acute infections, have their vaccines, while scientific sanitation eliminates tuberculosis, malaria and yellow fever. Only recently one of our colleagues privately announced a vaccine for acute articular rheumatism which acts like magic. So much for what the doctor has contributed toward his own elimination.

Consider for a moment how economic conditions have fostered the so-called medical abuses, dispensary and hospital abuses, the lodge and contract practise. While the doctor himself is responsible in part for the abuses we decry, yet the potent factor at work is an economic one.

In considering our dispensary and hospital abuses we have made a grave error in dividing the medical public into paupers and non-paupers, and saying that the free dispensary and hospital must not extend beyond the limits of the pauper, for herein we are failing to meet a pressing need for which some provision must be made. It must have occurred to those who ponder that there is a very large portion of our population in this great city who are not paupers, who are wage earners, who are self-supporting, but who are compelled to avail themselves of the charity provided at the dispensary and hospital. They pay their grocer and butcher; they cannot pay the doctor. What is there peculiar about the economic problem of this large class? This is the problem:

In a recent address by Dr. Bristow it was shown that the sum necessary in New York for a man, wife and three children to maintain a normal standard of living is $900 per annum. "Professor Chapin remarks that a family living on such an income in New York must economize in every way, especially in clothing, and must depend upon free dispensaries in times of sickness." If this be true of a family whose income is $900 per annum, what of that larger class whose incomes do not average over $500 or $600 per annum? These people are not paupers, but their income permits of no provision in time of sickness. They cannot afford luxuries, and the doctor is to them a luxury, though he is also an absolute necessity. What are these people to do? To deprive them of the dispensary and hospital would be to perpetuate a great social injustice.

And pertinent to this same economic condition is the so-called lodge and contract practise abuse.

It must be understood that lodge and contract practise is here and here to stay, because of an economic demand. Lodge and contract practise is a form of insurance adapted to the needs of the wage earner whose fixed charges leaves no adequate margin for sudden illness and who can thus by a small weekly premium provide for his family medical attention at home. Thus the poor man through the lodge and contract practise is using the principle of insurance in providing for his family just as you and I provide ourselves with an accident policy or a sick benefit policy; the principle is the same whether we pay a hundred dollars a year or ten cents a week.

Lodge and contract practise must and will continue until there is inaugurated some system of national or state medical insurance in this country, as has already been adopted in England. It will thus be seen that the doctor himself, together with modern economic conditions, conspires to minimize the demand for professional services that once existed.

How about the supply? The number of physicians in proportion to the population not only must decrease, but a hopeful sign is that it *has* actually decreased. There are 35 less medical colleges than there were ten years ago. There are 5,000 less medical students than there were ten years ago.

In the year 1912 there were 800 graduates in medicine less than in 1900, and this decrease notwithstanding the enormous increase in population.

In the United States there is about one physician to 500 of the population, while in Germany the ratio is about one in 2,000, and it is not improbable that this decrease in physicians will continue until the German ratio is more nearly approximated. For there will be still fewer medical colleges, the entrance requirements will be higher, and the course lengthened to five years. The future physician will be the product of a sound preliminary education plus his special laboratory and clinical training, which will evolve a higher type of practitioner and a safer and more valuable member of the community. I do not forget that the present conditions are by no means ideal. We of this generation are passing through a transitional period while new adjustments and adaptations of the social and economic status are being evolved.

I am not indifferent to the fact that in many quarters the shoe is pinching while the income is diminishing. There are real abuses which we as intelligent men should be able to correct, and which I am hopeful may be corrected through effective organization. The American Society of Medical Economics has started out with a splendid purpose and a practical program. With hearty co-operation it should be able to mitigate many of the abuses which now exist to our discredit.

We must, as citizens as well as doctors, note that the call of the twentieth century is to social service and in the direction of social equilibrium. During this century what has been regarded as the radicalism of the socialist will become a part of the organic law of the land, and in this new order the doctor cannot be an unimportant factor. For with his unexampled altruism, his fitness for social service and his example of true democracy, he has unconsciously through the ages, by precept and practise, preached the gospel of equality and fraternity, and thus made the earth a better place in which to dwell.

# QUARANTINE IN RELATION TO THE PANAMA CANAL.

By Joseph J. O'Connell, A.M., M.D.,

Health Officer of the Port of New York.

THERE is much discussion at the present time over what national honor and national prosperity demand of the national government with regard to the operation of the Panama Canal from a military and a commercial standpoint. To the thoughtful American who has reflected upon the subject, is would seem clear that the fortification of the canal by the United States is a national obligation to which we are constrained by the law of self-preservation. To leave the canal without gun or battlement under present political conditions would be to rely upon an altruism which, much as we may deplore the fact, does not exist. This republic means too much to humanity to leave exposed to attack one of its frontiers. Such foolhardiness, in view of the possible consequences, would be criminal upon our part. The proper course with regard to commerce is unfortunately less clear. There is much to be said on both sides of the question at issue, but I think we shall be safe in leaving it to the authorities having jurisdiction to determine wisely and justly, and bring out of the confusion now existing a solution that will keep our faith unbroken and at the same time involve no sacrifice of one of the essentials of sovereignty.

There is another aspect, however, in which this canal must be considered, and fortunately there is no confusion as to what our rights are in this respect. Nor can there be much controversy as to what are our obligations as a civilized state. No student of the history of this stupendous undertaking, from that remote day in the sixteenth century when Charles V had a survey made for a canal from the Chagres River to the Pacific, to the present hour, can escape a realization of the tremendous part which sanitation played in the successful execution of the project. Nor can any man, particularly if that man be a physician, consider the future of the great waterway without a realization of the vast possibility of sanitary service open here to the American republic. Our duty is so perfectly plain, our right so obvious and indefeasible, that on this point there will be no protest against the establishment of a world quarantine at Panama.

Sanitary science has the right to demand this of the government of the United States. Political conditions make it possible to demand it of no other power, for on this strip of territory our government exercises exclusive and supreme jurisdiction. Sanitary science can truthfully say that without its help this canal would never have been constructed; that with its help the Spanish or the French could have constructed it long ago. Without subtracting one iota from the credit due to the splendid engineering ability displayed in this work, we must in justice give full credit to the sacrifice, the industry, the high scientific intelligence of the American medical men who cleared the field for the engineering forces. They made it possible for men to live on the isthmus and until that had been made possible the work could not have been carried on. They cleared up the swamps, they banished the yellow fever, the typhoid and the malignant malarial fevers. When I was in Panama last month I saw but one mosquito, so thorough have been scientific methods of the sanitary corps in ridding the isthmus of this old carrier of the yellow fever and malaria germs.

By right of service then the science that has done this may justly demand in the name of civilization a course on the part of the government to which considerations of pure humanity on the one hand and self-protection on the other conspire to direct it.

You know that in the East from time immemorial the dreaded epidemic diseases, cholera and plague, have had their home. You know, also, that South America, and before American scientists took sanitary measures Central America and the West Indies, were the home of yellow fever. That dread disease is still prevalent in South American ports and particularly in the ports of South America upon its Pacific coast. When we open this canal we shall admit into the Atlantic ships coming directly from all these ports of plague and cholera and yellow fever. Cholera we have the least cause to dread from this direction because the short incubatory period of this scourge makes the broad Pacific Ocean an almost impassable barrier toward the west. The migration of cholera is in shorter stages and the infection goes from port to port in Asia and in Europe and annually threatens our Atlantic rather than our Pacific seaboard. Plague, on the other hand, being transmissible by the fleas of rats which infest the holds of ships, will be much more to be dreaded when the new waterway affords a direct route to our own ports for vessels hailing from the Far East. The great coastwise trade with South America which will bring to us numerous vessels direct from the pest ports of the Pacific coast of the southern continent, will bring with it the danger of yellow fever infection.

These are dangers to which we shall be not only directly but reflectively subject. Ships will not only come to the American ports but will take the canal route to the great European ports which are in active and continuous commerce with New York. It may be asked why we should establish a quarantine for the protection of Liverpool, say, or of Hamburg. A little reflection will show that the infection of the port of Liverpool, or the port of Hamburg, or of any of the great ports of Europe, would have a disastrous effect upon the commerce of New York and would expose to real danger the public health of the United States. This is the selfish consideration involved There is another broader and higher consideration. Are we going to allow vessels which enter our jurisdiction in the Panama Canal Zone to leave that jurisdiction with sick persons on board and with the likelihood of the contagious and infectious ailments from which they suffer, being communicated to every one else upon the vessel in which they may happen to be? This is what it will mean not to have a world quarantine service established at Panama.

When I visited the isthmus I consulted with the authorities there on this matter and I examined the ground for the purpose of seeing how far physical conditions favored the establishment of such a quarantine as I have mentioned. I found these conditions ideal for the purpose. It will take twelve hours for a vessel to make the voyage through the canal. These twelve hours can be utilized for inspection and fumigation without interfering with the natural flow of commerce. There should be a boarding-station at each end of the canal and a fumigating boat at each such station. At the Colon end of the canal there should be a temporary reception hospital. At the Panama end there are groups of islands, and two of these, Flamenco and Perico, are admirably adapted for use as sites for detention pavilions and contagious disease hospitals, just as we use Hoffman and Swinburne Islands in our own harbor. Permanent hospital wards and detention pavilions should be here constructed. The entire service should be a part of the public health service of the United States.

The protection of the Port of New York or any other port is not alone in the diseased persons removed at the Quarantine Station, but in the care maintained at the points of embarkation where communicable diseases are segregated and none but healthy persons allowed to be transported. The ships entering any port bringing in persons suffering from infectious or contagious diseases are charged with their care while in detention, and frequently the ships are detained for several days under quarantine, which is a severe penalty to any steamship company, and they have established careful inspection stations at the various ports of embarkation in order to avoid this loss.

---

## REMARKS UPON THE RELATION BETWEEN THE PATIENT, THE PHYSICIAN AND THE SURGEON.*

### By Russell S. Fowler, M.D.,

Brooklyn, N. Y.

IN this paper the terms physician, general practitioner and surgeon are defined as follows:

*Physician.*—A graduate in medicine who limits his work to the care of medical cases. *General Practitioner.*—A graduate in medicine who cares for medical cases and in addition, such surgical cases as in his estimation are within his capabilities. *Surgeon.*—A graduate in medicine who by reason of special aptitude, opportunity and study limits his work to the practice of surgery.

There are, of course, hybrids of each class, *i.e.,* men known for their surgical work who also care for medical cases; physicians who do operations. The strictly honest class seem to be the general practitioner, who poses neither as physician nor surgeon, but who candidly state that they care for all cases which they feel qualified to treat.

The general practitioner is on the increase. Each year sees him better fitted to care for a larger proportion of both medical and surgical cases. Nevertheless there must always be a large proportion of surgical cases which can only be cared for by the surgeon, either because these cases are too poor to pay the general practitioner, or because they are cases which he honestly feels are beyond his limitation. With these conditions the surgeon should be content. After all, this is a question for the patient to decide.

The surgeon draws his work from three sources: first, from cases referred by former patients; second, from his friends, the physicians; third, from his friends in general practice. There is but a small percentage which come because of his special aptitude for certain work. The proportions are about as follows, though they will vary in individual cases and with the reputation of the surgeon: 50 per cent. of cases from former patients, 25 per cent. from physicians, 25 per cent. from general practitioners.

---

* Read before the Brooklyn Medical Society, April, 1912.

The field of medicine and surgery has become so broad that in a community of any size it is not right that men should practice both branches, for they cannot be proficient in both. To become proficient requires experience, and the ordinary span of life precludes the possibility of more than fair proficiency in one branch. We must all our lives be students, weighing the case records and results of others with our own work.

*The Responsibilities of the Physician and the Surgeon.*—In relation to the result, the physician's responsibility is fully as great as the surgeon's. Unfortunately, however, the mistakes occurring in emergencies, such as appendicitis, extra-uterine pregnancy, perforating ulcers, and the acute inflammatory lesions of the gall bladder, give the most immediately disastrous results. His responsibility is really greater, however, in the long list of less immediately dangerous diseases, such as carcinoma, cholelithiasis, the various mechanical disturbances and tuberculous affections. Here it is that the physician can save his patient years of suffering, and in many instances, as in carcinoma, give the patient the only chance for life by conscientious study and early diagnosis.

The surgeon shares the responsibility with the physician for the diagnosis and is entirely responsible for the technic of the surgical treatment. For complications of a medical nature developing during the course of the illness the physician should be responsible. When the case is returned to the physician they are again equally responsible until the surgical condition has been cured. Time does not permit me to cite examples, nor is it necessary, for every one of us has had his disasters. We may fail in diagnosis, our treatment may result badly, but the point is, have we done our best? Have we, physician and surgeon, in each case used every means at our command to arrive at a correct diagnosis? Have we, as surgeons, used every means to insure asepsis; was each step at the operation performed properly; in the disastrous result either as regards life or limb, where was *our* error either of omission or commission? Our conscience will answer these questions in the negative or affirmative. We know when we have been lacking in foresight. We may, if physicians, try to excuse ourselves by saying Dr. So-and-So says so many cases of appendicitis get well without operation, so my case stands a good chance; or that the tumor of the breast which has been allowed to grow for months did not at first present definite signs of malignancy; or, if surgeons, that in the case of secondary hemorrhage from a slipped knot, or a hernia following an operation done by an interne, was done just as we would do it.

It is interesting to note the change that has taken place in the course of time in the relationship between the physician and the surgeon. Time was when the surgeon was a very small personage, one who was called in to do manual work at the direction of the physician and who was rather looked down upon. Nowadays the surgeon takes at least equal rank with the physician and is called in not only for his skill in performing operations but for his skill in diagnosing obscure conditions. More and more responsibility has been shifted to his shoulders. The real keynote to the surgeon's rise in this respect is his practical knowledge of living pathology. His knowledge of cases is based not only on the physical finding before operation, but upon the relationship existing between the findings and the actual pathologic conditions exposed at the operation. To the majority of us, physicians and surgeons alike, the most interesting part of our work is that which deals with diagnosis, the keystone of successful practice.

Every once in a while it is stated by a physician that he does not send his work to a certain surgeon because he does not receive his patients back again. This should not be so, and it can be guarded against by the surgeon by a very simple expedient. In the first place the patient should understand that he has been placed in the surgeon's care for the purpose of being treated for the surgical disease or complication from which he is suffering, and that when the need of the surgeon's special care in dealing with this has passed away he will be returned to his family physician for whatever medical care or further minor surgical care his condition requires. Whether the case has been referred by the family physician or not, the physician's name should be ascertained and recorded. Because Dr. X does not refer his case to a certain surgeon is no reason why that surgeon should return the case to any one but Dr. X.

When the patient is in condition to return to his physician he should be told to return to him for such further treatment as is indicated, and the physician should be notified. If the case is one in which special care is needed to guard against some complication, brief notes in this regard are added to the letter to the physician. A final examination by the surgeon can be arranged at the same time.

By following out this plan as a routine everyone concerned with the care of the patient, as well as the patient, knows just what is expected.

Patients will almost invariably follow the directions of the surgeon in regard to whom they shall submit themselves for their after-care. It occasionally happens that patients desire to be cared for by the interne who has done their dressings at the hospital. Such requests must be met by a firm denial and insistence be made that the case return to the physician. This sets a good example for the interne whose ideas of professional etiquette are apt to be moulded by the behavior of his chief in hospital work. The surgeon should impress upon the patient the physician's responsibility in the case and whenever possible strengthen the patient's confidence in the physician.

The charge is occasionally made that the surgeon assumes the care of the case without the instruction of the physician. This charge is undoubtedly true in many instances in office consultations; more rarely in the examination of patients in their own homes. As an example in office practice, Surgeon A is consulted by a patient who has been referred by the physician to Surgeon B for an operation. The patient for some reason does not care for Surgeon B and wishes Surgeon A to operate. Certainly Surgeon A would not be justified in refusing but he should notify the physician and should return the patient to him when the surgical treatment has been completed. This last Surgeon A should do even though the physician has belittled Surgeon A in comparing him to Surgeon B. Coals of fire are occasionally beneficial.

More frequently it happens that the patient consults the surgeon without being referred to any particular surgeon so that the course to be followed is even clearer and devoid of the possible unpleasantness of the first instance.

In the matter of house calls it is not difficult for the surgeon to decide a consistent course of action. His office should be instructed that, being a surgeon, he takes only surgical cases, whether for treatment or operation. The person answering his door and telephone should be particularly instructed to impress this on patients and their friends. Having ascertained that the case is a surgical one, the next question should be, "Who is your regular physician?" If there is no physician in the case the surgeon may, with propriety, assume charge of the patient. If there is a physician, however, the patient or the person applying for him should be told that the surgeon will not see the case except with the physician, and that application for the surgeon's services should be made through the physician. Sometimes patients wishing to save expense will prevaricate, saying that no physician has been in attendance, or may even prevaricate concerning the nature of the case. In such an instance the question, "How long has the patient been ill?" will show that some one must have been in attendance. The surgeon should insist on the physician's attendance with him at the examination. This is for the patient's best interests as well as the physician's and surgeon's. It simplifies the examination of the case, safeguards the patient's interests and saves time. If the case is an emergency, such as a hemorrhage or a recent fracture, of course the surgeon will respond at once, later notifying the physician of his action in the matter and assuming charge of the case with the physician if mutually agreeable. If in spite of all precaution, through the prevarication of the patient or his representative, the surgeon finds himself in the dilemma of seeing a physician's case without the physician, he can do only one thing, meet the indications there are for surgical treatment and explain his position at the earliest possible moment to the physician. Some physicians think that a consultation belittles them in the eyes of the patient. Such physicians are apt not to be more than moderately successful.

One of the objections which surgeons have to referring cases back to their physicians for minor surgical treatment is the fear that the physician may not understand the surgical indications. This is obviated to a great extent by the plans for formal notification which have been outlined, supplemented by such additional directions as the nature of the case indicates and by an occasional visit to the surgeon.

*Attendance of the Physician at Operation.*—The attendance of the physician at the operation is desirable from the patient's viewpoint as well as from that of the physician and surgeon. The patient is better disposed toward the physician who shows such interest in the case and more readily submits to the physician's future care of the case realizing that the physician has seen what was done. The physician who has the patient's best interest at heart will make every effort to be present at the operation in order that he may use the knowledge thus obtained in the future care of the case. The surgeon is benefited by the physician's presence in that the details of the case are apt to be discussed and their relation to the pathological condition found more firmly fixed. Should the physician not be able to be present he should request such information from the surgeon. Whenever possible the physician should follow the after course of the case in the hospital, so as to be better prepared to take up the subsequent care. The patient's circumstances permitting the physician should charge for the time spent in witnessing the operation and in subsequent visits to the hospital as this work is for the patient's benefit.

The physician should inform the surgeon of any variation from the normal in a patient's condition following discharge from the hospital and should ask the surgeon's co-operation in the treatment of any surgical complication. The physician should remember that it is the surgeon's reputation that is at stake in this regard as well as his own. In the event of an unfortunate complication such as delayed union or wound healing or latent infection in scar tissue or late or impaired functional results, the patient will blame either the surgeon or the physician's after care. Such complications are best met in their incipiency by the co-operation of the physician and surgeon.

It has seemed to the author that a great deal of very valuable information might be obtained by the practitioner of general medicine, particularly in the line of diagnosis and after treatment if advantage were taken by them of a few hours weekly study of cases as seen and treated in a general hospital. In appendicitis, for example, there is yet much to be desired in the matter of early diagnosis and the early selection of cases necessitating urgent operation. It is our belief that the majority of operating surgeons would welcome the attendance of the general practitioner at the clinics and during the rounds, and I know of no way in which a wide experience in diagnosis can be more quickly obtained. As to acquiring knowledge of operative technic, that can only be obtained by a prolonged and arduous relation as assistant to a master. While it may not be a popular note to sound, yet it is well that the occasional surgeon should confine himself to the minor operations which present in his general practice and develop himself more along the lines of diagnosis and preventive medicine, which, after all is said, are the more interesting as well as of more benefit to mankind.

## THE BULLETIN.

Beginning with the current number of the *Journal,* the Medical Society of the County of Kings has arranged to publish in its pages the monthly notices hitherto published separately by the Society in its BULLETIN. As a result of this arrangement the *Journal* will be sent to all members of the Kings County Medical Society. It is hoped that this arrangement will be mutually advantageous inasmuch as the *Journal* benefits by its increased circulation, while the BULLETIN assumes a more permanent form. The *Journal* is the only medical periodical of its kind published on Long Island and as such should be the medium of communication for all Long Island physicians—not only for publication of scientific material, but for items of general and local interest as well. With the growth of population proceeding at its present rate, Long Island will, before many years, become the residential, if not the commercial center of the Eastern States, and the importance of a united medical profession in this center cannot be overestimated. It is the hope of the Associated Physicians of Long Island to make the *Journal* an active factor in this unification, and the present co-operation of the Medical Society of the County of Kings is hailed as an important step in this direction.

# EDITORIAL

## WHO ARE THE UNFIT?

UNFITNESS is a very relative term, though we have developed a vicious habit of talking very dogmatically about it. We are really on very dangerous ground when we attempt to characterize definitively such types of humanity as fall short of obviously gross unfitness. There are degrees of degeneracy, decadence and criminality still leaving traits that are admirable, often undiscernible to such sensationalists as Nordau, such pseudo-scientists as Lombroso, and such people as the extreme, fanatical eugenists, bent upon "standardizing" the race. The only individual in history who was wholly damnable was Judas.

We ought to get past the attitude that the so-called unfit are any different from ourselves essentially. Properly viewed, the unfit are the unfitted. Such an attitude is not based on sentimentalism, but upon sympathetic understanding of other people and of the hard facts of life. It is the unfitters who deserve study—and sterilization. The burning at the eugenic stake of the products of our vicious social order is a remedy unworthy of a high civilization.

The born criminal is a rare bird and a late hatching when he does exist. Feeble-mindedness, also, is too often the result of generations of industrial slavery and bad hygiene. A Russian investigator recently found the antecedents of five hundred insane people whom he studied to be practically as good as those of five hundred sane men and women.

We confess a sneaking liking for the Alfred Jingles, Dick Swivellers, and Micawbers of the world. We are not for the unsexing of potential Rousseaus. If the "defective" boy Oliver Goldsmith were living today we should be the last to recommend him for observation as a near-imbecile. Nor would we feel any eugenic prejudice against such an "impenetrably stupid" boy as Richard Brinsley Sheridan. We protest against the condemnation by a board of eugenics of all the delightful vagabonds whose lives divert us and themselves. Through what prescience could such a board guarantee that no Colonel Mulberry Sellers would suffer at its ruthless hands? Such a board would probably include no humorist, and in this connection we should like to record our conviction that total lack of the sense of humor is the greatest earnest of unfitness that we can think of, more indicative of the need of sterilization than any other form of deficiency. What defective would be more of a menace than a eugenist endowed with power but lacking this sense?

We very much fear that in the eugenist's Utopia only the poor would continue to be exploited. The capitalist who works children all day and women all night, the demagogue, the smug philanthropist, builder of "model" tenements, constructed with money which in its

149

accumulation has caused more tuberculosis than it will ever cure—
would they take precedence of the idiot? Would such a type as the
man who corners a necessary of life in the market be arraigned by
a eugenic board before a low-grade imbecile? Would the embryo
Swifts, De Quinceys and Poes be wholly safe in its hands?

One so-called degenerate like Rousseau is worth all the enthusiastic and fanatical eugenists who are now filling the air with their advice. There will be no beloved vagabonds like Francis Thompson,
"the greatest achievement of nineteenth century Catholicism," no
John Synges, no Villons, no Masefields, no Levers, if they can help
it. The "half scholar, half vagabond" who interested the young
Lincoln in Burns and Shakespeare would never have received the
endorsement of a board of eugenics. Such a board would find no
solace or justification in the contemplation of the tramp in Synge's
"Shadow of the Glen," or of the picturesque vagabond in Gals-
worthy's "The Pigeon," or of the vagrant in Yeat's "A Pot of Broth."

Holbrook Jackson makes a bid for sterilization when he insists
that vagabondage is but the abjuration of the upholstery of civilized
life, which is but a distorted reflection of life itself. The truth is that
the vagabond is not nearly so mysterious, freakish and unaccountable
a figure as the one-idea'd eugenist, steeped in propaganda forever—
and the same propaganda; "devoted" to something eternally and
everlastingly; bent upon cheating himself and others of life and upon
establishing a régime of disgustingly sane people, absolutely moral—
according to Philistian concepts—and wholly "efficient" as regards
work-a-day, engineering standards.

Suppose the eugenist's dream were to be realized (there is no
danger of it, after all)? What then? Would we see the vision that
the soul of man yearns to encompass? Would anybody worth his
salt wish to live in the eugenist's world? Would he be happy? Could
he realize the greater possibilities of life and express them? What
would there be in such a world to inspire the Carlyles and Ruskins
and Emersons, much less to create them? What would be the final
outcome of such a society if not degeneracy—real, sordid decadence
of the worst possible sort?

If genius derives from certain of the unfit, pray God to conserve
a sufficiency of that element against the maraudings of these bulls in
the human china shop, that His purposes may be served and con-
summated.

ARTHUR C. JACOBSON.

---

## PERNICIOUS LEGISLATION.

A S a result of recent police activity supplementing reports received through the agencies of organized charity and private
observation, there has of late been an active awakening of
public interest in the abuse of narcotic drugs, especially cocaine, as
indicated by the accounts in the public press, which have portrayed
a condition of affairs almost beyond belief. The amount of cocaine
consumed, and particularly the youthfulness of its habitués, has
aroused an earnest and laudable determination to put a stop to the
degradation that regularly follows cocaine abuse. Singularly enough,
it is not from the medical profession, who should know most about

the matter, but from lay sources that the first efforts at control have come, and the legislation proposed is so restrictive in the limitations it places on the possession, sale, use, and prescribing of cocaine and other narcotics as to arouse an instant storm of indignant protest from physicians everywhere, and especially from the large class who specialize in diseases of the eye, ear, nose and throat. Assembly Bill No. 692, drawn by Mr. Delehanty of the New York County district attorney's office, is the particular red rag that has inflamed their ire, though Senate Bill No. 52 is not far behind as an irritant.

In the main, the objections that are to be urged against these bills lie in the restrictions placed upon prescribing and in the privilege bestowed upon the authorities to enter without warrant any physician's office at any time by any agent of the state for the purpose of inspecting the physician's stock of cocaine and his record of the quantity used. It is pointed out that the tenor of the bill is such as to brand every physician as presumably dishonest because a few have been convicted of unprofessional conduct in the sale and distribution of narcotics. If we estimate the public temper aright, some legislation along these lines is bound to be passed, but it is sincerely to be hoped that the bills may be recast in such a way as to call forth the co-operation of the medical profession rather than its antagonism. It is proper and feasible that some record of the amount purchased, its source and destination should be available, for only in this way can illicit trade in the drugs be traced. But it must be remembered that the administration of such a law is difficult, especially when we appreciate that the present cocaine law calling for certificates from druggists to consumers is largely disobeyed. The particular provision requiring a physician to keep an account of minute doses administered directly to patients is a hardship and seems unnecessary, as it would require for its careful observation an amount of time and bookkeeping that would be burdensome. Further, until an active co-operation can be established with neighboring states, such a bill would fall short of accomplishing its purpose, as it is a simple matter to obtain a supply from any one of our immediate neighbors.

The right of search claimed by Great Britain led to the War of 1812, and the principle established at that time has since been carefully respected both in public and private life. There can be little objection to a periodical report showing the purchase and disposition of narcotic drugs, but indiscriminate inspection at will constitutes a violation of private right that calls for vigorous opposition. Before any of these bills are finally adopted they should receive most careful deliberation and be so framed as to place the least burden upon those who are most nearly affected, the body of medical practitioners.

H. G. W.

---

## THE TURNING OF THE WORM.

MANY years ago, Bishop Berkeley, of sainted memory, wrote a prophetic poem whose last stanza is perennial inasmuch as it seems to apply to each new happening of the newer world:

"Westward the star of empire takes its way,
The first four acts already past;
The fifth shall close the drama of the day,
Time's greatest offspring is its last."

Which, being interpreted, is to say that the State of Colorado now harbors the greatest monument of potential medical legislative folly, if we are correctly informed, and we fear we are.

A physician, a member of the Colorado legislature, has introduced a bill into that august body the purpose of which is to encourage appendicitis. Apparently this disease is becoming so scarce in Colorado that it must be regulated and preserved, and as medical means seem to have been inadequate, legislative enactment is to be resorted to to curb the epidemic which threatens to rob the State of Colorado of its last appendix. How is this to be brought about? Forsooth, by fining the doctor who removes an appendix which, on submission to a jury, shall in their opinion fail to show sufficient evidence of crime. What a picture! There lies the victim writhing in the anguish of green apple colic! The hastily summoned surgeon looks wise, touches the spot, and says "ah-ha." Do they then proceed to operate? No. They first choose a jury of three unprejudiced physicians who are to umpire the game. Before their watchful eyes the original surgeon nervously proceeds to make good his diagnosis. The incision is made, the field is opened up, the appendix is identified, and, if the surgeon feels the courage of his convictions, the offending organ is snatched out and passed over to the jury for their verdict. If they are friendly to the surgeon, they shake their heads and congratulate him and the patient that the wretched organ has been so quickly and skillfully removed. But suppose they are not friendly, what then? They have but to shake their heads, say "this looks to us not to be diseased," and the surgeon not only forfeits his fee, but is liable to a heavy fine in addition for operating needlessly. As Mulvaney would say, "t'is is a joole av a law." Its evident absurdities stamp it as the product of a mind that is too narrow to understand the true cause of things—a sort of mental acrobat who would endeavor to prevent floods by legislative enactment regulating the rainfall.

Truly we live within the reign of law. As physicians we are regulated at both ends. We must have certain requirements as candidates, and having qualified to meet these requirements, we are to be regulated not by our trained judgment, but by the whim of every addlepate with a fad. We must not touch pet dogs and cats; we must not prescribe drugs; we must accept as equals the members of any sect that has been legislated into medical practice through cheap by-ways and short-cuts; and now the vermiform appendix has asserted itself—the worm has turned, so to speak. One is tempted to sympathize with Mr. Tony Weller in that moment of disgust and depression when he threatened to give up coaching and "go and keep a pike."

H. G. W.

DEPARTMENT UNDER THE CHARGE OF WILLIAM SCHROEDER, M.D.

## ERNEST PALMER, M.D.

Dr. Palmer was born in New York City in June, 1850, and died in Brooklyn, New York, January 30, 1913. He was the son of William Pitt Palmer, A.M., M.D., the poet, a graduate of Williams College and the University of the City of New York, who published three volumes of poems, "Ode to Light," "Orpheus and Eurydice," "Echoes of Half a Century." He died in Brooklyn, N. Y., May 2, 1884.

Dr. E. Palmer was educated at the Polytechnic Institute, after which he went West and attended lectures at the Toland Medical College. Returning to New York, he completed his medical education at the College of Physicians and Surgeons, New York, receiving the degree of M.D. in the class of 1879. During his professional life he was Sanitary Inspector for the Health Department. From 1884 he was Surgeon to the Long Island College Hospital and Consultant to St. John's, Kings County and Jewish Hospitals. He was a member of the Medical Society County of Kings from 1880, Associated Physicans of Long Island from 1899, American Medical Association, Brooklyn Gynecological Society and the Alumni of St. Mary's Hospital, The Sons of the American Revolution, Society of Colonial Wars, Montauk Lodge No. 286, F. & A. M., Crescent and Reform Clubs of New York, Rockland County Fly Fish Club and the Parkville Angling Club of Pennsylvania.

In 1877 Dr. Palmer married Miss L. L. Nicholson, of Brooklyn; a daughter was born of this union, Natalie, who, with his second wife, Florence L., survive him.

The funeral services were held at the Masonic Temple, Brooklyn, N. Y. W. S., Sr.

## TREADWELL LEWIS IRELAND, M.D.

Dr. Ireland was born in 1826 and died February 5, 1913, at Roslyn, L. I. He was one of the oldest physicians on Long Island, being graduated from the University of New York with the degree of M. D. in 1846. He practiced medicine during his professional life at Greenport and Roslyn, Long Island, and for a number of years was Coroner of Suffolk County. W. S., Sr.

## GEORGE CLINTON JEFFERY, M.D.

Dr. Jeffery was born in Albany, N. Y., in 1852 and died in Brooklyn, N. Y., February 11, 1913. He was the son of Reuben Jeffery, a former pastor in this city. His medical education was received at the Pulte Medical College in Cincinnati, Ohio, where he was graduated in 1875. He was a member of the American Institute of

Homeopathy and the County and State Homeopathic Societies. Dr. Jeffery is survived by his widow, Amanda W., a daughter, Mrs. Edgar R. Van Buskirk, and a son, George Clinton, Jr. Dr. Jeffery was interested in fraternal organizations, his membership being as follows: Philadelphia Council, R. A.; Brooklyn Lodge, B. P. O. Elks; Anglo Saxon Lodge, F. & A. M.; Orient Chapter, R. A. M.; Clinton Commandery, K. T.; Kismet Temple, A. A. O. N. of M. S.; and the Forty-seventh Regiment Veterans' Association.   W. S., SR.

## WILLIAM FOSTER GANSTER, PH.G., M.D.

DR. GANSTER was born in New York City on July 2, 1867, and died in Brooklyn, N. Y., February 11, 1913. He was the son of George Peter Ganster and Theresa Paul. His early education was received at St. Paul's Parochial School and St. Vincent College, Pennsylvania. He then entered the Philadelphia College of Pharmacy, receiving the degree of Ph.G. in 1889. His medical education was under the direction of Henry Noss, M.D., graduating from the Long Island College Hospital in the class of 1896. He practiced medicine in this city during his professional life. He was a member of the Medical Society County of Kings from 1906, American Medical Association and the Associated Physicians of Long Island from 1912.

Dr. Ganster was married on May 25, 1890, to Ellie Wynn at Reading, Pa. His children are Paul Vincent and Florence Georgianna Ganster.   W. S., SR.

## WILLIAM JAMES CALLAN, A.M., M.D.

DR. CALLAN was in the practice of medicine in Brooklyn, New York, for a number of years. He died at St. Joseph, New York, February 13, 1913. He was educated at Manhattan College, Fordham University and St. Francis College. His medical education was received at the Long Island College Hospital, receiving the degree of M.D. in the class of 1892. He was a member of the Medical Society of the County of Kings, 1889-1900.

For many years Dr. Callan was professor of Elocution and English Literature at St. Francis College, Brooklyn; St. Joseph's Convent, Brentwood; St. Joseph's Seminary, Dunwoodie, and St. Peter's College, Jersey City. He was a member of Morning Star Council, K. of C.   W. S., SR.

## WILLIAM ARTHUR LITTLE, M.D.

DR. LITTLE was born at Langford, Ireland, in 1849. He died in Brooklyn, New York, February 24, 1913. His medical education was received at the University of New York, where he received the degree of M.D. in 1878. He was in the practice of medicine in this city during his professional life, and for many years connected with the Bushwick Hospital. He was a member of the Medical Society County of Kings from 1879 to 1910, the Brooklyn Medical Society from 1895 to 1913, Hill Grove Lodge, F. & A. M.; DeWitt Clinton Council, R. A., and Central Congregational Church.

Dr. Little leaves a widow, Sarah Hale, and a daughter, Jeanne.
   W. S., SR.

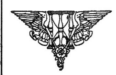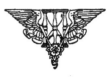

# Society Transactions

## TRANSACTIONS OF THE BROOKLYN PATHOLOGICAL SOCIETY.

*Stated Meeting, January 9, 1913.*

The President, PAUL M. PILCHER, M.D., in the Chair.

**The Value of the Gonorrheal Complement Fixation Test and the Wassermann Reaction in Determining the Fitness of a Person to Marry.**

DR. MAX LEDERER read a paper with this title. (See page 102.)

DR. WILLIAM LINTZ, in discussion, said:—'Dr Lederer has well emphasized the point in regard to a negative Wassermann reaction in cerebro-spinal syphilis. It is a rule in fact to get negative reactions in blood in cerebro-spinal syphilis. He also emphasized very well the fact that no reaction is complete until you have examined not only the blood but also the cerebro-spinal fluid. In cerebro-spinal syphilis you are most likely to get a good positive reaction with the cerebro-spinal fluid and not with the blood.

"An additional point to be emphasized is that in examining for cerebro-spinal syphilis, it is not sufficient to use 2/10 c.c.; we must use more, because otherwise the number of positive tests will be almost as low as, or perhaps lower, than that of the blood of the same patients. But if we use increasing quantities, say, up to 1 c.c.-1½ c.c. of the cerebro-spinal fluid, instead of 2/10 c.c., you will be surprised to see that the positive reactions reach almost up to 100 per cent. in some of the forms of cerebro-spinal syphilis.

"Another point well emphasized is the gonorrheal complement fixation test, especially in the late stages of gonorrheal infections. In these cases the use of vaccines of several strains as a rule will result in a negative reaction.

"There is one more point to which attention should be called and that is this: the gonorrheal complement deviation test does not become negative at once, after the patient is cured. The point to be emphasized is, that the gonorrheal complement deviation test will be positive for about three or four months after the patient is cured, and a positive reaction at the end of three or four months does not necessarily mean that the patient has active gonorrheal infection, but simply that his immunity is still present and will deviate the complement. However, after the complement fixation test persists at the end of four months without treatment, then it means that gonorrheal infection is still present."

DR. BURTON HARRIS, in discussion said:—"That is a question which had occurred to many of the genito-urinary surgeons, but to Dr. Keyes belongs the credit for making the first attempt to obtain reliable data. Failing to get the consent of his non-gonorrheal patients to submit to the experiment, he had the test made on a specimen of his own blood. The report being negative, he took four injections of polyvalent gonococcus bacterin (P. D. & Co.) twenty, forty, fifty and sixty millions at intervals of one week. His blood continued to show a negative reaction.

"When weighed in conjunction with the data obtained by a careful local examination, which should include repeated microscopic examinations and cultures of all the secretions, I am of the opinion that the complement fixation test will prove to be of value. For, the reports of Schmidt, Gradwohl, Swinburne, Gardner, Clowes and others who have had the good fortune to work in conjunction with expert laboratory men, show that the test is positive in a large percentage of chronic cases. One author reports five cases of urethral stricture, one of which was traumatic and gave a negative reaction. In the other four cases the test was positive and the patients all gave a history of gonococcal infection.

"The point mentioned by Dr. Lederer concerning the probable value of the test in cases of suspected gonorrheal arthritis is well taken; for it is often difficult to obtain a history, and, in women, impossible to make a local examination.

"Did I understand you to say, Dr. Lintz, that if a normal individual is treated with gonococcus bacterin he will develop a positive complement fixation reaction?"

DR. WILLIAM LINTZ (answering Dr. Harris' question), said:—"If a patient is under treatment for gonorrhea with vaccine, he invariably has the complement deviation test for gonococcus. That, of course, merely refers to a patient with gonorrhea. I have never experimented with perfectly normal individuals to ascertain the effects of gonorrheal vaccines. It has invariably been with gonorrhea-infected individuals. I cannot answer the point you have brought out."

DR. ROBERT L. DICKINSON, in discussion, said:—"This report is very welcome to the gynecologist, because our smear and culture methods have been such a disappointment. The results which the microscope promised have practically been such that it cannot be used in the office with any quick and simple and positive answer. A clue to one of the obstinate pelvic problems would be of the greatest value. For instance, we have in many sterility cases a history of gonorrhea sufficiently clear, or adhesions about the tube sufficiently definite to make it easy to say that the closed tube is the cause of the sterility. In no small number, however, with normal semen and with indefinite history or findings of gonorrhea it is impossible to know whether the sterility is from closed tubes or whether we dare hold out hope to the family. Here the complement fixation test will tell."

### Examination of the Semen with Special Reference to the Lesser Defects.

DR. WILLIAM H. CARY read a paper with this title.

DR. ROBERT L. DICKINSON, in discussion, said:—"On the practical application of Dr. Cary's work, which has been very painstaking and conducted under difficult conditions, I wish to say that it has had a very useful side to it, in that it enables us to predict results that we might not be otherwise able to do. These defective specimens may sometimes be enormously improved. For instance, take the obese man: he may, by training, develop himself to such an extent as to have a nearly normal semen, and the 'broken semen' of the neurotic individual is also susceptible of the amount of improvement which I spoke of just now. Therefore, it is not simply a scientific research, but has a very practical side."

### Preparation for Marriage; Instruction, Examination, Certificate.

DR. ROBERT L. DICKINSON gave an outline of a study he is making, of which the following is a summary:

Looking toward the time when law and custom will require the exchange of certificates of physical and mental soundness before marriage is permitted or even finally pledged, and with the character of the examination for such certificate standardized, he urged that the profession should get ready by formulating the type of the examination and certificate.

He suggested that a systematic attack on the problem involved:

I. *Clinical study of fitness as generally found*—a. physical fitness, b. mental fitness, c. moral fitness, d. preparedness—i. e., previous education or instruction bearing upon marriage, upon maternity.

II. *Standards of fitness and preparation*—a. ideal conditions and preparation, b. minimum requirements to be advocated at present.

III. *Examination for fitness*—a. heredity, b. personal history, c. physical examination, d. special instruction.

IV. *Certification*—Forms, simple, complete.

The speaker stated further that he had been collecting data for some years on the matters of preliminary instruction and the knowledge that his patients had received before marriage, and their later opinions as to what they should have been told. He has also faithfully tried for several years to properly instruct his patients, using, in general, the method he outlined in the LONG ISLAND MEDICAL JOURNAL in January, 1908. His experience has led him to believe that some such preparation was necessary and desirable. He was gratified to see evidences of the quick response to the claim for such certificates from men and women before marriage, and he suggested as a basis for discussion the two following forms:

### SIMPLE FORM.

I certify that I have, with due care, questioned and examined ...........
...............................; that to the best of my information and belief
neither heredity, habit, congenital or acquired defect or disease incapacitates
her for marriage or for maternity.

Dated at                , this           day of           , 19 .

(Signed)                                  , M.D.

### COMPLETE FORM.

I certify that I have carefully questioned and examined ...............
........................., and to the best of my information and belief,

I. There is nothing in her heredity, or personal history, or present condition, in the way of insanity, tuberculosis, or crime, neither habit nor chronic invalidism, nor congenital nor acquired defect or disease that will incapacitate her for marriage.

The only condition calling for special note is the following:

II. There is nothing in the history or examination to lead me to believe her incapacitated for maternity.

The only condition calling for a special note is the following:

III. She is a virgin.

Dated at                , this           day of           , 19 .

(Signed)                                  , M.D.

## Ante-Marital Examination and Instruction of the Woman.

DR. VICTOR A. ROBERTSON, in discussion, said:—"I remember apropos of this very subject which Dr. Dickinson has treated so admirably, years ago a young man of handsome physique who had a neurotic personal history and came of a neurotic family. He was apparently in perfect health, but was afflicted with what might be termed *petit mal*. In the course of conversation his head would drop and for a second or two he would become unconscious of his surroundings and then that condition would disappear. For a long time he did not realize what his ailment was. Now, this thing occurred during my hospital experience some twenty-five or six years ago. One morning I picked up a newspaper and found that this young man had committed suicide in the Grand Central Hotel on Broadway and had been taken to St. Vincent's Hospital. I was shocked, of course, not hoping but fearing it was perhaps the individual whom I had known under happier circumstances. I went to the hospital and found it was really the man I had supposed. He had just been taken to the morgue. I hardly recognized him from the fact that he was very much disfigured. He had shot himself in the right side of his head, and, furthermore, as he was exceedingly handsome and was always clean shaven, but had allowed a growth of a week or so of beard to accumulate on his face, he was hardly recognizable. What had happened, as I had afterwards found out, was this: He contemplated marriage and at last had recognized the gravity of his trouble. He had many worldly advantages, social position, money, and everything the world could give. He thought that this ailment possibly should be looked into. He went to a number of specialists in New York and they all told him the same thing, that this affliction was probably incurable. He left home and was away for five or six days, and finally summoned up resolution to take his life, a most unfortunate thing, but it was perhaps well that he did so and did not enter into the marital state and convey this affliction to his offspring."

DR. JACOB HOROWITZ, in discussion, said:—"I have been much interested in this social question. I believe it is the duty not only of the physician but also of the people to certainly see that the human species should propagate in a healthy and fitting way. I do not think that the physician is in position to go to work and remedy this thing, because I believe the people won't let him. I believe that if people want to get married as they are doing now, it is the duty of the government to look after this thing, and the government should see that when people apply for a license to marry, no license should be issued unless they have a certificate of health showing that they are fit to marry. The physician can make one step and the people will translate it in an entirely different manner and will think the physicians are looking for trade. I think it is the duty of the physicians as a body, as a medical society, and as a state society, to introduce a measure of this kind and have it enacted into a law, and that they should show the lay people that they are not working in the interest of the pocket, but rather in the interest of the community, and in that way I believe we will be able to bring about some benefit."

DR. WALTER TRUSLOW, in discussion, said:—"I think there is no question but that we realize the importance of this subject. Personally, I am of the belief that the laity are thinking much more of this subject and looking much further in the directions of this paper than perhaps we imagine. I think that they will increasingly make demands on us to show our ability to answer the questions that are before us. I can tell you that I know of cases where husbands or wives, who have had the advantage of just such premarital advice as has been spoken of, become in a very definite and a very real way true missionaries and that they are telling their most intimate friends of the advisability of this premarital information."

DR. MICHAEL A. COHN, in discussion, said:—"There was one thing which was not mentioned by Dr. Dickinson and that was the question of the general condition of women as regards the heart or lungs. I often see cases of this kind and at the present time have under treatment a beautiful young lady who is suffering with a bad heart—mitral stenosis and regurgitation. She gave birth to a child about five weeks ago and is now in a dying condition. I told her folks it was too bad she had not consulted a physician before, and had she asked my opinion beforehand she would never have been married, and had she married she would never have had a child, if I had any influence over her. I think it also wrong that women suffering from laryngeal and pulmonary tuberculosis should marry and give birth to children, and I can see the advisability of Dr. Dickinson's suggestions regarding the proposed examination of candidates for marriage.

"I would also like Dr. Dickinson to tell us about marriage among relatives. What is the concensus of the profession regarding relations—for instance, cousins? I remember having read Spencer on this question, and he seems to think, as do a great many other sociologists, that there is nothing wrong about near relatives marrying and that the question is overrated. In this regard I also want to speak of the case of a nephew of mine. He married a young lady and found out too late that intercourse was impossible, there being no vagina. Of course, she had not been examined beforehand, and after living together for a while they separated. She is now away in another town and wants him to divorce her, but he has refused to do so and says that he intends to let her wait a little while before he gives her a chance to deceive another victim. I do not think that lady ever menstruated. She is good looking and well developed. She probably never knew herself that she could not get married.

"Now, as to the question of prevention of pregnancy, Dr. Dickinson says that pregnancy should be regulated. It is a pretty hard thing to regulate pregnancy, because the law prevents us from giving advice as regards prevention; but I think it is a very vital question indeed. What should the physician do? And something should be done to enlighten the public at large and teach the people whenever it is absolutely necessary for their health and welfare not to marry, when not to intermarry in the same families, and how and when to prevent conception."

### Hereditary Traits and Defects of the Nervous System, Which Contraindicate Marriage.

#### *Discussion by William Browning, M.D.*

The subject of the evening is of course one of great interest to us young bachelors!

As indicated by Dr. Dickinson, there is little use attempting to discuss the subject medically unless in a frank manner.

The first thing is to define just what is meant by marriage. Many so-called marriages at the present day are not such in any real sense. If the term is applied in that loose way, there is not much to the purpose that I can say.

*Marriage is for the orderly propagation of the race.* All other factors are to be considered in their relation to that one prime function. A due recognition of this axiomatic fact would also contribute much to moral and social welfare.

We might classify our material in various ways:

I. Those who don't consult us. We cannot do much for absent sinners.

II. Those who do consult us. But if we reason only on the basis of such as we have seen, though many in total, our view will be limited.

Some of our nouveau scientists have wished to discover for us here a new field—it is quite as old as any of us have been in practice.

These matters come before us in every kind of way and shape. Often it is practically settled before we are consulted; and by that time it may be risky to object.

The fond mother often thinks her girl too frail to marry. Yet many a slip of a girl becomes the mother of vigorous and admirable children. Or, again, the fair maid is overcome with premonitory fears. If merely morbid, and not a settled state of alienation, these also usually turn out well.

A better division of the matter is into:

I. The most suitable mates. If this question could be answered, it would constitute the most important phase of the whole subject. It is the positive side. But here our scientists as yet give scant data to aid us in advising. We may have to do the gathering of facts, statistics, material and interpretations for ourselves.

II. Those who should not marry at all. On the theoretical side this negativ phase covers about the extent of our present advising.

Here, I think, a general rule can be propounded: *Neuroses that are either primarily degenerative in character or are hereditary in kind constitute a warrantable objection to marriage.* This applies first to the applicants and their ancestry, less binding if in collaterals.

The difficulty, as always, is in applying the rule. And any such rule should not as yet be considered as hard and fast, but as only an aid that needs judgment and wisdom in its application.

That the weak-minded and epileptic should not marry, we have long known and advised. The investigations of Goddard and others have now made this course imperative. With these should be put dementia præcox.

The inebriate is a separate problem, as such stock is sometimes the source of an intellectually superior line.

Some things, as the familial myopathies, Huntington's chorea, etc., will probably only be expunged by slow marital exclusion.

Of the non-dementing psychoses, paranoia falls distinctly under the ban. Manic-depressive insanity comes partly under the rule, and consequently requires careful consideration in the individual case.

I should like to add a word regarding a point brought up by one of the discussers.

Let the profession teach and advise here as freely as you will. But the actual control in these affairs should not be attempted by the law, certainly not be placed in the hands of every licensing clerk. These things can better be regulated by parents and the church, by social or other private organizations, by certificates or whatever process is found best. In the first place, too much legal interference with the free action of the individual is un-American in principle. That is the danger of our laws at the present time. But it has also been found to work badly in practice. As a concrete illustration I might cite a certain foreign city where at one period, as I have been informed, certain conditions for marriage licenses were left to the will of the licensing authorities. It matters little what the conditions were. As a result the time came when a majority of the inhabitants were illegitimate. The people paired and were as truly monogamous as ever. But they were not prepared to meet the requirements and so lived outside the law.

---

# TRANSACTIONS OF THE BROOKLYN SURGICAL SOCIETY.

*Stated Meeting, December 5, 1912.*

The President, RICHARD W. WESTBROOK, M.D., in the Chair.

### Astragalectomy.

CHARLES DWIGHT NAPIER:—"I thought it might be interesting to show a few cases of Whitman's operation for astragalectomy in various stages.

"As you know, in many of these cases of deformities following infantile paralysis we get an unstable foot; we get perhaps, a dangle foot with no power at all, or a paralysis of either the adductors or abductors of the foot, or paralysis of the calf muscles with calcaneus and a large heel. So Dr. Whitman brought out this operation of removing the astragalus in order to give a stable foot for walking and in his hands it has been successful especially for calcaneo-valgus, for which he first introduced it.

"The very bad deformity which is illustrated by this plaster (exhibited) represents the foot of Case IV before operation. The very large heel, the valgus or rolling of the foot inwards, and pes cavus, give an unstable support, and such a foot would have to be held with a brace forever, or the shoe would have to be repeatedly reinforced and made over constantly in order to give proper support to the leg, unless something radical were done. Dr. Whitman brought out astragalectomy first for this condition of calcaneo-valgus and he found the results so uniformly good (100 per cent.) that he extended the operation to cover many forms of foot condition, except, of course, certain cases where he could transplant muscles and get a satisfactory result; but in dangle foot as well as calcaneo-valgus, this operation was found very successful.

"I may say, first, that the operation is rather a simple one. The incision is made,—with, of course, an Esmarch bandage,—on the outer side, just below the external malleolus, coming out forward, not quite up to the tendons of the dorsal flexors of the foot, curving around under the external malleolus and up posteriorly towards the tendo Achillis. The external lateral ligaments are divided and the peronei tendons are followed down and divided to whatever length is desired, the foot is forcibly turned over and the ligaments cut around the astragalus which is then removed. The important point which Dr. Whitman makes is thus: he places the leg bones forward, so that instead of straddling the posterior portion of the os calcis, they straddle the junction of the os calcis and tarsus. That brings the weight a little nearer to the center of the foot.

"After the astragalus is removed, the tendons of the peronei are placed in the tendo Achillis. That was done in all the four cases shown. They are made short enough so that they give some support as ligaments to the foot, even if there be no power in the peronei they can take the place, to some extent, of the tendo Achillis. The wound is entirely closed without drainage."

### Report of Cases and Presentation of Patients.

CASE I.—"This little girl of five years had a simple dangle foot. The operation was done on October 23d, and the first dressing was made only yesterday, approximately six weeks later. The first dressing is usually at the end of three weeks, so that the foot may be changed a little in position if it be not quite right. There is no pain in it now and there is motion, although some of the joint cartilage and the malleoli have been removed. The foot is put up not quite at right angles, but about 10 degrees below in order to get a better balance of the foot by keeping the heel up and allowing the tendo Achillis and other tendons posteriorly to shorten up and give better support to the heel."

CASE II.—"This boy of eight was operated on a year ago last June. Of course, he is still paralyzed to a certain extent in his leg, but he has a stable foot. It used to roll inwards. The power seemed to increase, although there was very little before the operation."

CASE III.—"This girl, age 9, was operated last July for paralytic varus. The second plaster for six months, allows development of the bones and shortening up of the ligaments. They walk with the plaster within three or four weeks after the operation. In the first plaster, with the knee at right angles, the patient is kept in bed for a week with the leg elevated, supported by a bandage strung from the head of the bed to the foot. A great deal of cotton is used around the foot to allow for swelling, which is very apt to take place."

CASE IV.—"This little boy had considerable paralysis and had to go through a good deal of manipulation. I first saw him when he was about three years of age and he had very slight, if any, power of the calf muscles, so that he developed a marked calcaneo-valgus. This operation was done about three years ago. With the Whitman operation the foot was held in good position in plaster for six months, a brace for another six months holding it until it was strong enough, and now he has a very firm foot to walk on. The heel is still large, but I am inclined to think that that will show less in another five years.

"His other leg was considerably paralyzed. He has a little power, but very little, of dorsal flexion of the foot. He had no power at all in the quadriceps extensor, and the flexor muscles of the knee were weak. He wore a long brace for a long time in order to protect the knee joint and keep it in good position and prevent deformity, while the muscles were being developed.

"The operation done in this case consisted of transplanting the sartorius and semimembranosus and sewing into the tendon of the quadriceps, the silk sutures going into the tissues firmly attached to the patella so as to get a good grip, as they are apt to pull out if sewn into a paralyzed tendon. He has some power, as you can see, of extension, not full extension. There is,

I think, perhaps five or ten degrees more than there was a year ago, but even if he fails to get any more it seems that the operation was well worth while. He will now be able to wear a short brace on the foot to give support, unless something possibly be done with that foot also. One does not like to urge too many things, but he is in much better condition than he was. It was important to keep on the long brace in order to protect these tendons.

"I might add that in transferring tendons you may get a very beautiful result at the end of one year, but cases should never be shown at that time, while at the end of two years one is liable to have a poor result, because of paralyzed tendons, or failure to support them while developing them."

## Tendon Transplantation.

DR. J. M. CLAYLAND, in discussion, said that he endorsed Dr. Napier's statement and emphasized the fact that weak muscles cannot be efficient substitutes for strong ones, while improvement in some degree was all that should be expected.

## Carcinoma of Penis.

*(Reported by Wm. H. Rankin, M.D.)*

"I would like to report another case of carcinoma of the penis. It had been amputated out west and he came on here and became very much neglected. The sore was a horrible stinking slough; the cord was involved and the scrotum on one side also. I incised the cord and closed the ring, incised the testicle and transplanted the urethra, and he has since regained his weight. He was a patient of Dr. Kerr's and he is now robust and quite well and healthy."

## Duodenal Ulcer.

*(Reported by Wm. H. Rankin, M.D.)*

DR. T. B. SPENCE, in discussion, said:—"Dr. Rankin spoke of the subject of duodenal ulcer as threadbare. I do not think that is so. There has been and there is going to be a great deal of discussion on this subject for many years. The gastro-enterologist and general practitioner have far from made up their mind that the surgeons should have these cases.

"Mr. Lane, of London, has recently thrown a bomb among us by stating that they are due to Lane's kink. It is for us to determine whether that is true or not, and if it is, we are talking from an entirely wrong viewpoint.

"It is foolish to do a gastro-enterostomy if the trouble is down at the ileocecal junction. I have had only one case of that sort since I heard Mr. Lane speak and I was very careful to investigate the ilium and I am pleased to say that I found no evidence of any obstruction down there whatever and am hoping that my gastro-enterostomy will prove a means of cure to the man.

"My experience, which does not extend back very far in these cases, makes me feel that this is far from a threadbare subject. It leads me to believe a gastro-enterostomy is going to help a good many of these people. I have a number of cases which I hope before the end of the year to present to this society and which I consider very successful indeed, and yet the gastro-enterologist is not at all willing to accept the statement that operation is The Thing !"

DR. WM. LINDER, in discussion, said:—"For the last year and a half I have been keen on this subject, and since seeing Mr. Lane in London and having had a personal talk with him, I have examined every case to see if we had a Lane kink, to try and substantiate his claim that the ulcer was secondary to the intestinal sepsis, and in no case which we would consider as coming under the head of a gastro-enterostomy incision have I found it; but in six cases I found probable Lane kinks where the patients had decided stomach symptoms, four of whom were operated upon for ulcer of the stomach; where I found no ulcer, but there were not sufficient adhesions about the cecum and distant angulation of the ilium to cause distress, and yet in those cases I found a marked degree of gastric ptosis and all were relieved by liberating the ilium and also doing a Robsinck's operation for gastric ptosis.

"I could not see the rationale of his argument, and, as I said, I failed to find a given case of ulcer associated with this kinking of the ilium, and, therefore, I still think gastro-enterostomy, or excision of the ulcer, will have to be performed as we did heretofore."

## Amputation of Hip-Joint.

### *Discussion.*

Dr. ALEXANDER P. RAE, in discussion, said:—"In two cases of that kind, secondary operations at the hip-joint, for the control of hemorrhage, we used the old French hemostat with the thumb-screw arrangement over the femoral artery and it worked as well as any means we have yet had for controlling the hemorrhage. It was applied with the screw down tight, with a sterile bandage, held by an assistant so as not to slip. An incision was made and the operation was practically bloodless; so some of the old means of controlling hemorrhage are still in vogue."

Dr. R. W. WESTBROOK, in discussion, said:—"In amputation of the hip-joint I have used Wyeth's pins with much satisfaction. In the case of Dr. Rankin I was glad to note that he left the head of the femur in the acetabulum, as it seems to me that this does away with a difficult enucleation."

Dr. WM. H. RANKIN, in closing the discussion, said:—"I would like to change the expression 'threadbare' to perhaps 'a little timid;' as the subject has been discussed so frequently before, I considered that they were rather anomalous cases, and I therefore venture to do so.

"I am in accord with those gentlemen who believe that not all stomach symptoms are caused by Lane's bands. I remember, and I think Dr. Kirk recalls very well, the case of a man who had a very extraordinary condition in that a loop of the ilium was fastened in the pelvis by a reflected fold of the perineum and this finally got up an intestinal obstruction, but never in his life did he have any stomach symptoms. Practically the last six inches were bound down in his pelvis all his life and he never had any stomach symptoms except the belching of gas.

"I believe that with the happy results we secure after operation there is no reason why the operation should not be continued."

"In regard to the point mentioned about leaving the head of the bone in the acetabulum, this was simply done to get rid of that fold and have enough drainage or we would have to leave the acetabulum empty, and also because one gets a primary union and no hemorrhage."

## Appendicitis.  Thrombosis of Mesenteric Vessels.  Gangrene of Intestine.

### *Discussion.*

Dr. JOHN C. MACEVITT reported the case of a young woman of 26 upon whom he performed a laparotomy for the relief of pelvic distress. Upon opening the abdomen there presented a dark spot about 6 cm. across that suggested to the doctor and his assistants the presence of an ectopic gestation. Upon inspection this was found to be a portion of the small intestine which was of a dark slate color. After some hesitation it was decided not to operate upon the intestine, though both tubes and ovaries were removed. The abdomen was flushed with saline solution and the wound closed without drainage. No history of previous intestinal symptoms was obtained. The patient recovered. Upon subsequent consideration, while in some doubt, he was inclined to believe that a mesenteric thrombosis might have been the cause.

Dr. J. A. LEE, in discussion, stated:—That because of a case of mesenteric thrombosis that he had previously reported to the Society, he had been led to review the literature, in particular an article by Dr. Eliot, on this subject. He quoted Dr. Eliot as showing that one frequent cause of thrombosis is a preceding acute infection of the abdomen, such as appendicitis. He summarized the history of his case as follows:

"The patient entered the hospital with the diagnosis of intestinal obstruction. Neither gas nor feces had passed the bowel. There was no temperature. Pulse was normal. There was comparatively little tenderness to pressure, but the abdomen had a doughy feel. There was no previous history of pain or of accident or injury. Upon operation it was found that a thrombosis of the mesenteric vessels of the small intestines had produced gangrene of about two feet of the gut. The patient succumbed a day after an attempt at resection."

From this experience, as well as Dr. Eliot's paper, Dr. Lee concluded: First that diagnosis before operation must of necessity be infrequent. Second that if operation is attempted it should be merely to remove the gangrenous portion, leaving the cut end of the gut in the wound for subsequent anastomosis.

REPORT OF CASES.

*By Alexander Rae, M.D.*

Mr. B., age 65. Received in hospital 7.30 P. M., June, 1911. History: No movement of bowel for two days; vomited before coming to hospital; not fecal. Moderate fullness of abdomen but no tension; moderate pain in umbilical region; enema after entering hospital, no result. Respiration normal. Pulse 84, of good quality. No evident signs of shock.

Operation 8.30 P. M. ¬Anæsthetic, ether and oxygen.

As incision through skin was made, patient ceased breathing and in spite of all efforts could not be revived. After twenty minutes, there being no doubt that he had passed on, operation autopsy was preceded with. On opening abdomen there came into view a coil of small intestine, about four inches of which was gangrenous, with a well-marked line of demarcation at each end of this segment.

Incision enlarged downward; cæcum and appendix brought into view; the appendix from tip to base was jet black and without luster.

No history of an attack of appendicitis had been obtained. The sequence of events seemed to have been, inflammation of appendix, thrombosis of a mesenteric arterial branch, and resulting gangrene of segment of bowel.

The case being suggestive in several directions, and thinking it might interest the Society, I venture to report it.

Shock in obstruction of the bowels is often underestimated, and a sufficient degree of concealed shock may be present to account for a sudden exit. It is not difficult to understand the gangrene of the intestine as a result of the thrombosis. It is more difficult to understand how the attack of appendicitis passed without compelling the patient to seek relief.

This demonstrated condition suggests two possibilities. Assuming the sequence—appendicitis, thrombosis, gangrene—to be correct, a corresponding condition might occur:

1st. In developing an appendix by finger dissection in a mass of adhesions and in an altered circulation containing thrombotic veins. A thrombus might be set free which, lodging in a mesenteric arterial branch, would produce gangrene which would cause symptoms three or four days after operation, with a rapid collapse and fatal issue.

2nd. A thrombus might be detached spontaneously from the impeded circulation in the region of the appendix, and a similar issue result.

May not this sequence account for a fatal outcome in some cases?

DR. WM. LINDER, in discussion, said:—"About two years ago I was summoned to a patient about 22 years of age, with severe abdominal symptoms and vomiting, but no cecal pain in the right iliac region. I made a tentative diagnosis of appendicitis. On bedside examination I had felt a mass that was not present when examined under ether at the hospital. I began to look for a possible kidney that had slipped up, but couldn't get it down. This patient had very similar conditions to those mentioned by Dr. Rae. Two constricting bands were found and a portion of the ilium was involved. I had in mind a thrombosis but the question at that time was left unsolved and remained so until about six months after, when I was summoned to a child who had distinct onset of intestinal intussusception. This child was an early case, only six hours from the time of onset of severe pain and vomiting and rectal tenesmus. I felt a suspicious bulging in the rectum. The child was put under anesthesia and the abdomen opened and I saw the ilium just about to pass out from the cecum, which caused the trouble. In this latter case there were two distinct constricting bands. The second case explains the etiology of the first case. Both have recovered.

"To my mind, those two cases prove that if we find blackening of a small portion of the ilium near the ileocecal junction and there are no bands to explain it, we should consider the probability of a thrombosis of the mesenteric vessels or an intussusception which has relieved itself."

DR. H. B. DELATOUR, in discussion, said:—"I agree with Dr. Linder as to the probability of the cases cited being gangrene following an intussusception which had been relieved. I have seen one or two cases like them, and cases of intussusception where the gut has been withdrawn at the time of operation will give exactly the same appearance as he described. In cases of thrombosis of the mesenteric vessels the symptoms come on acutely, generally indicating acute intestinal obstruction. This is due to the fact that the portion of bowel which becomes rapidly gangrenous loses its muscular tone and loses power to empty itself, and that section becomes a closed part of the canal.

"Dr. Lee has given us a very gloomy picture of these cases, but I think that if he will look into the literature he will find he is mistaken. There are a number of cases of recovery reported.

"The tendency in doing a resection is not to go far enough beyond the line of demarcation, for if you go up close to the apparent gangrene you are very likely to have further sloughing take place. In a case of gangrene following constriction, as in hernia, you have an absolute point of demarcation due to pressure. Where you have gangrene due to thrombosis, the amount of involvement depends on the distance from the intestine that the vessel is blocked. In thrombosis you cannot be sure that the apparent line of demarcation entirely covers the area involved in the lack of blood supply; so, therefore, we must go well beyond the gangrene in making our anastomosis, otherwise a fatal result will follow due to gangrene taking place at the point of operation.

"I would feel very strongly in any case against operating in the small intestine and bringing the free ends out on to the abdomen. I have seen three cases of this character and they rapidly died because of starvation. I believe that, serious as these cases appear to be, if the patient is sufficiently strong to submit to primary operation at all, we should do a complete operation."

DR. ALEXANDER RAE, in closing the discussion, said:—"I am very much pleased that the report has brought out so much discussion.

"It remains to call attention to this possibility. Having dealt with the gangrenous intestine, the chances are many that the abdomen would have been closed, without discovering the lesion in the appendix. In this instance, complications must have resulted in a few days, attributed wrongly to the intestinal condition, and a fatal result ensue. Hence, examine carefully the appendix in all similar cases."

DR. JAMES P. WARBASSE, in discussion, said:—"If I may be allowed, Mr. President, I would like to endorse the suggestion made by Dr. Lee. There are cases, with a lesion high up in the small intestine, in so desperate a condition that resection means death.

"It is true, as Dr. Delatour said, that these patients are apt to die of inanition if enterostomy is done. One of the German surgeons, whose name escapes me now, has reported his treatment of just such cases wherein he collected the discharge from the proximal end of the small intestine, and reinjected it into the distal segment of the small intestine, and thus prevented the condition which Dr. Delatour has alluded to."

### The Anatomy of the Patellar Ligaments.

*By James P. Warbasse, M.D.*

*(See page 135.)*

DR. H. B. DELATOUR, in discussion, said:—"I think this is a very fortunate matter to bring before us. Those of us who have operated and observed cases of fracture of the patella feel that, as Dr. Warbasse has said, it is a very important surgical and anatomical matter. If we take a case of direct fracture of the patella by injury, by direct blow, the patella may be broken into a number of fragments and still the patient will be able to get up and walk. If the patella is broken by indirect violence, by muscular contraction, it is seldom that patient has any power to support himself on the affected limb. The reason for this is that in a direct fracture the bone is broken by the impact of the blow, and only the bone itself is broken, whereas in an indirect one there is a tearing of the lateral ligaments or expansion of the vastus muscle as it passes down on either side of the joint. I do not mean to convey by these remarks that in direct fracture of the patella the patient can always walk, but we can have the patella broken into a number of fragments by direct injury without tearing the lateral ligaments.

"The necessity of operation, to my mind, consists in the ability of the patient to use the limb. If we find the patient has been able to stand and support himself, or herself, on the leg after the injury ,we can be practically satisfied that there is no lateral tear and that the bone alone is involved, and in these cases many excellent results are obtained without suture. Where the tear comes laterally, the continuation down of the vastus muscle, then operation is certainly indicated and operation is absolutely of no value unless the tears are sutured, and if you will follow down you will find the tear passes well back, often to the posterior ligaments of the knee-joint. It has been my custom for years to rely almost absolutely on the lateral sutures for bringing the bone in position. I use always a chromicized catgut and the sutures are simply of the fibrous covering. As Dr. Warbasse has stated, I believe the suturing of the bone is much less important than the suturing of the lateral expansion."

DR. ALEXANDER RAE, in discussion, said:—"That presentation of this subject was fortunate, inasmuch as it brought out the value of bony crepitus as a diagnostic sign, for he believed that it was safe to treat cases in which crepitus could be elicited by simple approximation, while the absence of crepitus indicated a considerable tear of what some anatomists call the supernumerary extensor apparatus, which, when present, allows the soft parts to fall between the fragments and demands careful anatomic repair in order to assure bony union."

DR. N. P. GEIS, in discussion, said:—"The point regarding the relations of the patella, lateral ligaments and vastus muscle has been taught in the Department of Anatomy at Long Island Hospital for some years.

"Regarding the question of suture when crepitus is elicited, I recall a case where we got crepitus very easily; the patient was thrown from a wagon and landed on his knee—evidently a direct break; we got crepitus easily and I operated and found the lateral ligaments torn, as Dr. Delatour said, down almost to the posterior aspect of the knee-joint; we sutured that up, not interfering with the bone at all except to clean it out and bring it as near as possible by suturing the ligaments. Three months later he broke it again by muscular action, but not where the bony union had taken place, half an inch above that, and the ligament was torn above the place where it united before. This latter break, as I said, was by muscular action and we got no crepitus."

DR. R. W. WESTBROOK, in discussion, said:—"It would seem to me from Dr. Warbasse's description of the diagram shown, that the vastus and rectus ligamentous expansions are not so firmly united to the patella as I believe they must be. They are certainly in a measure practically inserted into the patella, for otherwise I do not believe that it would be possible to fracture the patella by muscular action.

"I have dissected quite a good many patellas also, and I have operated on a good many, and always paid great attention to the suturing of the lateral tears, the necessity of which Scudder pointed out quite a number of years ago. It seems to me those ligamentous attachments are very firmly adherent to the patella. Perhaps I have misunderstood Dr. Warbasse in the impression that they can be so readily separated from the patella proper."

DR. W. A. SHERWOOD, in discussion, said:—"I would like to ask how many cases of rupture of the quadriceps extensor tendon the members of this Society have seen? Until last week I can't recollect having seen but one and that was a case of Dr. Royale H. Fowler's. I find, on looking it up, that it is a very rare accident and very little is said about it in the literature. I would be interested to hear how many cases the members of this Society have seen."

[NOTE.—A gentleman in the first row stated he had had one; Dr. J. P. Murphy stated he had had three last month (November, 1912); Dr. Alexander Rae stated he had had two, and Dr. R. W. Westbrook stated he had had several that might be added to the number.]

DR. JAMES P. WARBASSE, in closing the discussion, said:—"I do not know that I may add anything of interest, except to correct the impression of the President. The ligamentous structures in front of the patella, as we all are aware, are very closely adherent to the patella. However, the two structures may be observed in the ordinary transverse fracture. You will recall, in fractures of the patella, the torn-out, ragged ends of the fascia. The fibres which represent the continuation of the rectus tendon, lying close to the bone, are glistening and ragged. The aponeurotic part of the prepatellar ligament is usually torn more cleanly across and has more the character of fascia or aponeurosis. These two structures are easily distinguished in the ordinary transverse fracture; both of them tend to curl backward. It is in the rectus tendon that it is difficult to make a suture hold. Any suture will be seen to pull out that the surgeon attempts to introduce without making a mattress suture. It is not my intention to discuss the treatment of fracture of the patella, as I have discussed that so frequently here already."

5

# edical Society of the County of Kings

## MONTHLY BULLETIN TO MEMBERS

NDER the direction of the Council this Bulletin is issued every month (except July, Aug. and Sept.). It is the purpose of the Council, rough this medium, to keep the members advised all matters pertaining to the Society's work, its rious activities, its membership, and other subjects general interest.

Items of general interest to the Society and pernal notes concerning its members are invited and ould reach the Secretary not later than 4 P. M. the 20th of each month. Address all communitions to the Society's Building, 1313 Bedford Ave., rooklyn, N. Y.

### MEDICAL SOCIETY OF THE COUNTY OF KINGS.

313 Bedford Avenue, Brooklyn, New York.

Telephone: 126 Bedford.

---

HE Medical Society of the County of Kings (organized 1822) owns its plant, valued at $100,000, and located at 1313-1315 edford Avenue. In addition to an auditoum (seating 400) and various smaller meetg rooms, offices, etc., the greater part of the iilding is devoted to the Society's medical brary of 60,000 volumes. There are only iree larger medical libraries on this continent. 1 the ample reading rooms over 600 current edical journals are regularly on file.

Through its public and scientific meetings, s Library, its Milk Commission, and its manild activities for the spread of medical knowlge, the promotion of scientific education, the nity of the medical profession, and the safeiarding of the public health, the Medical Soety of the County of Kings should enlist the :tive support and co-operation of every putable physician in the county who is enaged in regular practice.

### MEMBERSHIP.

*Qualifications for Membership.*—Extracts om the Constitution and By-Laws governing iembership (Chapter XVI) are as follows: Sec. 1. Membership in the Society may be )tained by physicians in good standing, residig in the County of Kings, and duly licensed id recorded in the office of the County Clerk f Kings County, in the following manner: ec. 2. Applications for membership shall be ade on blanks furnished by the Medical Soety signed by the applicant and endorsed by vo members of the County Society. Such anks shall be sent to the Secretary, who shall :esent them to the Board of Censors for inistigation and report. Sec. 3. If the candi-

date be accepted the Council shall so report to the Society at a stated meeting, and after the next succeeding stated meeting the President shall declare said candidate a member. Sec. 4. Every person thus admitted resident member shall, within three months after due notification of his election, pay an initiation fee of five dollars and the assessment of the Medical Society of the State of New York for the current year, sign the By-Laws or forfeit his election."

*Blank Application Forms for Membership* may be obtained on request at the Society's Building. This form should be filled out by the applicant, signed by him, his proposer and his seconder, and returned to the Secretary.

*Dues.*—New members pay an initiation fee of $5 plus $3 (the State assessment for the current year) and are exempt from the payment of further dues until the next annual meeting after their election.

The regular annual dues are $10 plus $3 (the State assessment for the current year), payable on the first day of February. All members who have not paid on or before the first day of May shall be placed on the list of members in arrears and so reported to the Society, and shall not receive the publications, or notices of meetings, or defense for suits for malpractice until their dues are paid. All members who fail to pay their arrears on or before December 31st shall be dropped from the roll of membership (Chapter XV of By-Laws).

*Advantages of Membership.*—Affiliation with your confreres in the representative medical organization of your County, participation in the Society's meetings and varied activities, and proprietary interest in its property and magnificent library, membership in the Medical Society of the State of New York and the Second District Branch; monthly receipt of the *New York State Journal of Medicine* and the Society's own publications, a copy yearly of the *Medical Directory of New York, New Jersey and Connecticut;* free defense to the court of last resort of all suits for alleged malpractice; eligibility to membership in the American Medical Association.

---

### STATED MEETINGS.

Regular stated meetings of the Society are held in the Society's Building, 1313 Bedford Ave., at 8.30 P. M., on the third Tuesday of every month (except July, August and September). Light refreshments are served at the social hour which follows the scientific program of each meeting.

## THE LIBRARY.

The Library (60,000 vols.) of the Society is open daily (Sundays and Legal Holidays excepted), from 10 A. M. to 10 P. M. For the purposes of reference it is free to the public. Members of the Society have the privilege of borrowing books. Trained librarians are always in attendance to help and direct readers who desire such assistance.

## DIRECTORY FOR GRADUATE NURSES.

For the benefit of the profession and the general public the Society maintains a Directory for Graduate Nurses, where reliable graduate nurses (male and female), masseurs and masseuses may be procured. There is no fee for securing a nurse through the Society's Directory, which is always open, day and night. Telephone 126 Bedford.

## THE COUNCIL.

*President*—JAMES M. WINFIELD, 47 Halsey St.
*Vice-President*—J. RICHARD KEVIN.
*Secretary*—CLAUDE G. CRANE, 121 St. James Pl.
*Associate Secretary*—BURTON HARRIS.
*Treasurer*—JOHN R. STIVERS, 180 Lefferts Pl.
*Associate Treasurer*—STEPHEN H. LUTZ.
*Directing Librarian*—FREDERICK TILNEY.

### Trustees.

ONSLOW A. GORDON, *Chairman,* 71 Halsey St.
JOSHUA M. VAN COTT.    JOHN O. POLAK.
JOHN C. MACEVITT.    ELIAS H. BARTLEY.

### Censors.

JOHN A. LEE, *Senior Censor,* 23 Revere Pl.
WALTER A. SHERWOOD.    JOHN G. WILLIAMS.
CHARLES EASTMOND.    J. STURDIVANT READ.

## CHAIRMEN OF STANDING COMMITTEES.

*Membership*—EDWARD E. CORNWALL, 1218 Pacihc St.
*Directory for Nurses*—CALVIN F. BARBER, 57 So. Oxford St.
*Entertainment*—ALFRED POTTER, 491 Eighth St.
*Historical*—WILLIAM SCHROEDER, 339 President St.
*Legislative*—HENRY G. WEBSTER, 364 Washington Ave.
*Public Health*—J. M. VAN COTT, 188 Henry St.
*Visiting*—JAMES W. FLEMING, 471 Bedford Ave.
*Milk Commission*—ALFRED BELL, 37 Linden St.
*Attendance*—ALBERT M. JUDD, 375 Grand Ave.

In the conduct of the affairs of the Society the officers hope that they may have not only the frequent suggestions of members, which are heartily invited, but also their practical and loyal co-operation.

*Supt. and Librarian*—ALBERT T. HUNTINGTON.
*Counsel*—WILLIAM E. BUTLER, Esq.
*Prosecuting Attorneys*—Messrs. ALMUTH C. VAN DIVER and JOHN G. DYER, 34 Nassau St., New York City.

## MINUTES OF STATED MEETING MARCH 18, 1913.

The President, Dr. James M. Winfield, the chair.
There were about 80 present.
The meeting was called to order at P. M. and the minutes of the previous meet were read and approved.

*Report of Council.*

The Council reported favorably upon following applications for membership:

William Murray Ennis, 31 First Pl.; gradu of Fordham Univ., 1910; proposed L. J. J. Commiskey and second by A. Judd.

Gustav Adolf Mäusert, 687 Bushwick A\ graduate of Univ. Giessen, 1899; propo by C. W. Stickle and seconded by J. Sheppard.

Jacob Sarnoff, 1819 85th St.; graduate N. Y. Univ, 1908; proposed by E. Mayne and seconded by Memb. Com.

Henry L. Wagner, 468 12th St.; graduate Univ. and Bell., 1911; proposed by N. Beers and seconded by R. W. W\ brook.

## ELECTION OF MEMBERS.

The following, duly proposed and accep by the Council, will be declared elected active membership at this meeting:

William H. Best, 1198 Bushwick Ave., gra ate of Univ. of Penn., 1909; proposed J. M. Winfield and seconded by E. Cornwall; December, 1912.

Isidor Betz, 108 Harrison Ave.; graduate L. I. C. H., 1910; proposed by E. E. Co wall and seconded by Memb. Com.; cember, 1912.

Eugene S. Dalton, 694 E. 5th St.; graduate Syracuse, 1908; proposed by E. E. Co wall and seconded by C. G. Crane; Ja ary, 1913.

Francis B. Hart, 812 Lafayette Ave.; gradu of P. and S., N. Y., 1905; proposed E. E. Cornwall and seconded by Me\ Com.; December, 1912.

Benjamin Koven, 1521 Eastern Parkway; gr uate of Univ. and Bell, 1908; proposed S. R. Blatteis and seconded by Me\ Com.; December, 1912.

Hyman S. Shlevin, 161 No. 6th St.; gradu of Yale Med Sch., 1892; proposed by E. Cornwall and seconded by Memb. Co\ November, 1912.

## APPLICATIONS FOR MEMBERSH

Applications for membership were recei\ from the following:

Edward B. Haslam, 71 Oakland St.; gra ate of N. Y. Univ., 1897; proposed T. H. McKinnon and seconded by Me\ Com.; March, 1913.

Harlan E. Linehan, 74 Norman Ave.; graduate of Baltimore Med. Coll., 1907; proposed by T. H. McKinnon and seconded by Memb. Com.; March, 1913.

Julius M. Nova, 1 Hanson Pl.; graduate of L. I. C. H., 1902; proposed by E. E. Cornwall and seconded by Memb. Com.; March, 1913.

Henry Wolfer, 678 Bedford Ave.; graduate of Univ. and Bell., 1908; proposed by T. Howard and seconded by J. A. Longmore; February, 1913.

2. Paper—"Vaccination and Anti-V tion" (illustrated by lantern s By Jay Frank Shamberg, State sioner ot Vaccination of P vania.
   Discussion by Mr. Frank W. and Dr. T. R. Maxfield, and by Dr. Shamberg.

A vote of thanks was tendered Dr. berg.

Meeting adjourned at 11 P. M.

CLAUDE G. CRANE, Secr

## EXECUTIVE SESSION.

The report of the Committee on the President's Address was read by Dr. Humpstone. The Committee presented eleven recommendations which were voted upon individually by the members. (The President's Address and the Committee report, together with the recommendations which ·were voted upon, will appear elsewhere in the JOURNAL.)

A letter was read from Dr. Burton Harris, enclosing a check for $300 to establish a fund for the purchase of literature bearing on the Surgery of the Genito-urinary Tract. It was moved, seconded and carried that the foregoing amount be made the nucleus of a fund, to be known as the Burton Harris Fund for the Purchase of Literature Bearing on the Surgery of the Genito-urinary Tract.

The President announced that he had appointed on the Press Censorship Committee, Drs. McEvitt, Van Cott and Tilney.

The President stated that at the last meeting of the Council he was directed to appoint a committee on education and that he had appointed as Chairman Dr. Kevin, the other members to be announced later.

The President presented the report of the Counsel with a request for funds to carry on the work. It was moved, seconded and carried that a committee of twelve be appointed to solicit funds from those who did not contribute last year.

The President read the following Necrology:

Philip Hansen Hiss, Jr., February 27, 1913. Member 1906-13.

John Davies Trezise, March 4, 1913. Member 1908-13.

William Arthur Little, February 24, 1913. Member 1879-1909.

## SCIENTIFIC SESSION.

1. Paper—"Meningitis in an Infant Caused by the Typhoid Bacillus."
   By Harold W. Lyall, of the Hoagland Laboratory.
   Discussion by Frederick Tilney and closed by Mr. Lyall.

## REPORT OF THE PROSECU ATTORNEY OF THE SOCIE

*To the Council of the Medical Society of the County of Kings.*

GENTLEMEN:—We have the honor 1 mit herewith- a *résumé* of the work c Counsel for the period of time from F 14, 1912, to March 12, 1913.

This report is the third annual one re to the Council of the Society.

Your Counsel feels that the rigid in\ tion of midwives and druggists by the tigators has made them more careful i ing the public generally. Charges of fraud are not as frequently made to- they were some years ago. This is do due to the fact that the person who s violate the medical law realizes that h it at the risk of arrest and prosecution

The Federal authorities have wor conjunction with your Counsel. As a of this the arrest and holding for trial R. Curtis Gray, on a charge of imp using the mails, resulted. Dr. Gray is ing trial in the United States District It is claimed that he induced patients t to his office for the purpose of perf abortions upon them.

The Board of Health refers complai rectly to your Counsel for action.

Your Counsel desires to take this tunity to thank the Board of City Mag; of the Second Division, and the Justi the Court of Special Sessions, and the bers of the Detective Bureau and Poli partment for their interest in violati the medical law, and for the assistanc dered to him in prosecuting and pu them.

A great amount of time has been gi your Counsel and his investigators to jng accurate information concerning plaints sent to the office.

Many persons have been interviewed office and advice concerning the indiv particular case has been cheerfully give

Fines imposed and paid during th year have amounted to $250.

Your Counsel desires the Society to that some cases have required as many teen court appearances and the prepa and submission of briefs to many of the City Magistrates.

Your Counsel feels that the work of the Society in attempting to suppress quackery has a great preventive effect and is beneficial especially to the credulous and ignorant portion of the community.

A more detailed account of the work done is contained in the following summary:

PEOPLE vs. PETER MANISCALCO, ANGELO LICAUSI, and LOUIS ROBERTS.

The defendants in this case had their place of business at 5523 New Utrecht Avenue, Brooklyn. A complaint had been received concerning an advertisement which appeared in the Italian newspapers. This advertisement stated that Prof. Maniscalco had a magnetic sanitarium, wherein absolute cures for practically every known disease could be obtained either by consultation or by mail.

An Italian investigator and a woman investigator employed by your Counsel were directed to investigate Maniscalco.

Maniscalco and one Licausi examined the woman investigator and gave a peculiar treatment consisting of waving a glass globe filled with green powder before the eyes of the patient, and assuring the patient at the same time that she should sleep and think only of sleep and all her diseases would disappear. A handkerchief was placed upon the back of the patient's neck and Licausi blew his breath upon the handkerchief twelve times.

Licausi manipulated the spine and the ankle of the patient.

Roberts acted as secretary, took the money for the treatment and gave the receipt. He also informed the investigator that he financed the business.

Upon a warrant the defendants Maniscalco and Roberts were arrested and held, after the submission of a brief to the magistrate, for trial in the Court of Special Sessions.

The defendant Licausi escaped arrest and has not as yet been apprehended.

It is reported that while in jail Maniscalco attempted to take his life.

Finally, on January 22d, the defendants, after trial, were found guilty by Justices Collins and Salmon and Chief Justice Russell. The defendants were sentenced to serve three months each in the City Prison. The conviction of Roberts in this case was especially pleasing, inasmuch as he was the person supplying the money for the carrying on of the business, according to his own statement.

PEOPLE vs. LOUIS H. WARNER.

The defendant in this case had his office at 1078 Park Place, Brooklyn. Upon his prescription blanks and upon a sign in his window, he called himself Louis H. Warner, M.D. The defendant had a fine apartment in which he claimed that he maintained a laboratory for chemical research work.

One Flitcroft E. Evans, a resident of Brooklyn, complained of his treatment by Warner.

Warner examined him and took a blood prescribed for him and injected a liquid his body for either "scarlet fever or meas

A further investigation was made by woman investigator, from whom the defen also took a blood test and stated tha would send the result of the blood test to through the mails. The defendant did send the result of the blood test.

Many complaints had been received con ing the defendant for a period covering than two years, but evidence sufficient to tify his arrest had not been presented in case.

After examination in the Magistrates' the defendant was held to await trial ir Court of Special Sessions in $500 bail. He tried on the 6th day of March, 1913, b Justices Salmon, Zeller and Moss. The fendant entered a plea of guilty.

He stated to the court that he was a gr ate of Heidelberg, and that more than fi years ago he had gone to the office of Clerk of the County of New York, paid clerk there a quarter, showed his diplom him, and that from that time he believe was properly registered, although he hac taken any of the state medical examinati

The court, unfortunately not being position to know definitely and certainly facts other than the facts presented in complaint concerning the defendant, sente the defendant to pay a fine of $50 or to ten days in the City Prison. The fine paid.

Justice Moss dissented from the view o colleagues and stated that a more severe tence should be imposed. A convictio Warner was a pleasing one in view of the that the defendant had been practicing cine in the City of Brooklyn for the pas teen years, and that during the past three many complaints had been received concei him.

PEOPLE vs. CHARLES MILDENBERGER.

The defendant in this case had his offi No. 61a Palmetto Street, Brooklyn. He vertised himself as an osteopath. He convicted during the year 1911, and the r of his conviction was contained in the annual report of Counsel to the Society.

The defendant, despite his conviction turned to practice. Evidence against him obtained by the male investigator, to who gave a form of osteopathic treatment. defendant also prescribed medicine. Up card bearing his picture he advertised to practically every known disease.

In view of the defendant's age, the c composed of Justices Russell, Zeller McInerny, sentenced him to pay a fine of or to serve thirty days in the City Pr The defendant paid the fine.

PEOPLE vs. HENRY J. KEMPF.

The defendant in this case was a dru and the proprietor of the drug store a' corner of Seigel and Lorimer Streets and Broadway, Brooklyn. Many complaints had been received concerning him.

Evidence sufficient to justify his arrest was obtained by the male investigator. The defendant treated the male investigator for a supposed venereal disease. He prescribed medicine and also used an injection.

The defendant, after examination in the Magistrates' Court, was discharged by Magistrate Hylan on July 31, 1912.

### PEOPLE VS. FRANK A. URBAN.

The defendant in this case was a druggist with his place of business at 151 Metropolitan Avenue, Brooklyn. Several complaints had been received concerning him. Evidence sufficient to justify his arrest was obtained by the male investigator. He treated the male investigator for a supposed venereal disease.

After examination in the Magistrates' Court, the defendant was held to await trial in the Court of Special Sessions. The defendant, after much delay, was finally tried before Justices Steinert, O'Keefe and Collins. Justice Collins voted to convict the defendant. Justices Steinert and O'Keefe voted to acquit the defendant.

The defendant stated that he was a graduate of the Columbia College of Pharmacy, and that he had educated himself by his own efforts and that he was a medical student.

### PEOPLE VS. JOHN ARFMANN.

The defendant in this case was a druggist who had his store at the corner of Fifth Avenue and Bergen Street, Brooklyn. Many complaints were received concerning him. Evidence that he was selling drugs for the purpose of causing unlawful abortion was obtained by the woman investigator.

He waived examination in the Magistrates' Court and was held for trial in the Court of Special Sessions. The defendant pleaded guilty on November 13th before Justices Forker, Collins and Fleming. Justices Forker and Collins sentenced the defendant to pay a fine of $25. Justice Fleming dissented from the opinion of his colleagues, stating that a long prison sentence should be given to the defendant.

### PEOPLE VS. MANFRED BROBERG.

The defendant in this case was a mechanotherapist, who had his place of business at No. 49 Nevins Street, Brooklyn. A report of his case was contained in the last annual report.

On February 15, 1912, the Court of Special Sessions sentenced the defendant to pay a fine of $25 or to stand committed to the City Prison for thirty days. The defendant paid the fine.

A notice of appeal from the conviction was served upon the District Attorney. The appeal was not prosecuted by the defendant.

### PEOPLE VS. GIOACCHINO STABILI.

The defendant in this case was an unregistered physician, who had his office at No Crescent Street, Brooklyn. Complaints received that he was treating Italians i neighborhood. Evidence sufficient to j the arrest of the defendant was obtaine the Italian male investigator, and the de ant was arraigned in the Magistrate's C He was held to await trial in the Cou Special Sessions. His case is now pendi

### PEOPLE VS. LOUIS BELL.

The defendant in this case was the prietor of a drug store at 403 Myrtle Av Brooklyn. Many complaints concerning sale of abortion drugs by him had bee ceived. Evidence sufficient to justify hi rest was obtained by the woman investi to whom he sold drugs for the purpo procuring a miscarriage at about six of pregnancy. The defendant made and pared a special liquid which he guara would cause an abortion.

The defendant waived examination i Magistrates' Court and was held to await in the Court of Special Sessions. His has appeared upon the calendar four or times and has been adjourned at the re of the defendant. A vigorous defense i pected from the defendant in this case. case is set for trial on March 19, 1913.

### PEOPLE VS. EDGAR G. BRADFORD.

The defendant in this case had his at 32 Putnam Avenue, Brooklyn. He a tised himself as a physiological engine hygienic specialist and chiropractor. H sued flamboyant literature, advertising patients whose cases had not been cure regular physicians. Evidence was obt against him by the male investigator.

He was arrested and arraigned before istrate Hylan, of the Gates Avenue C After an examination, at which only the dence of the complaining witness was sented to the magistrate, and after the mission of briefs by counsel, at the re of the magistrate the case was dism Your Counsel does not understand wh case was dismissed. The facts were pres to the office of the District Attorney of County and an indictment of the defe requested. The case is now under consi tion by Assistant District Attorneys Eg ton and Kellogg.

Your Counsel expects that the defe will be indicted and tried before a jury i County Court.

### INVESTIGATIONS.

Complaints received concerning Mrs. drickson, 437 37th Street; Miss Steffin Eldert Street; Mary Basile, 518 Henry St Emma G. Damrau, Halsey Street, wer vestigated by the woman investigator.

The persons complained of were mid They refused to prescribe for the investi or to perform any illegal operations. No evidence sufficient to justify any action was obtained.

A complaint concerning one L. E. Ellis, a chiropractor at 195 Joralemon Street, was investigated. No such person was located at the address given.

A complaint against H. Lunz, 293 Thorpe Avenue, a mechano-therapist, was investigated by the male investigator. Lunz refused to treat.

A complaint that a Mrs. Levy, at 95 Boerum Street, was selling a special preparation for rheumatism, was investigated. Mrs. Levy denied that she had ever sold such a preparation.

A complaint concerning one Hirschner, 1391 Putnam Avenue, Brooklyn, was inquired into. Hirschner is a chiropodist. He referred the investigator to a medical doctor.

A complaint concerning a druggist, Greenspoon, at Georgia and Sutter Avenues, was investigated. He refused to prescribe abortion drugs and refused to treat venereal diseases.

A complaint concerning one Ernestus, a hypnotist, at 954 Broadway, Brooklyn, was investigated. This matter will receive further attention.

A complaint concerning a chiropractor, Flick, at 92 St. Marks Avenue, was inquired into. Mr. Flick appears to work under the protection of a registered physician. This matter will receive further attention.

A complaint concerning the Private Medical Bureau, 72 Havemeyer Street, was investigated. The premises are occupied by an Italian bank. Inquiry there revealed the fact that one Pasquale Gabrielli also had another office at 292 Third Avenue, Brooklyn. Inquiry

here showed that Gabrielli sells some ki a patent medicine. The investigators unable to meet Gabrielli.

One Smith, a druggist at 61 Sands' S refused to treat venereal diseases or t abortion drugs.

Arthur Borner, at 7108 14th Avenue, was convicted in New York City, stated he was now the agent for certain herb and other like medicinal preparations.

A druggist named Caputo, at the corn Franklin and Park Avenues, against wh complaint was made, is a medical studen

The above investigations are reported to the fact that complaints have been re more than once. It does not seem po to obtain evidence sufficient to justif taking of legal action in many comp sent to your Counsel.

The following is a list of conviction tained: Broberg, February 15, 1912, $ five days; Mildernberger, October 16, $150 or thirty days; Arfmann, Novemb 1912, $25 or five days; Warner, March 6, $50 or ten days; Maniscalco, January 22, three months; Roberts, January 22, 1913, months.

Defendants discharged in the Magist Courts: Kampf, July 31, 1912; Bra February 26, 1912.

Defendants discharged in the Court of cial Sessions: Urban, June 10, 1912.

Cases pending in the Magistrates' C Bell, Stabili.

All of which is respectfully submitted.

ALMUTH C. VANDIVE
*Coun*

JOHN G. DYER, of Counsel.

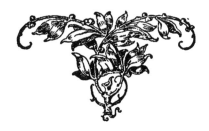

# CLINICS AT BROOKLYN HOSPITALS.

The following is a list of permanent Clinics supplied by the Clinical representatives various hospitals. Others will be added as soon as they are received by the Committ

R. L. DICKINSON, *Chairman*, } Clinical Committee, Medical Society County of Kin
W. A. SHERWOOD, *Secretary*, }

Daily bulletins of operations may be telephoned to the New York Academy of cine, where list will be posted.

**Telephone Numbers: 974 and 1304 Bryant**

## BROOKLYN HOSPITAL.

### General Surgery.
Dr. R. W. Westbrook, Tues., Thurs, Sat., 10-12
Dr. J. E. Jennings......Mon., Wed., Fri., 2-4

### Gynecology.
Dr. R. L. Dickinson....Mon., Wed., Fri., 10-12
Dr. A. A. Hussey ...Mon., Wed., Fri., 10-12

### Medical Clinic.
Dr. Glentworth R. Butler, or
Dr. Dudley D. Roberts ...........Thurs., 3

### Obstetrics.
Dr. R. H. Pomeroy....Mon., Wed., Fri., 10-12

### Ear, Nose and Throat.
Dr. C. Crane.....................Tues., 3-4
Dr. Shattuck ...................Thurs., 2-4

### Eye.
Dr. Jamieson ...................Thurs., 2-4
Miscellaneous, X-Ray, Laboratory, Diagnostic,

## BROOKLYN EYE AND EAR HOSPITAL.

### Eye.
Dr. J. S. Wood...........Mon. and Sat., 1-5
Dr. Snyder ......................Mon., 1-5
Dr. Waugh ......................Tues., 1-5
Dr. Meyer ...................Tues., Sat., 1-5
Dr. Bailey ......................Wed., 1-5
Dr. Ingalls ....................Thurs., 1-5
Dr. Simmons ..............Thurs., Fri., 1-5
Dr. Rushmore ....................Fri., 1-5
Dr. North ......................Fri., 1-5

### Ear.
Dr. Alderton ....................Mon., 1-5
Dr. Braislin ....................Tues., 1-5
Dr. Cox .........................Wed., 1-5
Dr. Shattuck ...................Thurs., 1-5
Dr. Lutz ........................Fri., 1-5
Dr. Collins .....................Sat., 1-5

### Nose and Throat.
Dr. Raynor ................Mon., Thurs., 3
Dr. Steers ............Mon., Thurs., Sat., 1
Dr. Arrowsmith .............Tues., Fri., 1.30
Dr. Tucker .............Wed., Fri., 1.30

## *BUSHWICK HOSPITAL.

## CONEY ISLAND HOSPITAL.

### Medicine.
Dr. Nash ......................Tues., 3.30
Dr. Hall ......................Tues., 3.30
Dr. Hegeman ...................Tues., 3.30
Dr. Byington ..................Tues., 3.30

### Surgery.
Dr. Fiske .....................Tues., 10.30
Dr. Bogart ...........Mon., Wed., Fri., 2
Dr. Murphy .............Tues., 10; Thurs., 3
Dr. Lack ..............Tues., 10; Thurs., 3

### Pediatrics.
Dr. Beck ..........................W
Dr. McQuillan ....................W
Dr. Pendleton .....................W
Dr. Van Wart .....................W

### Gynecology.
Dr. McEvitt .....................Thur
Dr. Mills .......................Thur
Dr. Mayne .......................Thur
Dr. Rankin ......................Thur

## CUMBERLAND STREET HOSPI

### Surgery.
Dr. R. F. Walmsley .........Mon., T
Dr. G. H. Iler .................Tues.,

### Laryngology & Rhinology.
Dr. Stewart .................Mon., T

### Oral Surgery.
Dr. B. F. Shea ..............Mon., F

### Ophthalmology & Otology.
Dr. Lloyd ....................Tues.,

### Gynecology.
Dr. W. H. Pierson, Wed.

## GERMAN HOSPITAL.

### General Surgery.
Dr. R. S. Fowler, Mon., Tues., Thurs.,
Dr. J. P. Warbasse.........Tues., Th

### Gynecology.
Dr. F. Weisbrod ..............Wed.,

### Ear, Nose and Throat.
Dr. J. H. Droge.................T

## *HOLY FAMILY HOSPITAL.

## JEWISH HOSPITAL.

### Gynecology.
Dr. A. M. Judd......Tues., Thurs., S
Dr. J. O. Polak .................Tu
No other entries.

## KINGS COUNTY HOSPITAL.

### G. U. Surgery.
Dr. H. H. Morton .................
Dr. H. Fraser ....................

### Obstetrics.
Dr. L. J. J. Commiskey..Tues., Thurs.,
Dr. A. M. Judd ...................Th

### Surgery.
Dr. A. T. Bristow......Tues., Thurs.,

### Dermatology.
Dr. James M. Winfield ..............

# LONG ISLAND
# MEDICAL JOURNAL

VOL. VII.          MAY, 1913          No. 5

## ®riginal Articles.

### THE THERAPEUTIC VALUE OF LUMBAR PUNCTURE.*

#### By Leon Louria, M.D.,
of Brooklyn, N. Y.

PERHAPS in no field of medicine are the clinician and the pathologist more intimately associated than in the study and observation of meningeal affections; and it is to the pathologist that the former is compelled to look to ascertain the true value of the information lumbar puncture may afford him.

In the discussion of the diagnostic and therapeutic value of lumbar puncture I shall pass briefly over the technic and application, which are so well known to you, and shall likewise say but a word on the pathological aspect of the cerebrospinal fluid, since not alone is this somewhat beyond my domain, but it has just been ably and comprehensibly covered by my predecessor of this evening.

As to the technic, I have found the left lateral prone position of the patient, originally recommended by Quincke, preferable, and deprecate the use of the sitting posture, in that the height of the column of cerebrospinal fluid causes it to gush out of the lumbar puncture and not alone gives rise to too sudden and extensive a drop in cerebrospinal pressure, as well as too great an evacuation of the fluid, but also gives the observer a distorted and erroneous conception of the existing spinal pressure.

Local anesthesia has always been employed in my cases excepting only in the cases of delirium, when the restlessness of the patient demanded otherwise.

As to the amount to be drained, 25 to 30 c.c. may be said to constitute a fair average, although in one of my cases of cerebrospinal meningitis even 220 c.c. were withdrawn at one time, and over 300 c.c. is recorded. However, the withdrawal of larger amounts than 30 c.c. is not usually warranted, for we do not seek to empty the cerebrospinal canal, but rather by the alleviation of pressure to break up the vicious circle of inflammatory reaction on the one hand, and the resultant over-secretion of cerebrospinal fluid and edema of the central nervous system on the other, which serve but to increase the intradural pressure, and by excessive pressure on the Pacchionian bodies in particular, prevent drainage.

In withdrawing fluid one should cease in the advent of sudden severe headache, collapse, fainting or marked drop in blood pressure.

---

* Read before the Brooklyn Pathological Society, November 19, 1912.

The use of the manometer in the determination of the spinal pressure is not needed for practical purposes, in that the apparatus is cumbersome, the *modus operandi* difficult, and moreover, a marked change in the propulsion of the fluid and decrease in the rate of flow are *per se* sufficient evidence as to when to cease tapping.

The use of the Sahli cannula to provide continuous drainage is rarely indicated, and similarly, the making of a crucial incision in the dura to provide patent drainage-way from the intra into the extra dural space and vessels.

The pathological examination of the spinal fluid embraces a chemical as well as a microscopical and bacteriological examination; whereas the former may be done immediately, the latter requires several hours to several days for complete cultural and morphological diagnosis. I shall add but a word to what Dr. Lederer has already told you of this interesting phase.

For practical and immediate purposes a chemical examination will throw material light on the character of the fluid. Whereas in health its reaction is alkaline or perhaps amphoteric, in disease it most often becomes acid, and with the Uffelman reagent one may readily demonstrate the presence of lactic (and allied) acids. The acidosis of the fluid is greater in severe cases, being in large part due to the edema of the brain and meninges. And though no parallelism has been shown to exist between the amount of acidosis and gravity of the condition, repeated observations have led to the belief that in general the higher grades of acidosis are found in the severer cases.

The diminution or absence of the Fehling reaction due to the disappearance of the carbohydrate components of the cerebrospinal fluid has been called to our attention by the previous speaker, and this is, perhaps, the earliest and most significant reaction from a clinical point of view. Much sooner than any other chemical changes take place the carbohydrates disappear from the fluid and their disappearance is constantly observed in cases of bacterial invasion of the cerebrospinal fluid, so that in the septic, pyogenic forms of meningitis the negative Fehling may be demonstrated even before the cultures and smears are positive. The Fehling reaction is negative in acute fulminant tubercular meningitis where the spinal canal is overwhelmed by the Koch bacilli, while in the insidious, slow developing, less acute forms of tubercular meningitis the Fehling reaction may be positive in the beginning of the disease, becoming negative later with the further invasion of the canal by the bacilli. The explanation of the foregoing chemical change is due to the fact that the carbohydrates of the cerebrospinal fluid are more easily broken up than other of its components, being used by the micro-organisms as a food. Therefore, the absence of the Fehling reaction is invariably the indicator of a bacterial meningitis, while in the toxic forms of meningeal inflammation the copper reducing bodies remain present. Here the changes in the meninges and the increased secretion are due to a chemical toxin which does not influence the carbohydrates. Continued observation of the Fehling reaction in the course of meningitis may also serve us as a basis for prognosis, for when on repeated puncture we find that the reaction slowly returns to normal, it may serve as an evidence of the abatement of the infection. I have dwelt at length on this simple reaction, within reach of every practitioner, because the possibility of early diagnosis and prognosis should not be denied to those who do not possess well equipped chemical and bacteriological laboratories at their ready disposal.

The increased amount of cerebrospinal fluid causes an increase of intracranial pressure. This is brought about by both the bacterial and toxic irritation of the meninges, which causes an increased secretion of the fluid, the outflow being impeded. As we know, the cerebrospinal fluid empties directly into the veins mainly through the so-called Pacchionian bodies, the intracranial pressure being slightly higher in health than the pressure in the veins, thus facilitating the outflow into the venous system. When the intracranial pressure is unduly raised, the organs which suffer from such an increased pressure are the blood and vascular system. The bones of the skull and spine do not give and the tissue of the brain, as we know, is not compressible, hence the result of the increase of intracranial pressure will be manifested in the altered cerebral circulation.

The interference with the cerebral circulation stimulates the medullary centers, inducing a rise in blood pressure to overcome the intracranial pressure, and the increased pressure together with the round cell infiltration of the Pacchionian bodies serves to make impossible proper drainage, and thus a vicious circle is established. Clinically such a process is manifested in the stimulation of the vasomotor, vagus and respiratory centers. Further clinical evidence is obtained by an examination of the eye-grounds.

We find the so-called edema of the papilla, which is due to the strangulation of the optic nerve by the cerebrospinal fluid, endeavoring to escape along the dural sheath. This condition of papilledema must be differentiated from the so-called choked disk, which is a later development and the evidence of continued compression. The edema of the papilla is an early symptom which disappears readily with the release of the cerebrospinal fluid.

The rise of the blood pressure can be easily ascertained by the sphygmomanometer and it parallels the variations of the intracranial pressure. With the diminution of the cerebrospinal pressure there occurs a fall of blood pressure, and simultaneously we notice the amelioration of the symptoms of the disease. The metabolic products of bacterial activity are poisonous toxins, and they produce a toxic effect on the nerve centers so that the clinical picture of meningitis is composed of symptoms due to the anemia of the brain on the one hand, plus the toxic effect on it by the metabolic products of bacteria on the other; but while the toxemia plays an important role in the composition of the clinical picture, the symptoms are mainly due to the anemia of the brain brought on by compression. This mechanical explanation, which has been ably demonstrated experimentally, is fully borne out by clinical and therapeutic observations. Therefore, the recognition of these facts determines the therapeutic value of lumbar puncture. It is impossible to divide the importance of lumbar puncture for diagnostic purposes from its therapeutic efficiency, for we know that the symptoms of meningitis are frequently identical irrespective of the causative organism. The meningococcus, pneumococcus, streptococcus and other pyogenic micro-organisms give clinical pictures which vary very little from one another, and only through the bacteriological examination of the contents of the cerebrospinal fluid are we in a position to make a correct etiological diagnosis. Upon the etiology will depend the prognosis and future treatment. We are all thoroughly familiar with the phenomenal successes attained by the injection of the anti-meningococcus serum in cases of epidemic cerebrospinal meningitis. The mortality of 75 per cent. has been reduced to about 30 per cent. since the introduction of the anti-meningococcus serum. Attempts have been made with the injections of a pneumococcus serum in cases of meningitis caused by the diplococcus pneumoniæ, and in three out of seven cases so treated recovery followed. Still less encouraging are the sero-therapeutic results in streptococcus meningitis. But in spite of the undeniable therapeutic value of the anti-meningococcus serum the majority of observers are of the opinion that the therapeutic effect is due in even larger extent to the repeated lumbar punctures. In the recent epidemic of cerebrospinal fever in Texas, much smaller quantities of serum were used than formerly. The amounts injected were always considerably below the quantity of fluid removed and it is interesting to note that the injections into the spinal canal were controlled by blood pressure readings. The intention of the observer was to keep the blood pressure continually at a lower level than it was before treatment was begun. The same observations have been made in the treatment of other forms of meningitis and it is a fully established fact that while the antitoxins are not to be denied their specific value, the main reliance in the treatment of meningitis must be placed upon repeated lumbar punctures and the reduction of intracranial pressure.

In cases of bacterial invasion of the meninges the lumbar puncture gives us a possibility of making a causative diagnosis and instituting a specific treatment, but in cases of meningitis due to non-bacterial toxic irritation of the meninges, the lumbar puncture has a direct curative effect. Take, for instance, cases of the so-called meningitides, where the pathologist fails to find any bacteria, but the cytology of the fluid shows a lymphocytosis, globulin is present and the amount of fluid is largely increased. In these cases the withdrawal of 30 to 40 c.c. of fluid is followed by an immediate improvement of the symptoms. I have in view here the familiar forms of serous meningitis frequently observed in the course of acute infectious diseases such as typhoid fever, pneumonia, general sepsis and so forth. The severe headaches, restlessness and delirium frequently disappear like magic after one lumbar puncture. These cases of serous meningitis should be differentiated from the so-called meningisms of acute infections. In cases of meningisms the cerebrospinal fluid may be slightly increased in amount, but does not otherwise show any pathological changes, while in serous meningitis there are definite changes testifying to the existence of an inflammatory process. Shott-muller in his studies of infections has found at autopsy in some cases of serous meningitis an invasion of the nerve centers by bacteria, while the meningeal sack remained sterile and the fluid free from bacteria; he suggests for this group the name of circumscribed serous meningitis to differentiate them from the general serous meningitides —for instance, a tubercular one where the fluid presents a definite bacteriology. In these cases of serous meningitis lumbar puncture has a direct curative effect. In some cases, especially those which develop during the course of an acute infectious disease or complicating acute intestinal intoxication, one lumbar puncture often suffices; in others, if the indications for relief of intracranial pressure persist for a long time, repeated lumbar punctures are needed to insure a cure. In one case, for instance, we performed six punctures, the case lasting four weeks. Those cases where careful bacteriological examinations and serological tests were repeatedly negative, while the cerebrospinal fluid showed distinct chemical evidence of cerebral inflammation, we were compelled to regard as belonging to the group of serous meningitides.

I shall not burden you with the details of the history of individual cases, but shall mention that we have at times had to perform several punctures before the symptoms abated, so that we shall not be discouraged if the first puncture does not give permanent relief. In tubercular meningitis, the most fatal of all meningitides, lumbar punctures repeated at short intervals has effected a cure in the hands of some observers, the presence of tubercle bacilli in the fluid leaving no doubt as to the diagnosis. Their success was due to the fact that the lumbar puncture was used not only for diagnostic purposes but as a therapeutic agent, death being considered as due mainly to the continued high intracranial pressure. Further, if the diagnosis is made early and the lumbar puncture repeated at short intervals, time may be gained for the application of tuberculin which may assist in the ultimate results of the treatment. In another form of fatal meningitis, that due to the pneumococcus, the literature records the recovery of ten cases in which no sera were employed, but the treatment directed against the meningitis consisted solely of repeated lumbar punctures, a signal record of the therapeutic value of repeated rachicentesis. These encouraging reports, though few in number, should stimulate us to a more active treatment in these fatal forms of meningitis.

In polioencephalitis, particularly in the meningeal forms, we have on several occasions had opportunity to observe the beneficial effect of lumbar puncture; while it did not prevent the development of paralyses or influence the existing ones, it invariably relieved the cerebral irritation, the headache, the stiffness of the neck, and so forth, as are seen in these meningeal forms of encephalitis.

The distinct cytology of the cerebrospinal fluid in syphilitic and parasyphilitic affections of the brain and cord has been pointed out to you by the previous speaker; a Wassermann may be negative in the blood and yet positive in the cerebrospinal fluid. Apparently the specific anti-bodies of lues were stored up in the spinal canal while the blood contained them in such quantities as to give a negative or at least doubtful reaction. In one case under my observation the patient complained of persistent headaches and dizziness, which later were followed by convulsions; her past history was negative; she had had several children and grandchildren, and in none of them could any evidence of specific disease be found. Lumbar puncture was made here mainly for therapeutic purposes, to relieve the above symptoms. The fluid withdrawn was examined, and the findings reported by Dr. Lederer were a great surprise to the attending physician and myself. Even though the therapeutic effect of the lumbar puncture was immediate, in that the headache was relieved, dizziness slowly disappeared and the convulsions did not return, its further diagnostic value was the means of establishing a rational therapy. The examination of the fluid indicated the treatment, for in this particular case, though the blood was negative, the fluid gave a strongly positive Wassermann. Specific treatment was instituted and the patient completely recovered. I may add, in connection with the parasyphilitic lesions of the brain, that the spinal fluid obtained through the lumbar puncture has been used for curative purposes. The hypodermic injections of this luetic fluid has produced an apparent improvement in cases of spastic paralysis and tabes. This method of treatment has been applied to too few cases as yet, and the future will show the value of autoserotherapy in these diseases.

Tumor and abscess of the brain increase the intracranial pressure by increasing the volume of the brain. The amount of cerebrospinal fluid may not be increased, and hence the lumbar puncture must be done with great care. This applies also to distension of the ventricle with closure of the foramina communicating with the intradural space. In this particular group of cases the lumbar puncture is attended with an element of grave danger. The cerebrospinal fluid forms a "water bed" between the cranium and the brain and rapid withdrawal of the cerebrospinal fluid may cause the jamming of the brain into the foramen magnum. In cases where we suspect any of the just mentioned conditions, lumbar puncture must be performed cautiously and only a small quantity of fluid slowly removed for diagnostic purposes. It is self-evident that in these cases we are unable to reduce the intracranial pressure by the withdrawal of the fluid because we are dealing with an increase in the volume of the brain itself. I had once the misfortune to suggest a lumbar puncture in a young woman who presented very indefinite meningeal symptoms. She had persistent headache, lasting a week or more, slight fever, marked rigidity, a positive Kernig and Babinski, and thought she did not present a picture which would fit into a definite type of meningitis, I was of the opinion that the withdrawal of cerebrospinal fluid in her case might bring relief and at the same time clear up the diagnosis. Lumbar puncture was performed carefully and 43 c.c. of cerebrospinal fluid removed under increased pressure. The fluid showed a three millimeter ring of albumen and positive globulin. The Fehling reaction was positive, the bacteriology was sterile, and the cytology, while not very abundant, showed 48 per cent. of polynuclear cells. The character of this cerebrospinal fluid suggested a reaction to some pyogenic process in the brain substance proper. Almost immediately after the lumbar puncture was performed the patient developed dyspnœa, a rapid pulse, pallor of the face, great anxiety, symptoms of sudden pressure on the medulla, and she expired in about half an hour after the lumbar puncture was performed. This was the only case in my personal experience where I could ascribe the fatal issue directly to the lumbar puncture. I wish to add that in this case the patient's history did not give me any clue as to the diagnosis. Similar cases have been reported in the literature and must serve as a warning in those cases where we suspect a neoplasm or formation of pus in the tissue of the brain. We had not suspected any of these in our patient and proceeded with the withdrawal of the fluid until its rate slowed down to normal. Apparently too much fluid was withdrawn—and a smaller quantity might not have produced a fatal result. Sudden death following lumbar puncture has been reported in a case where after the withdrawal of the fluid an intracranial hemorrhage occurred. At autopsy a ruptured aneurism was found, the rupture occurring where the wall of the vessel was most thinned out—another extraordinary instance where lumbar puncture was followed by an unexpected fatality. Here the lumbar puncture led to an intracranial hemorrhage, but in apoplexy when the hemorrhage has caused an increase of the intracranial pressure, the withdrawal of the fluid may be considered for the purpose of giving relief, although it must be kept in mind that the drop of pressure may increase the hemorrhage. In traumas of the head the lumbar puncture not only serves to establish the diagnosis of sustained fracture—in these cases the fluid frequently contains blood—but also affords relief for headache, drowsiness, restlessness and other meningeal symptoms due to increased intracranial pressure.

Lumbar puncture, while it finds its therapeutic application mainly in diseases of the brain and meninges, has proven its value and usefulness in other morbid conditions where the inflammatory changes in the meninges are lacking, but the clinical symptoms present evidences of irritation of the central nervous system. In uremia, especially in the cerebral forms, lumbar puncture on many occasions has served me well, the nervous phenomena promptly abating after the withdrawal of the cerebrospinal fluid. In scarletinal uremia lumbar puncture has been tried with success by French pediatrists. Good results have also been reported in convulsive seizures of whooping-cough, and even the persistent headache of chlorotic girls has yielded to lumbar puncture; and it has also been efficacious in cases of tinnitus aurium and Meniere's disease. A case of diabetes inspidus has been reported where the withdrawal of lumbar fluid has reduced the daily amount of urine from 10 liters to normal.

A survey of literature and our own clinical observations permit us to conclude, therefore, that lumbar puncture has a decided therapeutic value. It is indicated in all cases where there is an inflammatory condition of the meninges, or where symptoms of cortical irritation are present, and except in the very small group of tumors and abscesses of the brain and distension of the ventricles with occlusion of the foramina communicating with the arachnoid space, rachiocentesis is free from danger, is easily performed, gives invaluable diagnostic information and provides a potent therapeutic measure.


## THE CLINICAL VALUE OF DELUSIONS.*

### By Elbert M. Somers, M.D.,

of Brooklyn, N. Y.

IT probably would be better to approach the subject of this paper by considering for a few moments the mechanisms of the normal mind, since the vagaries of the healthy mind help us to best understand departures from certain rather wide and permissible methods of reasoning which we finally recognize as absurd or abnormal.

All of our perceptions are the result of the proper elaboration by the central nervous system of one or more of our senses which have been stimulated. Through no other sources can mental elaboration come about. The sixth sense, a term common enough among the laity, simply means the utilization of the material so gained and pre-eminently belongs to the highest type,—man. Our experiences coming to us through the various senses as the result of apprehension and attention, are clarified and selected, and form a basis for further intellectual processes.

The higher mental activities depend, to a great extent, upon memory. Impressions coming through our consciousness leave some

---

* Read at the April meeting of the Brooklyn Society for Neurology.

registration, but whether strong enough to be recalled, depend upon the intensity and the interest excited.

Most of our ideas are heterogeneous and only certain experiences impress themselves upon us and stand out clearly, whereas other impressions are soon relegated to the background because they lack permanancy due to imperfect assimilation. It is the utilization of oft repeated impressions that results in the formation of concepts and allows reproduction in the form of ideas, which are, of course, copies of impressions, and may or may not be accurate, depending upon the faithfulness of our memories.

This constant training permits us to develop still more complex mental products in the form of judgment and reasoning, since we have the means through perception, memory, formation of concepts and the valuable gift of associating ideas—all of which allow us to draw inferences accurate, inaccurate or incomplete.

Information that we gain comes to us in two ways. One is through experience and the other by the free action of the mind or imagination. Empirical knowledge is experience and is differentiated from pure belief which arises from the recasting and interpretation of experience.

Our wildest thoughts employ material gained from experience, and on the other hand, empirical knowledge is rarely free from more or less preconception. If the experiences we gain are scanty and unreliable, imagination comes in to fill the field with the products arising from the free action of our own minds. In children, invention and experience are hard to differentiate. The older we grow, the more we are able to draw distinctions.

There are as many grades of intelligence as there are persons, but given a certain sameness of nature and nurture, a considerable number will appear to be roughly alike as to view points, conclusions, and mental attitude, since they have been cast in the same mould on account of the similarity of the original stock, the environment, education, training, etc. This accounts for the difference in the mental levels which we experience daily in our intercourse with a variety of folks.

Mental differences are accounted for much as those purely physical. In both, hereditary virility and functional education play an important role.

We find that if we put certain people to the test of direct experience, the line between this and invention becomes very clearly defined. Those of the higher intellectual order have naturally more accurate judgment and reasoning because they have permitted experience to supplant purely primitive thought. They do not draw their inferences from insufficient data, and the imagination does not allow ignorance to carry matters too far. Nevertheless, even among the cultured, there are beliefs and traditions which experience or argument cannot shake.

It is a well known fact that untrained people do not draw the distinction between actual knowledge and belief. They credit their mystical ideas to direct experience. Hence, superstition survives among those not cultured. However, it is equally true that dogmatic opinions and fixed ideas occur among us all, even though we are educated and have more accurate habits of thought, and these opinions cannot help but mould our experience along the lines of prejudice. As instances, certain political, religious and social convictions, supposedly dependent on rational elaboration for their content, are well known to be inaccessible to opposition and argument. We may show good judgment and good reasoning in the ordinary events of life, but in these matters which we vigorously defend, there is an emotional significance which does not permit us to utilize fully the usual avenues of experience in coming to certain sweeping conclusions.

We could use further illustrations by designating at length many of the superstitions which are held by those more limited in thought, and even among our own kind. It is a well known fact that among the negroes in the South it is the feeling of helplessness and insecurity in the presence of the unknown and mysterious, which supplies the fertile soil for the various unwarrantable deductions which are tenaciously held. Again, the question of spiritualism, mental telepathy, etc., are matters of belief among some, while ridiculed by others. To us, maybe, they seem more questions of good judgment than the problem of the revision of the tariff. The one cannot be settled because it is inaccessible to final conclusion by argument, whereas the other can be, since it arises out of common experience and can, therefore, be settled some day by demonstration.

We permit the widest possible latitude in the matter of beliefs, conclusions and notions before we decide that ideas are unsound or abnormal. Something more is required to characterize a belief as a delusion. A delusion is simply the belief in something which does not exist in experience. A false notion does not arise from experience and deliberation. It arises from the erroneous interpretation of events within the person's own imagination or ideation. Sweeping conclusions are drawn from insufficient data. We therefore can see that even false beliefs or delusions may not necessarily be insane beliefs. Something more is required than the mere entertainment of an idea which may be in conflict with evidence. These false ideas have to possess individuals in such a way as to result in a morbid change in that person's mentality, after taking into consideration his mental level, training, environment and usual habits of thought.

A person can hold certain strange ideas or beliefs, but they do not take such possession of him that he is not in other respects quite on a par with his usual mode of thought and action, although he may, from an academic standard, be deluded along these lines. He is not, however, a potential lunatic. In other words, these ideas may not medically be classified as insane delusions, and very often we find that the legal view of insanity would not consider such ideas as necessarily indicating insanity. It is only where the person cannot perceive the contradictions between his fancies and former experiences, and allows his mental condition to influence his ideas to such an extent that he becomes incapable of using the function of judgment, that we then can consider the person insane. In health we are accustomed to judge all our fancies according to the standard of our own experience, and to regard as invention that which does not conform to knowledge. Clearly, we have not lost the power to oppose, correct and suppress wrong inferences. In other words, we reason from sufficient data. Our emotional side does not override our ability to come to a sound conclusion, at least for very long. We do not fail to correct the matters ourselves, or to see things in the right light after a certain amount of argument. We dispose of these things in such a way that they do not put us out of joint with our environment, whatever it may be, whether we be of limited mental calibre or otherwise. We do not act upon these ideas to the extent of attracting attention by talk, or bizarre conduct. We do not allow these ideas to morbidly effect our mood.

To be insane, one has to show a radical intellectual departure of thought, feeling and reactions from what was his normal self, of course after taking into consideration his natural makeup and the result of the nurture which has been given him.

It is hardly necessary, in this paper, to go into the general description of the question of what may be insanity, since time will not permit of an explanation as to how a person can be insane without having demonstrable delusions, but it is rather to show the clinical value that delusions may have.

Probably all delusions center in the self or the ego. They are either depressive or expansive in character, but depressive delusions stand the closest to normal life. Many normal people torment themselves with the belief that they are unlucky. It is but a step to carry such beliefs further, to the idea of unworthiness or ruin, and then to borrow further by considering that they have committed crimes, are irredeemable, refuted by God, and the accompanying emotional reactions readily supply further conclusions as to punishment. On this basis, the patient easily develops ideas of suspicion, of nihilism, of fear, or refers to everything as having a meaning. Or, the departure from the normal may be along hypochondriacal lines, with all sorts of somatic ideas regarding one's physical state.

Likewise, expansive delusions can be of all grades, even to the transformation of one's own personality.

When evidences of further mental weakness occur, fantastic and absurd notions of a depressive or exalted nature appear. The varieties are innumerable and may embrace the widest range of morbid reasoning.

Delusional reasoning processes of any type are always in proportion to the intellectual capabilities of the individual. A man of limited calibre will have a relatively simple and rather narrow, circumscribed trend, whether it be of a depressive or of an exalted type. The one with a previously higher developed mentality may or can embellish his reasoning processes to a profound degree, and although reasoning from false premises, will do so logically and clearly. In the latter case the person can draw from a greater fund of memory pictures than the one who has always utilized only a limited amount of mental timber.

Clinically, delusions are classified variously. Wernicke classifies concepts as to whether they relate to the outside world, to the individual's personality or to the individual's body, and speaks of the ideas respectively as allopsychic, autopsychic and somatopsychic. Delusions of persecution are referred to conditions without. The belief that one has committed an unpardonable sin is an autopsychic concept, whereas the belief that no stomach exists is a somatic affect.

Now, delusions can also be fixed, or changeable. That is, systematized or unsystematized. The fixed, or systematized delusions take their origin from actual occurrences and show a deep disturbance of reasoning process, and form a motive power for queer actions, and these actions center, more or less, about the dominant trend of whatever sort it may be. The subject regulates his life accordingly, either to avoid persecutors or to assume the characteristics of a fanciful personage. Should he be suspicious of food, he carefully investigates. He goes to infinite pains to shut out noxious vapors. His explanations are logical and the reasons are interminable.

Unsystematized or changeable delusions are not as fully assimilated. They do not enter into the organic makeup of consciousness to such an extent; and since the beliefs are unstable they do not specially control conduct for long; the subject simply makes the assertion of a belief without cogent argument, and may soon abandon it for a notion quite unrelated.

To barely touch upon paranoia (which in derivation simply means wrong thinking)—this possibly can be best disposed of by quoting from White's "Outlines of Psychiatry." At first he goes on to say that a psychosis may develop about a centralized event, and that the beliefs may be fairly well circumscribed; "but it is only by taking a view that an idea is a thing apart without organic connection with the personality of the individual that we can conceive of a person with a single wrong, delusional idea, yet perfectly all right every other way. The formation of an idea is dependent upon too many processes and cannot spring into being independently of them, and if it is itself pathological we must look to the mechanism of its growth for its explanation."

To further quote, Mercier says: "The delusion is not an isolated disorder. It is merely the superficial indication of a deep-seated disorder. As a small island is but the summit of an immense mountain rising from the floor of the sea, the portion of the mountain in sight bearing but an insignificant ratio to the mass whose summit it is, so a delusion is merely the conspicuous part of a mental disease, extending, it may be, to the very foundations of the mind, but the greater portion of which is not apparent without careful sounding. Precisely how far this disorder extends, beyond the region of mind occupied by the delusion, it is never possible to say; but it is certain that the delusion itself is the least part of the disorder, and for this reason, no deluded person ought ever to be regarded as fully responsible for any act that he may do. The connection between the act and the delusion may be wholly undiscoverable, as the shallow between two neighboring islands may be entirely hidden by the intervening sea. But nevertheless, if the sea stood a hundred fathoms lower, the two islands would be two mountain peaks connected by a stretch of low country; and, if the hidden springs of conduct were laid bare, the delusion and the act might be found to have a common basis."

In the main, we might say that a delusion is, in quite a number of forms of insanity, the unimportant question. It is rather what is the underlying intellectual disorder, as in mania, the reactions, the activities, bizarre conduct, and emotional changes are of far more importance. The delusions are simply the very commonplace evidences of a psychosis. They are fleeting, of practically no importance, and in five minutes or less may disappear. Again, to show that the delusional content is not necessarily a guide to an accurate diagnosis, we find that in cases of general paralysis the delusion is often not grandiose, but depressive in nature. These expressions may be self-accusatory or somatopsychic, and if we rely upon the delusional expression, and fail to test for memory defects, change of personality and organic physical alterations, we get an erroneous clinical picture and might on this basis just as well classify the case as one of melancholia, hypochondria or manic depressive insanity. It would be of the same value as making an accurate diagnosis of abdominal disease, simply because of the patient's general expression of pain anywhere in his belly.

In taking any classification of mental diseases, one can readily see that the same sort of delusions may occur in a variety of forms of mental diseases. In the deliriums we have delusions, but the confusion, the disorientation, the clouding of consciousness, are the leading features, and the delusional expressions are not alike in any two cases. In dementia præcox the impairment of attention, the evidence of dilapidation and the emotional tone are the guides to prognosis. In melancholia and in the depressive form of manic depressive insanity, it is rather the disturbance of the trend of thought, the clouding of consciousness and the painful concentration of the mind that permit of giving the diagnostic name. In paranoia it is the marked alteration of the personality, without disturbance of the coherence of thought, the retrospective falsification, and the systematized delusional trend which render these individuals dangerous, since they are chronically in an attitude of self-defence and are looking for evidences to support their beliefs and even force them upon others to their peril. Their beliefs are not like the beliefs of a harmless crank at large, since they dominate the personality and make them unsocial individuals, but just where the dividing line may be is often unfortunately only found out too late, just as in the case of a general paralytic who has squandered a large portion of his money before the relatives, through pride or ignorance, get ready to deprive him of his liberty.

Briefly, we may conclude that a delusion of itself, which is simply a false belief, may have no pathological significance, since a man can believe today is Sunday rather than Monday. This has only the significance of a mistake, and the reasons are hardly worth while following up. We would not dwell in argument with that individual, any more than we would take time today to explain why we differentiate between a lie and an insane delusion. A woman who states that her husband is untrue to her has not expressed anything which, on the face of it, is impossible. It may not be out of harmony with her education and environment. If we run down the origin of the belief, find upon what foundation it has been erected and if she gives reasons which are not logical, we will then be able to conclude that she has not only a false belief, but not a sane one. She may be safe to leave at home because her notion is a benign one, or the idea may possess her in such a way that she is a potential lunatic, because of collateral expressions, actions and conduct, attitude and manner, which render her unsafe to herself or others, and warrant incarceration. After being in a hospital, she might take up the subject of spiritualism and believe in it. It might be a further evidence of mental weakness, but though still existing, should she right herself as to the other beliefs, she would be discharged recovered.

Clinically expressions which are out of the ordinary, even if they be queer and absurd are of themselves of little value unless they be supported by some additional evidences of insanity.

It is true that some expressions are at once recognized as intrinsically insane in nature, but the point made in this paper still applies, since the more insane the utterances the greater is the insanity.

# OUR PRESENT CONCEPTION OF HYPERTHYROIDISM.

## By William H. Lohman, M.D.,

of Brooklyn, N. Y.

FROM the days of Parry,[1] the old Bath physician, who in 1815 first described cases of "Enlargement of the Thyroid in connection with Palpitation of the Heart," down to the present time, the study of exopthalmic goitre has been a favorite field for physicians with a speculative or investigating turn of mind.

Theories as to the causation of the disease or various of its symptoms have been innumerable, but during the last few years, the efforts of a host of scientists have revealed so many hitherto obscure, anatomical, physiological and chemical facts regarding this interesting affliction, that our concept of it has become fairly definite.

There is now no further room for doubt that the symptoms of Basedow's disease are due to an excess of thyroid secretion in the blood as Moebius was the first to suggest.

The investigations of Roos[2] and Oswald[3] proved that the active principal of the thyroid gland was iodothyreoglobulin. They proved that thyreoglobulin, which is formed in the cells, is physiologically inactive until it becomes iodized, which it does from the blood.

Oswald[3] states that it is the condition of the thyreoglobulin which determines the changes in the gland substance. Thus, when it is not iodized it accumulates in the cells and causes them to undergo colloid degeneration producing simple colloid goitre. Whereas an excess of iodin stimulates the cells to hyperplasia, giving the picture described by himself, Halstead,[4] McCallum[5] and Wilson,[6] in exopthalmic goitre, of alveoli surrounded by several layers of columnar epithelium, instead of the normal single layer of cubical epithelium. These several layers of cells may be heaped up projecting into the lumen of the alveolus in a manner suggesting adenoma and sometimes entirely obliterate the lumen.

The effect of the escape into the blood of the excess of thyroid secretion has been amply demonstrated experimentally and clinically. Briefly it may be said to produce a general stimulation of peripheral nerves, and an increase in metabolism, causing the breaking down of tissue proteids, especially of muscle proteids. This tallies perfectly with the clinical picture of Basedow's disease.

In considering the *pathology* of Basedow's disease we have to take up principally the changes in the thyroid. Other attendant lesions are uniformly found in the lymphoid tissue, thymus, eyes, muscles, nervous system and skin, but these appear to be of secondary importance.

The thyroid is usually uniformly enlarged; it may, however, present appearances of simple, cystic or adenomatous goitre and in the atypical forms (*formes frustes*) it may not be larger than normal. The superficial veins are very large and thin, and before operation, congested with blood. After a portion of the gland has been removed the vessels in the excised portion collapse and the cut surface shows the tissue to be hard, rigid and pale. These changes are usually diffuse throughout the entire gland, but they may occur in patches in an otherwise normal gland, or in a gland that is otherwise in a state of simple colloid degeneration. In either case the characteristic patches of Basedow's disease are readily distinguished by their dry granular and opaque appearance from the glairy colloid tissue surrounding them.

Microscopically is found the change which appears in the experimental compensatory hyperthrophy first described by Halstead.[4]

The fibrous tissue bands are much more abundant than in the normal gland. The alveoli instead of being rounded, filled with colloid and lined with a single layer of cubical epithelium, are mostly irregular and small. Occasionally a large alveolus may be seen. The lining epithelium is columnar in shape and made up of several layers. It encroaches on the lumen of the alveolus and (especially so in the acute severe cases) may entirely fill the lumen. Occasionally the epithelium may show considerable desquamation and the cells may be enormously swollen and irregular in shape. Sometimes where the alveoli are larger, the heaped up layers of cells project into the lumen giving an adenomatous appearance to the picture.

The colloid in these glands is subject to considerable variation, but is generally much reduced in amount and much more faintly staining than normal colloid. Most observers agree that the iodin content is likewise much reduced.

In cases of Basedow's disease supervening upon simple colloid goitre, the histological picture is as follows: We have the usual enlarged alveoli of simple goitre filled with deep staining colloid and lined with a single layer of flattened cubical epithelium and scattered through this are opaque areas of hyperplasia with the characteristic changes above described as indicative of Basedow's disease.

A characteristic of almost all the exopthalmic goitres is the presence of numerous masses of lymphoid tissue scattered throughout the thyroid. It is far in excess of the amount found in normal glands.

### Changes in other organs.

There is present a well marked general enlargement of the lymph nodes, especially in the neck and pharynx, but also in the thoracic and retroperitoneal regions (McCallum).[5]

The thymus has been found to be enlarged by many investigators. The changes found in the cervical sympathetic ganglia and the central nervous system are not uniform and need further study. They are not suggestive of any specific gross abnormality. The heart is hypertrophied, the aorta and carotids are enlarged and, according to Marine and Lenhart,[7] both carotids seem to terminate in the superior thyroid arteries.

Askanazy[8] has called attention to the general disturbance in the nutrition of the skeletal muscles. He found a marked atrophy of the fibers and a loss of normal striation. He also found fat deposits in and around the fibers which he thought resembled the fatty metamorphosis seen in the progressive muscular dystrophy. This condition has also been found in the muscles of the eye. Profound muscle weakness which is sometimes present without reduction of muscle bulk may be in some way due to this fatty change.

Blood: Little change is found in the red cells although there may be some anemia. The white cells, however, constantly show an increase in the large mononuclear lymphocytes. Marine and Lenhart have found this increase closely parallels the extent of active lymphoid and thyroid hyperplasia and hence is a fair index of the severity of the disease.

When we come to a consideration of the *etiology* of Basedow's disease, we find that there is a great diversity of opinion. Where we have definite symptoms of the disease the characteristic change is always found in the thyroid. This change corresponds to hypertrophy and it is currently accepted that it is this hypertrophy and over-activity of the gland which produces the symptoms of the disease. But if this is so, what is the cause of the hypertrophy? This is not so clear, and there are many theories to account for it. Those most favored at present are (1) the nervous hypothesis; (2) the thyroid hypothesis.

The nervous hypothesis scarcely explains the cases whose origin lies in excessive doses of thyroid extract, the surgical cures, or the constant presence of hyperplasia of the thyroid gland.

Those who maintain that Basedow's disease is a disease of the thyroid gland alone must, according to Crile[9] "be at a loss to explain the frequent cure by physiological rest, and the relapses that may occur after an apparently sufficient amount of gland has been removed if the patient is again submerged in the environment that originally produced the disease," also, it fails to account for the cases induced by nervous strain.

To harmonize these inconsistancies, Crile[9] has put forth what he calls the Kinetic theory. He holds that "Graves disease is not a disease of a single organ or the result of a fleeting cause," that its "excitation is through either some stimulating emotion intensely or repeatedly given, or some lowering of the threshold of nerve receptors thus establishing a pathological interaction between the brain and the thyroid."

Etiological factors are:

*Sex.*—Basedow's disease is much more common in females than in males; 20-1 Osler.

*Age.*—Probably eighty per cent. of the cases occur between the ages of 15 and 45 years, the period of greatest sexual activity in the female.

*Heredity.*—Family predisposition may exist and several members of the same family may be affected.

Hirschfelder[10] gives the following table of predisposing factors.

|  | Cases |
|---|---|
| Gradual onset with etiological factors unknown.... | 28 |
| Pregnancy | 10 |
| Chlorosis | 7 |
| At first menstruation | 6 |
| After fright, shock or grief | 5 |
| After fatigue | 8 |
| Infectious diseases (influenza alone 7) | 13 |
| Old simple goitre | 5 |
| Sojourn at high altitude | 2 |
| Heredity | 1 |
| Appendicitis | 1 |
| Total | 86 |

It will be noted that infectious diseases (especially influenza), pregnancy, menstruation and nervous disturbances are the most common causes.

*Symptoms.*—The severity of the symptoms seems to depend upon the degree of vascularity of the gland and the extent of the hypertrophy, some small but very vascular glands being attended by very severe symptoms.

Osler speaks of acute and chronic forms and relates a case with gastro-intestinal symptoms, tachycardia, exophthalmos and thyroid enlargement with symptoms becoming rapidly more severe; death taking place on the third day.

The writer recently observed a case in which the patient, a woman of 35, had suffered with mild Basedow's disease for some months. She was sent to the hospital for treatment of an old hip disease. Shortly after the application of a Bucks extension her pulse rate rapidly increased to 160 and she became delirious. After twelve hours coma supervened and the patient died on the fourth day. The pulse rate continued around 160 to the end. The thyroid which previously had not been palpable, was noticeably swollen during the attack.

W. J. Mayo[11] recognizes three clinical types of the disease (1) vascular type, (2) hypertrophic type and (3) the cases where hypertrophy develops in patients with pre-existing goitres.

Most of the cases come on gradually, oftentimes with periods of exacerbation and improvement and show the characteristic symptoms of tachycardia, exopthalmus, enlargement of the thyroid and tremor. In addition there may be attacks of vomiting and diarrhœa, loss of weight, psychic disturbances and flushing, sweating and pigmentation of the skin.

*Cardiac symptoms.*—The *tachycardia* results from the stimulation of the accelerator nerves of the heart. The average pulse rate in most cases is from 90 to 120 per minute and this elevation in the rate is usually continuous. Any slight reflex disturbance may cause a great increase in the tachycardia.

The maximal blood pressure is apt to be high, the minimal about normal giving an increased pulse pressure and an increased systolic output.

There is usually an enlargement and hypertrophy of the heart with a very forcible impulse over the precordium.

After the disease has persisted for a time, signs of serious cardiac overstrain may appear and we then have dilatation, with relative insufficiencies of the mitral and tricuspid valves. Murmurs are often heard even before the heart is much enlarged. They are usually systolic in time and may be heard at the apex or base. They are sometimes very loud.

*Ocular symptoms.*—The *exophthalmos* is very characteristic. It is caused in part by protrusion of the eyeballs and in part by retraction of the lids. When the eyeball is moved downward the upper lid does not follow it as it normally should, Graefe's sign, while the widening of the palpebial aperture is known as Stellwag's sign. Moebius' sign is the inability to converge the two eyes in looking at a very near object. There may be pigmentation about the eyelids (Jellinek's sign).

*Struma.*—In the majority of cases *thyroid enlargement* will readily be recognized. It is usually uniform, but one lobe may be larger than the other. The enlargement is not as a rule extreme. On palpation in the acute cases the substances may feel softer than normal while in the older and more chronic cases the consistence is much more firm. The characteristic feature is the granulation of the surface due to the lobular hyperplasia. A typical feature of these glands is their vascularity. There may be recognized a visible pulsation, a palpable systolic expansion, a palpable thrill, or a bruit, which is heard best at the entrance of the thyroid arteries.

It must be born in mind that many cases of hyperthyroidism exist where the thyroid is not palpable.

*Muscular changes.*—A fine *tremor* of the fingers has been designated by Marie as the fourth cadinal symptom. There are 8 to 10 contractions per second. It is undoubtedly due to the over-stimulation of the peripheral nerves. The tremor may involve all the extremities and the muscles of the neck and trunk. The increased metabolism with the breaking down of muscle proteids is the principle cause of the loss of weight which may reach from 30 to 50 pounds.

*Psychic manifestations.*—These are often pronounced. Feelings of restlessness, discomfort and anxiety are quite common. Irritability of temper, insomnia and general neurasthenic symptoms may be the most pronounced features early in the disease and cause the patient to seek medical advice. *Other symptoms* are attacks of vomiting and diarrhœa, flushing of the skin, sweating, transitory œdema, and fever. The blood shows a slight leucocytosis with a relative increase in the large mononuclears (8 to 16 per cent).

*The diagnosis* in typical well developed cases is very easy. It is in the very early and atypical cases *(formes frustes)* where difficulty may arise. Some cases undoubtedly occur without ocular symptoms and some without noticeable thyroid enlargements. These patients should be carefully watched, especially around menstruation when ocular or thyroid signs may be observed.

In the atypical cases one or more of the symptoms may persist with great severity and may resemble a cardiac neurosis, a psychosis, a chronic enteritis, a progressive inanition or a mild relapsing fever. The other symptoms may be very mild and only when the suspicions of the examiner have been aroused by some slight staring of the eyes or tremor of the fingers will a careful examination reveal the true nature of the disease.

The differential leucocyte count, showing a high precentage of mononuclears, may be of some assistance in diagnosis, as may also the cautious administration of thyroid extract or iodothyrin, when a prompt aggravation of the symptoms will appear in cases of hyperthyroidism.

*Treatment.*—Where a disease is subject to so many variations and may have so many spontaneous exacerbations and remissions as the one under consideration, it is very difficult to accurately determine the value of any given plan of treatment. There are certain principles, however, which experience has shown, may be safely followed, greatly to the benefit of sufferers from Basedow's disease, and an effort will be made to outline them, leaving the details of their applications in individual cases largely to the good judgment of the physician in attendance.

There are two general groups of therepeutic measures, first: those directed toward the correction of metabolic disturbances, especially those of the nervous system, and second: those directed toward reducing or counteracting the thyroid secretion.

I. Beginning with the measures directed toward the metabolic and nervous disturbances it is of primary importance that a careful history be obtained in order to ascertain if there be any underlying nervous exhaustion, irritation, worry or overwork. A history of infectious diseases should be carefully noted especially of recurrent infections such as tonsillitis. Gastro-intestinal disturbances may be prominent. Where any such underlying cause is present, measures should immediately be instituted to remove it.

*Rest.*—This is immediately suggested by the enormous increase in tissue waste, and the over-stimulation of the peripheral nerves which are such constant factors in this disease. The rest should be both mental and physical and is of the greatest importance. Indeed much of the improvement which has followed surgical removal of a portion of the gland has been ascribed to the prolonged rest which most surgeons insist upon both before and after the operation.

It is desirable above all to obtain mental rest, and we should bear in mind that mental rest is not necessarily associated with the mere restriction of physical activity. As a rule a change of environment is necessary and this may best be obtained by removal to a hospital or sanatorium. The tastes and means of the patient should be consulted, the object being to get her in surroundings where her mind is tranquil and her body inactive.

In the mild and improving cases, moderate exercise may be allowed, preferably out doors.

*Diet.*—Is of importance second only to rest. An effort should be made to overcome the tissue waste and loss of weight, with good wholesome food. As the appetite usually remains good a generous mixed diet containing proteids, fats and carbohydrates should be allowed. Alcoholic stimulants, tea and coffee should, of course, be forbidden.

The value of *suggestion* is universally admitted and the physician should take advantage of every slight improvement to impress upon his patient that recovery is taking place. Baths and massage may be used both for their tonic effect and for the effect on the patient's mind.

*Drugs.*—Many drugs have been recommended for the regulation of the cardiovascular system. They are of very doubtful value. For the tachycardia there is nothing so satisfactory *as rest in bed with an ice bag over the heart.* Late in the disease when there are signs of heart failure digitalis, strophanthus or other cardiac stimulants should be used to meet the indications.

The administration of sodium bromid gr. V or X three times a day is often very useful for controlling nervousness and insomnia and sometimes causes an amelioration of all the symptoms.

Opium, bearing out the experiments of Reid Hunt,[12] is not well borne by these patients and it should be used cautiously.

Iron and arsenic may be indicated to overcome anemia and proper measures used to control attacks of vomiting and diarrhœa.

The administration of thyroid extract and iodine preparations are held by most clinicians to be harmful, but Marine and Lenhart hold that small doses will hasten the degeneration of the thyriod hyperplasia to colloid, bringing about in this manner a physiological cure. When used at all, the effects should be carefully watched. There may be a positive indication for the use of thyroid extract in those cases that are associated with symptoms of myxoedema.

II. Measures directed toward reducing the thyroid secretion. *A.* Surgical measures.—A survey of the brilliant results obtained by such operators as Kocher, Halstead, the Mayos and Crile would almost lead one to believe that exopthalmic goitre is purely a surgical disease. But a more careful study of the facts will not justify such a conclusion. The principal objection urged against medical treatment, namely, that the cases do not stay cured and are subject to relapses, may also be urged, with considerable truth, against operative cure, as many cases undoubtedly relapse after operation. Furthermore the cases which resist medical treatment are the ones in which surgery is apt to fail, and we should bear in mind that the cases which are operated on successfully are always subjected to long periods of medical treatment both before and after operation. However, the partial removal of the thyroid in suitable cases gives such a high percentage of cures (75 to 90 per cent.) and the mortality in the hands of skillful operators is so low (about 5 per cent.), that in the absence of contraindications, operation should be advised in all cases where the medical treatment does not result in marked benefit after a trial of two or three months.

The atypical cases (*formes frustes*), the very early and the mild cases will rarely need operation being mostly all amenable to less radical treatment.

The contraindications to operation are: serious permanent complications, especially cardiac or renal; very feeble heart, or very high pulse frequency; and pronounced nervous excitation. All very acute cases stand operation badly, and any acute exacerbation in a more chronic case is best treated medically until a period of remission sets in.

Among the positive indications for operation are: Mechanical pressure of the enlarged thyroid on the trachea, and thyroid tremors.

*B. Serum treatment.*—Only two forms need be considered. The serum of Moebius made from the blood or milk of thyroidectomized animals, and the cytotoxic serum of Rogers and Beebe.

The Moebius preparations have been widely used, but while good results have been reported, the general opinion is very contradictory.

The Rogers and Beebe serum is prepared from the blood of rabbits and sheep which have been inoculated with the nucleo proteids and globulin of a human thyroid gland. Good results have been reported in the early and acute cases. Beebe[13] claims favorable results in from 75 to 80 per cent. of all uncomplicated cases. It is to be noted that he combines other measures such as rest, diet, etc., with the serum and insists on its use for at least a year. It is rather doubtful if such good results can be ascribed entirely to the use of the serum.

*C.* Finally the X-ray should be mentioned. This has been used for the purpose of inhibiting thyroid activity and reports of cases where the thyroid diminished in size after its use have been fairly common. Whether this is actually the effect of the X-ray on the gland or due to its profound effect on the mind has not been settled, but its use seems indicated where other means have failed or are not available.

## REFERENCES.

1. Parry: Quoted from Dock, G., *J. Am. M. Assoc.*, 1908, li, 1119.
2. Roos, E.: *Ztsch. f. Physiol. Chem.*, Strassb., 1896, xxi, 19.
3. Oswald, A.: *Arch. f. Path. Anat.*, Berl., 1902, cixix, 444.
4. Halstead, W. S.: *Johns Hop. Hosp. Rept.*, 1896, i, 373.
5. MacCallum, W. G.: *J. Am. Med. Assoc.*, 1907, xlix, 1158.
6. Wilson, L. B.: *Am. J. M. Sc.*, 1908, cxxxiv, 857.
7. Marine and Lenhart: *Arch. Int. Med.*, 1911, viii, 265.
8. Askanazy: Quoted from Marine and Lenhart.
9. Crile, G. W.: *Am. J. M. Sc.*, 1913, cxlv, 28.
10. Hirschfelder: Dis. of Heart and Aorta, 2d ed., 683.
11. Mayo, W. J.: *J. Am. M. Assoc.*, 1907, xlix, 1323.
12. Hunt, Reid: *J. Am. M. Assoc.*, 1907, xlix, 1323.
13. Beebe, S. P.: Hare's Modern Treatment, Vol. II, 492.

# DIRECT TRANSFUSION FOR HEMORRHAGIC PURPURA.

## By Warren L. Duffield, M.D.

A S the treatment of hemorrhagic purpura is so ineffectual and the prognosis so grave, in the severe forms, it would seem that the following case report might be of some interest particularly as no record can be found of a transfusion performed for this condition.

Miss 19042, eighteen years of age, was admitted to the Jewish Hospital on January 10th, 1913, suffering with hemorrhagic purpura; her temperature was 103⅖, pulse 140 and respirations 36; there was profuse bleeding from the nasal mucosæ which could not be controlled by anterior and posterior tamponade; her face, arms, neck and chest were covered with an extensive petechial eruption; a urine examination was negative and an examination of the blood revealed 50 per cent. hemoglobin, 3,800,000 red cells and 6,600 white cells with 50 per cent. polymorphonuclear.

She had a tuberculosis of the right hip joint beginning at age of eighteen months with a discharging sinus which persisted until two years ago. She had previously been in the hospital for five weeks under treatment for a petechial hemorrhagic purpura but two days after her discharge had had a recurrence of the petechia and was treated at home for ten days when a profuse nasal hemorrhage rendered a return to the hospital necessary. Upon her readmission 45 c.c. of human blood serum were injected and calcium lactate one dram to the pint was administered by continuous Murphy drip. Ten minims of adrenalin three times a day were also given.

The day following her admission, Dr. Londoner, under whose care she had been, requested us to do a transfusion which was immediately performed, her brother acting as donor.

A one-half per cent. solution of novocain was used as a local anæsthetic and the radial artery of the donor and the basilic vein of the recipient were exposed and immediately anastomosed by the aid of an Elsberg canula. Blood was allowed to flow for 45 minutes during which time the blood pressure of the donor fell from 140 to 120. Immediately following the transfusion there was a fall in pulse, temperature and respiration followed by a rise the next day and a subsequent return to normal within thirty-six hours. In forty-eight hours hemorrhages had completely ceased, the petechia had faded fully fifty per cent. and the general morale of the patient was excellent.

Though the outcome in this case was ideal it raises the question whether in these little understood hemorrhagic conditions it would not be wise to obtain as a donor one who was not a blood relation assuming that there might exist in an entire family a predisposition to like conditions in which event the transfused blood might have the opposite effect from the one desired.

# EDITORIAL

## MEDICAL PUBLICITY.

THE Council of the Medical Society of the County of Kings have recently taken a step the full consequences of which are as yet not entirely evident, although some of the immediate results are bearing fruit.

At a recent meeting a committee was appointed whose function is to censor the publication of medical matters intended for the lay press. The appointment of this committee is the direct outcome of the appearance in certain newspapers of interviews that have been granted by physicians in Brooklyn upon medical topics which seem to have contravened the established code of ethics. These have included full page illustrated articles describing medical and surgical procedures the apparent intention of which was to bring the physician in question before the general public, as well as less offensive interviews carrying authoritative information on recent advances in medical and surgical treatment and varying from the extreme of fulsome self aggrandizement to the moderate dignified expression of personal opinion.

The physician who permits himself to be interviewed on any topic of a medical or surgical nature lays himself open to misrepresentation at the hands of the interviewer. While his remarks may be correctly reported it has nevertheless happened that at times the interview takes the form of erroneous impressions interpreted through the interviewer's imperfect comprehension of what he may have been told. Nor has the physician any control over the comments of the reporter who often has made the mistake of adding a flattering personal notice of the physician's professional position and acquirements. This least offensive form of public statement may and often does place the physician who has granted an interview in a peculiarly unenviable light. The readers of a widely circulated newspaper cannot help but attach importance to the utterance of a man who is stated to be professor of such and such a subject, attached to a variety of institutions and stated to be an authority on the subject under discussion. At the least, this is an unfair position for him to assume toward his fellow practitioners, however worthy his motive may have been. Little need be said of the man who willfully prepares a so-called interview and provides a portrait and illustrations to eke it out—by their works ye shall know them. This is as true now as two thousand years ago, nor is it yet possible to gather figs from thistles.

The craze for sensationalism continues to grow, fostered by the unfortunate spirit that activates some newspapers whose object seems to be not to instruct and uplift their readers, but to stir their emotions rather than to cultivate their intellect.

Apropos of this subject we recall the witty rejoinder of a well-known editor to the impassioned oratory of the representative of one of the yellow press who had proclaimed that the policy of his paper was not to try to reach down and draw up the individual but to get under and shoulder up the masses from the mud of ignorance and vice. "Why," he replied, "having shouldered them up do you still continue to wallow in the filth?" The physician who willfully aids and abets in this effort to further sensationalism is not only myopic but has a moral squint as well. It is the purpose of the Publicity Committee to provide correction for such visual errors.

The plan is that the physician who is asked for an interview shall either refer the interviewer to the committee, who remaining anonymous, are expected to give a conservative, dignified and authoritative opinion; or else to submit to them a written interview for their approval such as upon publication cannot lay him open to criticism from his fellows. He is thus guarded against misrepresentation and misunderstanding. The immediate result of this action has been a local newspaper disturbance, which will, of course, quiet down. The ultimate effects are by no means easy to foretell. There can be no doubt from the standpoint of medical conservatism of the necessity for curbing the tendency to undue publicity. On the other hand there comes from other quarters a cry for more enlightenment. Education is the slogan of today, but it depends largely upon the interpretation of that word how far it is safe and proper to publish medical facts indiscriminately. The science of medicine, being the study of human ailments, belongs in some measure to every one in proportion as he or she is a sufferer. We cannot have experience without resulting knowledge, and the science of medicine is the accumulated experience of the ages clarified and reduced to system. If everyone by virtue of suffering is entitled to possess medical knowledge and therefore should receive instruction in medical matters, it nevertheless is true that the act of suffering befogs the judgment and makes the sufferer the one least able to weigh and judge his personal needs. Physicians have always differed as to the amount of information that should be imparted to those who are not trained in estimating the value of symptoms. We are, however, becoming more and more preventative rather than curative in our practice and knowledge widespread and broadcast is the surest factor in fostering prevention. It would seem that what we believe to be the established facts of medical science should be as widely known and appreciated as possible. As these facts are common property and for the common good they should be so published as to carry conviction, and should, therefore, issue from an authorative source.

Viewed from this standpoint any pronouncement backed by the Society's committee on press censorship should turn out facts that are not easy to controvert. The influence of the committee should also tend to minimize the harm that comes from the public braying of individuals with partly developed reason, especially such as air in the public press personal grievances that come not from the attitude of society toward them, but from their attitude toward society. There have always been objectors and objectors there will always be. Society needs them. It is objectors like Luther and Wesley and Paré who have shaken ancient error and brought about substantial progress. But the objector is not always sane in his public utterance; he is more apt to appeal to the hysterical and emotional among the people and thereby provoke hasty and ill-considered legislation that may undo the real progress of fifty years of enlightenment. This is especially true of the art of medicine where suggestion plays so vital a part;

the public which cannot swallow a capsule of castor oil, let us say, can yet gulp down with the keenest enjoyment sensational impossibilities, chaff by the bushel, legislative monstrosities. If the reading public could be assured that whatever appears in the public press without the sanction of some representative medical body is as yet of doubtful and unproven value, they would be less prone to rush blindly to every new cure that is not a cure, to champion each new fad that is but the resurrected shell of yesterday's error and to squander money for husks.

If the effort inaugurated by the Kings County Society can be kept above partisanship; if the committee can continue to represent broad and liberal views; if the petty jealousies which are so prone to develop among physicians can be kept out of sight, we believe that publication of medical knowledge under the sanction and seal of so influential a society will go far toward increasing public health and combating misconception and error.

H. G. W.

## PUBLICITY COMMITTEE.

A T the last meeting of the Council of the Medical Society of the County of Kings the president was authorized to appoint a committee of three members to seek co-operation with the editors of the press in order to devise some plan whereby articles and interviews on medical topics by members of the Society published in the daily papers should be truthfully and correctly reported. The Council received so many complaints from members of the Society practically accusing the Council of negligence in not meting out punishment to members guilty of unethical conduct in the matter of self-exploitation through the public press that the Council felt it necessary to have an advisory committee on publicity appointed.

At a meeting of this committee it was decided that its objects were as follows:

1. To prevent the publication in the daily press of misleading and erroneous statements on medical topics.

2. To prevent the publication of cures and surgical operations so exaggerated and false that mental anguish, physical suffering and expense would be imposed upon the sick and afflicted.

3. To prevent the reporting of ordinary medical cases and surgical operations of no interest to the profession which are misunderstood by the public and serve but to exploit the narrator.

4. To act as an advisory committee, if so desired, to members of the Society who contemplate publishing medical articles in the newspapers and who desire to conform to the code of ethics.

5. To further the publication of scientific articles on medical subjects relating to the public health.

6. To seek the co-operation of the editors to accomplish these purposes.

The committee desires it to be understood that they do not discourage publicity but, on the contrary, advocate the greatest publicity possible on the liberal, ethical lines of the American Medical Association, which encourages members of the profession to give as wide publicity as possible to all matters pertaining to hygiene, sanitation and the public health, but discourages all direct or indirect self-advertising. The committee recognizes the futility of any attempt on its part to dictate to the press what it should or what it should not publish. It is thought by the committee that the adoption of these suggestions will relieve members of the Society of any fear of criticism and will aid representatives of the press in securing interviews without difficulty.

The committee wishes it thoroughly understood that it will in no sense act as a complainant body against offenders, but will most willingly extend its advice to those who voluntarily seek its aid.

John C. MacEvitt, M.D.,<br>
Joshua M. Van Cott, M.D.,<br>
Frederick Tilney, M.D.

## THE GLANDULAR ORIGIN OF SECOND SIGHT.

OUT of the tranquil respectability of Montclair, New Jersey, comes the voice of one Trippet, proclaiming signs and wonders and literally speaking with tongues, for is he not conscious that this is at least his third appearance upon earth? It has not been granted us to speak with Mr. Trippet in the flesh, but through the published word only. Like Pharaoh's butler, he was troubled with a dream, not once, but many times; he himself hints at some relation between this dream and a quality of tobacco he had used, but it seems more reasonable to accept the ultimate belief that this vision was a vague memory of a former life revealed to him in the watches of the night. There is nothing in the gentleman's name or occupation to indicate his truly emotional nature, but if we remember aright, Mr. Kipling, always a veracious historian, found a similar experience in a prosaic bank clerk. With him the vista of the past opened in glimpses only; forgetfulness came when he fell in love. Will the parallel hold good for Brother Trippet? These nocturnal experiences have been woven into a book in which the curious may find set out at length all that the author has had revealed of his past.

Not content with psychic experiences only Mr. Trippet has further propounded a theory of dazzling possibilities. He has proposed to demonstrate to the scientific bodies of Montclair, Upper Montclair, Bloomfield, and the region thereabout, his conclusion that second sight is dependent upon an enlargement of the pituitary gland. He argues that certain fish found in the Mammoth Cave possess no eyes, but nevertheless find their way about quite comfortably without them. In these fish, obtained after some difficulty through government channels, he has found an enlarged pituitary body; what is more logical, therefore, than the evident conclusion that the pituitary body enables the eyeless fish to see, provides them in short with that strange sense by which certain human beings are able to delve into the past, present and future, to elucidate mysteries and cajole coin from the curious? Having found this remarkable power in the wife of one of his townsmen, he is even ready to demonstrate in her an enlarged pituitary gland and is doubtless hungering for the time when ocular demonstration may supplant surmise. The Academy of Sciences of Montclair, of which the postmaster, constable, two justices of the peace and the local veterinary are enthusiastic members, is ardent in its support of Mr. Trippet's theory. In point of fact, the last named expert is now at work elaborating his investigations into second sight in the cow, and it is feared that the researches of this scientific body are likely to promote a considerable mortality among the domestic pets in Montclair and may lead to a clash with the S. P. C. A.

We must confess to considerable disappointment in acknowledging that, as a result of careful reading of recent literature, we fail to find any reference to the effect of pituitrin in increasing the ability of obstetricians to foresee the outcome of their labors. Next in importance to the ability to predetermine sex we place the capacity for accurately foretelling whether it will be a boy or a girl. It is earnestly to be hoped that the possibilities of Mr. Trippet's theory will be appreciated and thoroughly investigated by the Obstetric Society with a view to utilizing the clairvoyant power for practical ends. We are looking eagerly forward to further inroads into the field of occult science by the gifted town-clerk of Montclair.

H. G. W.

## THE JUNE MEETING.

THE President, Dr. Samuel Hendrickson, announces that the Spring Meeting of the Society will be held at Cold Spring Harbor on Saturday, June 14, 1913. Among the attractions offered are opportunities to inspect the Fish Hatchery and Biological Institute. The latter establishment is a particularly interesting one, conducting investigations that will amply repay a visit. The Director, Dr. Davenport, has most obligingly offered to present some remarks on the work under his charge and will also be prepared to exhibit some of the records of the Institute. A new building for research work is under construction and should be open for work before the date of the meeting.

A clambake is also under consideration, and should prove a most delightful feature of the meeting.

Full information as to train service and a detailed program will be mailed by the secretary in due time.

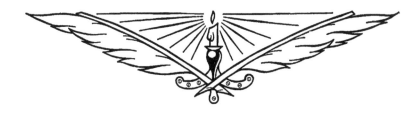

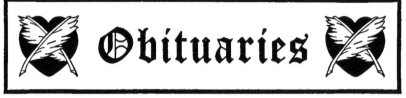

## ALGERNON THOMAS BRISTOW, M.D.*
### An Appreciation by William Francis Campbell, M.D.

ON March 26th, 1913, Algernon Thomas Bristow died of a septic wound inflicted during the performance of an operation; and thus was removed from our ranks a man of light and leading; a scholar of profound learning and great scientific attainment; a surgeon of conspicuous ability.

The passing of Dr. Bristow is surrounded with peculiar pathos if not a touch of romance.

There is a smug complacency that deafens its ears to the call of service and rests content in slippered ease far from the noise of battle. To such as this it may seem a prodigal waste that such a life at the full realization of its usefulness should be given a ransom that others less needed might survive. And yet he died as all true men would die—on the firing line with his face to the front. Where duty called he counted no cost and dreaded nought but cowardice. He realized that there was no great achievement without a great adventure, and no great adventure without a challenge to fate. "He heard the call of Tomorrow, and hastened to answer the summons of Destiny."

Dr. Bristow matured late. There was nothing precocious or callow in the unfolding of his life. The roots of his mind struck deep into the fundamentals of his art. Anatomy, physiology, chemistry, pathology, biology and botany were the springs by which it was fed; and the versatility, profundity and readiness of his knowledge were at once the wonder and delight of those who shared the intimacies of his mind. Thus upon a solid foundation was reared a superstructure of commanding proportions.

His mind was at once analytical and judicial. He marshalled his data, correlated his facts, and made his deductions with a convincing logic that rendered his conclusions invincible and unanswerable. Thus as a diagnostician he was superb because he was supreme.

He was a great teacher because he had a great passion for truth; he was a great surgeon because he had a great passion for perfection. He was a scholar because he never left school. He was always the student, ever graduating, not out but up, from one class to a higher class; recognizing in the larger relationships, that life is the school, work the curriculum, character the diploma.

Our noblest impulses and finest thoughts he crystallized into words. Honored with a position of commanding importance as Editor of the State Journal, he employed its columns for the instruction, the chastening, the defense and the uplift of the medical profession. His facile pen did valiant service, and through it he confessed himself.

---

* Presented at the Brooklyn Pathological Society, April 10, 1913.

His editorials showed depth of thought and beauty of diction. They scintillated with satire, and an aptness of quotation which showed an intimate acquaintance with the masters of literature. There was sometimes heat but always light. There was always breadth but never shallowness. We may have differed, but always with respect.

Through his leadership we have all gained a clearer vision and a larger outlook, for he trod the higher slopes.

Though profoundly respected and much beloved, he was much misunderstood. With an equipment so complete, yet his armor was vulnerable in its exquisite sensitiveness, and thus he was often wounded. With a large opportunity for moulding men it was much curtailed by a temperamental impatience with the apathy of others to appreciate what his alert mind so readily comprehended.

He had no patience with the cheap, the mediocre, the superficial, the bizarre.

He could not mingle with the multitude and thus for lack of sympathy the multitude misunderstood.

Sensitive as a woman, petulant as a child; he possessed a woman's tenderness and the child's open mind.

Not amid the turmoil and the strife was he at his best. He was too fine a fiber to bear unflinching the buffets of a coarse competition. At his own fireside, at the family altar whereon burned with steady glow his heart's purest affection: there amid the peace that passeth understanding his simple and gentle soul found its native clime: there in the family circle we often sat charmed by the beauty of his mind which never lost its power of leading us by an unspoken invocation "to a green field, ever kept fresh by a living fountain."

Faults he had—the heritage of our common humanity. Had he less we could not love him more. But above and beyond them all is the asset that survives. For in all that makes for manhood, for conscience and for character, in nobility of purpose, in lofty aspiration, in the larger vision, and in "the mighty hopes that makes us men," Dr. Bristow passed "Through all this tract of years wearing the white flower of a blameless life."

## PHILIP HANSON HISS, JR., A.B., M.D.

Dr. Hiss was born in Baltimore, Md., September 17, 1868, and died in New York City February 27, 1913. He was the son of Philip H. Hiss and Susan Shirk. He was educated at Johns Hopkins University, where he was graduated with the degree of A.B. in 1891. His medical education was received at the College of Physicians and Surgeons, New York, from which institution he received the degree of M.D. in the class of 1895.

During his professional life he was Professor of Bacteriology in the College of Physicians and Surgeons, Bacteriologist in the Health Department, Professor of Hygiene in the Women's Medical College, and was a member of the Medical Society County of Kings from 1906, American Medical Association, Society of Naturalists, Society of Bacteriologists, Association of Pathologists and Bacteriologists, Society of Experimental Biology, American Public Health Association, the New York Pathological Society, and Harvey Society. Dr. Hiss is survived by his widow, Carolyn Dow, and two children.

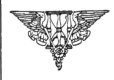 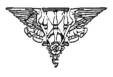
# TRANSACTIONS OF THE BROOKLYN SOCIETY OF INTERNAL MEDICINE.

*Regular Meeting, January 24, 1913.*

The President, DR. TASKER HOWARD, in the Chair.

*Executive Session.*

Remarks by President Howard:

In starting in the second year of the Society, I should like to congratulate the Society on the success of the last year under the skillful leadership of Dr. Cornwall. I congratulate him and the Society that he not only carried the Society with success through the first year but conceived the idea of having a Council to help out the President, to advise with him and talk over the matters of the Society. In this way I think he has gone a long way toward making for the success of the Society in the future.

I have asked to serve on the Council, Dr. Butler, Dr. Cornwall, Dr. Kerr and Dr. Lincoln, besides the officers of the Society.

There is one part of the program I wish we could enlarge a little, and that is the voluntary report of cases. Last year was the first year of the Society and perhaps the members did not know each other as well as they do now; but I hope as they come to know each other better, some one will make a break in volunteering to report cases. I hope members who have any cases which are interesting will bring them out and talk them over. Reports should not take over five minutes. I think that will make a very helpful part of the program. It would be a good scheme before bringing up a case in the Society, to notify either the Secretary or President of the Society of our intention to do so.

## Headache: Its Treatment.

*By William S. Hubbard, M.D.*

Probably no single symptom is more frequently noted in the history-taking than *headache,* and in a large number of cases it is the only thing complained of by the patient; but its exact significance is for the most part a matter of difficulty to determine, and to rid the patient of the distressing misery often baffles the skill of the physician, even of the one who was consulted after you were discharged from the case.

In this discussion of the subject I ask your pardon for dividing headaches into *several groups* according to several body regions:

1. Those whose causes seem to be in the region of the head, as head-headaches.

2. Those which depend upon circulatory and respiratory derangements, as thoracic headaches.

3. Those whose origin is in the digestive and eliminative system, as abdominal headaches, and,

4. Those which seem to bear some relation to the pelvic viscera, as pelvic headaches.

This is not a scientific classification, but aims to bring the subject under few heads for consideration.

To consider not all but some of the more common head-headaches, we shall think of migraine, neuralgia (including tic doloreaux), psychoneurosis, meningitis, tumor of the brain, infections of the various sinuses, and a number due to eye-strain and nasal deformity. Of these I omit the first, which has been abundantly treated by the first speaker.

Psychoneuroses—nervous headaches or imaginative pains in the head— form a very large class and include neurasthenic, hysterical and phychasthenic

196

types functional in kind and of great variety, defying classification as to topography, severity and regularity of incidence.

Some are frontal, some are vertical; others temporal or occipital, and these are diverse in kind and severity, from blinding to dull and from throbbing to boring. They often occur on rising in the morning and wear off as the day wears on. Again, they appear at night. They are complained of by people who give other evidence of nervous derangement. Trigeminal neuralgia and tic doloreaux are so clearly defined as not to need any remarks about location and paroxysmal seizures.

In meningitis and other infectious *headache,* though often the most pronounced, is but one of the symptoms presenting, while the headaches due to aural, nasal or ocular disease or deformity are often proven to exist only by careful examination when proper treatment relieves the suffering.

Syphilis, la grippe and typhoid are frequent causes of most severe headaches which sometimes fail of proper diagnosis.

Under the head of thoracic headaches are those referable to the cardiovascular apparatus, including the vasomotor system as well, and the headaches of pulmonary disorders, asthma and pneumonia.

Whether *anæmia* is to be accounted sufficient cause for headaches is a question, but we shall all agree that *hyperæmia,* especially venous, is a frequent cause of this symptom.

Chemical poisons entering the system by inhalation, as illuminating gas, marsh gas and other gases, give rise to headaches, and changes in the arterial caliber, especially within the cranium, may account for some headache and vertigo, and this is most surely the case when changes of a similar kind have invaded the renal vessels.

By far the largest class of headaches that I see are due to disturbances of the functions of digestion and elimination—abdominal headaches.

Gluttony, alcoholism, constipation, intestinal toxæmia and putrefaction, ptomaine and leucomaine poisoning, and other less well-defined chemicals—by-products of faulty metabolism—are among the established causes of headaches.

Other names, erroneously applied, such as lithæmic, rheumatic, gouty, are probably fully covered in the foregoing list.

(In many cases some one article of diet will so poison the blood as to cause violent headaches.)

Of pelvic causes we may say that, though often alleged, the causal relation is not so clear here as it might be, and many so-called reflex headaches are referred to disorders of the pelvic organs, which more probably arise from toxic substances carried in the bloodstream from the abdominal organs. But it is also equally probable that internal secretions set free at the time of great functional activity in the pelvic organs may account for the headache of puberty and the menopause.

Beyond and above all the so far classified headaches there are unquestionably many which are frequently listed as constitutional, hereditary, chronic, but which we may as well admit quite baffle our knowledge to define.

The treatment of this distressing malady is often an urgent matter and tests our ability to the limit. Many cases seek aid from widely advertised cures of questionable efficiency or dangerous composition, and, really, one can hardly blame the sufferers.

To treat successfully such cases, however, it is necessary, first, to study most carefully for the underlying causes as the main object to be obtained, and, secondly, to relieve the present distress at least temporarily, or else to give the patient a good reason for not doing so, making every effort to obtain and retain the patient's confidence.

These patients are often beside themselves and will do anything and take anything to obtain relief; it is therefore incumbent upon us to relieve them rather than to let them seek the aid of unknown remedies which may do untold harm if constantly employed. 'Tis not the drug that is at fault, but the manner of its use, and we are often forced to confess that the drugs which the laity get for themselves are the same that we would prescribe if called upon. I have found it useful in this connection, especially among neurotics, to prescribe two drugs to be taken alternately, one the potent drug and the other a placebo. There is nothing new in this idea, but it works on each new patient like the old joke on the newcomer and it at least diminishes the frequency of the depressing agent.

Very often in searching for the cause of headache we discover a surgical affection which *may* be the source of the trouble, viz., a nasal spur or a slight ocular deviation, and we advise an operation as the only permanent relief.

My own feeling is that we should exercise great care not to overdo the possibilities—to be sure by exclusion that there is no other cause for that particular headache before submitting the patient to the surgical procedure. No great amount of time need be lost in careful diagnosis, and we shall often find that there is another cause perhaps not quite so apparent to the head-light as the spur or other deformity. It must be admitted that all the anatomical asymmetries are known to exist without causing any trouble at all, and, on the other hand, we have all seen and cared for cases of neuropathic headaches which date from some surgical operation, more particularly in the field of gynæcology, especially before the days of more conservatism in dealing with the adnexa.

When surgery is needed there should be no doubt of that need and no hesitation in resorting to it, and the results here will prove the correctness of the diagnosis and advice; but where there is a question less harm is done, even if there is no symptom-relief, without resorting to surgery, than if the symptom persists after an ill-advised operation.

I am no foe to honest surgery. I know its great benefits, but I am confident that now and again surgery is called upon where greater care in diagnosis or better advice would work better results.

In the cardiovascular cases very particular attention must be paid to hygiene and diet and rest, to atmospheric conditions and to exercise.

In psychoneuroses much can be done to lessen the complaining, at least, of these headachers, by studying to interest these patients in things outside of themselves, often a most difficult thing, but most efficacious when accomplished. Attention to details, anticipating the expected headache of menstruation in neurotic women by vigorous catharsis and rest, will often break up a seemingly fixed habit.

In urgent cases of unknown cause a small dose of morphia and hyoscin hypodermically, or even a sterile water injection in cases unacquainted with the needle, or K I in small does, often repeated by the physician, using in conjunction the power of suggestion, have been followed by rapidly favorable results.

I have had but little good effect from either electricity or vibration, probably because I do not use them faithfully or skillfully.

When all is done that can be done there are some headaches which time alone will cure, and then some which nothing relieves till death comes to stop all pain.

### Headache, from the Standpoint of the Ophthalmologist.

Dr. B. C. Collins, in opening the discussion, said:—"That eye-strain may and does cause headache we all know. Every physician has had or heard of cases that have been relieved and cured of headaches and various reflex nervous disturbances by the use of glasses. The defects requiring glasses may be hyperopia, myopia and astigmatism, with their various muscular weakening, and presbyopia.

"Headache is much more often associated with hyperopia and astigmatism than with myopia. It is surprising to learn that many patients require careful correction of a slight refractive error and must wear their glasses constantly, while others may have a much greater defect, ignore correction, and be perfectly comfortable.

"The determination of the proper use of lenses for the improvement of sight followed closely upon the invention of the ophthalmoscope. No exactness in the determination of the value of glasses was possible until the lens, vitreous humor, choroid and retina could be in each case examined to determine if opacities or other changes existed in them. A few years after the ophthalmoscope came into use surgeons all over the civilized world were adjusting glasses for eyes given up as blind, or nearly so, and had been given over to the unscientific jeweler or optician.

"That the eye may give perfect distant vision and still be very defective we know, and this is the class of patients in which we have the headaches. In these cases the ciliary or focusing muscle is compelled to do too much work and strain is the result. To detect these defects in persons under 40 years a drug must be used to paralyze the ciliary muscle. The defects, in spite of many instruments recently devised, cannot be accurately determined in any other way, and this is the reason why the optician cannot relieve this class of cases.

"I may illustrate by this case:

"A boy, 12 years of age, came under my care two years ago. He was wearing glasses and had been confined in a home because he would not attend school or study. The school doctor advised the parents to have his eyes examined and they took him to an optician who prescribed O U plus 50 di. sph.

"His distant vision was 20/15 and he could not be made to attend school for more than three or four days at a time. He was sent to a truant home. He said he was uncomfortable when reading and would not do so.

"Tested under homatropin he showed hyperopia plus 4.50 ds. sph. A good result followed the glasses.

"For muscular defects I do not believe in a graduated tenotomy. Prisms very seldom.

"I believe that if our refractive errors are fully corrected the muscles improve also.

"Prisms may be used to strengthen muscles with good results.

"Presbyopia is often a cause of headache. A person passes 40 years and goes on reading as before. He or she may be very timid about their age and feel that they can see as well as ever and they put off their near glasses until headache causes them to seek relief from the oculist.

"Nasal accessory sinus disease is often cause of headache and must not be overlooked. Next to eye-strain I would place it second as a cause of headache.

"Then comes the ear. If the headache is associated with a chronic running ear look out for a brain abscess.

"This reminds me of the case of a school teacher who came to see me for an eczema of the auditory canal, and while treating this condition she said she would have to consult her oculist, as her headaches were returning. I asked her who her oculist was and she mentioned the name of one of the most prominent men in New York, who said she would have to have another graduated tenotomy done. She had had five already, but as her headaches were returning she decided to go over and have another tenotomy done. She consulted Dr. Hubbard, who cured her. That was in the days when we were all greatly alarmed by uric acid. Dr. Cornwall could tell you something about that. The cure in her case was a proper elimination and change in diet. I have had her under observation, as has Dr. Hubbard also, for thirteen or fourteen years. She has had her glasses changed for presbyopia three or four times during that period but has no more headaches as long as she attends to her diet.

"I think spurs may cause headache, but if more attention were given to nasal sinusitis more relief would be found in these chronic headaches, and when they have that they will not have a constant headache, but recurring headaches, and oftentimes you will examine any one of the sinuses and at that time you will find a mucous or muco-pus from one of the sinuses making its way into the nostril.

"I would place nasal accessory sinus diseases as probably second to the eye as a cause of many cases of chronic headache. Then we must not omit the ear. Take a case of chronic suppuration; you would be surprised to find, as Dr. Brush can tell you, too, that oftentimes a patient is suffering for years and years with a chronic brain abscess discharging into the auditory canal with no symptoms other than headache. Dr. Eagleton, of Newark, in a paper read at Atlantic City in the past fall related this and stated he had seen a number of cases, and that brought many men to their feet who had also seen cases of brain abscess when nothing was suspected. He mentioned a symptom that I saw in a case in July with recurring headaches of four or five years' standing and chronic discharge of eighteen years. In this man the only symptom was the headache, and it would come on at certain periods and last until, I presume, an extra amount of discharge from the ear relieved him, and he also had a slight facial paralysis that unless your attention was called to it you would hardly detect, and that was merely a twitching of his mouth. You would notice that in coming into the room or in speaking to you his mouth would turn to one side. Dr. Eagleton made the statement that if that symptom were present in any one he regarded it as almost diagnostic of brain abscess if associated with a chronic discharging ear on that side."

Dr. J. STURDIVANT READ, in discussion, said:—"Syphilis is often the unsuspected cause of headache. It is surprising how frequently this is forgotten. Many wide-awake physicians overlook it in women of fine morality and intelligence who have been infected in the marriage bed and who have never known it. Syphilitic infection in both men and women without their cognizance is possible. The initial lesion is so situated that it escapes notice; the secondaries so slight that they are overlooked. This explains why some honest and intelligent patients will deny any previous infection when tertiary lesions are present. In the past year I have seen three intra-urethral chancres. In these cases diagnosis of mild urethritis had been made.

"The character of syphilitic headaches varies. The intense meningeal type is easily recognized, or at least lues as a cause is early suspected. We should remember that this poison may be present in varying degrees and consequently the head pains are not always of this pronounced type. Any long-continued series of headaches which has resisted 'all treatments,' should have the possible basis of lues eliminated by blood examinations and therapeutic tests.

"Even in the presence of a negative Wassermann, in *tertiary* syphilis, we should not hesitate to try the therapeutic test, as the Wassermann is negative in about 15 per cent. of these cases."

DR. J. M. WALLFIELD, in closing the discussion, said:—"It seems to me that every part of the body was taken into consideration as producing headache, but the teeth were forgotten. I want to cite one or two cases where the headache was traced directly to an abscess at the root of a tooth which was crowned and where no pain was felt by the patient.

"My practice is located in a section and among people who are suffering a good deal with headaches. The Jewish race is usually nervous, especially the women. I have seen cases of syphilitic headaches, but they are more marked and can be more easily recognized than the headaches from other causes. Dr. Cornwall pointed out the slowness of speech in syphilis, the continuous headaches and the tendency to lie down.

"A couple of years ago a traveling salesman complained while in Buffalo of an earache and headache. The doctor there incised the drum, expecting to find pus. This did not relieve him. About four weeks later he happened to be in Pittsburg and was told that the mastoid was involved and he was advised to return to New York and be operated upon. Before going to the operation I was called in to advise him as to what he should do. I examined the ear but could not find anything. There was headache on the same side as the earache and I asked him if he ever had a pain in his teeth. He could not recollect that he recently had one, but about two weeks previous to the attack he had had pain for a day or two. On striking the teeth with a steel instrument I elicited pain in one of the molars and advised him, before having the mastoid operation, to have that tooth pulled. A few drops of pus were found and the headache and earache were relieved. Since then I make it a routine practice in my work to examine teeth by striking them before I come to the conclusion that the pain in the head is not due to the teeth.

"I was called in not long ago to see a young woman—a very nervous woman—with a history of headache for three months on one side, and after carefully striking the teeth I found a molar on the same side which gave her pain. I advised her to go to the dentist and the dentist claims that he allowed some gas to escape from the root of the tooth by drilling a hole there. She was relieved immediately.

"Dr Brush mentioned that Strumpel says he has never seen any results from any operative work on the nose in headaches. An old woman, 72 years of age, suddenly developed a headache which kept up for four months. It was a frontal headache. She went over to a surgeon in New York who told her that he could not do anything for her; that there seemed to be a growth in the head. She became so bad that her son-in-law, in whose charge she was, became frantic and ran for the first physician he could find and he struck me. I came up and on examining her could not find anything but an hypertrophied turbinate. To satisfy myself I took a few drops of adrenalin and applied them to the turbinates. She felt immediately somewhat relieved. I advised her to go over to a nose man and have them removed, and she was cured of the headache."

### Headache, from the Standpoint of the Gynecologist.

DR. WILLIAM A. JEWETT, in discussion, said:—"The symptom of headache is one of the most common that the gynecologist has to deal with, but, in my experience, the nature of the headache does not help very much in a diagnosis of the condition.

"The headaches due to pelvic disease are usually found in the vertex or in the occiput, according to the text books. I think that you find just as many attacks of migraine or a condition that I would call migraine. Frontal headaches seem to be just as common as those in the vertex and occipital region. The character of the pain and the severity and distribution are practically the same as in headaches, from any reflex cause. Headaches are more marked at the time of the menstrual period. The type that I speak of as migraine (I hardly dare use the term after hearing Dr. Brush's paper) will very often come before the menstrual flow. It may precede it for twenty-four or forty-eight hours. The pain will be more marked on rising in the morning and occupy the frontal region, not necessarily unilateral, though it may be more to one side than the other, and it is usually not very severe in type. The pain may be sharp; it may be stabbing; it may be of a boring character similar to those described in migraine. Usually there is some nausea or vomiting with the pain due to pelvic disease the same as in the attacks of migraine.

"Among our patients we meet with a great many neurasthenics and they are frequently patients who will attribute their headaches to some pelvic disorder though careful pelvic examination will reveal no abnormal condition that could account for it.

"We have to deal with cases of anemic headaches in girls just at the time of puberty where there is the frontal headache, pain in the orbits and vertex and occiput, and, in fact, pain all over the head which is quite severe. If the anemia is marked, as in extreme chlorosis, we have very severe headaches.

"The treatment for headaches of this character is to remove the cause; remove the anemia and you will remove the headaches.

"We have many headaches, following excessive menstrual flow, metrorrhagia or menorrhagia. The headache will be one of the symptoms due to the anemia and not to the pelvic disease itself.

"We meet many patients with so-called bilious headache due to constipation and disturbed digestive functions. A great many women in our clinics will have general enteroptosis, due to laceration of the pelvic floor and relaxed abdominal walls. This condition will cause constipation and absorption of toxins from the intestines with resulting headache. Laceration of the cervix will occasionally give rise to a reflex headache, usually vertical, and very often associated with neuralgias of other parts of the body. The laceration itself I hardly think is the direct cause of the headache, but the cervical laceration reduces the tone of the whole system, the patients' general health is impaired, and the headache results from that. Sometimes, in the cases of cervical laceration with erosion and endocervictitis, headaches will be relieved by the topical application of a 10 per cent. solution of cocain or 4 per cent. nitrate of silver solution. This latter tends to relieve the inflammatory condition in the cervix that has caused the reflex headache. Chronic endocervictitis acts in the same way. With an infected endometritis of the body of the uterus frequently is associated tubal and ovarian inflammation. These patients have headaches. Just what the relation between the pelvic condition and the headache is I do not know. I assume that it is due to the effect on the general health—the general depressed state of health that favors headaches. Sclerosis of the uterus, a chronic interstitial metritis, seems to give a very severe type of headache. The pain is located in about the same regions as other headache, but it is of a more severe type. It, of course, appears at the time of the pelvic congestion, at the menstrual period, and usually appears at the same time each month associated with backache and bearing-down pains in the lower abdomen.

"The posterior displacements of the uterus I think rarely cause any headaches unless the uterus is adherent. If we have a retroverted uterus that is adherent the patient will frequently complain of headaches. In those cases I think it is due to the inflammatory condition which is present and believe that that is more the cause of the headache than the displacement itself.

"The same would apply to cases of prolapse of the uterus. If the prolapse is the cause of a chronic pelvic congestion that will cause headache.

"Tumors of the uterus very rarely cause any headaches unless the tumors are of such a character that they give us a chronic congestion. If they do, we have the same cause that we have in the inflammatory conditions in the pelvis and we may have headaches. The treatment where headache is due to pelvic disease is the removal of the diseased condition; curettage in endometritis, repair of cervical lacerations with removal of the scar tissue, and breaking up the adhesions of an adherent netro-displaced uterus, etc., will cure many of these patients.

"We must be guarded in our prognosis. It is not possible to promise a cure by surgical procedure in every case, as Dr. Hubbard has said. Many times headaches and other pains are attributed to some pathological condition that is easily found in the pelvis and the general system is neglected in the examination."

DR. EDWARD E. CORNWALL, in discussion, said:—"Headache is, of course, not a disease, but a symptom, and a symptom found in very many conditions. A classification of headaches, according to the underlying pathological conditions which seems to me a natural and convenient one, is the following: 1. Organic, those caused by inflammatory or neoplastic conditions in the brain. 2. Circulatory, those caused by too much or too little blood in the brain. 3. Toxemic. 4. Reflex. These underlying pathological conditions frequently

4

exist in combination; the circulatory and toxemic conditions are often found together and with headaches of reflex nervous causation circulatory disturbances may be found.

"A large proportion of the headaches we meet have for an exciting cause a toxemia. Whether or not migraine can be classed as a toxemic headache is not altogether clear, but it would seem that a toxemic factor is often present. It has been suggested that the basis of migraine is a diathesis. What is a diathesis? I would define offhand a diathesis as a condition, congenital or acquired, in which are present one or both of the following things: subnormal resistance of particular tissues to particular poisons, and a subnormal protective mechanism. An inherited weakness of the brain and nervous system or a natural intolerance of the nervous and circulatory systems to certain poisons, might explain the phenomena of migraine with or without abnormally low functional power of the protective mechanism, a prominent element of which is the liver. The particular poison to which the nervous system may be intolerant, or with which the protective mechanism cannot deal adequately, may be uric acid, or putrefactive or other poisons from the intestines, or perversions of the internal secretions.

"With this provisional explanation of migraine we can proceed to discuss its treatment; and the most obvious rational therapeutic indications are, to lessen the work of the protective mechanism by diminishing the quantity of the poisons which are under our control, so that the protective mechanism, thus relieved, can devote its energies more to the particular poison to which the complaining tissues are intolerant. This we can do to a very large and often to a very effective extent by diminishing the quantity of the toxic substances which are introduced with the food or produced from the food; by substituting for the habitual diet another diet which will supply adequate nutrition with production of fewer toxic by-products whose neutralization would preoccupy the liver and other elements of the protective mechanism—in other words, we would substitute for the conventional diet, which is a relatively hard diet from the point of view of the metabolism, an easier diet which supplies sufficient nutrition with less strain on the mechanism.

"In connection with the subject of toxemic headaches, I would like to say a word about katzenjammer. How does drinking alcoholics produce a headache next day? Is it entirely a result of the action of the alcohol on the brain tissue? I think a good part of it is caused by the other toxins which escape destruction in the liver because that organ is so much occupied trying to destroy the alcohol. Perhaps in many cases katzenjammer is largely acute putrefaction toxemia of intestinal origin.

"Apropos of the subject of syphilitic headaches, I will briefly refer to a case of cerebral syphilis which came under my observation a few years ago This case is impressed on my memory because of the extreme severity of the headache, which became stupefying, and because of the treatment. I rapidly ran up the dose of the potassium iodide, so that the patient, a woman thirty-five years old, took an ounce of it daily for over two weeks. She recovered."

### A Case of Brain Abscess

*Reported by Dr. B. C. Collins.*

This is the case of a boy that I saw for the first time on Wednesday afternoon, about two o'clock, with a history of an attack of grip, two weeks previous, followed by an earache and discharging ear. My examination at that time revealed an abscess in the middle ear and a tender and edematous mastoid. There were no other symptoms except a subnormal temperature.

The family doctor had been in attendance practically two weeks and said that there had been very little pain and discomfort and he sent him to me on account of the swelling and tenderness of the mastoid. There had been no temperature during the two weeks at any time, though the doctor had taken it. The temperature when I saw him was 97. I advised operation for relief of the mastoid abscess and was surprised to find after clearing out the neurotic mastoid that the bone over the temporal region and behind and above the meatus was necrotic and covered an area probably the size of a half dollar. The dura was covered with granulations and foul-smelling pus. On exploration with the probe I found that the probe penetrated the dura to a depth of about one-half inch, and, curving my exploratory probe, it entered the sulcus between the cerebrum and cerebellum, with free flowing pus. I incised this dura freely and inserted gauze drains. In a previous case I put in a drainage tube which I found was not reliable as a drain for that location. Therefore, this time I put in gauze.

Of course, it is too early to tell of the result, but the patient is today in very good condition. Vomiting was constant all day yesterday; the pupil was dilated yesterday on the affected side and irresponsive to light, but today the pupil is contracted and responsive and vomiting has ceased. I think the indications for recovery are fair, but it is a little too early to tell.

### A Case of Gastric Tumor, Disappearing Spontaneously.

*Reported by Albert F. R. Andresen, M.D.*

Miss A. B., age 42, American, single, dressmaker.

*Family History.*—Father died of old age at 85; mother died of carcinoma of the rectum at the age of 67. Five sisters and two brothers, all living and well.

*Previous History.*—Had been nervous all her life; did not go to school until ten years of age; had scarlet fever at four years, followed by nephritis and "paralysis of legs;" at fifteen began menstruating; felt fine for three years; at eighteen began to get nervous again and lost weight and had severe pains in her right hip which kept her in bed for a long period of time; then began to have stomach trouble, and had a tape worm which was gotten rid of at twenty years of age and which never recurred.

As early as fourteen years she had suffered from car-sickness; she also vomited when she stood up too long, as for having a dress fitted on; had almost constant burning pain in the left side of the abdomen; abdomen was always tender; sometimes she vomited for weeks at a time and then had long remissions.

Twelve years ago she began treatment with a physician under whose care she remained until three years ago when he left town. At first she got much relief and was well for two years; then the pains returned and after a year she had severe vomiting spells followed by melena, nine years ago. Two years later she had another similar attack. After any exercise, especially lifting the left arm, she would get severe vomiting followed by diarrhea; patient never vomited any blood. For three years she had almost constant vomiting and repeatedly refused operation, which was advised. Finally, in March, 1910, a mass having developed gradually in the epigastrium, she was operated on at the Kings County Hospital by Dr. Calvin F. Barber.

When the abdomen was opened she was pretty weak and at the time went into a state of collapse and the abdomen had to be closed up almost immediately, there being merely time to inspect the stomach. The entire pyloric end of the stomach was found to be the seat of a hard, indurated mass, and the tip of the finger could with difficulty be inserted into the pyloric orifice. A carcinoma of the pylorus was diagnosed and the abdomen closed, it being considered inoperable. After the operation the patient was in bed three or four weeks and began to improve slowly. During the following summer she gained ten pounds, did not vomit, her bowels were regular and her only complaint was severe lumbar backache. In the autumn she had another spell of vomiting. Then followed a period of constant burning epigastric pain, which was very bad at night and was relieved by regurgitation of food or vomiting; also by taking sodium bicarbonate. Two more attacks of melena occurred before I saw her in March, 1911. She was then having a vomiting spell with severe epigastric pain; the extremities were cold, the face anxious, of high pallor, the vomiting greenish; she was emaciated and pale and there was a large, hard, nodular mass in the epigastrium, which seemed to be about four or five inches across and adherent to the scar of operation. During a few of these attacks only morphine seemed to relieve the spasms, and finally, the case being considered hopeless, I prescribed opium and belladonna suppositories to be used as required, thinking she was going to die. After this I did not hear from her for two years, during which time she improved in every way, gained fifteen or twenty pounds, was out walking and had no vomiting, except occasionally after marked indiscretions of diet. She still continued to have left-sided burning pain and nausea when the left arm was raised. She had been taking the opium every day although the dose had gradually been decreased. Last summer she passed per rectum a mass shaped like one-half of a small hollow rubber ball, tough and elastic. I did not see this, so do not know what it was. About one month ago I was called to see her in another attack of vomiting, this time not followed by tarry stools.

Examination disclosed a pretty well-nourished woman with a good color, the chest was negative and there were no glandular enlargements. The abdomen showed a fine narrow epigastric scar; slight tenderness in the mid-epigastrium and no sign of any mass whatever. No other abnormalities.

*Test Meal.*—An hour after ingestion brought up 150 c.c. well-chymified material, free hydrochloric acid 40, total acid 65. No evidences of stagnation. Urine was absolutely negative, stool contained no occult blood; hemoglobin as high as

95 per cent.; red and white cells count normal. She has improved considerably since then under suitable treatment, has been out of bed and is having practically no pain.

During the past month I have broken her of the mild opium habit which she had acquired and have treated her gastric ulcer. She is now doing very nicely, is having practically no pain, and feels well.

### A Case of Gastric Ulcer with Carcinomatous Infiltration.

*Reported by Dr. Albert F. R. Andresen.*

About a month ago I saw a case which reminds me strongly of the case I have just reported.

Mrs. M. W., American, about 42 years of age, widow, houseworker by occupation. Seen at Brooklyn Hospital Dispensary in January, 1913.

*Family History.*—Negative.

*Previous History.*—Ten years ago she had a fistula of the rectum, for which she had an operation, was cured and was all right after that. She was married twenty years; had one child after a year, which died of malnutrition at the age of three months; no other pregnancies; menstruation always regular. Last Christmas she was treated for pleurisy and since then she has dated her principal trouble, although for the past year she had moderate epigastric pains which occurred about an hour after meals and which were frequently relieved by vomiting or regurgitation. She suffered from constipation during that year.

*Present History.*—Since a year ago until Christmas, that is, in the course of eight or nine months, she lost weight to the extent of fifty pounds, coming down from 195 to 145. That occurred since the sorrow of losing her husband a year ago. Since Christmas her stomach symptoms have been much worse. At first there was a good deal of gas with regurgitation of clear watery fluid after meals, although pain was less severe. For six weeks before I saw her she had vomited food every two or three days, sometimes from two or three days before.

When I saw her she was vomiting every two or three days and was vomiting all food eaten for two or three days back. She said her appetite was good, but she was afraid to eat and was able to eat only soft food, but vomiting continued, being of coffee-ground character. There was severe constipation and the stools were very dark in color. She felt weak, but otherwise felt well enough to do some work.

*Examination* showed a woman who did not look particularly cachectic, but showed the evidences of loss of weight. Tongue coated; teeth bad; chest negative; skin inelastic; abdomen quite flabby and inelastic, with a small, hard mass the size of a walnut and freely movable to the right of the epigastrium, in the pyloric region, not tender and not moving with respiration. No other abnormal findings. She then weighed 131 pounds, which was 65 pounds less than a year before and 15 pounds less than six weeks before.

*Test Meal.*—An hour after taking regular test meal of 300 c.c., I got out at least 1,500 c.c. of dark material containing food which she remembered eating thirty-six hours back. It formed into three layers and yeast fermentation was evident from bubbling and beer-like odor. Free hydrochloric acid 10; total acid 24; yeast, sarcinæ and blood-cells found under microscope. Stool negative. Urine negative.

The large number of yeast cells and sarcinæ in the stomach contents is supposed to indicate an ulcer as a rule, and the large quantity of material indicated an obstruction of the pylorus.

After removal of contents a mass could be felt along the line of the lesser curvature and pylorus and the patient was referred to Brooklyn Hospital for operation for callous gastric ulcer of the lesser curvature and pylorus with possible malignant degeneration.

On the strength of the sarcinæ and yeast cells it seemed reasonable to think that this large mass was an ulcer, but there was, of course, the suspicion of malignancy. Dr. Westbrook, on opening the abdomen, found the hard, indurated mass lying along the lesser curvature and involving the pylorus. He did a resection of more than two-thirds of the stomach and posterior gastrojejunostomy. She was doing nicely at the end of a week, but suddenly died from an unknown cause, probably of cardiac dilatation. No autopsy was obtained.

The pathologist, Dr. Hulst, reported a carcinoma, probably of recent origin, and commencing in the base of the callous ulcer.

This case evidently must have had a mass there for a long time, probably as large as the previous case, before she had a carcinomatous degeneration there, so the presumption is that the first case must have been an ulcer also, although diagnosed as carcinoma.

## A Case of Chronic Dysentery.

### *Reported by Dr. Edward E. Cornwall.*

The patient, a man of 35 years, contracted dysentery in the Philippines last year. He was treated in the government hospital, and according to his statement, the ameba was found in his stools by the hospital pathologist. After a course of ipecac he recovered from the acute condition, but a chronic condition persisted.

He came under the writer's care about two months ago. A diet deemed suitable for chronic dysentery and colonic irrigations with quinine solution were prescribed. He improved greatly under this treatment, but still had occasional relapses. The writer then gave him colonic irrigations every other day with a weak solution of dextrose in normal saline solution, to which was added a culture of the lactic acid bacillus. Under this treatment he became apparently well, and two weeks ago reported that he was in splendid condition, had only one movement a day, and was gaining flesh. ·

### *Scientific Session.*

Dr. F. B. Cross, in discussion of his case of primary abscess of the lung, described a second case as follows:

F. H., male, German, aged 53, was seen December 5, 1912. Family history, negative. Past history, good health. Habits, heavy smoker; steady drinker up to four years ago.

In January, 1912, he had an attack of "pleurisy," which means that he may have had any condition from muscular rheumatism, pleurisy or bronchitis up to a lobar pneumonia. The exact diagnosis was not determined owing to the death of his former medical adviser. Since recovery from this acute illness, he has had cough, expectoration of thick, creamy, purulent material, and has lost flesh and strength.

Physical examination.—A thin, large-framed man of sallow complexion, whose loose-fitting clothes and weight of 155 indicated a loss of many pounds. His hands showed the chronic pulmonary osteo-arthropathy of Marie, which was suggestive of chronic indurative phthisis, bronchiectasia, chronic empyema, pneumonia with production of new tissue, or lung abscess. T. 100.4, P. 104. Heart negative. Arteries: marked sclerosis. Urine: heavy trace of albumin, hyalin and granular casts. Lungs: left lung negative except for signs of compensatory emphysema. Right lung: anteriorly at fourth rib and posteriorly at about level of scapular spine, dullness to flatness from this level downward. Voice distant, whisper almost absent, absence of vocal fremitus, no rales. Sputum negative to tubercle bacillus.

Throacentesis in the eighth interspace brought forth four ounces of thick, creamy pus of offensively sweet heavy odor, resembling closely the sputum raised daily or twice daily. ·

The patient was sent to the M. E. Hospital for two weeks. During his stay the temperature fell to normal; white blood cells 16,000, 85 per cent, polymorphonuclears. Patient was tapped twice, the first time with no result; the second tap, deep in the ninth interspace, yielded seven ounces. He returned to the hospital January 15th and was operated by Dr. T. B. Spence. The operation revealed adhesions between lung and chest wall. The lung was entered and drained, the abscess cavity being the size of a small grapefruit. In the eight days since operation, the temperature has been normal and the tube drainage of the abscess free.

The outcome of this case is by no means certain. We do not know at this time whether the abscess cavity will granulate and slowly fill, or continue as a chronic abscess. In either case we may expect shrinkage of the affected side of the chest. The age of the patient, 53 yars, necessitates a guarded prognosis.

Dr. Tasker Howard said:—"In regard to Dr. Cornwall's point on the prognostic value of the increased area of cardiac dullness, it is interesting to note that in the original description of percussion by Leopold Auenbrugger, published in 1761, that was one of the points he made. In pneumonia, or acute cirrhus of the lung, as he called it, when the area over the heart which gave a 'fleshy' note on striking was increased, the patient seldom lived long. Auenbrugger used immediate percussion, striking on the bare chest with the gloved fingers. The method was not taken up until fifty years after, when Courvoisier resurrected it, and added the important improvement of the method of immediate percussion."

Dr. F. B. Cross said he would like to ask Dr. Cornwall's opinion of the hypodermic use of camphor in the later days of a pneumonia with failing left heart.

# TRANSACTIONS OF THE MEDICAL SOCIETY OF THE COUNTY OF KINGS.

Stated Meeting, February 18, 1913.

The President, JAMES M. WINFIELD, in the Chair.

### Does the Girls' School Need the Doctor?

A paper with this title was read by Dr. McAndrews

DR. ELIZA M. MOSHER, in opening the discussion, said:—"I feel as if we have been going through an earthquake or a cyclone during the last hour, and that some of our familiar landmarks in education have been demolished. We have heard it predicting that such a shaking up of school methods would come sooner or later—must come. The speaker of the evening, by his clear showing of the needs of our girls, has precipitated it, for us at least. The remote effects of great upheavals are almost always beneficial, for they break up the ground and make room for new buildings on models better suited to the conditions of to-day. I am, therefore, sorry that the territory affected by this one is so limited. I wish it could have reached all the educators in the Borough of Brooklyn.

"Dr. McAndrews, by the pictures he has displayed here this evening showing the new method of teaching in the Washington Irving High School, has proved himself a good reconstructionist, a true medico-educational doctor, as well as a demolisher of old methods. If he could be permitted without hinderance to carry out the plans he has in mind in the fine new buildings which will soon be the home of the Washington Irving High School, we might hope for a splendid example of what can be done to suit the education of girls to their real needs as women and as mothers of our future citizens.

"The question, 'What is woman's mission in the world?' is answered by the fact that if no more children should be born for one hundred years, not a man, woman or child would be alive and all the cities of the earth would be desolate. If, therefore, the mission of the great mass of women is to co-operate with men in home making, child bearing, rearing and educating, it follows that our girls should be given such training in school as will make them able co-operators, good home-makers, the best possible mothers, and first-class educators. More than boys, girls need a liberal education, for what man on the street has to answer as many questions as does the mother of wide-awake children? Who, more than she, requires training in the natural sciences to enable her to meet the problems which arise in home making? And who needs the wide outlook on life acquired through the study of history and literature more than does the mother and teacher?

"Dr. McAndrews has made good progress in the art of combining the practical for girls with the technical, uniting the school interests with home interests. In avoiding mental strain for girls, and yet holding them up to strong intellectual work, what the Washington Irving High School has done other schools can do, and we, as a body of physicians, should endorse his work in all these directions unequivocally."

DR. EDWARD P. CROWELL, in discussion, said:—"I am sure that I have enjoyed exceedingly the lecture of Dr. McAndrews this evening, and I regret that there are not more of the good doctors of the city present here tonight to learn something of the changes that are taking place here in the matter of education.

"He has asked the question if the doctors are needed in the schools? I may say as a physician, as a member of this Society—I may say as a school man that the doctors are most decidedly needed, and the help of this Society in this borough can be of very great influence in many, many ways. I wish that our doctors were better acquainted with our schools; I wish that they would understand something of our difficulties, of our needs, for I know that they would come to our relief. Many, many times we are seriously hampered through inability to secure proper support, support that you doctors little realize. For example, it is a surprising fact, sir, that a doctor's certificate written here in Brooklyn, accepted in court, will not be accepted by the Board of Health. It is a surprising fact that you may give a certificate that a little child on your block is too anemic to attend school, but that certificate will not be accepted by the Department of Education. Are doctors needed in our schools? I think they are, and I look forward to the time when Dr. Bartley and our good Dr. Fairbairn over here will put on the fighting mask again and come out and give us some help."

Dr. ELIAS H. BARTLEY, in discussion, said:—'I rise to make a motion, that it is the sense of this meeting that we approve of the principles Dr. McAndrews has set forth here for the training of girls in high schools and of high school age."

(The above motion was regularly seconded and carried.)
Paper:

### Athletics a Factor in Sex Hygiene.

*By Henry S. Pettit, M.D.*

DR. EUGENE L. SWAN, in opening the discussion, said:—"It seems to me that after this clear, clean-cut, manly paper of Dr. Pettit's, there is very little for me to say except a very hearty Amen!

"I may say, however, that in the course of two years I have known about twenty-five athletes. Last year I was up at Red Top with the Harvard crew and I was also with the Yale crew for some time and with the Harvard track team, and I am absolutely as positive, as Dr. Pettit is, of the moral standing of those fellows in regard to this subject. One athlete in particular I have in mind at this moment and that is the captain of next year's Yale football team, Captain Ketcham. Ketcham is not only strong in regard to his convictions as to living a pure life, but he is carrying forward that propaganda in the preparatory schools. At my camp for boys in Maine, I have seen but one case that I knew to be a masturbator, and that was cured, I am sure, by athletic exercise and by putting him under a carefully directed diet. I would like very much, if I may take a few minutes, to interest you in the Renaissance that is sweeping across the country in regard to this matter of sex instruction. I have asked many physicians if they knew the proportion of women that have venereal infection—innocent women—and a very busy one said, 'I do, because I am a gynecologist,' but I do not believe that many physicians do. Do you know that of the babies born blind while we have been in this room, a large proportion have been born so because their eyes had been burned out by venereal infection? It is simply appalling. In regard to matters of sex hygiene and sanitary and moral prophylaxis, isn't it true, gentlemen, that too many of us diagnose carefully, guardedly prognose and treat our case of gonorrhea and syphilis, then smilingly, sometimes flippantly, dismiss it? Isn't it true that we do not warn the patient that years afterwards he may put out the eyes of his children, or may infect an innocent girl through a seemingly respectable marriage covenant? Eighty to 86 per cent. of the vigorous women that suffer major operations do so because of having been infected by their husbands. It is said that 230,000 cases of venereal infection will occur in men between eighteen and thirty years of age in this coming year. I feel very, very strongly that upon the conscience and the soul of the medical man there is a terrible responsibility to which he must answer. Who, if not the honest physician, is responsible for the physical morality of the community in which he lives, and who, of all mankind, has the splendid opportunity of carrying forward this work of creating 'a new conscience in an ancient evil?'

"I have made it my business to try and find out some of the conditions surrounding the social evil and I find that the average fellow claims 'sex necessity,' that it is necessary for him to have intercourse with women in order to be in good condition. If you can *prove* to him—not smile and laugh at him—prove to him that that is not true, citing instances of athletes, priests and others that we know live a continent life and yet remain in good health, I think you will be able to accomplish considerable. Now, the question naturally arises, what are the fellows working in the factory or in the office who cannot go to summer camps going to do to secure athletes as a factor in sex hygiene? For them there are your Y. M. C. A.'s, your rowing clubs, your various walking clubs, or you can take the trouble to point out some definite line of exercise which you might have been engaged in yourself. It is surprising the arguments they will put up; many of them say, 'I don't believe masturbation hurts anybody; there are your night losses, which are the same thing.' If you can show them the waste of real vitality or spermin in the one and that it is merely an albuminous fluid in the other, you will have been able to accomplish something in the way of prophylaxis and you have succeeded in answering him with a sane, helpful truth. It seems to me that even the laity are ahead of us in some ways. You can scarcely pick up a magazine or a newspaper that has not something of moral prophylaxis or sex hygiene in one of its branches.

"I believe, gentlemen, it's the biggest question on the top of the earth today. I do not think that there is any question, political or otherwise, that can compare with the fact that three-quarters of the women of the community who are operated on (50 per cent. some say), are operated as a result of venereal infection, and that there is a vast array of three-quarters of a million males are abroad in this country suffering from venereal infection. You go down in the drug store and you will find a little disc and you put in some money for the blind children. Would it not be a more broad-minded, far-reaching thing to place the truth in the minds of men? A well-known clergyman told me that he asked three prominent physicians to speak in his church, on this very subject, and they didn't *dare* do it. They said, 'It will offend the people that we treat; our patients would not like it.'

"I know that I have not added much—could not add much—to Dr. Pettit's paper, but if there is anything I can say to rouse up a flaming spirit and tremendous interest in this subject I shall feel that I have not taken your time in vain. If all the men in this Society should say, 'I will warn every boy of what he may do with his disease after he has left me and the subjective and objective symptoms have disappeared, that he must have microscopical and bacteriological examinations to be sure he is free from his disease,' and even then he may not be free, I think we would find a lot of fellows who would think twice; but, instead, we laugh and shrug our shoulders over and over again, in many instances.

"Over in New York, in the garment workers' strike, I found a lot of unfortunate, unhappy things—a lot of girls, foolish, overdressed, but not *bad* girls, arrested and locked up with streetwalkers and thrown into jail. They feel society is against them and they are sore and bitter, and the girl of the street tells her of an easy way to earn money, and finally this foolish, overdressed little garment worker out of employment drifts into a clinic with some venereal disease, not a bad girl, just a foolish girl, a poor girl, an unhappy girl. The doctor diagnoses her and treats her, but does he always warn her of the disease and point to a better, more useful life? It seems to me that there ought to be a Chair of Eugenics in every medical college. There is one in Oxford University. Every young physician should hang up his diploma with a solemn vow to do everything morally and professionally within his power to stamp out this 'Great Black Plague.' As you are aware, the Board of Health sent you postal cards in the last few days asking you to report the number of case of gonorrhea and syphilis you have seen in the last year. It would be interesting to know how many men in this audience have answered that question."

Dr. WALTER TRUSLOW, in discussion, said:—"I am sure we will all be interested to speak on this subject, because of its importance. I can simply add a little experience in the direction of the advantages of athletic life, on growing boys, who are attaining habits of laxity. When I had a camp for boys, occasionally during the first week we would find a boy in the corner bed or elsewhere, who liked to get by himself and who needed tactful watching. But the harmful habit usually lasted but a little time. The healthy outdoor life that they pursued was the thing that accomplished the results.

"Another phase of this subject should be considered, that is, the duty of fathers to talk with their boys on this great question of sex life. A parent came to me recently and asked if I would not have a talk with his boy, about fifteen years of age, about these questions. I said to that father, 'I should be very glad to if you wish it, but may I put it to you as a great privilege, that you are foregoing, of having that kind of an understanding, that close intimacy, with your boy, in yourself having this kind of a talk with him? If, after you do, you wish me to say something more, I should be very glad to do it.' It is a pleasure to report that the father told me sometime afterwards that he would not have missed that privilege for a good deal. I feel it is a great duty on the part of parents, as well as a privilege, to talk about these things with their own sons."

Dr. HENRY S. PETTIT, in closing the discussion, said:—"I have nothing more to add except to say that I had hoped to have heard from some of the doctors here whether their patients who were overexercised were gymnasts or athletes, because I am firmly of the opinion that the only proper way to develop a boy is first to develop his muscle, heart, lungs and nervous system in the gymnasium, putting him in such physical condition that he can undertake athletics, which is not a body builder or a restorer of health, but simply a developer of character, the weights for the muscle, the apparatus for the co-ordination and the athletics for the character. The question of informing the child regarding sex hygiene would come as an adjunct to character building. I think the best thing to do would be to inform or train the parent, because my experience has been similar to Dr. Truslow's. I have had a great many parents come to me and others call on the 'phone, asking me to talk to their boy regarding sex, stating

that they do not think they are fit to do it, that they do not think they understand it, and request me to impart sex knowledge that is and should be the duty
of the parent."

## PRESIDENT'S ADDRESS.
### By James Macfarlane Winfield, M.D.
#### *January 21, 1913.*

*Introduction.*—It is stated in the by-laws that the President may deliver an
inaugural address in January; this privilege has usually been honored in the
breach, but when I realized that I had been an elective officer of this Society
for about twenty years, I thought that I could venture to take this opportunity
to talk over with you some things which, from my experience, might tend to
advance our Society, and benefit the medical profession in *Kings* County.

During these twenty years I have seen many changes in our Society, as well
as in the methods, administration and entire outlook of the medical profession.

This century has ushered in an awakening to a keener sense of personal
obligation in our dealings with affairs; we are all vividly conscious of a deep
sense of responsibility in economics, politics, in civics, both local and national,
and in the methods of dealing with education and the cure and control of crime.

If the fifteenth century was the renaissance of art and letters, the twentieth
bids fair to bring to birth a new and intense sense of personal responsibility for
existing rights and wrongs, and a deep realization of human brotherhood; at
last we seem to be finding an answer to Cain's long unheeded question, "Am I
my brother's keeper?"

We are living in a transitional stage; all society is in a condition of fer-
ment; all avocations, and particularly medicine, are undergoing a critical inspection and revision.

*Secret Division of Fees.*—Various medical matters are being discussed and
agitated by all sorts of people both in and out of the profession, as, for instance,
the secret splitting of fees, which seemed so portentous a couple of year ago,
but which has been practically adjusted.

*Medical Economics.*—Just now it is the question of medical economics that
chiefly occupies medical minds. This is of considerable import. It is inevitable
that as time goes on this question also will be satisfactorily solved, but we individually and collectively can do much to hasten this solution.

There are many factors that combine to make the struggle of the physicians
arduous, the high cost of living, the necessity for physicians to appear prosperous, the well-known lax business methods of medical men, the non-enforce-
ment of existing medical laws, the inadequate medical laws regarding the conduct of dispensary practice, and the pernicious over-activities of the Board of
Health.

Right here, allow me to say, that I think it is time for the medical profession of the City of New York to take notice of what the Board of Health is
doing. Perhaps all of its activities are within the law, but the physicians of
the city are not being considered. I would suggest that a standing committee
of this Society be appointed, whose duty it shall be to keep close watch upon
the activities and intentions of the Board of Health.

The opportunity for obtaining free medical advice has never been as great
as it is at present, the Board of Health, the Board of Education, hospitals, dispensaries and other charitable organizations are all competing in their efforts to
help the sick poor; it is unnecessary for me to say how flagrantly these laudable
charities are abused, nor need I emphasize the danger that all this may further
reduce our already diminishing income. Do we realize that the average earnings
of our patients have increased from 25 to 50 per cent. over what it was a decade
ago, while the average medical fee is practically the same as it was fifty years
ago? Perhaps if these facts were recognized and physicians would agree to
value their services by present-day standards and stand together, much might be
done toward clearing up the economic question.

I do not believe in the multiplication of societies, nor do I think it wise to
create new organizations for the express purpose of dealing with this problem.
I think it should be taken care of by the already existing societies, county, state
and national, for anything that tends to benefit medical men is undoubtedly one
of the functions of the County Society; while it might be burdensome to deal
with these questions in open meeting, would it not be possible to have a special
committee of the Society appointed to devote time and energy to the subject
and work out a satisfactory solution?

*Medical Education.*—During the last few years a great deal has been written regarding medical education.  That it is of interest to the community at large is evidenced by the fact that laymen, sometimes in official positions and sometimes not, have assumed the *rôle* of advisors as to how a man should be trained for his medical life work.

There is no doubt that raising the standard of the preliminary education of medical candidates will produce beneficial and lasting results, but the fact should not be lost sight of that there is also a moral qualification necessary to make the true physician.  In olden times the family doctor, who knew all the young people in his families, was consulted when a young man thought he wanted to study medicine, and if this physician was a wise man, and he usually was, he would advise the young person regarding the matter, and by his tact and kindly criticism often eliminated many unfit for this exacting calling; now this is all changed; anyone who wants to become a physician simply applies to a medical school, and if he can pass the law's requirements in due time he is graduated in medicine; no one has advised him, no one has looked into his moral qualifications, and in spite of the higher educational standards, in every class graduated there is a certain per cent. of incompetents in the finer requirements that are as necessary to the true physician as is his scholastic knowledge.

The question of medical education has been taken up by the A. M. A., and as the County Society is a unit of this great body, would it not, perhaps, be wise if we took a more active interest in this matter, and as a Society kept in closer touch with our local medical school?  This could be done by a committee of the County Society on Medical Education.

*Press Notoriety.*—There is a subject that I consider I should allude to; that is, the ephemeral notoriety that has come to some medical men through certain articles on medical matters, printed in the public press.  Upon investigation it is often found that most of these articles were not instigated by the man or men who were advertised, but that these physicians were the victims of over-zealous reporters; on the other hand, articles have appeared as alleged interviews with medical men, under head lines so written as to give the laity false and biased views of the aims, actions and work of the medical profession.

The life of the physician is hard enough without this sort of misrepresentation; all will agree that this latter sort of article is beneath the dignity of the profession and a crass breach of ethics; we should do all in our power to stop the exploiting and lauding of operations, and the still more insidious articles which by innuendo appeal to the suspicion and distrust of the unintelligent public.

This is a commercial age, the old formal order of things is passing away, and the medical profession is being hard pressed by the change; everything is being exploited and advertised, and the newspapers are asking, "Why should not the important things of the medical profession be told to the world through the medium of the press?"

The question is, can those who still cling to the old and honored traditions be able to hold back the tide of modernism and keep the medical profession in the high and ethical status that it has always been, or will the spirit of modern commercialism prevail, and our profession become a trade pure and simple?  We as a profession must go forward, we cannot stand still; but we can do a great deal to prevent undignified exploitation by teaching medical ethics in the medical schools, by the example of the older doctors to the younger, and by frequent elucidation regarding what is and what is not becoming to the dignity of our high calling; if the whole medical profession rightly interpreted ethical questions twentieth century medicine might then become a business profession, and the unethical self-advertiser would cease to exist.

These, briefly, are the general medical questions before us for consideration today; now let us devote a few minutes to the discussion of affairs directly concerning our own Society.

*President.*—The office of President, in as important a society as ours, is one of great honor, but it matters not how brilliant and energetic the President may be, his administration cannot be a success unless there is perfect harmony in the organization and he has the hearty co-operation of all of its members.

One of his duties is to provide programmes for the meetings; at first sight this might seem a very simple matter, and although it is comparatively easy to secure readers from out of town, it is very difficult to induce our own members to present papers.

I take exception to the idea that the physicians of Kings County are in any way inferior to those of any other city or borough.

The trouble is we have all allowed ourselves to be eclipsed by our proximity to Manhattan, but the time is rapidly approaching when this borough will be the great residential and necessarily also the medical center of the city; now is the time to prepare for this; take your light from under the bushel and let it shine. If we all unite, we can make Kings County as great a medical center as any other city in the world.

*Vice-President.*—The Vice-President is elected to act for the President during his absence. I have noticed that frequently the relationship between these two officers is not very close. Since the precedent has been established that the Vice-President succeeds to the Presidency, it would seem that perfect understanding and team work should exist between these two officers. I would suggest that the Vice-President be made the presiding officer of the Board of Censors. Then each of the three governing bodies of the Society will have presiding officers who will rotate automatically.

The President presides over the whole Council, the Senior Trustee over the Trustees, and the Vice-President over the Censors.

*Secretary.*—The office of Secretary is the most arduous of all and in our Society it has always been filled in the most capable manner; there is one suggestion regarding the duties of the Secretary that I would like to make. I have noticed that there is no immediate recognition by the Society when one of its members dies. I think it would be proper if the Secretary, as soon as he becomes cognizant of the death of a member, were to extend immediately the Society's sympathy to the bereaved family.

*Censors.*—The most important of all the officers of the Society are the Censors, because they are intrusted with the duty of ascertaining the qualifications of perspective members. A candidate for election to our Society is proposed either by an individual or by the Membership Committee, the name is printed in the BULLETIN a certain number of times and then comes before the Board of Censors for action. If the credentials appear to be satisfactory and no objection has been made, the candidate is elected; it is not the duty of the Censors to do detective work, so it is unjust and unfair to criticise their action if, sometimes, an undesirable person is elected. The question is often asked, "Why is So and So a member of the County Society?" or it is declared, "Such a man should not be allowed to remain in the Society," or "How did Dr. Such-a-One pass the Board of Censors?" I can assure you that, generally speaking, the Censors are very critical and painstaking, and it would greatly aid them in their task if every member would remember that it is his duty and privilege to notify the Board of Censors when he sees a man proposed for membership whom he thinks would not be a creditable member of the Society.

*Membership Committee.*—The duty of the Membership Committee is to ask graduates in medicine to become members of the Society, but this Committee is not supposed to delve into the past history of candidates nor to act in any censorial manner; they simply collect and make the nominations, then the Censors admit or reject.

*The Directory for Nurses* was organized to be helpful to the members of the Kings County Medical Society and to the public at large, and it was the ambition of its founders to make it the great central bureau of exchange for nurses in Kings County. At first, before private registries were organized, this bid fair to be the main medium of exchange, but latterly it has been but little patronized by our members.

It is the hope of your officers and the Committee on Directory for Nurses that 1913 will be a banner year and every member will try to patronize our Directory and do his best to induce all eligible nurses to register with us.

I am sorry that time will not allow me to speak in detail of all of the different committees, for long observation has acquainted me with a number of things that might be spoken of to advantage.

*The Entertainment Committee* is the President's corps of aid-de-camps, the duties of its members are arduous, but they have the satisfaction of knowing that they preside over the pleasantest part of the monthly meetings.

I think one of the functions of this Committee is to greet new and shy members, receive, and to make them feel at home. I have the assurance of my Committee that they will carry out this programme.

*The Historical Committee* is very important, because it "marks time" in the history of our Society, and to it is given the task of annually paying the public recognition to the memory of our dead members.

I want to take this occasion to officially thank the Chairman of this Committee, who has held this office for a number of years, and should receive a life sentence, for the hard work he has done, and for the splendid collection of historical items he has collected and presented to the Society. These are already of great value and will continue to become more so as time goes on.

*Legislative and Public Health Committees* must be active committees, for there are many things of great importance in both legislation and public health that comes before these committees in the course of the year. The gentlemen making up these committee are active practitioners, and it might easily happen that many things regarding health and legislation could escape their notice; therefore, I most earnestly hope that the individual members of the Society will give these committees their aid whenever they can.

*The Visiting Committee* has been in existence but a few years; its members are expected to visit any colleague who is ill or in distress.

I think their duties could be enlarged to advantage by having them notify the President and Secretary of the illness or death of a member of the Society.

*The Milk Commission.*—It is unnecessary to dwell on the importance of the duties of the Milk Commission, for its efficient work all know well. There is one suggestion I would like to make. I think it would be proper if the Commission rendered a financial report to the Trustees, for while, in a measure, the Commission is an independent body, it works under the auspices of the County Society.

As to the duties of most of the committees are important, I would suggest that the By-Laws be so changed as to make the Chairman of each a member of the Council, and I further think that although the standing committees are the personal appointments of the President, all committees should receive the ratification of the Council.

A society as large as ours has outgrown the methods of the time (1822) it was created, and it might not be a bad plan to take steps now to reorganize all of the methods and machinery and bring it up to present-day standards.

*Directing Librarian and Board of Trustees.*—I have purposely deferred mentioning the Directing Librarian and Board of Trustees until the last, for neither are part of the ordinary County Society.

We occupy a unique position among county societies, we are the proud owners of a splendid library, and the possessors of valuable property; the scientific interest of our members centers around the library.

As an ex-Directing Librarian and now your presiding officer, I earnestly solicit your continued aid in building up here in Kings County a still more splendid library of medical research.

Nearly twenty years ago the Board of Trustees and the society at large were awakened to the fact that if the Medical Society of the County of Kings wanted to forge ahead and not sink into a state of complete lethargy, it was imperatively necessary to have new, modern and larger quarters; how faithfully and efficiently that need was met you all know and our present building attests.

History repeats itself; the building that seemed so large ten years ago is rapidly becoming overcrowded. The stack room is too small to hold the new accessions, the cramped quarters are beginning to hamper the administrative end. In short, we are in immediate need of more room, and this need must be met in the very near future, for if we expect to go forward and maintain the influence we have in the community we must be properly housed.

We are in immediate need of larger quarters and we also need an endowment of at least $2,000,000.

These are the facts, and if you wish your Society to again become revivified you must all get together and help me solve the problem.

When one realizes the manifold duties and obligations of an active County Society such as ours, he is surprised at the amount of work that must be done by those who have charge; the functions of a County Medical Society are educational, medico-legal and medico-political. We are expected to see that illegal practitioners are apprehended; we are supposed to take an interest in all things pertaining to public health and civic welfare, because we stand for education; all this and much more is required of the ordinary society, but in addition our Society, from its size and importance, must of necessity figure largely in national and state medical matters. We should make it a factor in scientific medicine; we have a medical library, the fourth largest in the country; we own valuable property, and as the possessors of this library and property we must constantly strain every energy to maintain it.

Some of our members who recognize our unique position among county medical societies have wondered if it might not be advantageous if a holding body was to be created, this body or organization to have charge of the scientific part of the Society's work, and to be responsible for the maintenance, etc., of the library and other property now belonging to the Society.

This new organization would admit to membership all reputable, scientifically equipped physicians. It would in no way interfere with the County Society, for the ordinary county society can be run with much smaller dues than can ours at present; consequently, if the new organization were to assume the burdens of the property and library, every man who is eligible for membership in the County Society and who is not a member because of the high dues, could belong, because the dues of the County Society would then be merely nominal.

Such a dis-association as spoken of would, at first glance, seem an ideal way to solve many of the questions that must constantly perplex us, but while some things might be made easier, is it not impossible that other perplexing problems would arise with the new order of things.

Progression we must have; the building of a great center of medicine here on Long Island is sure to develop, but all changes take time and must only be made after due thought and deliberation.

While the time of deliberation is passing, can we not all get together and do our utmost to wake up the Society and give it a new impetus?

I look to all the members for help in my administration. I invite your honest criticism.

I ask the advice and council of the older members, from the younger I hope to get the inspiration to help me see the way to accomplish all I hope to do in the year 1913.

### REPORT OF COMMITTEE ON PRESIDENT'S ADDRESS.

The Committee, appointed on the address which was made by the President to the Society at the January meeting, begs to offer the following report:

The Committee convened March 15th, 1913, and there were present Dr. George McNaughton, Chairman; Dr. McCorkle, Dr. Fairbairn, Dr. Henry A. Morton, Dr. Wm. Linder, Dr. Humpstone. The address was read and the various recommendations discussed with the following results:

*First.*—That the attention of the Legislative and Public Health Committee be especially called to the President's recommendation to closely observe the work of the Department of Health, the management of dispensaries and hospitals, and other civic matters of particular interest to the medical profession.

*Second.*—That a committee be appointed to revise the fee-bill, which was printed and distributed for the guidance of the members of the Society about fifteen years ago.

*Third.*—The Committee commends the President's remarks on medical ethics and recommends that the Society publish in one of the numbers of the monthly BULLETIN a copy of the Code of Ethics of the American Medical Association; in this way a copy will reach each member of the Society. The Committee recommends that each member of the Society carefully peruse this honored document. The Committee is informed that the Long Island College Hospital proposes to offer a series of lectures on medical ethics. This advance step in medical education should be commended.

*Fourth.*—The Committee considered the duties of the Vice-President as well as those of the senior Censor, and it is the opinion of the Committee that it would *not* be wise to change the By-Laws in reference to the duties of either of the officers mentioned.

*Fifth.*—We endorse the recommendation of the President that the Secretary be authorized, on behalf of the Society, to at once take cognizance of the death of a member by sending a communication to the family of the deceased.

*Sixth.*—The President, in his address, called attention to the fact that each member of the Society has a right to object to the election of a candidate for membership in the Society, if such a candidate be for any reason undesirable. In this way only can our membership be carefully safeguarded.

*Seventh.*—The attention of members of the Society is directed to our Directory for Nurses, which is maintained at considerable expense for the convenience of the public and the profession, and for this reason should receive the support of the members of this Society.

*Eighth.*—With the President, the Committee believes that the Milk Commission should render an annual financial report to the Board of Trustees.

*Ninth.*—The business of the Society has been in the past carried on in such a satisfactory manner that this Committee hesitates to recommend any change in its form.

*Tenth.*—The Committee heartily endorses the suggestion of the President, as to the need of more space in the care of the library and for the development of other features of the Society; and that such efforts may be quickly instituted we recommend that the President appoint a committee of fifty to consider ways and means to solve the problem.

*Eleventh.*—The Committee believes the time inopportune to consider the formation of a holding company; but suggests the reference to a committee of the question of classifying the dues, so as to enable young men to join our Society without undue burden.

GEO. McNAUGHTON.
JOHN OSBORN POLAK.
J. A. McCORKLE.
HENRY A. FAIRBAIRN.
HENRY H. MORTON.
WILLIAM LINDER.
O. P. HUMPSTONE, *Secretary.*

# edical Society of the County of Kings

## MONTHLY BULLETIN TO MEMBERS

NDER the direction of the Council, this Bulletin is issued every month (except July, Aug. and Sept.). It is the purpose of the Council, h this medium, to keep the members advised matters pertaining to the Society's work, its s activities, its membership, and other subjects neral interest.

ns of general interest to the Society and per- notes concerning its members are invited and reach the Secretary not later than 4 P. M. e 20th of each month. Address all communi- s to the Society's Building, 1313 Bedford Ave., lyn, N. Y.

## MEDICAL SOCIETY OF THE COUNTY OF KINGS.

Bedford Avenue, Brooklyn, New York.
Telephone: 126 Bedford.

E Medical Society of the County of ings (organized 1822) owns its plant, alued at $100,000, and located at 1313-1315 ord Avenue. In addition to an audito- (seating 400) and various smaller meet- ooms, offices, etc., the greater part of the ing is devoted to the Society's medical ry of 60,000 volumes. There are only larger medical libraries on this continent. e ample reading rooms over 600 current cal journals are regularly on file.

rough its public and scientific meetings, ibrary, its Milk Commission, and its mani- activities for the spread of medical knowl- the promotion of scientific education, and the of the medical profession, and the safe- ling of the public health, the Medical So- of the County of Kings should enlist the e support and co-operation of every able physician in the county who is en- 1 in regular practice.

## MEMBERSHIP.

alifications for Membership.—Extracts the Constitution and By-Laws governing bership (Chapter XVI) are as follows: 1. Membership in the Society may be ned by physicians in good standing, resid- a the County of Kings, and duly licensed ecorded in the office of the County Clerk ings County, in the following manner: 2. Applications for membership shall be on blanks furnished by the Medical So- signed by the applicant and endorsed by members of the County Society. Such s shall be sent to the Secretary, who shall nt them to the Board of Censors for in- ation and report. Sec. 3. If the candi-

date be accepted the Council shall so report to the Society at a stated meeting, and after the next succeeding stated meeting the Presi- dent shall declare said candidate a member. Sec. 4. Every person thus admitted resident member shall, within three months after due notification of his election, pay an initiation fee of five dollars and the assessment of the Medical Society of the State of New York for the current year, sign the By-Laws or forfeit his election."

*Blank Application Forms for Membership* may be obtained on request at the Society's Building. This form should be filled out by the applicant, signed by him, his proposer and his seconder, and returned to the Secretary.

*Dues.*—New members pay an initiation fee of $5 plus $3 (the State assessment for the current year) and are exempt from the pay- ment of further dues until the next annual meeting after their election.

The regular annual dues are $10 plus $3 (the State assessment for the current year), pay- able on the first day of February. All mem- bers who have not paid on or before the first day of May shall be placed on the list of mem- bers in arrears and so reported to the Society, and shall not receive the publications, or no- tices of meetings, or defense for suits for mal- practice until their dues are paid. All mem- bers who fail to pay their arrears on or before December 31st shall be dropped from the roll of membership (Chapter XV of By-Laws).

*Advantages of Membership.*—Affiliation with your confreres in the representative medical organization of your County, participation in the Society's meetings and varied activities, and proprietary interest in its property and magnificent library, membership in the Medical Society of the State of New York and the Second District Branch; monthly receipt of the *New York State Journal of Medicine* and the Society's own publications, a copy yearly of the *Medical Directory of New York, New Jersey and Connecticut;* free defense to the court of last resort of all suits for alleged malpractice; eligibility to membership in the American Medical Association.

## STATED MEETINGS.

Regular stated meetings of the Society are held in the Society's Building, 1313 Bedford Ave., at 8.30 P. M., on the third Tuesday of every month (except July, August and Sep- tember). Light refreshments are served at the social hour which follows the scientific program of each meeting.

## THE LIBRARY.

The Library (60,000 vols.) of the Society is open daily (Sundays and Legal Holidays excepted), from 10 A. M. to 10 P. M. For the purposes of reference it is free to the public. Members of the Society have the privilege of borrowing books. Trained librarians are always in attendance to help and direct readers who desire such assistance.

## DIRECTORY FOR GRADUATE NURSES.

For the benefit of the profession and the general public the Society maintains a Directory for Graduate Nurses, where reliable graduate nurses (male and female), masseurs and masseuses may be procured. There is no fee for securing a nurse through the Society's Directory, which is always open, day and night. Telephone 126 Bedford.

## THE COUNCIL.

*President*—JAMES M. WINFIELD, 47 Halsey St.
*Vice-President*—J. RICHARD KEVIN.
*Secretary*—CLAUDE G. CRANE, 121 St. James Pl.
*Associate Secretary*—BURTON HARRIS.
*Treasurer*—JOHN R. STIVERS, 180 Lefferts Pl.
*Associate Treasurer*—STEPHEN H. LUTZ.
*Directing Librarian*—FREDERICK TILNEY.

### Trustees.

ONSLOW A. GORDON, *Chairman*, 71 Halsey St.
JOSHUA M. VAN COTT.    JOHN O. POLAK.
JOHN C. MACEVITT.      ELIAS H. BARTLEY.

### Censors.

JOHN A. LEE, *Senior Censor*, 23 Revere Pl.
WALTER A. SHERWOOD.    JOHN G. WILLIAMS.
CHARLES EASTMOND.      J. STURDIVANT READ.

## CHAIRMEN OF STANDING COMMITTEES.

*Membership*—EDWARD E. CORNWALL, 1218 Pacific St.
*Directory for Nurses*—CALVIN F. BARBER, 57 So. Oxford St.
*Entertainment*—ALFRED POTTER, 491 Eighth St.
*Historical*—WILLIAM SCHROEDER, 339 President St.
*Legislative*—HENRY G. WEBSTER, 364 Washington Ave.
*Public Health*—J. M. VAN COTT, 188 Henry St.
*Visiting*—JAMES W. FLEMING, 471 Bedford Ave.
*Milk Commission*—ALFRED BELL, 37 Linden St.
*Attendance*—ALBERT M. JUDD, 375 Grand Ave.

---

In the conduct of the affairs of the Society the officers hope that they may have not only the frequent suggestions of members, which are heartily invited, but also their practical and loyal co-operation.

---

*Supt. and Librarian*—ALBERT T. HUNTINGTON.
*Counsel*—WILLIAM E. BUTLER, Esq.
*Prosecuting Attorneys*—Messrs. ALMUTH C. VAN DIVER and JOHN G. DYER, 34 Nassau St., New York City.

## MINUTES OF STATED MEETING APRIL 15, 1913.

The President, Dr. James M. Winfield, the chair.

There were about 85 present.

The meeting was called to order at 8 P. M. and the minutes of the previous meet were, on motion, accepted as printed in LONG ISLAND MEDICAL JOURNAL.

*Report of Council.*

The Council reported favorably on the f lowing applications for membership:
Harlan E. Linehan, 74 Norman, Ave.; gra ate of Baltimore Medical College, 19 proposed by T. H. McKinnon and seco ed by Memb. Com.

*Election of Members.*

The following, duly proposed and accep by the Council, will be declared elected active membership at this meeting. (Subj to Chapter XVI, By-Laws):
William Murray Ennis, 31 First Pl.; gradu of Fordham Univ., 1910; proposed by L J. Commiskey and seconded by A. Judd.
Gustav Adolf Mausert, 687 Bushwick Av graduate of Univ. Giessen, 1899; propo by C. W. Stickle and seconded by J. Sheppard.
Jacob Sarnoff, 1819 85th St.; graduate N. Y. Univ., 1908; proposed by E. Mayne and seconded by Memb. Com.
Henry L. Wagener, 468 12th St.; graduate Univ. and Bell., 1911; proposed by N. Beers and seconded by R. W. Westbro
*Applications for Membership.*
Applications for membership were recei from the following:
George Francis Hoch, 523 Throop Ave.; gr uate of Cornell, 1910; proposed by J. Fitzsimmons and seconded by G. L. Bui April, 1913.
Thomas Joseph Kearns, 1490 Pacific St.; gr uate of Cornell, 1906; proposed by J. Scannell and seconded by E. J. McEnt April, 1913.
Edward Vincent McGoldrick, 115 Russell graduate of L. I. C. H., 1902; propo by T. H. MacKinnon and seconded Memb. Com.; April, 1913.
M. P. Blaber, 203 18th St.; graduate of and S., N. Y., 1910; proposed by Ha W. Lincoln and seconded by Memb. Co April, 1913.

*Executive Session.*

The Council presented the following cc munication:
The Council has unanimously agreed t the following statement of facts be made the enlightenment of the members, who h read in the public newspapers certain garb and inaccurate accounts of a recent meeting the Council.

A county medical society is a unit of state medical society, the state medical soci is a unit of the American Medical Association which proscribes certain rules and regulations for the guidance of its members.

Each state medical society applies these rules to its own use, as far as they are applicable under the circumstances; each county society bases its own by-laws on those of the state medical society; thus each county society throughout the United States is guided, in matters regarding ethics, by the American Medical Association.

The Council of a medical society is the executive committee of the society, and is composed only of its elective officers.

The Council of the Society transacts its business, and reports all important matters at the regular meetings of the Society.

It often occurs that the Council has to consider various complaints that are brought to its notice.

Each individual member of the Society has the right to complain about anything that seems to him to be irregular, either in the administration of the Society's affairs or the unethical conduct of any member.

When the attention of the Council is called to anything that might be construed as a breach of the by-laws and ethics of the Society it becomes the duty of the Council to take cognizance of the complaint, and if the complaint is well founded the Council makes certain recommendations.

This is in accordance with the By-Laws, Chap. XIII, Sec. 9, which says: "It shall be the duty of the Council to take cognizance of breaches of the precepts of medical ethics, which shall be laid before it, and it may report the results of its preceedings thereon to the Society, if it think proper."

When the Council receives a complaint of any sort it must investigate it; there is no alternative, the by-law is mandatory.

If the complaint is against a fellow member it is the custom for the Council to ask the alleged offender to meet it in a friendly conference. Its action regarding these matters is seldom, if ever, reported to the Society at large, because usually the complaints are ill-founded and are made against members who are innocent of wrong intent; up to the present time it has never occurred that the proceedings of a gentlemanly conference have been made public through the medium of the press; there is neither reason nor excuse for anyone telling of the proceedings of the Execuitve Committee of this or any other organization.

Recently complaints were received regarding four members of this Society. They were, according to custom, invited to meet the Coun-

cil and explain; two of the gentle knowledged their errors, were adm( and the matter was closed. The third was found entirely innocent of wrong in fact, he knew nothing about the pub of the newspaper article which was th of the complaint, and the Council is mous in regretting the inconvenience a savory notoriety into which he has bee lessly drawn.

As the fourth gentleman did not giv isfactory explanation, his case is still consideration and will be definitely d of at the convenience of the Council.

It was moved, seconded and carried t name of the member who had been exo by the Council be presented to the So

The President stated that Dr. LeGrar was the member who had been entirel erated and that the Council regrette much that Dr. Kerr had been subje unwarranted notoriety.

It was moved that the name of th ber who had not been exonerated be pr to the Society. Motion not seconded.

It was moved, seconded and carried t communication from the Council be r and placed on file.

The President announced the Commi Education: Dr. J. Richard Kevin, Cha Dr. Edward P. Crowell, Dr. Walter 1 and Dr. George D. Hamlin.

The President read the following nec Algernon Thomas Bristow, A.B., Member 1876-1913. Died March 26, 19 Frank Little, M.D. Member 18 Died April 4, 1913.

Eugene Joseph Carolan, M.D. 1 1880-1902. Died March 14, 1913.

John Herman Droge, M.D. Membe 1897. Died March 15, 1913.

*Scientific Session.*

1. Paper—"The Pneumococcus in .the and the Role of the Intesti Acute Lobar Pneumonia." By Anthony A. Rutz, M.D.

2. Paper—"Observations and Suggestic garding Lobar Pneumonia." By Edward E. Cornwall, M.D.

3. Paper—"The Important Surgical of Pneumonia." By William Francis Campbell, M Discussion by Henry A. Fairbairn J. M. Van Cott, M.D., B. M. M.D., H. B. Delatour, M.E closed by Edward E. Cornwall,

Meeting adjourned at 10.30 P. M.

CLAUDE G. CRANE, *Secre*

# LONG ISLAND MEDICAL JOURNAL

| VOL. VII. | JUNE, 1913 | NO. 6 |

## Original Articles.

### THE USE OF DIGITALIS IN DISEASES OF THE MYOCARDIUM.

### By T. Stuart Hart, M.A., M.D.,

of New York City.

IN practically every case of cardiac insufficiency, some preparation of digitalis or its allies, strophanthus and squills, has been our chief dependence, yet every practitioner of medicine is impressed with the variable outcome he has obtained with digitalis in these conditions. The really brilliant results we all have secured in certain cases are interspersed with frequent failures. One case seemingly hopeless in its outlook is rescued to comparative health, another with superficial appearances less grave proceeds on its downward course in spite of all our efforts. In our endeavor to solve these failures we have offered various explanations; sometimes we have thought that the preparation of digitalis was at fault; perhaps it had never been active or had been kept so long that it had lost its activity: or we did not, or could not use a dose of digitalis sufficiently large; perhaps the patient had an irritable stomach and could not retain any considerable amount. Certain other cases we were content to assign to a group which had passed beyond a point where any therapeutic measures were of avail; degenerated muscle cannot be regenerated by drugs. So we explained our failures and successes with digitalis and no doubt in many instances our explanation was correct.

Be this as it may, there has come to us in recent years through the newer methods of the study of cardiac function by graphic means a light which has penetrated some of the dark corners. These new methods have cleared up a few of the mysteries of digitalis action and have permitted us to reform our groups of heart cases on a basis of abnormal cardiac function in a manner which has hitherto been impossible. This new knowledge is not only of academic interest but also of great practical importance. It has taught us to treat our cases more intelligently and has in a degree at least shown us the kind of case in which we may expect satisfactory results from digitalis. It has differentiated certain groups in which digitalis is of very little assistance and others in which its action is distinctly harmful.

*Fundamental Properties of Cardiac Muscle.*—To have a clear concepton of the data which serve to segregate the functional dis-

2

orders of the heart into groups it is necessary to consider the fundamental physiological properties of heart muscle as formulated by the studies of Gaskell and Engelmann. These observers have shown that the heart is an automatic organ whose muscle fibres have five distinct functions: (1) stimulus production, (2) stimulus conduction, (3) irritability (the capacity of responding to stimuli), (4) contractility, and (5) tonicity.

In the normal heart the properties of stimulus production and irritability seem to be most highly developed at a point near the junction of the great veins with the right auricle; this is, therefore, the most rhythmic part of the heart and is commonly known as the "pace-maker." A stimulus arising at this point is *conducted* over the auricles thence through the bundle of His to the ventricles. As the stimulus reaches the muscle fibres of each chamber, these being normally *irritable,* respond and a coördinated *contraction* of each chamber results.

In the abnormal heart one or more of these fundamental prop-

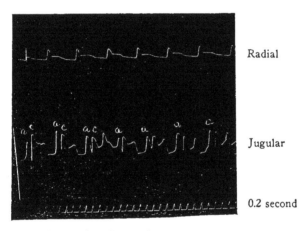

Radial

Jugular

0.2 second

FIGURE 1.—NORMAL POLYGRAPH.
*Note.*—Regular radial and jugular pulse.
Rate 75. *a* wave present in jugular tracing.
*a-c* interval normal, less than 0.2 second.

erties may be disordered and it is the discovery of such disorders that permit us to group our cases in accordance with the function at fault. For example *conduction may be impaired* so that the stimulus instead of occupying its usual time in traveling from the "pace-maker" to the ventricle is delayed and passes very slowly. Of this defect in conduction we may have many grades up to a point when the conducting path is completely severed. Accordingly under the group of defective conduction we may have "delayed conduction," "partial block" and "complete block."

In another group of cases *irritability* is at fault. Some points of the cardiac tissue are excessively irritable and contract before the rhythmic stimuli from the normal pace-maker can reach them and as a result we have the premature beats and extrasystoles arising in the auricle or the ventricle.

*Effect of Digitalis on the Heart Muscle.*—When we come to study the effect of digitalis on these fundamental properties of cardiac muscle, two facts stand out very prominently, digitalis (1) decreases conductivity, and (2) increases irritability. If we give considerable doses of digitalis to a case in which conduction is impaired it will usually increase this defect. In nearly all cases if we give large enough doses of digitalis we can produce extrasystoles.

It is plain therefore that in cases of imperfect conduction and in cases of abnormal irritability (as evidenced by the occurrence of extrasystoles) digitalis is distinctly contraindicated.

*Auricular Fibrillation.*—Having briefly pointed out two groups of cases in which digitalis is distinctly out of place, let us turn our attention to that functional condition in which beyond all others digitalis is indicated. This is the condition now recognized as auricular fibrillation. In this condition there is no contraction *en masse* of the auricle, the wall of this chamber is in unceasing activity, but this activity consists of a series of incoördinated movements of its

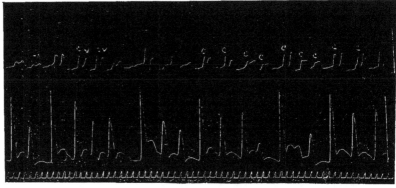

Jugul

Brac

0.2 se

FIGURE 2.—AURICULAR FIBRILLATION.
*Note.*—Complete irregularity of brachial, irregular in time and force, rate 90. Ventricular form of jugular tracing, absence of *a* wave, complete irregularity.

muscle fibriles, giving an undulatory motion to the auricular surface which has been likened to the squirming of a bunch of worms. As a result of this activity the junctional tissues are bombarded by a shower of stimuli and the ventricle responds at irregular varying intervals in a series of arhythmic contractions.

Auricular fibrillation is a clinical entity very frequently seen and hence of great importance. Before the recognition of its nature it passed under many different names, "delerium cordis," "the mitral pulse," "nodal rhythm," "pulsus irregularis perpetuus," etc. It is the most common of the cardiac irregularities comprising at least one-half of the arhythmias of cardiac insufficiency. The recognition of the true nature of this condition is mainly due to the brilliant electrocardiographic investigations of Rothberger and Winterberg and of Thomas Lewis working simultaneously and independently. Of the minute pathology and the underlying causes we are still in doubt. We know that it is a common occurrence in hearts damaged by rheumatic attacks, it is an exceedingly frequent accompaniment of mitral disease and that it is rarely met with in cases of pure aortic disease, it may occur with no discoverable valvular lesion. It has been produced experimentally in animals by frequent induction shocks applied to the exposed auricle, and by overdistension of the auricle.

Once established it usually continues uninterruptedly to the end of life, having been known to continue for twelve years. The heart may, however, revert to a normal rhythm; among 150 cases of auricular fibrillation which I have studied by graphic methods there were nine in which the rhythm returned to the normal.

*Graphic Records of Auricular Fibrillation.*—The graphic records of the heart and blood vessels in auricular fibrillation are quite characteristic (figures 2 and 5). The radial pulse (figure 2) shows a "complete irregularity," that is the pulse is irregular both in time and force; large and small beats separated by time intervals of unequal length succeed one another in a haphazard way "without rhyme or reason." The jugular pulse shows a corresponding irregularity and in addition the *a* wave, which in the normal jugular

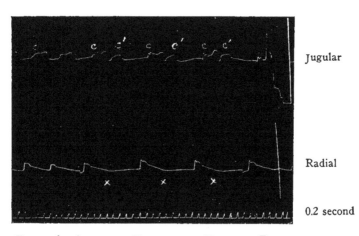

Jugular

Radial

0.2 second

FIGURE 3.—AURICULAR FIBRILLATION, DIGITALIS EFFECT, COUPLED BEATS.

*Note.*—Complete irregularity, rate 60. *x* Indicate ventricular extrasystoles which barely reach the radial. Jugular tracing shows absence of *a* wave, ventricular form of venous pulse, complete irregularity, coupled beats.

tracing precedes by 0.2 second the waves (*c* and *v*) referable to ventricular activity is absent. The jugular pulse is of the ventricular type, *i. e.,* all the positive waves occur during the time of ventricular activity. Occasionally when the heart action is slow a series of small undulations are seen in the jugular curve during the diastolic period. These are believed to be due to the fine undulatory activity of the auricle.

The electrocardiographic records, which have been the most important means in the discovery of auricular fibrillation in the human subject, are also quite characteristic. In the normal electrocardiogram (figure 4) the auricular activity is represented by the *P* wave, the ventricular activity by the *QRST* group of waves, the diastolic pause is represented by the horizontal line from *T* to *P*. In auricular fibrillation (figure 5) the *P* wave is absent, the ventricular complexes *QRST* follow each other at irregular intervals but are normal except that they are distorted by the small undulations *ff* which represent the fibrillary activity of the auricles and which continue uninterruptedly through both systole and diastole.

*Clinical Recognition of Auricular Fibrillation.*—As a rule these graphic records are unnecessary for the detection of auricular fibrillation, the trained eye, finger and ear are quite sufficient to differentiate this complete irregularity from the other common arhythmias, indeed my house physician is usually able to make the diagnosis on admitting a patient to the hospital without employing instruments of precision other than those with which nature has endowed him. The pulse shows a complete absence of rhythm of any kind, large and small beats follow one another helter-skelter. The same haphazard sequence of ventricular contractions is detected on auscultating the heart. When a visible jugular pulse is present the only visible wave is synchronous with the apex impulse, the normal presystolic wave *a* is absent. If the heart is rapid and decompensated many of the ventricular contractions fail to give a perceptible wave in the radial artery. I have frequently counted the apical beat at 140 a minute while a radial count taken simul-

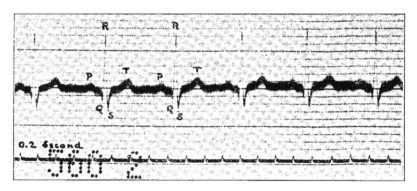

FIGURE 4.—NORMAL ELECTROCARDIOGRAM.
*P* wave represents auricular complex. *QRST* represents ventricular complex. Horizontal line from *T* to *P* represents the diastolic rest.

taneously showed a pulse not over 80, thus showing a "pulse deficit" of 60 per minute.

A further means of corroborating the diagnosis is the therapeutic test. Rest and the administration of a reliable preparation of digitalis in sufficient dosage usually produce a marvelous improvement and such a one as follows the treatment of no other cardiac abnormality with which I am familiar.

*Clinical Recognition of the Extrasystole.*—Cases showing the defect of increased irritability as evidenced by extrasystoles may also be recognized by the finger and ear. Here the fundamental rhythm of the normal pace-maker is usually present, this is inter-

rupted at more or less frequent intervals by a pulse wave which
occurs too early to fit into the fundamental rhythm, this wave is
too early, smaller in volume than the normal waves and is followed
by a pause before the first beat of the resumption of the fundamental rhythm, the beat immediately following the pause is as a
rule a little greater in volume than the average normal wave. At
times the small extrasystolic waves cannot be detected in the radial
pulse and the finger appreciates only the long pause so that the
condition simulates a "dropped beat." By auscultation of the heart
the extrasystolic contraction, which may have been too weak to
open the semilunar valves, and the succeeding pause are even more
easily recognized.

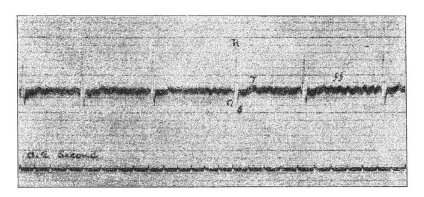

FIGURE 5.—AURICULAR FIBRILLATION.
Complete irregularity. *P* wave absent. *QRST* complex normal. Continuous
small waves (*ff*) of auricular fibrillary activity.

It would lead us too far to discuss the clinical differentiation
from auricular fibrillation of those rare cases of arhythmia which
occasionally puzzle those with the best trained powers of observation. Some of these are easily assigned to their proper group by
a study of the polygraphic records, a few can only be solved by the
aid of the electrocardiographic records and there is an occasional
case which in the present state of our knowledge eludes even these
means of analysis.

*The Treatment of Auricular Fibrillation* consists of absolute rest
and the administration in large doses of an active preparation of
digitalis. The best preparation is a fresh and properly made infusion (the infusion will retain its full activity for only three or four
days and should therefore be ordered only in small quantities). In
a case with marked decompensation and a rapid pulse an active
infusion may be administered in two dram doses every six hours.
The tincture may be given in ten drop doses every four hours.

The beneficial action of digitalis in these cases is probably due
to its interference with the property of conduction (see above). By
establishing a partial functional block a part of the numerous impulses from the auricle are impeded so that the ventricle has a
longer time to recuperate and its individual contractions become
more efficient.

One usually expects to see a decided improvement following

such therapeutic measures in three or four days. When digitalis has been continued for some time its toxic effects may become manifest, such as headache, nausea, vomiting, diarrhœa and a slow pulse. Sometimes the overdosage is indicated by an increase in ventricular irritability which is evidenced by the occurrence of ventricular extrasystoles; this can be detected by palpation and ausculation as a "coupled rhythm," that is one can perceive a series of two beats occurring close together followed by a considerable pause (figures 3 and 6). Graphic records show that the second of the coupled beats is a ventricular extrasystole (figures 3 and 6). Any of the above signs indicate that digitalis must be withdrawn.

A much better way to follow the effect of the administration of digitalis is to record the "pulse deficit," that is the difference in the number of beats per minute as obtained by palpation of the radial and auscultation of the apex. As the deficit gradually disappears and the heart becomes slower the digitalis should be cut down and just enough should be given to keep the pulse at about 70 with a deficit of not over 5 a minute. Such a dose may be continued daily for years with beneficial effect. The observation of

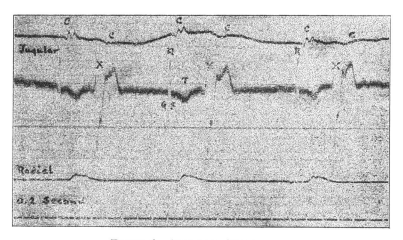

FIGURE 6.—AURICULAR FIBRILLATION.
Digitalis effect. Coupled beats. Every other beat is an extrasystole (*x*) which does not reach the radial and is only faintly seen in the jugular record. The *a* wave is absent in the jugular record.

the deficit also affords valuable information as to the amount of physical exertion which should be permitted. I have found that if one watches the pulse rate and the deficit in this manner, the toxic symptoms above described are practically never seen and the physical limitations and necessary dosage of digitalis may be nicely adjusted to the needs of the individual patient.

*Conclusions.*—1. Success or failure in digitalis therapy depends mainly on the nature of the cardiac disorder in which it is employed.

2. Digitalis is particularly useful in cases of auricular fibrillation where the establishment of a partial functional block is desirable.

3. Digitalis is contraindicated in cases of delayed conduction and in many cases where cardiac muscle irritabilty is increased.

# DOES THE GIRLS' SCHOOL NEED THE DOCTOR?

## By William McAndrew,

Principal of Washington Irving High School, Manhattan.

(With Lantern-slide Demonstration.)

IN Detroit, where I used to live, we had an electric sign on the City Hall, "Welcome"! Detroit aspired to be a great convention city, and in order to give the personal touch to the different associations that came there would be added to this sign when the convention was meeting in town the name of those that were the city's guests. Tonight you would read, "Welcome, Women's Christian Temperance Union!" and tomorrow night you would read, "Welcome, Association of Brewers and Distillers!"

The arrangement of this program tonight suggests as violent a change in its last half from the first half as those signs did in Detroit. Such an important and fine impression has been created by the paper of the first part of the evening that my heart has gone down to a place that no intelligent physician expects to find a heart, for it is impossible for me to continue in any way or carry out in any manner the suggestions of the first part of the evening. Suffice it to say that my impromptu remarks were prepared before knowing what the whole program was going to be. My subject is "Does the Girls' School Need the Doctor?" I am in the unusual position at this moment of consulting a hundred eminent specialists, and I am without any idea of paying a fee. I am to ask you questions, to state problems to you. In order that it may be kept within the bounds of propriety, I will ask the president to lend me his watch.

Now, think of the difficulty that we are in, doctors, a moment. We who are in the public schools are working with an organization that was planned for something that dates away back to the middle ages when books were few and knowledge was small. The guardians of those books united themselves into schools and undertook to impart that knowledge. The system of schooling which they devised is the system which was passed from Europe over to America, so that every school that I know anything about, and every school possibly that you know anything about, is based on the idea of transmitting knowledge. Yet all the theory of education set forth in professional books or preached by eminent educators is a different theory from that. The present doctrine is that education is not for the purpose of transmitting knowledge; it is not for the purpose of giving information, but it is for the purpose of changing boys or girls from what they are to what they ought to be. We must dismiss from our minds the idea that we who are teachers are such for the purpose of transmitting information from a book or from ourselves to young and growing intelligences. This new idea seems to be a necessary theory for American education. In 1776 there occurred in this country an event which has affected all the life of this nation and all the common interests of it. It was so complete a change that it went under the name of Revolution with a large R. It was a decision by the founders of this country that royal roads and royal lighthouses and

---

*Read before the Medical Society of the County of Kings, February 18, 1913.

royal mails and royal everything which had been done for people in Europe before was now to be done by the people for themselves. Government undertook to manage all those common interests which had been managed before by superior people who belonged to the ruling class, to the court or to the church. For us to attempt to run on the old European basis a common interest in this country is to lose sight of the fact that we are a country by ourselves and have our own history and own ideals. Among the very first things this country undertook was to say that what things people could do for themselves in common better than could be done by one man or family should be done in co-operation. Thus arrangements were made by which such things as lighthouses, as roads, as mails, as the provision for water supply and all things of that sort should be done in common by the people themselves. Persons who undertook to do these things became the agents of the people and were delegated to carry out the measures of the people of this country. One of the most important things the founders of this republic undertook to say should be done in common was the education of children. Therefore I can not see how working back to our situation historically, we can get at any other idea than that the schoolmaster and school teacher are delegated agents of the whole people of this country, to do that which the people alone would do. It is true, is it not, that the unit of government is the family? What the family itself would want done for the boy or for the girl must be the thing that the school should do for the boy or the girl. Is that true? Is it? I am consulting you, dear doctors, and I ask you is this a proper diagnosis or prognosis or post-mortem statement of the reason for public education at public expense? [Voices: "Yes."]

Good! On this the doctors agree. We accept that in America because of our essential principles of government, because of the tremendous fact of 1776, the public school system is politically and morally bound to do that for children which the best type of parent wants done for his own offspring. Consider the case of a daughter. What is the natural, instinctive and proper hope of a parent for a girl child? What is yours for your daughter? What was, ladies of the association, your mother's hope for you? Was it, and is it that a daughter shall grow to be a healthy, handsome, pure-minded, successful, noble woman? Yes? Is there any other desire more current or more to be approved? No? We are still agreed.

And this is exactly what all the writers and speakers on schools say that education is for; not for information, but for power; not for knowledge, but for nobility; not for courses, but for character.

But why is it that all the schoolmasters say these personal powers are the chief end while maintaining a form of organization and a method of everyday work that neglects these things? We say the purpose of a girls' school is a healthy, happy, handsome, noble woman. We have no organization based on this purpose.

Instead of selecting persons expert in the growth of girls from girls to women, we select experts in traditional knowledge. Anybody who prepares to be a teacher does not specialize on the things that make fine women; on health, intelligence, industry, courage, patriotism, consideration for others, and all those qualities which, if you could get school out of your mind, you could put down as being the characteristics of the fine woman. There isn't anybody in the teachers' training school specializing on that. A person specializes

on a part of knowledge, physics; he specializes on a piece of information, English, or algebra. The whole basis is that which all the
educators say education is not. The whole scheme is to take pieces
of knowledge and divide them and have them passed about and applied today and tomorrow, to prepare portions of a course of study.
If the teacher succeeds hour by hour in getting that portion of
knowledge out of her system and succeeds in getting the idea talked
about by herself and the children, it is considered that the day has
been well spent.

The school publishes its purpose as not to centre upon knowledge, but to train efficiency, but it sees no broad ideals of efficiency
and makes no plans to realize them; does such a school need a doctor? The school declares it has discarded the old European purpose
of imparting information but maintains the old European organization; does such a school need a doctor? The girl's school announces
itself as desirous of realizing the parents' hope of healthy, handsome, happy, noble women, but it uses for this purpose a machine
designed to drive mediæval scholarship into boys. What does such
a state of affairs require? [Voices: "A doctor;" "an insane asylum."]

Now, let us see what is done in girls' schools. [Lantern slides
illustrating: Latin, algebra, effects of state examinations, amount
of home study, loss of sleep, formal and unproductive exercises in
physical training, exclusion of music in favor of grammar, together
with attempts to graft upon the mediæval trunk exercises based upon
girlish instincts and intended to educate through interest and happiness.]

I have taken you into the girls' school of today. You have seen
the work with your own eyes. What do you think of it? It seems
to me one of the most chaotic and absurd propositions of any period
of our history. What should be done is simple and big and inspir-
ing. What is being done is weak, sapless and pedantic. Can't you do
something about it? You say and you write that the girl of thirteen
is just entering a period when changes within her begin which are
portentous of her happiness or sorrow, her health or debility, the
virility or degeneracy of a coming race. You say she needs the fresh-
esh blood, the calmest nerves, the soundest sleep, the serenest content
throughout this period. This, you say, should be her easy time. But
what you say to me, a schoolmaster—what you say without any variation—is that we are making this the young girl's hardest time, annoying her, irritating her, loading her with tasks, robbing her of
sleep, shattering her nervous system with the excitement of examinations, prize systems, promotions and fool inventions for the benefit of
the school's system, not for hers. I am tired of the futility of it.
The things it produces are not, as it seems to me, what parents want
nor what the world needs. There is no quality now more wanted
than youth. It is the one great demand, the very essence of progress.
It is no pretty sentiment, but a big and gripping fact. If he loses
it at fifty or eighty or ninety, the man becomes dead weight. I have
seen high schools drive it out of women at twenty. Nothing can, in
my mind, compare with the service of passing up to the waiting world
strong, radiant women ready for a robust, progressive life. If girls'
schools will not do this, if girls' schools put up requirements that tend
to deterioration of health and vigor and to succeeding generations
of weaklings, then they need, and need exceedingly, a strong, decisive.
determined doctor of many ills.

# IMMUNIZATION AGAINST TYPHOID FEVER.*

## M. L. Ogan, M.D.,

Department of Health, New York City.

### Brief Synopsis of Immunity Types

I MMUNITY to disease may be natural, as when the normal animal organism produces antibodies sufficient in amount and power to neutralize toxins developed by bacteria or capable of destroying the bacteria themselves.

A similar immunity may be brought about passively by introducing from without antibodies elaborated in the blood serum of an immunized animal, as in the injection of diphtheritic antitoxin.

An active acquired immunity may be produced by an attack of the disease or it may be artificially acquired by the introduction of bacteria or their products into the body (as in vaccination for variola).

### Former Conception

Immunity to disease was formerly thought to be due either to insufficient culture media within the body or to the production by the bacteria themselves of materials which checked their further growth.

### Development of Present Conception
### Metchnikoff Theory

While other observers had noticed the ingestive faculty of leucocytes through their ameboid movements, Metchnikoff first credited the body cells with the ability to digest or destroy bacteria, which he believed they did by virtue of enzymes produced by their own synthetic processes. Furthermore, he taught that through cellular disintegration these enzymes were liberated in the tissue juices, which then became endowed with the same power possessed by phagocytes. These ferments were then further credited with ability to neutralize toxins thus endowing them with power to destroy not only bacteria but bacterial products.

### Ehrlich's Theory

Ehrlich's side chain theory differs from this in that he conceives the complicated cellular protoplasm as possessing innumerable nascent molecular side chains with specialized affinities for corresponding molecules. These are called receptors. Through these metabolic processes are carried on and through them the cell may also be attacked by the deleterious products of hostile bacteria.

In either the Metchnikoff or Ehrlich theory the normal cellular content of the fluid tissues is held to be considerable enough to meet what may be termed the average normal exposure. Whenever the organism is attacked in force, however, these defensive elements are increased through the phenomena of inflammation.

### Wright Theory

Wright and his followers accepting the Metchnikoff theory of phagocytosis have shown that the body fluids are of equal importance with leucocytes. The latter may ingest and destroy bacteria but only after they are attenuated by partial digestion or solution through the agency of ferments in the serum. These ferments or enzymes he

---

* Read before the Brooklyn Pathological Society, February 13, 1913.

terms opsonins (from the Greek meaning to "prepare food for"). Wright holds therefore that immunity is dependent on the opsonic content of the serum and has devised his formula called the opsonic index.

It was Wright's belief that "the protective substances which were involved in the case of disease and that were present in considerable quantities in the blood were to be regarded as produced by internal secretions." He "did not know where they were produced in the body." The researches of Sajous and of a number of independent workers indicate that the thyroid, adrenals and pancreas are the source of these ferment-containing secretions.

Whatever their origin, bacterial inoculation stimulates their production and has proven its worth therapeutically to some extent, but more particularly as a preventive.

Its efficacy has been demonstrated in the establishment of immunity from typhoid fever as shown by its use in army barracks and camps where typhoid incidence has been reduced to a remarkable extent.

### Typhoid Immunization
### Historical Note

Inoculation against typhoid was begun in 1893 by Fränkel and has been continued and developed by many others using various cultivated forms of the bacilli typhosis until at the present time the killed but untreated bacteria are utilized in preference to all other preparations.

### The Culture

The Health Department culture is produced in the following way, which is practically identical with the method of other laboratories. A laboratory culture of typhoid bacilli which has lost its virulence through long artificial cultivation is used. Large surfaces of agar in Blake bottles are inoculated from fresh agar cultures. After 24 hours growth at 37 degrees C. the bacteria are washed from the surface of the agar with normal salt solution. The suspension is then standardized by counting the bacilli, by the Wright method. This is done by mixing an equal part of blood and the bacterial suspension. Smears are made from this mixture and stained. The number of bacilli and red cells are then counted under the microscope, going over about twenty-five fields. The proportion between the two being determined, the number of red cells being known, the number of bacilli per c. c. can then be estimated. This suspension is then heated one hour at 56 degrees C. to kill the bacilli. After heating, the sterility of the suspension is tested by inoculating generous amounts into media and incubating these under aerobic and anaerobic conditions. If no growth occur, 0.25 per cent. of carbolic acid is added to the suspension and the suspension diluted with 0.25 per cent. carbolic acid in normal saline solution so that one c.c. contains the appropriate dose. It is then bottled for distribution.

### The Injection and Reaction

For the injection of one individual the necessary three doses are supplied in individual vials. Where several are to be injected at the same time the vaccine is distributed in 10 c.c. vials.

A large experience has shown that these three inoculations are necessary and that they should be given at intervals of seven to ten days. The emulsion is given subcutaneously over the deltoid muscle after properly cleansing the arm, for which we use tincture of iodine, which penetrates quickly to the deeper layers of the skin, especially if the oily secretions are first removed with alcohol or ether. A needle of ordinary calibre should be used as this is sufficient to admit the bacteria in suspension and occasions little wounding. If the needle has extra length and is inserted parallel with the surface there is little likelihood of any portion of the emulsion escaping. The several doses had better be introduced at points about one inch apart and no covering is required for any of the punctures. Following the injection and after a lapse of several hours a local and general reaction may develop. There is frequently a red and tender area seldom exceeding three inches in diameter and generally considerably less. This reaction may, however, be more severe, and the local lymph nodes may become enlarged and tender. The general reaction consists of headache, malaise or even a rise of temperature, possibly accompanied by backache, nausea, vomiting, herpes labialis, or rarely albuminuria, but this complex symptom is exceptionally infrequent, and any appreciably general reaction is absent in most cases.

One series of observation covering 31,000 inoculations showed no untoward results, and it is claimed by those of large experience that the ordinary reaction is not to be compared in severity with that of smallpox vaccination. All unite in saying that the severest types subside within forty-eight hours, usually within twenty-four.

This accords with our own experience since beginning inoculations on January 1st covering a total number of seven hundred.

It may be remarked that the greater portion of persons inoculated in the preceding figures were men selected for military service. Included among them, however, even in military circles are many women and children of posts and garrisons. Children are reported to tolerate the injections exceptionally well.

Over five hundred female patients in the Richmond, England, Asylum were injected during an epidemic in the wards. Not one showed constitutional symptoms severer than those previously described. In this number but one per cent. developed typhoid, whereas among the nurses, orderlies and medical staff, the members of which received no such treatment, 14 per cent. became infected.

### The Negative Phase

For a long time the belief in a negative phase acted as a deterrent in the proper adjustment of doses and the earlier results were therefore not so brilliant. Wright himself held tenaciously to the conception of such a phase and even advised that soldiers entering an epidemic area be not treated within several weeks of such time.

It seems now there is no negative phase in any material sense and that the fear of such probability has been a great obstacle in the development of this type of prevention. Many now doubt any increased susceptibility even during a severe reaction, and it is confidently held that the danger of contracting typhoid on exposure to a case in a household, ward or in a community where the disease is prevalent exceeds the danger of susceptibility during the twenty-four to forty-eight hours of reaction following an injection. Injections are therefore performed in the immediate presence of typhoid just as serum immunization is practiced in the presence of diphtheria.

If the inoculations were composed of attenuated but living bacilli this susceptibility might be considerable through the simultaneous assault of virile organisms whilst the defenses were engaged in attacking the weaker and comparatively harmless bacteria.

As it is these immunizing bacilli are presented to the serum and tissue fluids of the body ready for solution. They offer no resistance; they cannot multiply, they simply afford in their decomposition typhotoxin which stimulates a livelier production of typhoid destroying emzymes, agglutins, lysins, etc.

### Results of Immunization

Without referring to the earlier work which was necessarily crude, but which nevertheless afforded stimulatingly favorable results, I will review briefly some figures beginning with 1908.

In this year in a division of the English Army 5,473 inoculated men developed twenty-one cases of typhoid. Among the remaining 6,610 uninoculated there were one hundred and eighty-seven cases. That is among the immunized or partially immunized there were only 3.8 cases per thousand, as compared with 28.3 cases per thousand among the others.

Some protection is established with one dose and it is increased by the second and third and becomes stronger with a lapse of time up to undetermined limits, but is said to be at its highest at the expiration of ten to twelve months and endures for several years.

Major Russell remarks that he has not found any diminishing force after four years. The same authority states that among 58,000 troops under observation in 1912 there were but fifteen cases of typhoid, whereas in 1901 among 26,000 soldiers, under older methods of prophylaxis there were 250 cases, that is 2.6 cases per ten thousand as compared with 96 cases in 1901. In the southwest 60,000 doses were served to a body of 20,000 men within twenty days, and although the soldiers "mingled with the people of San Antonio and other cities where sanitary conditions were not always of the best in food supplies, water, or surroundings, and where typhoid prevailed as a general thing, there were few cases in the army, whereas in the Spanish-American war one-fourth to one-third of the men were affected."

I think there were in fact just two cases in this Division, one being an unvaccinated teamster and the other one probably in the period of incubation at the time of treatment. He ran a very mild course.

Does it not seem likely in this large body of men exposed as they were to typhoid that there were others in the incubation stage whose onsets were prevented?

Other convincing statistics are available from civil life, but those given should suffice especially as nowhere have there been any contrary experiences. The elaboration of proof is no longer necessary. This is the time for propaganda.

### Routine Procedure of the Department in the Matter of Immunization

On receipt of a report of a case of typhoid the reporting physician is called on the telephone and his permission solicited to offer immunization to members of the family. It is explained to him that if he prefers to attend to the matter himself we will equip him with a series of doses for each one exposed or contiguous to the case. In the event that he elects to make the injections we ask him to report to us the dates of the various treatments and the character of the reaction. In many instances the physician responds with alacrity. In quite a few instances he temporizes, stating that he will think over the matter, consult the family himself and advise us of the result. Almost without exception this is the last we hear from him. Not infrequently we find on our routine investigation of the typhoid case itself that nothing has been said to the family, or that if it has been presented to them it is supplemented by disapproval on the part of the practitioner. It seems to us that this is wholly unworthy; quite akin to the ancient antipathy to smallpox vaccination and diphtheria immunization.

If typhoid is preventable let us use every agency to wipe it out. Sanitation problems are difficult in so rapidly growing a community as the City of New York with its mixed population. Secondary cases occur frequently in some portions of the city which are preventable through this measure. Since beginning this work we have had secondary infections where we have done no immunizations. Up to the present time, however, no such cases have occurred where we have been permitted to inoculate. In one family nine were exposed to typhoid, eight accepted. The one who refused developed typhoid. When we obtain consent or where the indifference of the physician inspires no further interest on his part, and if the family are favorable to it we feel that we should be at liberty to perform this service. Presuming that the field is clear the inspector on visiting the premises for the routine inspection made in every case of typhoid, offers to inject the members of the household, and if their consent is obtained proceeds as follows: The arm is sterilized at the insertion of the deltoid, the injection is made subcutaneously and the report of the name, age, address is forwarded to the Central Office. He revisits the family at an appointed time usually on a Saturday afternoon from four to six o'clock, in order that the reaction if any occur may take place while the person is in bed. If there is no contrary reason the visits are made at intervals of ten days.

The inspectors make a report of each reinjection and at the conclusion of the series a final report covering the history of the case. The only contra-indication considered is a definite case of tuberculosis or the presence of other debilitating diseases, or of course in the case of infection.

We do not offer inoculation as a therapeutic measure, nor do we advocate it. This lies without our domain and might constitute an encroachment.

It is not unlikely that this movement will meet with considerable opposition. We would be content could we induce the physicians in charge to immunize the family and give us reports. Indeed it is very difficult for the Department to keep up with the burden entailed by our determination to effect for typhoid a situation similar to that attained for smallpox, but we feel it is incumbent upon us to speedily place this great community in an approximate position to that enjoyed by the United States Army and Navy today. Let me respectfully request or even urge you to propagate the good doctrine of immunization. This body represents, I am sure, that element of our profession keenly interested in prevention.

# ATHLETICS—A FACTOR IN SEX HYGIENE.*

## By H. S. Pettit, M.D.,

of Brooklyn, N. Y.

A GOOD athlete is the product of something more than the mere running of a race or the playing of a game. He is the result of a course of years systematic training in the gymnasium and on the athletic field. Pulley machines and mechanical devices for exercise such as are found in the gymnasium develop muscle, correct deformities, remove the effects of bad habits of posture, and raise the standard of health. This is acknowledged by every one who has had any experience in a gymnasium. Such exercise has no psychological value beyond the fact that by improving the health a beneficial influence is produced on the mind. The boy or man who devotes his time exclusively to muscle building machines will certainly develop large bulky muscles; he will also become slow and awkward. He will attain strength but will not know how to put that strength to practical purposes. There will be plenty of muscle but no co-ordination or initiative—a truck horse type of athlete.

The gymnast and acrobat devotes his time to exercise on the various pieces of apparatus with which a gymnasium is equipped, such as horizontal bar, parallel bars, horse, rings, mattresses, etc., and not only develops muscle but acquires grace, skill, agility, strength, muscular control, physical courage and steadiness of nerve. The gymnast has a great respect for his body and is continually striving for symmetrical development. He realizes that certain things weaken and enervate. With him a better condition of health and symmetrical development becomes an obsession. There is ever present a sense of duty to care for the body so that it may always be at its best. There results a more perfect control of the muscular system by the brain and a strengthening of the heart, lungs and nervous system. We have now developed muscle by means of the machines and by means of gymnastics acquired control of that muscle. We have worked to the point demanded by Cicero who said: "The body ought not to be neglected, but by exercise brought to such a frame and condition, as that it may be able to obey the prescription of the mind, in performing that business and bearing those fatigues which are required of it."

If we stopped at this point, however, we would stop short of making a manly man. As yet practically nothing has been done to develop the emotions and it is in this respect that athletics holds such an important place in a course of physical training. The athlete exercises principally out-of-doors practicing and playing all kinds of games such as baseball, football, tennis, rowing, running, jumping, and all the track and field events. Games played in teams develop in a marked degree self-control, self-reliance, quickness of perception, reasoning and judging, physical courage. They tend toward making one gentlemanly, courteous and honorable. In other words a good sportsman. The good sportsman can take the hard knocks as well as give them. He is a good loser as well as a good winner. He can subordinate individual impulses and selfish desires. In team work the ego is lost sight of. The players are a unit working together for

---

*Read before the Medical Society of the County of Kings, February 18, 1913.

mutual benefit. The team may be compared to a wheel. If one cog is defective the wheel loses in efficiency. This teaches discipline—the value of co-öperation, necessity of obeying orders and the power of combination.

The boy who specializes in athletics and excludes gymnastics is making a sad mistake for, strange as it may appear, the man or boy who suffers pulmonary, cardiac, circulatory or nervous disturbances from over-exercise is not the boy who works indoors in the gymnasium practicing gymnastics or acrobatics but the athlete or out-of-door man. I would like to emphasize this statement. The boy who practices gymnastics or acrobatics arrives at a far better physical condition than does the boy who practices athletics exclusively even though in the case of gymnastics the exercise is in the gymnasium and the athlete is out-of-doors. The ideal is to combine the two—first build up the body by gymnastics and then finish the development by athletics. I hope that every doctor here will go over in his mind any patients he may have had who have been injured by over-exercise and then say whether the patient was an athlete or a gymnast.

True education is physical, mental and moral. Physical education is the real education, it teaches "how to live." In school the boy receives book knowledge but in his play he acquires real education. Just as our schools recognize the importance of developing the physical as well as the mental and moral. So physical training would be a failure if it neglected to evolve the mental and moral as well as the physical. The object of physical training is to make a strong healthy boy—and by strong is not meant the ability to raise a heavy weight or to perform any feat of strength that requires the training of a particular group of muscles, but strong in the sense of a sound body, one symmetrically developed, one in which all the organs and muscles are able to perform their functions normally.

This can be attained by any boy who is not actually suffering from structural disease. Keep him at the pulley machines until the muscles grow strong. He will then show an interest in gymnastics and acrobatic exercises. There will be the incentive of learning something new, something requiring skill. The boy is now deriving pleasure from the training, improvement will be noticed almost daily as some new "stunt" is learned. The mind has become master and can readily control muscular action. We have now a fine animal—strong, healthy, graceful and with a high degree of co-ordination, but something more is demanded than the creation of a beautiful animal—we are anxious to produce a manly man. As yet nothing has been attempted to develop character. It is as a psychological factor that athletics or team games are so vastly important, and not as a body builder or health restorer. Take as an example a game of basket ball which develops and strengthens qualities that are the very basis of character. A ball is passed through the air. A good player must be quick to notice while the ball is in the air whether it will be caught by a companion or an opponent. If by a companion he rapidly eludes his guard and places himself in a favorable position. He must anticipate plays. If his perception has been good, his reasoning accurate and his judgment correct, his team will probably score a basket. In the play of the game, which is exceedingly rapid, there are many petty annoyances and aggravating situations which demand to a remarkable extent absolute self-control and self-restraint. The player may receive a slap in the face, a punch, a push, a hard fall, which may or may not

3

have been delivered intentionally. If the boy loses control, is unable to restrain his passions and retaliates by intentional roughness or use of his fist, he will be removed from the game, an inferior player will be substituted and his team will lose in efficiency. A player who has suffered this penalty learns self-control.

No faculty develops except through the performance of its special function. Athletics afford constant and ample opportunities for such practice, with the result that the intellectual faculties, quickness of perfection, reasoning, judging, and the emotions of self-control, self-restraint and self-reliance are wonderfully developed.

In my experience as a trained athlete and gymnast (1882-1888) during youth and early manhood, I never saw, or rather have never seen, a boy masturbate. I cannot remember that my companions ever mentioned the subject. It was not until I began the study of medicine that I realized it was such a universal practice and it was not until I began to teach and study boys that I learned to what extent boys formed clubs for this purpose. I know positively that my athletic friends respected their bodies and would think twice before attempting anything that would tend to impair force or vitality.

An experience of 21 years of teaching high school boys at the Adelphi Academy in physical training has convinced me that the school boy who does not attend the gymnasium or take part in athletics has a great deal of idle time, much of which he spends with some companion telling immodest, obscene stories or in the company of a sensual girl, fondling and caressing her day after day. Many of these boys spend their afternoons on Fulton street in the neighborhood of the large department stores meeting and scraping acquaintances with girls who are out for the same purpose. This class of boy finds relief from his sensuous imaginings by masturbation and some suffer mentally because of frequent nocturnal emissions. There are boys who do not enter the boys' sports or attend the gymnasium who are mentally and morally sound. The non-athlete is not necessarily of a prurient mind. This sort is polite and a good student but he is only an apology for what a boy stands for and will develop into a nice lady-like man.

For 17 years I have conducted summer camp work with boys ranging from 8 to 25 years of age. Last summer there were 88 boys at camp for 10 weeks. At camp I see the boy all day and watch him during his sleep. We eat, sleep and play together and I learn to know the boy much better than does his parent. When a boy is at his play he is natural and off his guard so that his characteristics may be studied under favorable conditions. Masturbation is not common at camp, but when present it is always discovered the first week of camp and eliminated, or rather never again detected. During these 17 years I have watched my campers grow to manhood, graduate from high school and college, I have noted the wonderful change that takes place in a boy as he becomes fond of healthy sports. He becomes more manly, more alert and wide-awake, right habits of living and thinking become inculcate. He becomes a hero-worshiper of a strong, healthy, virile manhood, a "good mixer" and a stronger character.

I have among my camp councillors for 1913 ten prominent college athletes who have been with me 3, 4 and 5 years. We have eaten, played and slept together. They do not smoke or drink, are pure minded and have never had sexual intercourse with women. They are not exceptional. My experience is that the majority of prominent athletes are clean, healthy specimens of manhood, sound mentally and morally. The more sports a boy participates in the stronger his character.

The ardent zeal for athletics is a safety valve whose value cannot be cherished too highly. The good results far outweigh any possible harm that may follow from over-exercise or physical injury. Nerve energies are used up in safe channels, objectionable emotions are restrained.

Sedentary occupations and idleness are dangerous especially during the period of growth from childhood to manhood. A boy is skeptical. He demands material proof. He says, "show me." He can be led and not driven. He is a hero-worshiper and demands an ideal. It is folly to suppose that education will strengthen character. Boys and men govern their conduct by emotion rather than reason. Distinct knowledge of the evil consequences of certain acts will not restrain when environment and strong emotions are at work otherwise a medical man would never become addicted to the use of morphine or cocaine. The poor man knows when he drinks to excess that he will ultimately lose his position and his family will suffer privation, yet he will continue to get drunk. The fact that a young man has suffered venereal disease will not restrain from continued illicit sexual relations. Fear is not a preventive.

It is necessary to cultivate the emotions of self-control and self-restraint in order to elevate the moral sense, to check dissipation and evil doing. These emotions which are the very basis of character are direct results of athletics properly conducted.

Herbert Spencer says: "Whatever moral benefit can be effected by education, must be effected by an education which is emotional rather than intellectual. If, in place of making a child *understand* that this thing is right and the other wrong, you make it *feel* that they are so. If you make virtue loved and vice loathed, if, in short, you produce a state of mind to which proper behavior is natural, spontaneous, instructive, you do some good. But no drilling in catechism, no teaching of moral codes can effect this." Knowledge may be pumped into a boy in school but he gets his real education through contact with the other fellows and in his games.

Dr. Grassman of Munich in a paper read before the Educational Committee of the Medical Association says: "The backbone of the sexual training of the individual is and remains the formation of character. More energy must be thrown into our efforts in this direction. Sexual pre-occupation of the mind must be antagonized on the principle of displacement. The readiest means for this purpose are body exercise and rational physical training."

In closing I would enter a plea for properly conducted athletics, and no matter if the games are more dangerous than they should be. The indisposition or disability that may result from a fracture or dislocation, or sorrow and loss from an occasional death are insignificant alongside of the excellent qualities developed.

# EDITORIAL

## THE ETHICS OF THE CASE.

IN the last issue of the JOURNAL editorial comment appeared from two sources in regard to the newly appointed committee on medical publicity. Among the statements made of the purposes of the committee was one to confer with the editors of various newspapers, in order, if possible to arrive at some sort of co-operation so as to regulate and insure correct reporting of medical matters. Shortly after the publication of the JOURNAL a news item in a Brooklyn daily appeared, telling at some length of a communication sent to the Kings County Society in which more than forty practitioners of medicine in this borough were accused of unprofessional conduct. The article further quoted from the JOURNAL'S editorial, choosing for the purpose isolated phrases so arranged as to give an impression exactly contrary to the spirit of the editorial. We cannot believe that this is wilful misrepresentation, but prefer to think that the mental bias of the person who contributed the news item prevented a proper appreciation of both the subject and the editorial point of view. This furnishes further evidence of the absolute need of greater conservatism in talking about medical matters. The public washing of dirty linen, domestic, fraternal or corporate betrays a spirit of pettiness that the educated physician should feel is beneath him. Surely a profession that for nearly four thousand counted years has been honored for the good it has done for humanity, for its self-sacrifice and constant striving towards higher ideals, should, by its environment, elevate its members above mean jealousies, recrimination and narrow mindedness. The practitioner of medicine who finds time to quarrel with his fellows in the newspapers can hardly appreciate the harm that he is doing himself as well as the profession to which he owes his daily bread. Advancement in medicine in the long run depends upon conscientious, painstaking study, the strictest application to professional work and the demonstration of personal fitness to meet responsibility. "Bluff" may and often does carry one rapidly to a measure of financial success, but in the long run, unless backed by ability, it is inadequate to raise one to a position of respect and dignity in the profession. The man who does not abide by the code of ethics, sooner or later suffers in proportion as he fails to live by its teaching. Unhappily there seems to be a disposition to regard the code of ethics as the arbitrary ruling of a majority of physicians based upon time-honored custom and medieval dogmatism. Actually the code of ethics represents the golden rule of medicine crystalized out of the bitter experiences of generations who have found that courtesy, unselfishness, honesty and common sense are the foundation stones best suited to support a profession that more than any other is dependent upon fraternal co-operation. Inability to perceive that common sense is the real basis of ethical living and failure to apply the test of common sense in weighing one's own actions may be taken as proof that something of unworthiness is present in the practitioner of medicine who neglects the cardinal rule of Plato's teaching, "know thyself."

The question may be frankly asked whether inability to obtain hospital experience or even to make a reasonable living is not primarily the fault of the individual. It is incomprehensible that all the physicians of a locality or of a country should be banded against one unless there is in that one some fault that makes him an Ishmael. To live at peace with one's neighbors, to get the best out of life, one must recognize the good that is in everyone and must equally appreciate where he himself errs. The neighbors will complain if one practices too persistently on the cornet before an open window. This is a free country which recognizes a man's right to play upon a cornet, but the persistent abuse of that harmonious instrument infringes on the rights of the neighborhood which may justly declare that volume and persistence of sound do not constitute music. In the same way the persistent use of the lay press for the airing of minority grievances in time reacts upon the aggressor. If one is sensible that a wrong has been done, common sense should teach that the first thing to do is to call upon your neighbor and in a frank and manly way, without heat or passion, discuss the question from all sides; this promotes a happy understanding more quickly than if one first bangs his neighbor with a club and then asks him to reason peaceably.

We confess to have wandered somewhat from the original purpose, but in extenuation would point out that these thoughts, rambling though they may be, naturally grow out of a consideration of the turmoil that is now agitating the medical profession in Brooklyn. H. G. W.

## "SIMILIA SIMILIBUS CURENTUR."

THROUGH the courtesy of a committee of the American Institute of Homeopathy the JOURNAL has been furnished a copy of a communication to be presented to the American Medical Association at its meeting at Minneapolis on June 17, 1913, asking a "joint investigation of the scientific merits of the method of drug selection expressed by the formula 'Similia similibus curentur.'" The reasons for this request, quoted from the letter, follow:

"This rule has governed the selection of drugs in the treatment of disease by a considerable number of medical practitioners for over a century. We feel that the time has come when this formula should be brought before the whole medical profession, carefully investigated by modern scientific methods and a determination made of the exact value of this method in the practice of medicine. We seek this

"1st—Because the voluntary testimony of a large number of physicians who do not understand the correct application of this method indicates their desire to make use of it.

"2nd—Because a large number of men who attempt its use ought to be able to get a better understanding of its true significance.

"3rd—Because we believe a large majority of the medical profession would have their usefulness and their power to benefit the sick largely enhanced by a thorough knowledge of this method.

"4th—Because we believe that suffering is lessened and sickness more speedily and comfortably terminated through drugs administered according to the rule of similars.

"5th—Because we feel that a careful investigation of this subject belongs to the whole medical profession and not to a single branch of it.

"6th—We feel that such research regarding the formula of similars is desirable. Because the exactness of modern science with the present means of investigation, together with the accurate observation of the subjective as well as the objective symptoms, make it expedient to investigate the action of many drugs coming into use at the present time, as well as to re-examine those long proven.

"For the above various reasons we pray that your organization appoint a committee of five to meet a like committee from the American Institute of Homeopathy to discuss this subject with a view of attempting a demonstration of the accuracy of the theory of similars, or of proving its falsity.

"It seems to us that its joint investigation should be made under the auspices of some research laboratory like the Rockefeller Institute of New York or the McCormick Institute of Chicago. These institutions have the experts necessary for such a test; with trained eyes they could follow its course from start to finish. Whether the result of the particular investigation should prove satisfactory or not, the effort would not be wasted because a list of drugs in common use among the members of your association as well as ours can be selected for this study of their physiological action. These accurate observations would be of permanent value to both schools.

"After careful investigation of the effects of these drugs in different strengths upon the human body, as well as observing their poisonous effects in animals, an extensive trial of their therapeutic efficacy should be made in some of the large public hospitals to test the action of these remedies in exemplifying this theory of drug administration.

"In recent years every effort has been made to unite the medical profession. A large number of legal practitioners is kept from affiliation because of its belief in a method of drug selection, the truth of which is questioned by the majority. Let us make a thorough test of this hypothesis. If it be proven true, humanity will be benefited by the enlarged and improved armamentarium of all physicians; if it be disproven, the last obstacle to medical union will have been removed."

The goal toward which every open-minded physician should strive is essential unity, and this step on the part of the Homeopathic practitioners should be met as frankly as it is made, for it heralds the beginning of an undersanding that will go far toward breaking down an artificial and needless barrier. Mutual understanding begets confidence, and mutual confidence is a grand thing, as big John Brodie explained to David Copperfield. By all means let us have a thorough investigation with a fair field and no favors shown.

H. G. W.

## "FOR MARRIAGE FIT."

IF he be correctly reported a clergyman of Newburg, New York, has fearlessly announced at the beginning of his ministry his intention of uniting in marriage only the physically fit. In this stand he follows the pronouncement of the Chicago Ministerial Association, who, in turn, have fallen in step with a number of well-known divines whose stand upon this matter has been announced in the last few months. This is only another evidence of the determination to aid in the physical uplift of this country. The eugenic movement seems to have taken vigorous hold upon the imagination of a large number of thinking people. They have been told, and it is true, that idiocy, criminality, immorality and insanity upon the mental side, and some forms of disease upon the physical, may be visited upon the children unto the third generation; and this seems to them a practical way not merely to check the growth of decadence but to spread abroad the idea of its prevention, for the refusal of one clergyman to unite an unhealthy couple is not limited to this specific case, but is talked about and commented upon as the ripples spread when a stone is thrown into a pond. If all the clergy of all denominations can be brought to stand firmly together, their attitude in time will accomplish much for the physical betterment of the race.

But what of the vast number of civil marriages? So far little has been done to surround this form of marriage contract with safeguards that may be considered adequate. May not the church by an insistence upon this rule impel those who are physically unfit to seek a civil marriage? The marriage relation is based not upon moral or intellectual choice but upon the physical impulse common to all animate creation. Social convention has proved the wisdom of our present attitude toward marriage. In their last analysis the cogent reasons that support the marriage contract are essentially economic—utilitarian if you please. The instinct that urges man to wed is far removed essentially from the rules and regulations with which man has chosen to surround himself. The eugenic standpoint seems to overlook this primal fact. It is Homer who said: "As long as a youth and a maiden sit on a moss-covered log beneath the stars, so long will love spring up and flourish," and depend upon it what was true beneath the walls of Troy is true to-day and, fit or unfit, men and women will mate and children will be born. In so far as serious minded people may, their crusade for healthy marriage will help to bring to the thoughtful the need of keeping themselves in health or, conversely, of keeping their diseases to themselves; but not until moral education has raised every last son of Adam to a high degree of self-abnegation will marriages among the unfit cease to be.

Underlying this great problem is a deeper and a darker one that concerns physicians in particular. How shall we stamp out syphilis, interlocked as it is with the inherent sexual craving? How many physcians are giving to this problem, which they know so much about, the thought that it deserves? Are we safeguarding our own children as we should? If we are to hold our place in the foremost rank of those who are striving to better the health of the country, and through bettering its health, to better its morals, :it is essential that every man who calls himself a physician should keep this problem constantly before him, and strive by co-operation as well as by individual effort to hasten the time when the need for a certificate of good health shall have passed away.

H. G. W.

## ILL-ADVISED THERAPEUTIC AND DIAGNOSTIC ZEALOTRY.

A T the risk of courting an indictment for heresy we are going to set down some thoughts about prevalent professional customs which, though enjoying the sanction of the rank and file, are nevertheless, from certain points of view, more or less indefensible.

The fact that an individual has albumin in his urine, or that a murmur is discovered in his heart, is very often no good reason why he should be informed of the fact and made to change radically his mode of living. It has often seemed to us that the rules that are laid down for the guidance of those whose health is not perfect (whose health is?) make their lives hardly worth the living. Many of the people whose blood pressure is regularly taken and who look forward to perhaps twenty years of life providing they do certain things would be happier and longer lived if they were not painfully aware that their vessels were slightly arteriosclerotic or their hearts "weak." High blood pressure is a compensatory phenomenon commonly, and we are glad to note an increasing disposition on the part of our clinicians to let such drugs as the nitrites rather severely alone. We once derived much satisfaction from the reading of a paper of Osler's in which he set forth the "advantages" of a little albumin in the urine of elderly men. We were recently consulted by a girl who was greatly perturbed about her health because an eminent man had told her that she was "nervous," which she had never imagined herself. Here was a neurasthenic in the making—and the artificer a physician! How many neurasthenics owe the initial impetus to the doctors themselves?

There is undoubtedly an unwarrantable amount of tinkering with the organs of people. There are unquestionably many persons who are regarded as tuberculous for no very sound reasons. It is almost in the nature of things that such crazy cults as Christian Science should be founded. They at least furnish a haven for the many who resent the constant suggestion of bad health. It is as much the function of the physician to suggest good health as it is to treat actual disease. We should never have permitted the freak cults to secure such a lead as they have in the matter of psychotherapeutics. Good health doesn't interest us nearly so much as departures from it.

We hold no brief for the careless physician. No one can be too well equipped in the art of diagnosis. But there is a deadline. Even the physician should take good health for granted sometimes.

Some one recently raised the question as to whether the tinkerings of "medical gynecologists" with the cervix uteri and its canal contributed to cancer of the womb. This is a little far fetched and yet suggestive withall. Doubtless gynecologists with no sense of humor will resent the imputation utterly.

ARTHUR C. JACOBSON.

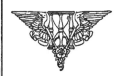 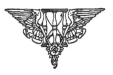

# Society Transactions

## TRANSACTIONS OF THE BROOKLYN GYNECOLOGICAL SOCIETY.

*Regular Meeting, January 3, 1913.*

The President, CARROLL CHASE, M.D., in the Chair.

### Scientific Section. Presentation of Specimens.

DR. ALBERT M. JUDD presented a specimen of fibroid tumor of the uterus.

DR. JUDD:—I removed this growth this morning. It is not particularly interesting except in the technique of the operation. It was one of those cases of intramural fibroid of considerable extent, with another large fibroid developing subperitoneal, the whole practically filling the true pelvis and making it difficult to manipulate. It was very troublesome to pull up the tumor and to get hold of the uterine arteries, and this was accomplished by making a peritoneal flap. In this case I was able to get the best peritoneal flap that I have ever obtained in a similar operation from the posterior surface for covering the stump. The patient was 51 years of age and had had menorrhagia for two years. The flow would come on every two months and last from ten to fourteen days; she was anemic, with a percentage of hemoglobin of 45.

DR. POLAK asked if in operating in such cases of fibroid Dr. Judd has cut directly across the cervix and by drawing the parts aside with a vulsellum forceps exposed the uterine arteries?

DR. JUDD:—I studied over this case many nights to see how I could proceed without severe hemorrhage. With the method I used we get a good peritoneal flap without buttonholing it. Lower down the adhesions would be found too solid.

DR. C. R. HYDE presented a specimen of cystic ovary.

"The patient from whom this specimen was removed was operated on for a large pyosalpynx and ovarian abscess on the right side. I was not allowed to remove the left tube and ovary by agreement prior to the operation. The left ovary, which was normal in size, was bound down with adhesions. After freeing the ovary from its bed of adhesions it was tacked up to the broad ligament. The patient did well after the operation but three weeks later was suddenly seized with acute pain in the left side, in the ovarian region. Her condition becoming worse I operated again, and found this large cystic ovary which, as you see, is about four times the size of a normal ovary. The case is unusual, in my experience, in that a cystic ovary could develop so rapidly. The question arises as to the possible cause, whether due to a twisting of the ovarian ligament and consequent shutting off of the circulation with acute production of a cystic condition."

DR. HYDE also presented a specimen of uterine fibroid.

"The patient was 66 years of age and had carried this growth for nearly thirty-five years. During the recent illness of Dr. Palmer the case had come under the care of Dr. Hyde. Seven days before the operation the patient developed an obstruction of the bowels. This was not at first diagnosed, as she had been in the habit of going three to four days without a movement. Her condition growing worse, the case was diagnosed as intestinal obstruction, probably due to the presence of the fibroid. She was removed to the hospital for operation. Laparotomy was performed and this large fibroid was removed. In exploring for the obstruction the cæcum was found enormously distended with a rupture at the hepatic flexure through which fæces was oozing. Opposite this rupture, at the mesenteric attachment, the wall of the cæcum was partially ruptured. Both were closed by a double row of lembert sutures. While exploring in the true pelvis, a carcinomatous area was felt in the rectum. Exsection was performed with end to end anastomosis by bagenstecker suture material.

"There are two points of interest in this case. In the uterus the tumor was found to be a large sub-mucous fibroid which had undergone calcareous degeneration, as you can see; and yet, with this kind of a fibroid, which usually gives menorrhagia or metrorrhagia, there were no menstrual disturbances. The periods were normal and she passed the climacteric easily. As regards the obstruction, the interesting point is whether the uterus, by its size, pressing against the rectum for so many years, and with obstinate constipation always present over a long period of time, produced sufficient irritation to make the rectum undergo cancerous degeneration. The rectum was obstructed so much that the lumen of the gut would admit only an ordinary lead pencil. The symptoms of this obstruction—dilatation of the intestine—were referred to a point well back from the obstruction, as is common, i. e., the gut in obstruction is usually distended at a point some distance removed from the obstruction itself. I would like to ask if anyone present can give any reason as to the possibility of constant pressure on the rectum for a period of years being sufficient reason for the production of cancer? Dr. Murray reports true adeno-carcinoma of the rectum.'"

DR. POOL:—May I add another case, one in the course of which I did some plastic work upon the right ovary and suspended it after the Gardner method, letting it lie between the tube and round ligament, in the fold of the broad ligament. The patient did nicely and made a good recovery. At the end of two and one-half weeks I found a tumor on the right side, at the side of the uterus, which was evidently this suspended ovary. I was at a loss to account for the sudden enlargement, but Dr. Hyde's case is enlightening. At the time I thought it was due to interference with circulation, because of constriction or torsion of the pedicle which might occur in this particular form of operation. The patient was symptomatically cured, and not having heard of her in some time, I trust that the swelling has also disappeared.

DR. JUDD:—I have seen a number of cases of sudden cystic degeneration of ovaries within a few months after operation by puncture for cyst or resection, from an appreciable size to that of an orange. I now do no conservative work on the ovaries unless there are particular reasons, as in young women who wish to take the risk of pregnancy, and, if possible, let the ovary absolutely alone.

DR. POLAK:—This case of Dr. Hyde's is interesting. I reported a case I had at the Woman's Hospital to the Society a couple of years ago with a similar history. It was a woman in whom I resected an ovary and a week afterwards she developed an acute abdominal condition causing an obstruction of the bowels which necessitated opening the abdomen. By that time a cyst had formed on the ovary about the size of a lemon, and this in the interval of a week. The point that Dr. Hyde brought out is the basic principle. Anything that disturbs the circulation is apt to be followed by trouble. Suspension operations, unless they are done on an anatomical basis, and I doubt if Gardner's operation is entirely so, are apt to be followed by annoyances. If you disturb the afferent and efferent circulation you lay the foundation for possible degeneration. It is not uncommon to find a resected ovary as large as an egg shortly after the operation and later to find it down to normal or even smaller. No matter what you do when you change its position, if there is an interference with its blood supply it is bound to swell and the further development of the condition depends upon whether the ovary is in bad company or out of trouble. If it is free from peritoneal irritation it will go down in size, particularly if it is the right ovary. We feel, as Dr. Judd has said, that true conservatism is to leave it alone. It is never the same in other operations about the uterus, we rarely get secondary enlargements following removal of dermoids or fibroids. In these plastic operations we must go deeply into the tissues and make the apposition as near to its natural form as we can. The apposition can be had by the use of fine catgut and if properly done the ovary does not swell. I believe there will be little trouble if we place the broad ligament in an even line of suture where we have made extensive resection.

DR. O. PAUL HUMPSTONE presented two X-ray plates of a case of a chondroplasia fœtalis.

DR. HUMPSTONE:—The subject of fœtal pathology is a neglected one and more reports on it should be made. Modern investigation is enlightening the causes of its many phases. The woman from whom this specimen was removed was a colored multipara with six normal children, followed by two abortions, and now presenting a positive Wassermann. She had the largest abdomen I ever saw, from a polyhydramnios; we took away more than five gallons of fluid and then delivered this specimen by version. Some difficulty was encountered in recognizing feet from arms. The characteristics of these cases are shown very beautifully in these plates, viz., the shortening of the long bones, with the widening of their ends, and the increased distance between the ends of the bones, and the shape of the head and the extremities. This condition was formerly called fœtal rickits. Investigation into the causes of these conditions is practical in that it gives opportunity for prevention. If this woman had been under antisyphilitic treatment she most probably would not have given birth to this monster. Every case of suspected syphilis should have active treatment during pregnancy.

Narration of cases:

DR. BEACH:—I wish to present the case histories of two patients. The first: Mrs. D., aged 21 years, was delivered by me one and one-half years ago by high forceps through a 9 cm. true conjugate, causing a perineal laceration; this was drawn together by chromic gut in the vagina and silkworm gut in the skin, which resulted in primary union; the bowels moved on the tenth day. The baby died of a septic condition at the end of two weeks from a condition which began as a skin infection of the neck and legs; the child also suffered from malnutrition. This woman came under my care pregnant a second time and was due November 10th. She passed that date and on November 15th, in view of the increasing size of the baby and the pelvic contraction, I decided to induce labor. She was taken to the hospital and prepared for delivery. When I attempted to introduce a bougie into the uterus it met resistance; taking it out partly and trying again, again it met resistance; a third attempt resulted in passing the bougie, but at once there occurred a profuse hemorrhage, so profuse that I at once ruptured the membranes, and this stopped the bleeding temporarily; it was a good stream of blood, sufficient to require serious attention. I used a large-sized Voorhees' bag, and packing and thought it would go through, but the hemorrhage commenced again and soaked through the packing, down to the bed and through everything. I took out the packing and tried pressure, but without result. There was no placenta previa; I examined carefully to ascertain this point. The bleeding continued, the patient's condition became weak, pulse 128, and I determined to do an abdominal operation. She was taken to the operating room and was delivered of a child weighing 9 pounds 15 ounces. To me this case was very instructive and I wish to express my condemnation of the use of bougies to induce labor in such cases. There is no doubt that the bougie in this case produced a marked placental separation, and I believe that the woman would have bled to death had she not been operated on. I should prefer the use of the bag or a large rectal tube.

The second case was that of Mrs. B., aged 47, had been married twenty-four years, and had five children. Her history shows that she was operated on ten years ago after the delivery of her third child for prolapse symptoms, perinorrhaphy and right öophorectomy. Four years ago, after having had another child, she was operated on again, this time for the same symptoms, a perinorrhaphy and ventrosuspension. Two years ago I delivered her of a seven months' child, the delivery being complicated with a profuse hemorrhage due to separation of the placenta in which a bag relieved the condition and spontaneous labor resulted, the baby being born dead. Nine months later I saw her again; she had no headache, no backache, no leucorrhœa, but was nervous and said she had hot flashes; she had gained twenty-five pounds in weight. She had seen no blood since the delivery of her last child. I made a diagnosis of probable menopause. I made an examination and found the uterus in the anterior position. I saw her twice after that at intervals of one month, and then she began to complain of bachache, pelvic pains anteriorly, and frequency of urination. I recommended operation at this time but it was refused. On August 19th, *e. g.*, two years after the last labor, I was called to see her at her home. She had taken a great deal of exercise and done a great deal of ocean bathing and thought she had taken cold. She had been suffering from cramps very acutely, in the lower abdomen; there was no increase in temperature but a marked median hypogastric tenderness. Vaginal examination was unsatisfactory. She was given codia, and ice bag applied, and rest advised, but the pains increased. Two days later I was called, when she said: "Last night something came away from me that was bloody and my pains ceased; it was dark fluid and there was about a quart of it." She remained in bed about a week and felt well when she got up. She had never had a trachelorrhaphy. The condition had gone on for two years. The cramp-like pains had come on at more or less regular intervals, and were of a menstrual type, the intervals being perhaps five, six or seven weeks apart. On October

19th I saw her again. She had had another attack of cramp-like hypogastric pains lasting two or three days but no blood, and it was probably an attempt at a period after the hematometria. The condition was evidently a hematometria, and I should like to ask if any of the gynæcologists can explain it in any other way. What is to be done in this case, amputation of the cervix or hysterectomy?

Dr. HUMPSTONE:—In Cæsarean section for bleeding, either from placenta previa or accidental hemorrhage, we have always to deal with a much softer, flabbier, unresponsive uterus than in the ordinary cases of Cæsarean for distocia. It is particularly in this condition that pituitrin in Cæsarean is useful, in my experience. The result is very prompt, particularly if the pituitrin is injected directly into the flabby uterine muscle, as I used it in one case.

Dr. JUDD:—I have used pituitrin in these cases, but prefer to use a large dose, and find that 4 c.c. works well. I used it the other night for a Cæsarean; there was less bleeding and less trouble in handling the uterus.

Dr. HUMPSTONE remarked that earlier he had recommended larger doses, 4 c.c., because of the weakness of that particular preparation, but the preparation is now stronger, each c.c. representing 2 decigrams of the active principal, instead of the former 1 decigram to the c.c., and 2 c.c. is now an ample dose.

Dr. POMEROY:—The use of the Cæsarean delivery for unusual cases leads to a broad discussion of indications. Classically we still carry the thought that it should be resorted to only in the presence of bony obstructions. I wish to speak of a patient whom I delivered two weeks ago for retraction ring by Cæsarean section. The subject of retraction ring distocia has not yet been thoroughly worked out. This patient had been delivered spontaneously of a living child which weighed six and one-half pounds after a twenty-hour labor at her first confinement and it is always a presumption with me that if a patient has been delivered in such manner it is to be considered in her favor at the next confinement. I saw this patient about two weeks before the date of her expected confinement and found the head above the brim. The pelvis was a slightly flattened justo-minor. A week later I decided to interfere and stripped the membranes. She had pains for some hours but failed to go into active labor. Five days later the membranes ruptured spontaneously early in the morning and without pains. Pains followed later, continued irregular and cramp-like during the day but with no progress and I advised removal to the hospital; this was after the membranes had been ruptured ten hours. The cervix was soft and I could insert three fingers without difficulty. There was a distinct retraction ring which I am positive was not the internal os. I gave her 2 c.c. of pituitrin and when I saw her later it apparently had had no effect. About 11 o'clock that night I introduced a four inch Voorhees bag above the retraction ring and left it in for four hours. The patient had a great deal of tenesmus, irregular pains, discomfort, and became decidedly frantic on the subject of the bag, and we took it out. The cervix remained soft but the retraction ring in front of the head persisted. I then gave the patient a 1/20th gr. of strichnia and she promptly went to sleep for two hours. Examination thereafter showed no descent of the head, and a distinct caput had formed. The fœtal pulse would run up as high as two hundred beats to the minute. We decided upon operation and she was delivered by me by Cæsarean section, the child weighing seven pounds and four ounces. At the request of both parties I tied off and sectioned both tubes. The child lived and the mother made an uneventful recovery.

Dr. HUMPSTONE:—It is my opinion that women have increasing size babies, and the experiences of those in hospital work with the difficulties that follow these cases will bear me out in the statement. Such cases require the Cæsarian operation, and they should be recognized. In a case at the Jewish Hospital only two weeks ago such a condition arose. A retraction ring developed that was so tight around the neck including the arm in its grasp that in getting it out the arm was broken.

Dr. POLAK:—I want to report very briefly the case of a woman who was under my care at the hospital recently. This woman had a very large fibroid and had been bleeding for a number of months almost continuously. She had become greatly weakened and anemic and her hemoglobin had been reduced to 25 per cent. Packing in the hospital had no effect upon the bleeding and I did a hysterectomy. Previous to her entrance to the hospital there had been a history of glycosuria, but in the later examinations of the urine there was an entire absence of sugar. After the operation an examination of the urine disclosed the presence of acetone and diacetic acid and sugar. She began to show symptoms of coma, and this condition became deeper and she became more and more drowsy. We infused this patient with a five per cent. solution of bicarbonate of soda, giving her 500 c.c. in a forty minutes period. The reaction was almost miraculous. I have seen bicarbonate of soda used in such cases but have never seen the patients come out of the coma. The acetone and diacetic acid disappeared but the sugar remained. Another interesting point was that immediately after the operation with the appearance of the acetone and diacetic acid she ran a high temperature with a pulse between 80 and 90, and the pulse did not go above 100. Two days after the infusion of the bicarbonate of soda solution the temperature kept between 105 and 106. I should like to know if it has been the experience of the members that such flights of temperature are usual in these conditions. I am sure it was not due to infection.

Another case I should like to report was that of a woman upon whom we operated at the hospital yesterday morning; a woman who had been operated upon four years ago for a retro-displacement by a distinguished New York surgeon. She complained continually of a pain on the left side but examination showed the uterus to be freely movable. In examining her it was noticed that the uterus would spring over to the left side, and it showed some tendency to sinister-version. The diagnosis made was that there had been a suspension, and the surgeon had done a Gilliam operation, the left side had been successful but the right side had resulted in a slipping of the ligament and the uterus had been swung up at one corner, and this was confirmed by the operation.

DR. CARROLL CHASE:—I should like to ask Dr. Polak if his case of glycosuria showed any evidence of pancreatic disease. The presence of pancreatic disease in these cases has been of great interest to me.

DR. POLAK:—The patient did not show any such symptoms.

DR. POOL:—Dr. Polak's case recalls one I had in which I was less fortunate. It was a woman who I saw at my office suffering from a procidentia. The urine showed nothing abnormal and she was operated on at the hospital. Two days after the operation she developed a glycosuria and passed 80 ounces of urine, increasing to 120 ounces. She passed rapidly into a moderately comatose condition. The same treatment as that employed by Dr. Polak was used but the coma deepened and the patient died on the eleventh day after the operation. This woman showed no symptoms of the glycosuria, local or general, before the operation but I should think that she must have at some time previously suffered from this condition.

The paper of the evening was then read by Dr. Paul Pilcher, "New Growths of the Bladder," exhibiting the use of the monopolar and bipolar current in the treatment of these conditions.

The president stated that through a misunderstanding Dr. Dickinson of the committee appointed to discuss the paper was not able to be present, and the two other members, Dr. Maneke and Dr. Baldwin were also absent. The paper was open for general discussion.

## TRANSACTIONS OF THE BROOKLYN SURGICAL SOCIETY.

*Stated Meeting, January 2, 1913.*

The President, R. W. WESTBROOK, M.D., in the Chair.

*Program.*

I. Report of Cases.
    *a.* Fracture of Pelvis with Complete Rupture of the Urethra. (Paper.)
    *b.* Punctured Wound of Abdomen with Protrusion of Intestine. Patient. (Paper.)
    *c.* Compound Fracture of Skull. Laceration of Lateral Sinus. Patient. (Paper.) By Eugene W. Skelton, M.D.
    Case *a* discussed by Dr. H. B. Delatour, M.D.
    Cases *b* and *c*, no discussion.
II. Report of Cases.
    *a.* Cholelithiasis. (Paper.)
    *b.* Epispadias. Patient. (Paper.) By L. W. Pearson, M.D.
    No discussion on either case.
III. Report of Cases.
    *a.* Peritonitis and Colloid Carcinoma of Rectum (in a Boy of Fifteen). (Notes.)

b. Syphilitic Endarteritis. (Notes.) By R. M. Rome, M.D.
Case *a* discussed by Dr. R. W. Westbrook. Discussion closed by
Dr. R. M. Rome.
Case *b,* no discussion.
IV. Report of Cases.
  a. Multiple Vesicle Calculi Complicating Hypertrophied Prostate.
  (Notes.)
  b. Three Cases of Angulation of the Sigmoid. (Notes.)
  c. Carcinoma of Esophagus. (Notes.) By Walter A. Sher-
  wood, M.D.
  Case *a,* no discussion.
  Cases *b* discussed by Dr. H. B. Delatour, Dr. R. M. Rome, Dr.
  T. B. Spence and Dr. R. W. Westbrook. Discussion closed
  by Dr. W. A. Sherwood.

### Fracture of Pelvis with Complete Rupture of the Urethra.

*Reported by Eugene W. Skelton, M.D.*

F. H., aged 9, was admitted to the hospital on November 27, 1912, with
the history of having been struck by a large motor truck while crossing the
street. He was brought to the hospital by the ambulance and examination
showed skin and mucous membrane pale with no dyspnœa, cyanosis or rigidity
of the abdominal wall. There was no pain on pressure of the abdominal wall
when admitted. The house surgeon noted a fracture of the pelvis on the right
side and on being catheterized it was found that only a few drops of urine
were obtained and quite a little blood. I saw the boy about four hours after
the injury and he was in marked shock at the time and had passed no urine.
His abdomen was then very tender and a peculiar mass on the left side about
the size of an orange was noted and outlined. This abnormality was not
accounted for at the time, but the boy had the typical facies of one suffering
from a severe injury of the abdomen. It was thought best to do an immediate
exploratory operation and the patient having been prepared was then anæthet-
ized. Some difficulty was met in entering the abdomen by reason of a large
amount of edematous tissue just above the pubes. The incision was carried
higher up on the left of the median line and the contents of the upper abdomen
explored. There was no evidence of injury here and the entire intestinal tract
was then examined; this was also normal. As the lower quadrants were
explored a fracture on each side of the symphisis pubis was found. The
bladder was also found to have been torn from its anterior attachments so
that the examining finger could be passed under the pubic arch. I then realized
that the urethra had been torn from the bladder at the sphincter, which had
retained its tonicity and, retaining the secreted urine, formed the mass on the
left side as noted. A steel catheter was then passed through the meatus and
anterior urethra, only to find the free end coming into the pelvic cavity just
internal to the arch. It was found to be impossible to enter the bladder through
the abdominal route, and the boy's condition not warranting any extensive or
long time effort to restore the continuity of the parts, I decided that the best
chance was in doing a perineal section. This was followed out and having
identified the posterior urethra, I opened it and passed a catheter into the pelvic
cavity, but it was impossible to go on into the bladder, which had been torn
away as stated above. I then opened the bladder through what had been the
space of Retzius, and passed a steel catheter from within out through the
sphincter of the bladder and by means of a silk ligature tied on to the steel
catheter and the proximal end of the rubber catheter, it was drawn back into
the bladder and the secreted urine drained out through the perineal wound by
means of the rubber catheter, which was sewed in situ for continued drainage.
I should have stated that before I opened the bladder I brought it into as
normal a position as possible and closed the upper part of the incision and
then walled off by sponges any communication with the peritoneal cavity. The
bladder was then closed in the regular manner and the rest of the abdominal
incision closed by layer suture of chromic gut and silk. The pelvic fracture
was retained in place by wide adhesive straps and the boy placed in bed with
proper stimulation and in the Fowler position. As in most of these cases,
the wound became infected in the lower angle and has formed a sinus from
the abdominal side through to the perineum which is closing in at the present
time. The catheter has been out several times but on only one occasion was
there any difficulty in replacing it, and the bladder has drained well. The boy,
being particularly restless, has displaced the fractured end so that at some
future time when the suppuration has entirely cleared up, the bones will have

to be readjusted and the bladder connected up to its natural outlet. I report this case with interest, as it appeals to me that in the presence of shock, etc., it is far better to relieve these cases by a perineal drainage and later on do a complete restoration, although I recognize the difficulty that will be met in doing the later operation.

### Punctured Wound of Abdomen with Protrusion of Intestine.

#### *Patient. Reported by Eugene W. Skelton, M.D.*

Fred S., aged 30, admitted to the Norwegian Hospital on October 10, 1912, with the history of having received a severe blow on the abdomen while shifting a belt from one wheel to another, the stick having been caught in the wheel of the block and forcibly thrown against him. The ambulance surgeon found him without much evidence of shock or pain, but examination revealed a punctured wound of the abdominal wall in the center of the lower right quadrant. About twelve inches of the small intestine protruded through this traumatic hernia and the intestine was of a dark-red color and congested, due to the constriction. The patient was taken to the operating room and immediately anæsthetized. The intestine, which had become mixed in with the pubic hair, was then carefully protected by towels on the abdominal wall and saline irrigation poured over them. They were then wrapped up in large lap sponges and the abdominal wall thoroughly prepared, after which the punctured wound was enlarged and the cavity explored for further injury and the intestines carefully looked over. The protruded intestines were then replaced and a small cigarette drain placed in the lower angle of the wound to remain in situ for five days, after which time, there being no evidence of internal injury, the wound was allowed to close in. The patient has made a good recovery.

### Compound Fracture of Skull. Laceration of Lateral Sinus.

#### *Patient. Reported by Eugene W. Skelton, M.D.*

Boy, A. S., aged 6 years, was admitted to the general service of the Norwegian Hospital on August 17, 1912, with the history of having been struck while crossing the street by a motorcycle. The blow was received on the left side of the head, just posterior to the mastoid process. When admitted he was in an unconscious state with bleeding from the left ear and nose. He vomited some blood, which evidently had come from the posterior nares. Mark of contusion over the frontal eminence on the left side. There was a soft mass on the left side behind the mastoid process and also a depression. After being prepared and placed under anæsthesia, an incision was made over the depressed part and some comminuted bone was taken out at the point where the blow had been received. The surrounding bone had been depressed from the injury, but on removing the loose bone a profuse hemorrhage from the lateral sinus followed. This was controlled by packing with iodoform gauze and the skin incision partly closed. On two subsequent occasions on removing the gauze, the hemorrhage started again, but after a wait of ten days from the last attempt it was removed without further trouble. The depressed bone was then elevated and the boy made a good recovery, aside from one tender point behind the ear.

### A Case of Cholelithiasis.

#### *Reported by L. W. Pearson, M.D.*

Mrs. B., 75 years old. Had chronic indigestion for years with occasional attacks of colic. For the past seven years these were unmistakably due to gallstones. Her general health for many months has on this account been poor. I was summoned July 5, 1912. She was suffering considerable pain; was intensely jaundiced and exhibited a typical gallstone paroxysm. Notwithstanding her greatly impaired physical condition operative measures were strongly urged. This advice having been rejected, palliative treatment was employed. For three days she suffered very much, her condition continually becoming worse, until I no longer urged an operation and stated frankly to the family that she would possibly, even probably, die on the table if it were resorted to. The following day, the 9th of July, permission was asked to have her old family physician, a distinguished member of this Society, see her. Cheerfully I assented; glad to have his advice and moral support. He insisted that an operation offered the only hope, giving a very grave prognosis. The next morning, July 10th, with the assistance of Drs. Sheehey and Susman, I operated on her at the Samaritan Hospital. A Mayo-Robson incision gave us ready access to the gall bladder region. Adhesions were so firm and the viscera so matted together it was impossible to indentify anything. The gall bladder was neither visible nor palpable. The patient's condition was so critical that it was important to save every minute. It occurred to me that a finger introduced through the foramen of Winslow, then directed towards the gall bladder region, might be of service. By this means the gall bladder was discovered at once and the stones palpated. Pressure forward brought the offending organ near the surface, permitting ready access. It was quickly incised and the stones and friable lithic material easily removed. It was one of those old, contracted organs that had been a long time affected. A rubber tube was inserted, the walls of the gall bladder infolded about it and the operation hurriedly concluded. I regret to add that the patient's vital powers were too feeble to sustain the ordeal.

I report the case because of the ease with which the offending organ was located, by passing a finger through the foramen of Winslow. I have a hazy idea that I have somewhere read of this device, but when or where I cannot say, or even if I have done so at all. However, that is but a little matter. The main thing is to disseminate it that it might be serviceable to some other when sorely needed.

## Epispadias.

### Patient. Reported by L. W. Pearson, M.D.

How often little things give the most trouble! In one sense this is not such a little thing, yet it has caused us much worry. When I first saw Mr. B. with Dr. Raub some three years ago, the urethral canal terminated at the glans penis and was devoid of covering throughout its distal half. During erection it was deflected dextrally and altogether a most unruly member. Our first object was to form a channel through the glans. It was done after the manner of Thiersch. Two longitudinal incisions were made on the dorsum, converging ventrally, and a strip along each denuded. A soft rubber catheter was depressed between them and enclosed by linen sutures. No pins were used. This was healed within ten days. The second step was effected three weeks later and consisted in forming a roof for the distal half of the urethra. This, too, was after the manner of Thiersch. The third step, the closing in of the defect at the proximal margin of the glans, was done by making a transverse incision through the redundant prepuce at the frænum, through which the glans was drawn. This gave enough material for our purpose and we sutured to the glans and the newly made urethral roof. Although this readily healed, orifices no larger than a pinhead appeared at three or four places and gave much trouble before they were all obliterated. With the second step of the operation an attempt was made to overcome the lateral deviation during erection. Fibrous bands were found and divided and restraining bands arising about the pubic ramus were severed subcutaneously and the apparently freed organ deflected to the opposite side and there retained, but all to no purpose. This deflexion has been lessened, but by no means overcome; and it was to obtain suggestions upon this point that led me to bring the patient here, as well as to show what has been accomplished. He came to me with a greatly defective organ, and now behold it! "a thing of beauty," and, I hope, "a joy forever."

### Carcinoma of the Rectum in a Boy of Fifteen.

### Reported by R. M. Rome, M.D.

Francis St. C., aged 15, was admitted to the Kings County Hospital October 18, 1912, complaining of abdominal pain.

Family history: Negative as to hereditary diseases.

Past history: Enjoyed fair health; usual diseases of childhood.

Present illness began about one month ago with abdominal pain; never vomited, but has had a bloody rectal discharge for the past two weeks; at first diarrhea, subsequently constipation.

Rectal examination: About two inches within the anus an obstruction was met with, which proved to be a tumor, completely surrounding the bowel, of indefinite extent, but apparently having its origin anteriorly. The examining finger cannot be passed through the stricture without undue violence. No bleeding upon examination. Inguinal glands slightly enlarged on both sides.

In order to relieve this obstruction a right-sided colostomy was done and the peritoneum found to be studded with what are evidently tubercles; some fluid in the peritoneal cavity.

Microscopical examination of a piece of peritoneum containing these tubercles proved the condition to be carcinoma. Examination of a section from the rectal mass was carcinomatous.

## Syphilitic Endarteritis.
### *Reported by R. M. Rome, M.D.*

Patient, Charles T., 24 years of age, born in Jamaica, West Indies, was admitted to the Kings County Hospital September 12, 1912, with the following history:

Syphilis three years ago. No treatment. One year ago the patient gave evidence of disturbance of circulation in his hands and feet. There were cold, prickly feelings, considerable pain and some edema. In this condition he entered the hospital. Since his entrance all the signs of gangrene have appeared in all his four extremities with marked lines of demarcation in his legs at the junction of the middle and lower third and in his arms about three inches above the wrists. In the middle of December both legs were amputated just above the knee, but the gangrene has recurred higher up.

## Case of Multiple Vesicle Calculi Complicating Hypertrophied Prostate.
### *Reported by Walter A. Sherwood, M.D.*

L. D., a Frenchman, aged 79, came under my care and was admitted to the hospital on the 12th of August with the following history:

For the past ten years the patient has been addicted to the continual use of the catheter in order to empty his bladder. For the last year there has been increasing pain in the passage of the catheter and the urine has been of foul odor, contained much thick, white sediment and sometimes blood.

Rectal examination revealed a much enlarged, soft and tender prostate, the gland being about the size of a small orange. No attempt was made at instrumentation because of the serious traumatism already inflicted. A permanent catheter was introduced, the bladder irrigated twice each day, a 20 per cent. solution of argyrol being left in the bladder every second day, and large doses of urotropin were given. This treatment was continued until there was a marked improvement in the cystitis and in the function of the kidneys. On August 26th, under ether, a rapid suprapubic cystotomy was done and seventeen stones of varying size were removed from the bladder. No attempt was made at this time to interfere with the prostate, which was further examined with the finger inside the bladder. Proper drainage was established and the bladder irrigated daily until September 18th, when, through the suprapubic opening already made, the prostate was rapidly enucleated. Hemorrhage, which was considerable, was controlled with hot saline irrigation and gauze tampons. The subsequent history of the case was uneventful, although his complete recovery and wound healing were somewhat tedious. The sinus gradually closed and at the end of his discharge from the hospital, early in December, he was able to control his urine perfectly, it was passed without difficulty, and he was able to hold it from five to six hours at a time. For the first time in ten years he was freed from the use of the catheter, he had no pain, his urine was clear, and he has since taken up his occupation as a metallurgist.

This case is cited to illustrate the fact that with proper precaution and sufficient time for preparation in a man of such advanced age, a surgical procedure offers the only hope of relief in these aggravated cases of prostatic obstruction, and that in two stages the operative work can be done with comparative safety after first controlling the infection and re-establishing a fairly normal kidney function.

## Carcinoma of Esophagus.
### *Reported by Walter A. Sherwood, M.D.*

This case is reported because of some interesting features in the history and the discrepancy which existed between it and the physical findings at autopsy.

A. W., aged 59, German; family and previous personal history negative; admitted to the hospital on November 7, 1912. His chief complaint was inability to swallow. Three months previously, while eating and without any previous trouble, the patient experienced a sudden and very severe pain in the left hypochondriac region; he felt as if he had swallowed some sharp foreign body; on attempting to swallow some water it was promptly regurgitated. Since this time he has had increasing difficulty in swallowing and for the past two weeks has been unable to get any nourishment into his stomach. When he attempts to swallow milk or water it is regurgitated almost immediately, unchanged except for a few streaks of blood. During the last six weeks he has lost between thirty and forty pounds. The general appearance of the patient, in spite of his loss of weight, showed that he was well nourished and had no cachexia.

4

Abdominal examination was negative. He was examined with the Killian esophogoscope by Dr. Sturgis, who demonstrated a malignant growth beginning 5 or 6 centimeters above the cardiac orifice of the stomach. It was impossible to permeate the growth with the smallest bougie, the entire lumen being occluded, even though most of the growth appeared to be situated on the posterior and right lateral wall of the tube.

On November 11th, a gastrostomy was done after the method of Kader. Through the tube thus introduced the patient was fed at regular intervals and although for a few days he seemed to be doing well, he gradually became weaker and died six days after operation, apparently from inanition and starvation.

At autopsy the esophagus was found to be the seat of an extensive malignant growth which began 5 centimeters above the cardiac end of the stomach, involving the entire lower segment of the tube, the posterior wall of the stomach, the liver, the kidneys, the spleen and the omentum, all of which contained numerous metastatic foci of carcinoma.

The rapidity and suddenness of the onset of this condition, resembling the history of foreign-body obstruction, together with the unusual findings at autopsy in a man who showed so little external evidence of malignant disease, seemed to make the case of sufficient interest to report.

## Angulation of the Sigmoid.
### Reported by Walter A. Sherwood, M.D.

Several cases of angulation of the sigmoid have been reported by members of this Society, notably by Dr. Delatour, who, several years ago, was first to call attention to this subject in a paper read before the Brooklyn Pathological Society. If I remember correctly, these cases have all been of the acute type with the symptoms of acute intestinal obstruction, for which immediate relief was demanded. In reporting briefly three cases I refer not to the acute angulation, but to a kinking of the gut due to perisigmoid adhesions with sufficient disturbance of the continuity of the canal to produce a definite train of symptoms, namely, those of chronic obstruction or intestinal stasis with all of its various phases.

CASE I.—W. L. D., aged 33. One year ago this patient consulted me complaining of obstinate and increasing constipation, pain and discomfort in the lower left side of the abdomen. On examination a mass was found in the left inguinal and iliac region, somewhat sausage-shaped, about 3½ or 4 inches in length and 1½ inches in width. This mass was somewhat tender and was always present at repeated examinations and did not seem to be relieved by thorough movements of the bowels. The patient was kept under observation for several months. He lost some flesh and under treatment there was no improvement in his constipation or his pain and no disappearance of the mass. Operation was advised and accepted.

Operation showed a distinct angulation in the sigmoid about 3 inches above the recto-sigmoidal junction. This angulation was due to a distinct band of adhesions which held the gut close to the lateral wall of the abdomen and produced a right angled kink. This band of adhesions was freed, the raw surfaces were closed over with catgut and the wound was closed in the usual manner. The patient made an uneventful recovery and has been entirely relieved of his constipation and his pain and repeated examinations have failed to reveal any evidence of a mass in his left iliac fossa.

CASE II.—This case was referred to me by Dr. Webster with a diagnosis of probable malignant growth of the lower bowel.

C. L., aged 68. His chief complaint is obstinate and increasing constipation with low abdominal pain. For the past year this constipation has increased to such an extent that even with the strongest cathartics and enemata he is unable to obtain a satisfactory movement of the bowels, sometimes going for three of four days without any bowel movement. With the constipation he has pain and severe burning sensation across the lower abdomen which is relieved when the bowels are moved. The stools are hard. At times he has passed small quantities of blood. He never has passed mucus. He has no vomiting. He has lost some weight and looks cachectic.

Examination of the rectum, both digitally and with the proctoscope, fails to reveal any evidence of a tumor. The passage of a bougie, however, seems to meet an obstruction about 7½ inches from the anal orifice. Examination of the abdomen reveals a mass 5 by 2 centimeters, palpable, in the left iliac region, following the course of the sigmoid. An X-ray plate, taken by Dr. Wallace, reveals a distinct angulation in the sigmoid near the recto-sigmoidal junction.

With this history and in the absence of any demonstrable evidence of malignant growth, a diagnosis of angulation of the sigmoid was made, for which operation has been recommended but not yet accepted.

The case will be reported at a later date.

The third case, a young woman aged 22, a pupil nurse in the hospital, who gave the following history:

Operation for appendicitis seven years ago. For the past year the patient has been constipated. This constipation has been growing gradually more obstinate until now it is impossible for her to obtain a movement of the bowels without large doses of cathartics or the frequent use of enemata. For the purpose of experiment the patient has on one or two occasions gone for ten days or two weeks without a bowel movement. For the past month she has had almost constant and severe pain in the lower left quadrant of the abdomen, vomiting has been frequent and persistent, and she was, at the time she came under my care, unable to retain the simplest kind of nourishment on her stomach. For the past month or six weeks the patient has been under medical observation in the hospital, during which time she has had a constant elevation of temperature of from 99½ to 100 or 101, and her pain is always worse at the time of her menstrual periods.

She was examined pelvicly and this examination failed to reveal any abnormality of the uterus or of the uterine adnexa.

Examination of the abdomen revealed a mass which could be distinctly felt, somewhat sausage-shaped, in the lower part of the left iliac fossa, corresponding to the situation of the sigmoid flexure. This mass was distinctly tender.

Examination of the urine and blood were negative.

Operation December 23, 1912. A left rectus incision was made and the same condition as described in Case I was found, namely, the sigmoid was tightly adherent to the left side of the abdominal wall and held there by several dense bands of firm, white adhesions. Another angulation was present lower down where the gut had become adherent to the left tube and ovary, causing a distinct right angled twist in the lumen of the gut. These adhesions were separated with considerable difficulty, the adhesions above were clipped with the scissors and the raw surfaces were covered over with sutures and catgut. It was seen that the sigmoid now followed its normal course. Nothing further was done, the wound was closed and the patient has made an uneventful operative recovery except for an intestinal paresis which persisted for the first two or three days following the operation. She is now up and around, is free from pain, has a good appetite, no nausea and her bowels are moving with fair regularity, occasional recourse to mild cathartics being necessary. According to the patient's statement, she feels better than she has in years, she is gaining weight, has no fever and seems to be markedly benefited by the operation.

In this case it is evident that, in addition to the chronic obstruction, causing pain and constipation, she was suffering from an auto-intoxication as evidenced by vomiting and a persistent temperature and loss of weight.

*Discussion on Fracture of Pelvis with Complete Rupture of the Urethra.*

Dr. H. B. Delatour opened the discussion and said:—"This is an exceedingly interesting case and it is interesting in that we have had cases occurring of the same sort in the past. Dr. Bristow had one, I had one, and the one Dr. Skelton has reported. They all occur from crushing injuries and the urethra is torn off directly at the bladder—squarely across at the bladder, but the sphincter has remained intact and there is no leakage of urine. They are very difficult cases to handle because as a rule the local injuries are so great. Dr. Bristow, I think, reported his case to this Society last spring. He had a great deal of difficulty in that case in connecting up the urethra to the bladder after suppuration had ceased. Dr. Skelton has not been able yet to make that communication, but I think that in his case it is not going to be so difficult as I have had the opportunity of observing the same.

"In my case I immediately passed a catheter through the urethra, opened the bladder, passed a sound directly through the bladder into the wound and with this was able to direct the catheter and bring it into the bladder, and then by fastening the end of the urethra to the catheter I was able to bring the urethra up against the bladder wall and place a suture there. It was not difficult and the operation did not take very long, but the man was in bad general condition from the severe crushing of the pelvis and the amount of blood that he had lost before he had been brought to the hospital. He died about twenty-four hours after. The interesting part of these cases is the fact that you have no leakage of urine into your wound and you can make the diagnosis almost on that fact alone."

*Discussion on Peritonitis and Colloid Carcinoma of Rectum.*

DR. R. W. WESTBROOK, in discussion, said:—"I would like to hear from the men here in Brooklyn as to their observation of cases of carcinoma of the rectum in early age. I have seen one case. I do not remember the exact age, but it was somewhere between sixteen and eighteen."

*Discussion on Three Cases of Angulation of the Sigmoid.*

DR. H. B. DELATOUR, in discussion, said:—"This subject interests me very much, inasmuch as I described it, I think, originally in 1897 or 1898. I reported a number of cases before the Pathological Society. In these cases the diagnosis was not confirmed by operation. The condition was described as being a probable one and a number of cases were cited, as Dr. Sherwood has said, of rather a chronic nature, giving rather acute symptoms but with chronic history. Subsequent to that paper I operated and demonstrated several cases and in the last few years I have had a number of them.

"There is no question whatever but that we have occurring in the sigmoid an angulation due either to ptosis of the sigmoid into the pelvis or of angulation by adhesions, and it is a condition which gives just the symptoms Dr. Sherwood has given us here tonight—obstinate constipation and more or less pain in the abdomen, particularly the lower abdomen, and frequently referred to the left side. Very frequently the sausage tumor can be made out. Sometimes it is not low down in the pelvis. I had a case recently in which it lay so high that I was in doubt as to whether or not I had a movable kidney that was low down in the pelvis.

"What shall we do with these cases from the operative standpoint? If we have adhesions the first thing to do is to divide them and see the position of the intestine afterwards. It may be necessary to remove the adhesions, but in those cases where the sigmoid becomes unduly elongated and you have a long line of intestine dropping down into the pelvis, something more has to be done. I have tried four different procedures in these cases. In the first I simply brought up the intestine out of the pelvis and sutured it to the lateral abdominal wall. I did two such cases and the immediate results were good, but unfortunately they were hospital patients and I have not been able to trace them, but the result anatomically, when it was finished, was not perfectly satisfactory, because the intestine was not made into a straight line or giving a condition which you could be sure would remain permanent, and the adhesions produced by the suturing were liable to spread and give us a recurrence. Whether there was any recurrence or not I do not know. In one case I resected the sigmoid and did an end to end anastomosis with perfect result. That man suffered the most excruciating acute pains at times previous to his operation, so much so that he gave symptoms of acute intestinal obstruction. After the operation his symptoms entirely disappeared. I am sorry I did not bring the X-ray plate of that case with me because it is an exceptionally good one. It was taken by Dr. Eastmond and showed the position of the sigmoid very beautifully and the subsequent straightening out of the intestine after operation. Recently I had two cases in women where there was a very long sigmoid dropping down into the pelvis, each limb being from 6 to 8 or 9 inches long, making the entire length of the sigmoid somewhere between 15 and 18 inches. In the first I did a lateral anastomosis between the two limbs, but when it was finished I was not perfectly satisfied with the procedure because it did not seem to give as direct and straight a line between the descending colon and rectum as I should like. In the second case I made the anastomosis with the Murphy button. The sigmoid dropped over the edge of the pelvis down into the pelvic cavity in a large loop. In the first case I made an anastomosis between 2½ and 3 inches long. This patient was greatly relieved by the operation. In the next case I put a Murphy button in also.

"It is absolutely impossible, I believe, in the majority of cases, to make a satisfactory anastomosis close enough up to the side with sutures. In this case the button came away on the seventh day and the patient has been perfectly comfortable. It is now only about four weeks since that operation was done and her symptoms have been very much relieved.

"One of the difficulties of these cases is to get the lower intestine free of fecal matter so that you have a good, clean, intestinal tract to work with. This loop will hold fecal matter against almost any kind of irrigation.

"I believe a great many of the cases of chronic intestinal obstruction and of the auto-intoxications, etc., are due to angulation of the sigmoid at the point where it passes into the rectum."

DR. R. M. ROME, in discussion, said:—"This subject is interesting to me because of the fact that there was a case of this kind in my own family. My brother-in-law for some fifteen years had suffered with chronic intestinal stasis with marked auto-intoxication and suffered from frequent and severe attacks of gout. One year ago a diagnosis of sigmoid trouble was made. The sigmoid was looped down in the pelvis and about 10 inches were resected. He has not had an attack of gout since the operation, no evidence of intoxication, and his constipation is very much improved and he has only occasionally to use a cathartic."

### Discussion on Peritonitis and Colloid Carcinoma of Rectum.

Dr. R. M. Rome, in closing the discussion, said:—"With reference to some statistics with regard to the occurrence of carcinoma of the rectum in early age: the literature gives various ages, but in the majority of cases the seat of the trouble is not given. There are a few collections in which there are no cases under twenty years, and there is another collection of 13 cases, but they do not give the seat of the carcinoma. There were reported cases of children of thirteen and eight years and a patient the age of fifteen and another in a patient the age of twelve."

### Discussion on Three Cases of Angulation of the Sigmoid.

Dr. T. B. Spence, in discussion, said:—"Some years ago I reported a case before this Society in which a little different procedure than that described was pursued. This man had an angulation of a little different sort. The loop that came down was drawn back again so that it made a double loop and it was held there by the shortened piece of meso-sigmoid. This man also had a good many adhesions of his descending colon and it was supposed that possibly they might be causing the trouble and for that reason I did a short circuiting and anastomosed the ileum to the lower limb of the sigmoid and that relieved him completely. He stayed well. I think it is four or five years since that was done."

Dr. R. W. Westbrook, in discussion, said:—"This subject has interested me a good deal since Dr. Delatour described his case a number of years ago. I have seen a number of cases of acute obstruction which I felt were due to that cause, one in quite an elderly individual and two in younger individuals, one a young man, I think, of twenty, who had suffered from constipation for years and had attacks of partial obstruction, but never laying him up. A very vigorous catharsis usually cleared him up, but when I saw him he had an acute attack of intestinal obstruction. There was no further intestinal content procurable through the rectum and I did the operation for intestinal obstruction and on making a long incision and finding the obstruction in the vicinity of the sigmoid I merely lifted it out. The sigmoid was very much distended with the descending colon very much distended above it. I passed a long rectal tube up the anus and rectum and an enormous quantity of content began to discharge through the tube and I milked him out in that way and then sutured this greatly distended bowel to the abdominal wall. That was some seven years ago, I think. I have heard from him at different intervals and also within a few months and he has been practically well since except for a little difficulty with his bowels, but he has been so well that he has not considered it necessary to consult a physician and has been recently married.

"I have seen another almost exactly similar case and have seen cases diagnosed as volvulus, but they were not, to my mind, demonstrated to be volvulus at operation and I believe they were practically an angulation of the sigmoid not due to adhesions but to a very greatly elongated and relaxed sigmoid."

Dr. W. A. Sherwood, in closing the discussion, said:—"I would like to say that in the third case I reported—the case of the young lady—I mentioned the fact that for a definite length of time previous to operation she had been running a temperature of 99½ to 101 or over, but since operation this temperature has stayed practically at the normal point. I think this pretty definite proof that her temperature was due to intestinal stasis.

"I would like to emphasize the fact that these cases are not simple cases of constipation which we can discard by recommending cathartics or enemata, but they have a definite line of symptoms—a train of symptoms which I do not believe can be relieved medically.

"I am not willing to accept all of Lane's ideas on the subject of intestinal stasis, but I do believe this is one class of cases which demands some very definite surgical procedure for their relief.

"I am glad to hear Dr. Delatour's experience, which has been very much more extensive than mine. The only cases I have had were due to adhesions, causing a distinctly angulated sigmoid. The simple division of these adhesions seemed to be sufficient to relieve their symptoms."

# edical Society of the County of Kings

## MONTHLY BULLETIN TO MEMBERS

NDER the direction of the Council this Bulletin is issued every month (except July, Aug. and Sept.). It is the purpose of the Council, rough this medium, to keep the members advised all matters pertaining to the Society's work, its rious activities, its membership, and other subjects general interest.

Items of general interest to the Society and pernal notes concerning its members are invited and ould reach the Secretary not later than 4 P. M. the 20th of each month. Address all communitions to the Society's Building, 1313 Bedford Ave., rooklyn, N. Y.

### MEDICAL SOCIETY OF THE COUNTY OF KINGS.

313 Bedford Avenue, Brooklyn, New York.

Telephone: 126 Bedford.

HE Medical Society of the County of Kings (organized 1822) owns its plant, valued at $100,000, and located at 1313-1315 edford Avenue. In addition to an auditoum (seating 400) and various smaller meetg rooms, offices, etc., the greater part of the iilding is devoted to the Society's medical brary of 60,000 volumes. There are only ree larger medical libraries on this continent. the ample reading rooms over 600 current edical journals are regularly on file.

Through its public and scientific meetings, s Library, its Milk Commission, and its manild activities for the spread of medical knowlge, the promotion of scientific education, the nity of the medical profession, and the safearding of the public health, the Medical Soety of the County of Kings should enlist the tive support and co-operation of every putable physician in the county who is enaged in regular practice.

### MEMBERSHIP.

*Qualifications for Membership.*—Extracts om the Constitution and By-Laws governing embership (Chapter XVI) are as follows:
Sec. 1. Membership in the Society may be otained by physicians in good standing, residg in the County of Kings, and duly licensed d recorded in the office of the County Clerk Kings County, in the following manner:
Ec. 2. Applications for membership shall be ade on blanks furnished by the Medical Soety signed by the applicant and endorsed by o members of the County Society. Such anks shall be sent to the Secretary, who shall resent them to the Board of Censors for inestigation and report. Sec. 3. If the candi-

date be accepted the Council shall so report to the Society at a stated meeting, and after the next succeeding stated meeting the President shall declare said candidate a member. Sec. 4. Every person thus admitted resident member shall, within three months after due notification of his election, pay an initiation fee of five dollars and the assessment of the Medical Society of the State of New York for the current year, sign the By-Laws or forfeit his election."

*Blank Application Forms for Membership* may be obtained on request at the Society's Building. This form should be filled out by the applicant, signed by him, his proposer and his seconder, and returned to the Secretary.

*Dues.*—New members pay an initiation fee of $5 plus $3 (the State assessment for the current year) and are exempt from the payment of further dues until the next annual meeting after their election.

The regular annual dues are $10 plus $3 (the State assessment for the current year), payable on the first day of February. All members who have not paid on or before the first day of May shall be placed on the list of members in arrears and so reported to the Society, and shall not receive the publications, or notices of meetings, or defense for suits for malpractice until their dues are paid. All members who fail to pay their arrears on or before December 31st shall be dropped from the roll of membership (Chapter XV of By-Laws).

*Advantages of Membership.*—Affiliation with your confreres in the representative medical organization of your County, participation in the Society's meetings and varied activities, and proprietary interest in its property and magnificent library, membership in the Medical Society of the State of New York and the Second District Branch; monthly receipt of the *New York State Journal of Medicine* and the Society's own publications, a copy yearly of the *Medical Directory of New York, New Jersey and Connecticut;* free defense to the court of last resort of all suits for alleged malpractice; eligibility to membership in the American Medical Association.

### STATED MEETINGS.

Regular stated meetings of the Society are held in the Society's Building, 1313 Bedford Ave., at 8.30 P. M., on the third Tuesday of every month (except July, August and September). Light refreshments are served at the social hour which follows the scientific program of each meeting.

## THE LIBRARY.

The Library (60,000 vols.) of the Society is open daily (Sundays and Legal Holidays excepted), from 10 A. M. to 10 P. M. For the purposes of reference it is free to the public. Members of the Society have the privilege of borrowing books. Trained librarians are always in attendance to help and direct readers who desire such assistance.

## DIRECTORY FOR GRADUATE NURSES.

For the benefit of the profession and the general public the Society maintains a Directory for Graduate Nurses, where reliable graduate nurses (male and female), masseurs and masseuses may be procured. There is no fee for securing a nurse through the Society's Directory, which is always open, day and night. Telephone 126 Bedford.

## THE COUNCIL.

*President*—JAMES M. WINFIELD, 47 Halsey St.
*Vice-President*—J. RICHARD KEVIN.
*Secretary*—CLAUDE G. CRANE, 121 St. James Pl.
*Associate Secretary*—BURTON HARRIS.
*Treasurer*—JOHN R. STIVERS, 180 Lefferts Pl.
*Associate Treasurer*—STEPHEN H. LUTZ.
*Directing Librarian*—FREDERICK TILNEY.

### Trustees.

ONSLOW A. GORDON, *Chairman*, 71 Halsey St.
JOSHUA M. VAN COTT.   JOHN O. POLAK.
JOHN C. MACEVITT.    ELIAS H. BARTLEY.

### Censors.

JOHN A. LEE, *Senior Censor*, 23 Revere Pl.
WALTER A. SHERWOOD.    JOHN G. WILLIAMS.
CHARLES EASTMOND.    J. STURDIVANT READ.

## CHAIRMEN OF STANDING COMMITTEES.

*Membership*—EDWARD E. CORNWALL, 1218 Pacific St.
*Directory for Nurses*—CALVIN F. BARBER, 57 So. Oxford St.
*Entertainment*—ALFRED POTTER, 491 Eighth St.
*Historical*—WILLIAM SCHROEDER, 339 President St.
*Legislative*—HENRY G. WEBSTER, 364 Washington Ave.
*Public Health*—J. M. VAN COTT, 188 Henry St.
*Visiting*—JAMES W. FLEMING, 471 Bedford Ave.
*Milk Commission*—ALFRED BELL, 37 Linden St.
*Attendance*—ALBERT M. JUDD, 375 Grand Ave.

In the conduction of the affairs of the Society the officers hope that they may have not only the frequent suggestions of members, which are heartily invited, but also their practical and loyal co-operation.

*Supt. and Librarian*—ALBERT T. HUNTINGTON.
*Counsel*—WILLIAM E. BUTLER, Esq.
*Prosecuting Attorneys*—Messrs. ALMUTH C. VAN DIVER and JOHN G. DYER, 37 Wall St., New York City.

## MINUTES OF STATED MEETI

MAY 20, 1913.

The President, Dr. James M. Winfi the chair.

There were about 100 present.

The meeting was called to order P. M. and the minutes of the previous ing were read and approved.

*Report of Council.*

The Council reported favorably up following applications for membership:

George Francis Hoch, 523 Throop Ave.
Thomas Joseph Kearns, 1490 Pacific S
John L. Madden, 262 Schermerhorn St.
Luther F. Warren, Long Island College
pital.
Henry Wolfer, 678 Bedford Ave.

## ELECTION OF MEMBERS.

The following, duly proposed and ac by the Council, was declared elected to membership:

Harlan E. Linehan, 74 Norman Ave.

## APPLICATIONS FOR MEMBER

Applications for membership were re from the following:

Benjamin Aquaro-deodati, 637 Lorime
Univ. Naples, 1903; proposed by
Lewis; seconded by E. E. Cornwall.
Harry Cleveland Harris, 25 Stuyvesant
Jefferson, 1908; proposed by J. O.
seconded by R. M. Rome.
Samuel Linder, 1780 St. John's Place;
nell, 1910; proposed by E. E.. Cor
seconded by Memb. Com.
Joseph Rosenthal, 572 5th St.; P. &. S.,
1906; proposed by A. M. Judd; sec
by L. Louria.
Carl Schumann, 116 Prospect Place;
C. H., 1909; proposed by E. E. Cor
seconded by Memb. Com.
Walter T. Slevin, 65 Eighth Ave.; L. I.
1898; proposed by E. E. Cornwall
onded by Memb. Com.
Wm. Alfred Sprenger, 1106 Bushwick
Med. Chir., Phila., 1899; proposed by
Wade; seconded by E. E. Cornwall

## FOR REINSTATEMENT.

Geo. F. Buttschardt, 222 St. Nicholas
Univ. & Bell., 1902. Former me
Reinstatement.

## EXECUTIVE SESSION.

The President, Dr. James M. Winfiel quested Dr. Ludlum to present a report Milk Commission. Dr. Ludlum presen printed folder containing a report o work of the Commission to date.

## SCIENTIFIC SESSION.

1. Paper—"The Treatment of Chronic Cystitis."
    By J. Sturdivant Read, M.D.
2. Paper—"The Modern Treatment of Fractures," illustrated by lantern slides and patients.
    By J. Bion Bogart, M.D.
    Discussed by John E. Jennings, M.D., J. Beeckman Delatour, M.D., Wm. Linder, M.D.
    Discussion closed by Dr. Bogart.
3. Paper—"Clinical Observations on Acute Suppurative Pyelonephritis Due to Bacterial Infection."
    By Burton Harris, M.D. (Owing to the lateness of the hour Dr. Harris deferred reading his paper to a later date.
    Discussion by Edward E. Cornwall, M.D., Henry G. Webster, M.D.
    Adjourned 10.30 P.M.
        CLAUDE G. CRANE, *Secretary.*

---

## CALENDAR OF SOCIETY MEETINGS

### MEETINGS HELD AT 1313 BEDFORD AVENUE.

*June 19, Third Tuesday.*
MEDICAL SOCIETY OF THE COUNTY OF KING.—8.30 P. M. Stated Meeting.

*JUNE 24, Fourth Tuesday.*
SECTION ON OPHTHALMOLOGY.—8.15 P. M. Stated Meeting.

*JUNE 25, Fourth Wednesday.*
SECTION ON PEDIATRICS.—8.30 P. M. Stated Meeting.

*June 27, Fourth Friday.*
BROOKLYN SOCIETY OF INTERNAL MEDICINE. —8.30 P. M. Stated Meeting.

*June 4, First Wednesday.*
BROOKLYN SOCIETY OF NEUROLOGY.—8.30 P. M. Stated Meeting.

*June 27, Fourth Meeting.*
BROOKLYN SURGICAL SOCIETY.—8.30 P. M. Stated Meeting.

*June 6, First Friday.*
BROOKLYN GYNECOLOGICAL SOCIETY. P. M. Stated Meeting.

*June 10, Second Tuesday.*
HOMEOPATHIC MEDICAL SOCIETY.—8.3 Stated Meeting.

*June 11, Second Wednesday.*
Censors, 8.30 P. M.E shrdlu h mhm h
COUNCIL.—8.30 P. M., Board of Tr
Censors, 8.30 P. M.; Council, 9.00 P.

*June 12, Second Thursday.*
BROOKLYN PATHOLOGICAL SOCIETY. P. M. Stated Meeting.

*June 13, Second Friday.*
SOCIETY OF EX-INTERNES OF GERMA
PITAL.—8.30 P. M. Stated Meeting.

*June 16, Third Monday.*
SECOND DISTRICT DENTAL SOCIET P. M. Stated Meeting.

*June 20, Third Friday.*
PHYSICIAN'S LEAGUE.—8.30 P. M. Meeting.

---

## OTHER BROOKLYN MEETINGS

*June 16, Third Monday.*
WILLIAMSBURGH MEDICAL SOCIETY P. M. Stated Meeting. Held in th loughby Mansion, 667 Willoughby Av

*June 20, Third Friday.*
BROOKLYN MEDICAL SOCIETY.—8.30 Stated Meeting. Held in the Hart B 1030 Gates Avenue.

---

## AMERICAN MEDICAL ASSOCIA

*President:* Dr. A. Jacobi, New York
*Secretary:* Dr. A. R. Craig, 535 D Avenue, Chicago, Ill.
The next annual meeting will be Minneapolis, Minn., June 17-20, 1913.

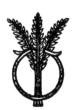

# LONG ISLAND MEDICAL JOURNAL

| VOL. VII. | JULY, 1913 | No. 7 |

## ®riginal Articles.

### THE X-RAY DIAGNOSIS OF GASTRIC ULCER.*

#### By Charles Eastmond, M.D.,

of Brooklyn, N. Y.

THE first part of the duodenum is embryologically, histologically and physiologically associated very intimately with the stomach, so I shall include disease of that part with and under the general heading of gastric ulcer.

The X-ray diagnosis of gastric ulcer is made by the proper interpretation of the pathological changes in the anatomy or functioning of the organ as learned from a study of the X-ray plates or the fluoroscopic screen. Each method of examination has its advantages and disadvantages, but these need not be considered here.

The difficulty or ease of the diagnosis is dependent upon the extent of the lesion, the duration of the disease and the degree of variation from the normal.

*Recent ulcer.*—Where the lesion is recent and slight in extent, amounting only to an erosion of the mucous membrane, the recognition of the condition may or may not be possible.

At times one is able to secure positive information by the deposition of a mass of bismuth on the ulcerated surface, this mass remaining after that portion of the stomach has emptied. Care must be exercised to differentiate such a spot from the normal deposition in the rugæ of the gastric mucosa. As a rule, the ulcer will extend over more than one ruga.

If the ulcer be located at or near one of the curvatures of the stomach, usually the lesser, within the contracting part, there is absence of peristalsis at that point. To determine such a condition, a large number of plates must be taken, usually over a dozen, to secure the necessary evidence.

Ulcer of the contracting portion of the stomach is most commonly overlooked when it is on one of the walls of the stomach, usually the posterior, for here it is obscured by the large mass of bismuth present.

*Old ulcer.*—Old ulcer of the stomach will present different appearances whether it be perforating or not.

In the presence of a perforating ulcer, when on or near the curvature, there is a small out-pocketing of the gastric outline, presenting like a diverticulum. In the apex of such a pocket there is

---

* Read before the Brooklyn Medical Association, March 12, 1913.

frequently a small bubble of air.    The German observers have laid great emphasis upon the presence of the air bubble, but in my own experience it has been seldom seen.    When the ulcer is on one of the walls, anterior or posterior, the only evidence may be a local area where the bismuth shadow is denser than in the surrounding parts. To obtain this, the bismuth meal must contain a small proportion of bismuth.    Frequently an oblique view of the stomach will present the condition when it can be obtained in no other way.

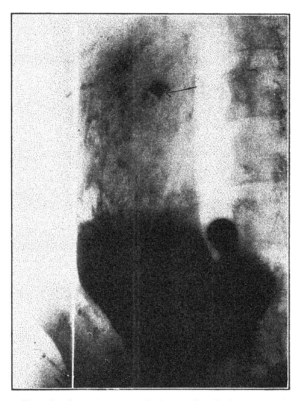

Fig. 1.—Recent ulcer of the wall of the stomach
showing the bismuth adherent to the ulcer.

In perforating ulcer adhesions may or may not be present.    As a rule, the position of the stomach is unchanged.

The essential points in the diagnosis of old ulcer, non-perforating, are referrable to the adhesions that are formed and the changes are dependent upon them.

In cases of ulcer with adhesions the general position of the stomach is usually altered.    It is displaced upward, often being as much as four inches above the umbilicus.    The pylorus is correspondingly elevated, and instead of being straight upward, it faces upward and to the right.

The distortion of position depends, of course, upon the site of the ulcer.    In the pars cardia, that part is drawn to the right; when in the pars media or pylorica, the affected part is drawn directly upward.    It is an axiom that peristalsis is absent at the site of any path-

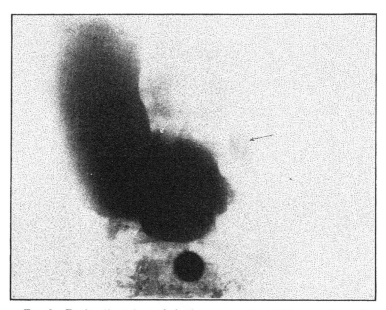

Fig. 2.—Perforating ulcer of the lesser curvature with secondary adhesions between the gall bladder and the outer side of the cap.

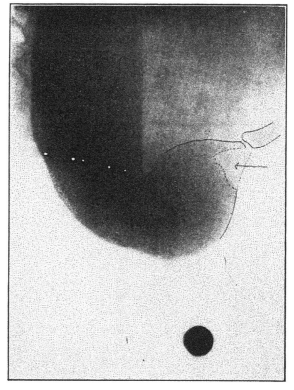

Fig. 3.—Stomach held above the umbilicus from adhesions dependent upon old ulcer near the pylorus. Dotted area shows the region of bismuth deficiency from the adhesions.

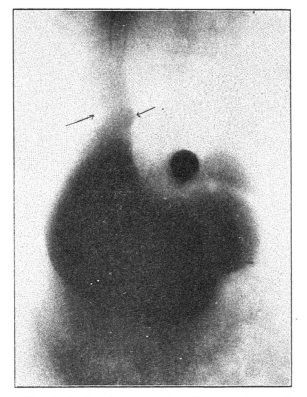

FIG. 4.—Perforating ulcer of cardiac end of stomach with spasm opposite the ulcer. The pouch of the perforating ulcer is seen on the lesser curvature, the spasm on the greater.

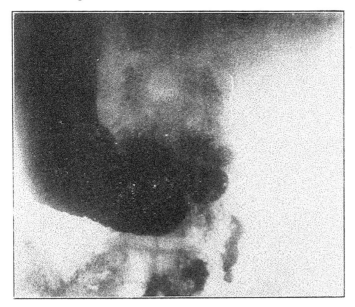

FIG. 5.—Marked constriction of the cap from old duodenal ulcer. The area of constriction is indicated by the bracket. Note the dilatation of the pyloric portion of the cap.

ological lesion of the stomach; consequently it will be found that the affected area does not contract.

When the lesion is at or near the pylorus, that is seen to be constantly open and the bismuth is seen to be passing through continuously. No evidence of the pyloric sphincter is present. On the other hand the lesion, by the formation of cicatrical tissue, may invade the lumen and produce obstruction. Cicatrization of the pars media may produce an hour-glass constriction.

Very frequently, in the presence of an ulcer of the pars cardia, whether perforating or non-perforating, recent or old, a deep indentation is seen in the greater curvature. This may be so marked as to practically divide the stomach in two. This is usually indicative of an ulcer at or near the lesser curvature opposite the site of the spasm. While such a spasmodic contraction is not pathognomonic of ulcer, the suspicion is so strong that every means of determining whether it is present or not should be used, even to having the patient return for a confirmary examination.

In duodenal ulcer, a recent lesion may give no discoverable evidence of it. When the ulcer is old the adhesions or cicatrization will produce a marked irregularity in the outline.

This irregularity is constant and persistent and is seen by preference on the left side in distinction to the right sided adhesions in gall bladder disease, but they may be general.

The extent and severity of the lesion will determine the degree of the irregularity.

The effect of these adhesions or cicatrization is to destroy the expansion power of the muscular walls, there is no restraint upon the pylorus, and the stomach empties with undue rapidity.

Should the contraction of the duodenum be very marked or the pylorus constricted, gastric retention and dilatation may be present.

In the final analysis, the X-ray diagnosis of ulcer of the stomach and duodenum is not and often cannot be made from the detection of any one point of evidence, but is deduced from a study of all the pathological lesions and changes in function presenting to the Rœntgenologist. One single feature may give rise to a suspicion, but it is the study of the whole that establishes the diagnosis.

---

# REFRACTIVE ERRORS IN CHILDREN.*

## By David T. Bishop, M.D.,

of Brooklyn, N. Y.

MY purpose in this short paper is to call your attention to some of the visual defects which are frequently met with in children, what they suffer in consequence of these defects, how they may be recognized, how best treated, and some of the results of neglecting treatment.

We are not concerned tonight with those visual defects which are dependent upon structural lesions, such as opacities of the cornea, lens and vitreous, inflammations of the choroid, retina and optic

---

* Read before Section on Pediatrics of the *Kings* County Medical Society, March 26, 1913.

nerve, and I shall do no more than mention them in passing. What we are interested in are the troubles produced by errors of refraction, and here the field is a large one.

Children present the same forms of refractive error that we encounter in adults, namely, hyperopia, myopia, and astigmatism, either simple or compounded in various ways. It is well known that among adults who have refractive errors the majority are hyperopic. This is even more true of children, and most of them carry it with them through life. In some cases, however, as the child grows the hyperopia gradually becomes less and less in degree, and the individual eventually becomes emmetropic; or if the change continue, it may pass into a condition of myopia. Of 50 cases which I selected as they came in the case files, and none of which was over 10 years of age, 41 were hyperopic, 5 myopic, and 4 had mixed astigmatism.

*Hyperopia,* as you know, is far-sightedness, and is due to either a short eye ball or a too weak refractive apparatus, so that images focus at a point behind the retina. A child with this condition, in order to maintain clear distant vision, must exercise sufficient accommodation to bring the focus forward to his retina and hold it there. To a child with only a moderate degree of hyperopia this is a matter of comparatively easy adjustment, because his muscle of accommodation, the ciliary muscle, is strong, and the lens soft and elastic. Such a child may show no signs of eye strain, and the condition may remain unrecognized. A child with a high degree of hyperopia must make a strong and continuous effort at accommodation, and the excessive strain that he labors under will manifest itself in one or more of the following ways. If the child has reached the school age he begins to have frequent headaches after using his eyes; he will complain that it hurts him to read and that the print blurs. His school work is very likely to be below the average, due partly to his poor vision, and partly to a disinclination to use his eyes for study. The continuous eye strain eventually causes a chronic hyperemia of the ocular structures, which is seen in the conjunctival injection, photophobia, marginal lid inflammations with the formation of large crusts in the cilia, and frequent styes. If the condition is one of less degree there may be no more than a frequent blinking of the lids. By far the most serious sign which results from this condition of hyperopia, however, is strabismus. We meet with it in persons anywhere from a year old to adults. It is usually found to accompany the higher degrees of hyperopia, and especially those which are astigmatic, but this is not invariably the case. One of my little patients, 2 years old, had an intermittent convergent strabismus and only one diopter of hyperopia in each eye, while another child, 5 years old, had 14 diopters of hyperopia in the right eye, 13½ in the left eye, and no strabismus.

There are several factors which enter into the production of convergent strabismus; the disturbance of the normal relationship of convergence to accommodation, the presence of a greater refractive error in one eye than in the other, causing a less distinct image in that eye, and most important of all, a faulty development of the power of fusion, so that there is not the normal tendency for both eyes to fix the same object at the same time. With a well developed fusion sense there may be a considerable amount of hyperopia and still no strabismus, and, on the other hand, a child with very little power of fusion may have a squint, even though the refractive error be a slight one.

When a child develops a squint he very quickly learns to suppress the image formed in the squinting eye, and thus avoids diplopia. The result of this, if long continued, is that the visual acuity in the squinting eye remains below normal, and the eye becomes either partially or completely amblyopic. If such a child could have his defect corrected early by the wearing of proper glasses, such a result might easily be avoided, and the child grow up with two good eyes instead of one bad one.

We sometimes have squinting children of 8 or 10 years of age, or older, brought to us with the statement by the parent that they had not bothered with the condition because the doctor said the child would outgrow it. If such a child is found amblyopic it is usually beyond relief. These children must be treated as early as possible to get the best results.

It is practically impossible to determine accurately the visual acuity of a baby of 3 or 4 years, or younger, as subjective tests are worthless. But the refractive error can be estimated with considerable accuracy by objective methods, measurement with the ophthalmoscope, and especially skiascopy, and this should always be done with the child under the influence of a cycloplegic.

*Myopic* children are met with much less frequently. Here the trouble, near-sightedness, is due either to an elongated eye ball, or a too strong refractive apparatus, and consequently the image focuses at a point in front of the retina, somewhere in the vitreous.

While, as already stated, a hyperopic child can obtain clear distant vision by accommodating, and so bringing his focus forward to the retina, a myopic child has no such relief, and is absolutely at the mercy of his error. He can see clearly only those things which are within the limit of his far point, and this is determined by the amount of his myopia,—beyond that his vision is blurred.

Here the chief complaint or symptom for which they seek relief is poor distant vision. They cannot see the blackboard in school is the usual story. Headache is also a frequent complaint, although not so constant as in hyperopia.

When a myopic child develops a strabismus it is usually a divergent strabismus, and for the following reason. A child whose far point is, for example, 5 or 6 inches from his eyes, in order to see an object at that distance with both eyes, must converge excessively. If this be maintained for any length of time the internal recti become fatigued, convergence is relaxed, and one eye swings outward. He sacrifices his binocular vision to his muscle comfort, and this occurs more easily if one eye is more myopic than the other.

Myopia is a far more serious condition than hyperopia because of the tendency it has to become progressive, the results of which may be extremely unfortunate. Such an eye becomes more and more stretched and elongated, areas of inflammation and degeneration develop in the choroid, with the outpouring of opacities in the vitreous, the vision gradually falls lower and lower, until the final calamity, detachment of the retina, brings about total blindness. For these reasons it is of extreme importance that a myope should constantly wear proper correcting lenses, and undergo regular periodic examinations that any change in the condition be promptly noted, and prompt relief measures instituted.

*Astigmatism* is the condition which perhaps more than any other causes people, children as well as adults to seek relief from eye strain. Thorington states that 80 per cent. of all eyes are astigmatic. With this condition the vision is blurred both for distance and for near, and nothing short of proper glasses will give relief. The defect may be either in the cornea or in the lens, usually the former, and is due to unequal lengths of the radii of curvature of the refracting surface in opposite meridia, the corneal surface being more sharply curved in one meridian than in the meridian at right angles to it. The condition is usually congenital, but may be due to contracting scars in the cornea, resulting from injuries, operations or ulcerations.

The varieties of astigmatism with which we meet are five in number: simple hyperopic, compound hyperopic, simple myopic, compound myopic, and mixed astigmatism, in which hyperopia and myopia are both present in the same eye.

The one symptom which is common to all the forms is blurred vision. Headache is a relatively constant symptom, and we also encounter the other signs of eye strain already mentioned.

The treatment for these various conditions is, first of all, properly fitting glasses. By their use the hyperopic child no longer has to strain his ciliary muscle in order to see clearly. He begins to get the benefit of a normal condition of things, and where school work was formerly the thing he hated most, he now begins to take an interest in it, because he can do so without suffering.

So also the myopic boy begins to see and understand things that are more than a foot or so from the tip of his nose. He has a chance to become less self-centered, and in many cases it is surprising what a change takes place in the dispositions of these children when their visual defects are neutralized.

If children with strabismus can be treated sufficiently early the glasses will often correct the condition, so that operative interference is unnecessary. As before stated, these cases of strabismus, however, are associated with a lack of development of the fusion sense, so that there is very little tendency for the eyes to maintain binocular vision, even with correct glasses. When this is so, careful attention must be given to the underlying cause, and correction of the refractive error must be supplemented by such visual exercises as will tend to develop the fusion centre.

There are certain conditions which may result from neglecting treatment in these children with refractive errors. Some of them are apparent during the childhood of the individual, others may not exert their influence until adult life is reached.

In the first place, the child who sees imperfectly, and with great effort, goes through life with a tremendous handicap. He makes frequent mistakes and his work is very likely to be of a low standard.

A child who has an amblyopia develop in one eye from neglect may get along fairly well with his one good eye, but he may some day be confronted with a situation similar to that which is now presented to a patient who recently came to Dr. Wood's clinic at the Brooklyn Eye and Ear Hospital. He is a young man of about 25 years of age, who came complaining that the sight in his right eye was getting bad. The vision in his right eye was two-thirds normal, and in his left eye one-tenth normal. The left eye he said had always been bad; he had never been able to see much with it. On examination, the left eye was found perfectly normal as to media and fundus, but there was a considerable degree of hyperopia, an eye which in infancy had been allowed to become amblyopic. In his right eye, which had always been the good one, we found a well developed brownish mass in the upper portion of the fundus, pretty well forward toward the ciliary body, with some associated detachment of surrounding retina.

Now here is a young man with an intra-ocular neoplasm, probably a melano-sarcoma of the choroid, in his one good eye, making the removal of that eye imperative. He will be left with only an amblyopic eye to use.

The over-development of the ciliary muscle in a hyperopic eye may in later years become a predisposing factor in the development of glaucoma. The hypertrophied muscle, appropriating to itself more space than nature intended it should occupy, crowds the base of the iris forward, and so renders a glaucomatous attack much easier of development.

As already stated, an untreated myopia may become progressive and eventually terminate in a useless eye. Unfortunately, in some of these cases, even the most constant and careful attention to the details of glasses, ocular hygiene and general health cannot check the degenerative process.

In conclusion, I wish to emphasize the fact that it is a mistake to think that children must wait until they are six or eight years old before they can wear glasses. The objection is sometimes made that it is not safe, as the glasses would be broken easily during play, and so endanger the eyes. As a matter of fact, this is a very rare occurrence, and there are many children as young as two and three years, and some even younger, who are wearing glasses with safety and great comfort.

It is necessary that these refractive errors should be corrected as soon as they can be diagnosed, for only by so doing will many of these children have saved for them vision which might otherwise be lost.

---

## REMARKS ON GASTRIC DISEASE.*

### By H. W. Lincoln, M.D.,

of Brooklyn, N. Y.

IN these days, when we are asked to believe that every case of chronic digestive disturbance means ulcer either of the stomach or duodenum (more frequently the latter), chronic appendicitis, gallstones, pancreatis, "Lane's kink," "pericolitis," or what not, in other words, all chronic cases presenting mainly symptoms of impaired digestion, either gastric or intestinal, should be promptly turned over to the surgeon, it may not be entirely out of place to look a bit carefully into the matter, and see if, in spite of all this surgical furore, there may yet be left some legitimate work for the man who claims to treat medically disease affecting the stomach and intestine.

In the first place, I believe that our most radical adherents of operative interference as a cure-all concede the fact that functional cases, more especially those having neurotic tendencies, make poor operative risks. Here, then, is one spot left for the medical man. Let us see just how small a spot this really is, judging from the experi-

* Read before the Brooklyn Society of Internal Medicine, March 28, 1913.

ences of some of our accredited authorities, not in gastro-enterology, but in general medicine, for no man is so well balanced to pass upon a case as to its medical or surgical needs, as the well-equipped medical man, because he is called upon to give opinion upon all classes of cases, while the vast majority of cases from which our operative statistics are gleaned are from the ranks of those who are either beyond question surgical, or beyond even the aid of surgery. Now, it is not for one moment to be supposed by any thinking man, that patients coming into the hands of such men as Deaver, or Murphy, for example, ever receive operation that is not positively indicated, but it is the impression made by the public utterances of these and other of our really great surgeons, upon the minds of others who are operating, that has done more or less harm. Such men have become imbued with the idea that we should simply make our diagnoses and at once call in some operator to cut something in order to save our patient from chronic invalidism or something worse.

Could we but once in a while hear of the abdominal openings made at which nothing abnormal was found, instead of being continually upbraided in lengthy discourses upon the cases which have "been treated for years medically, until at last they were permanently relieved by surgery," it might throw a more genuine light upon the condition of things.

We have been repeatedly told that the diagnosis of ulcer is a simple matter, yet in Cabot's series of 3,000 autopsies, it had been diagnosed correctly in but 36 per cent. of cases.

It is a well-known fact that even with the abdomen opened, and the diseased parts in hand, it is sometimes impossible to make a satisfactory diagnosis, or even to state whether ulcer is pyloric or duodenal. Why, therefore, must we be expected to make a diagnosis of organic trouble, and advise immediately surgical intervention every time a patient comes complaining of regurgitation of sour material, pain relieved by food or alkalies, etc.?

How many neurasthenics have been "explored," and in some instances, re-explored, and with no benefit!

I have in mind a very recent case, who has consulted a man in nearly every specialty in town. It is but a question of time when she will succeed in getting her "exploratory laparotomy." We must admit that we are all woefully ignorant when it comes to these cases; therefore it seems hardly the right thing to assume that simply because they may prove intractible to medical treatment, there is some trouble present requiring surgery. In this particular case no less than six most competent medical men, beside an equally able surgeon and a most experienced radiographer have made careful examinations, and the case is still without a satisfactory diagnosis. The one complaint is pain in the abdomen.

We must not mention hyperchlorhydria except as an indication for surgery. True in some cases, and yet there are patients complaining of sour eructations, gas and belching, who show an increase in both total and free acidity who have neither gallstones, ulcer, nor appendicitis, and who recover and remain well longer than some of our "successfully" operated ulcer cases, under purely medical and dietary management. You may call it hyperchlorhydria or whatever you choose.

Out of 100 cases taken as they came there were found seventeen cases, seven male, ten female, in whom the above symptoms presented and in whom there was no evidence of extra gastric disease (organic), and in whom there were not sufficient findings to warrant diagnosis of ulcer, gastric or duodenal, and in whom treatment proved the correctness of the above assertions.

In a recent paper in one of the medical journals (*A. M. A.,* March 8, 1913; W. H. Wathen; "When Is Operative Treatment Indicated in Chronic Dyspepsia") the following observations are made:

1. In 90 per cent. of cases of chronic dyspepsia there is no pathologic lesion in the stomach, and the conditions requiring operation in the entire gastro-intestinal tract and all structures in the abdominal and pelvic cavities do not exceed 30 per cent.

2. In about 30 per cent. the stomach trouble is caused by cardiac and kidney insufficiently, tuberculosis, arterio-sclerosis, tabes dorsalis, etc.

3. Another 30 per cent. is caused by congenital or acquired defects in the viscera of the abdominal and pelvic cavities plus gastro-intestinal neuroses—gastroptosis, enteroptosis, atonic dilatation of the stomach, etc.

We have here 30 per cent. which need operation, 30 per cent. where the trouble is organic, but outside of the abdomen, and still another 30 per cent. where the trouble is due to neuroses, ptoses, etc. Perhaps the other 10 per cent. might be placed in the category of cases which are opened for abdominal disease which upon opening the abdomen is found to be absent.

This same author observes further on, "It is probably true that some of the best known men in internal medicine, men who contribute much to medical literature, have seldom or never seen an abdominal operation on a living person."

I suppose there are some surgeons who would even go so far as to agree to a statement like that.

REMARKS UPON DISEASES OF THE STOMACH.

In December I was asked to look at a gentleman who gave a most graphic description of chronic ulcer of some fifteen years' standing. After treating him for a time, I learned that this diagnosis had been made by several surgeons here in town.

There was one, however, who took note of the fact that when upon his vacation, and free from the cares and worries of a busy professional career, this gentleman had scarcely any trouble, and he believed that the trouble was in part at least neurotic. During the short time which I observed this case the pain was at times intense, and was relieved only by medication directed to ulcer. I concurred in the diagnosis of chronic ulcer. There was a constitutional disease present, and the patient failed quite rapidly, until one night there was very copious bleeding, presumably from the stomach and the end came.

An autopsy was done. Absolutely no ulcer was found. No evidence of any previous ulceration was present in either stomach or duodendum, the blood having no doubt been due to degeneration of some minute vessel in the gastric mucosa somewhere.

In spite of all this, one gentleman of the surgical persuasion who had previously seen this patient states that he believes there was ulcer. It will be observed that the most conservative of all of us was the surgeon who took account of the neurotic element in the case.

A Second Case of Similar Findings.

Mrs. M., age 44, no children, passed menopause at 39 years, F. M., 1 B and 4 S., living in good health. One S died of heart trouble. Patient had scarlet fever and diphtheria as a child, no serious illness since, excepting pneumonia some fifteen years ago.

I first saw the case June 17th, 1912. She stated that she had been subject to so-called bilious attacks most of her life, but these would only come at long intervals, sometimes three years elapsing between attacks. Present trouble came on in April, 1912, with periodic vomiting. She has vomited brownish material which had a sickish decayed taste, and burned as it came through the nostrils. There has been absolutely no pain. There was some gas and belching. For the past three weeks solid food had refused to stay down. The weight which the patient stated in February, 1912, was 160 pounds, on June 17th, 1912, was 118 pounds.

Examination revealed what seemed to be a mass a short distance below the ensiform, and a point of tenderness further down and to the right of the mid-line. The stomach contents showed a total acidity of 44 with free Hcl. 12; some mucus, and some food from the previous 24 hours, but no occult blood.

The consensus of opinion of all who saw this case, including her family physician, a surgeon and myself, was that there was a beginning mechanical pyloric obstruction, probably malignant. The X-ray examination concurred in the obstruction view. The abdomen was opened by a most competent man and absolutely no lesion of pylorus or duodenum was found. Neither was there any disease of the upper abdomen, excepting that the liver appeared to be somewhat shrunken.

This patient went on and died about 10 or 12 weeks after operation, and unfortunately no post-mortem was permitted.

Here was a case which certainly showed unmistakable signs of pyloric obstruction, which could only be relieved by surgery. After a few experiences such as the above two cases one is apt to be a bit hesitant about making positive diagnosis of this, that or the other organic disease in the upper abdomen and urging immediate operation.

Ewald, Ed., 1896, p. 536, speaking of "neurasthenia gastrica," the existence of which disease is strenuously denied by some, says: "A correct diagnosis is possible only after a prolonged observation of the course of the disease, discovery of the causal factors, the failure of all measures directed toward suspected organic disease of the stomach and intestines, and a proper estimation of all the signs of neurasthenia which may be present."

It will be observed that even some seventeen years ago advice was here given to beware of arriving too quickly at a diagnosis of purely functional disease to the exclusion of possible organic trouble.

Yet we have been accused of calling everything "nervous."

Many quotations from recognized authorities, written in a similar vein, might be given.

Osler in his eighth edition (p. 509) observes "serious functional disturbances of the stomach may occur without any discoverable anatomical basis." I think most of us will admit that if there is an "anatomical basis" for trouble Osler would be quite as liable to find it as some of our surgeons who are emphatically proclaiming that there is no such thing as functional stomach disease, nervous dyspepsia, etc.

Fischer, *Med. Record,* February, 1913, in an article entitled "Remarks Upon the Gastric Motor Functions," says:

"As most cases of chronic dyspepsia are resolved by analysis to a basis of disturbed relationship between acidity and motility, the question always arises as to which function succumbed first. So heated was the discussion upon this subject at one time that the camp of gastrologists was fairly divided into obstructionists and non-obstructionists. Given advanced cases of hypersecretion with food retention, the primary disturbing cause was attributed to either one function or the other, according to the particular bent of the individual. The decision depended upon physiological or chemical mental tendency. Surgery always favored the obstructionist view, and indiscriminating gastro-enterostomy became the rage. Fortunately, a healthy reaction has set in, due partly to many recurrences of symptoms following operation, due also to a better knowledge of the regulating mechanism of the motor functions themselves."

Again, further on the author notes that "when we consider that 90 per cent, of our ordinary chronic dyspepsias possess a determinating neurotic element, that 90 per cent. of these neurotic elements are of the type known as anxiety neuroses, in which the emotional state is known to be markedly exaggerated, and, lastly, that 90 per cent. of these disagreeable sensations in the stomach experienced by these individuals are due to either increased or decreased muscular tone of the stomach, it becomes evident that the minor influences of everyday life must bear directly upon the muscular activities themselves, and that the determination of these activities, their present and past tendencies, is an item of considerable moment for a proper estimation of every case." This paper contains valuable material for, beyond any question, impaired motility of either stomach or intestine, whether temporary or continued, is the most dreaded dyscrasia with which we have to deal.

The advice of Deaver, in cases such as the majority which it is to be supposed he sees, to operate first and have the laboratory work done afterward is no doubt, from his standpoint, sound. Lives may have been sacrificed by undue procrastination on the part of over-conservative yet well-meaning medical men. On the other hand, it cannot be truthfully denied that many patients have been rushed to the operating table, and needless operations performed by over-enthusiastic surgical workers. For example permit a brief history of a case which came to my attention, but with which I was not professionally connected, some three or four years ago.

A gentleman was suffering greatly from what was subsequently found to be œdema of genito-urinary organs, retention partial.

A very well-known surgeon was called in consultation and advised an immediate operation, stating emphatically to the patient and his family that he should be at the hospital no later than 8 o'clock the following morning. The consultation was held late in the afternoon. This man had known me for many years, and after the surgeon left, he insisted that I come up and talk the matter over. I told him that if it were my own case, I should prefer to have somebody else see it before submitting to surgical intervention. I made a suggestion along these lines, which was accepted. This man was addicted to alcohol, that is, he was a steady drinker, never, however, to the extent of becoming intoxicated. The second consultation took place and the advice was that it would be entirely out of place to operate in the patient's present condition, but that after the alcoholic effects had worn off, if operation were at all necessary, it would be a simple affair and could be done with no particular trouble. This, as I stated, occurred several years ago, and the man has been in perfect health ever since. It is quite possible that should surgery ever be needed in that family, consultant number two will be chosen. I appreciate the fact that this is not in any sense a gastro-intestinal case, but I think it serves well to illustrate my purpose, namely, that some surgeons are fully as over-enthusiastic, as some medical men are hesitant, when it comes to the border-line cases.

In tabulating cases, I have chosen private, rather than hospital ones, because I believe one is better able to follow them.

I have avoided recording any with which I was unable to keep in touch in some way or other as time went on. The organic cases have been pretty well proven either by operation or by subsequent history. Those that I saw but once or twice and felt confident were functional, I have not included. Those seen once or twice, and that presented all signs pointing toward organic trouble have been included as such. That seems fair enough.

Of 800 cases gone over, there were 497 functional, or about 67 per cent., as against 303 organic.

Of the organic only those of some interest will be mentioned. Ulcer comprised 58 males, 35 female, total, 93.

Of these there were 47 duodenal; 32 male, 15 female.

The average duration of these 93 cases was 8.2 years.

Carcinoma was divided as follows: Stomach 20, sigmoid 4, rectum 1, liver (primary) 1, prostrate 1, œsophagus 2, hepatic flexure 2 (1 male and 1 female, the latter proven by operation).

Gall bladder: Gallstones, males 7; 1 operated and gall bladder filled with dark stagnant bile. Recovery to date. Females 12; 3 operated for gallstones with appendicitis, 2 operated for stones only. One case also showed no stones but stagnant bile. Percentage of female cases about 67.5. Average age of said females 46.75 years. Of the males there was one associated with chronic duodenal ulcer, one with marked hepatic cirrhosis. Two gave a very clear history of previous typhoid infection. Of the females there were three with chronic appendicitis.

Hepatic cirrhosis 25 cases; 23 male; 2 female, with an alcoholic history in most of the males and in both of the females, notwithstanding the fact that nowadays there is said to be not so marked a connection between alcohol and cirrhosis as was formerly taught. The Talma operation was done on one case, a male, 33 years of age, with a fatal termination about one week after operation. This case was not alcoholic.

Chronic appendicitis comprised 30 cases; 12 male, 18 female. So far as I am aware, but 9 accepted the advice to be operated during the interval. Of these one had ulcer as well as appendicitis, another had gallstones, and a third a cirrhotic liver.

Of syphillis there were 12 cases, none of which were active, 10 male, 2 female. Most of them came complaining of ulcer symptoms, and in all but one there was a marked increase in gastric acidity.

Tuberculosis was present in 9 cases; 5 male, 4 female.

Epilepsy 4 cases; 2 of either sex. Average age was 33 years.

There were five cases of chronic malaria; one gave a most typical history of chronic duodenal ulcer, and was promptly benefited by treating the malaria and ignoring the ulcer idea. The plasmodium was found, and the patient is still well, some three years after treatment.

Two cases of pernicious anemia presented themselves, both females. One was some five months pregnant, and, through the very careful management of her physician, went to term, and is now apparently well, a year and half later. The other case is still under observation, improving on large doses of Hcl. Both patients were, as is usual, achylic.

The remainder of the organic conditions encountered included those of heart, kidney, circulation, etc.

Of the secretory stomach troubles, the only one worth mentioning was achylia gastrica, which occurred in but 20 instances. This does not, of course, refer to the atrophic gastritis coincident with carcinoma. Some claim a more frequent occurrence of this deviation from the normal.

The great deviation from the present claim by surgeons of the comparative frequency of duodenal over gastric ulcer may be accounted for in part by the fact that some which I called gastric may have been duodenal, for I most emphatically deny the simplicity of differential diagnosis professed by some men.

The finding of occult blood in the stools, I have not been as fortunate with from a diagnostic standpoint as some claim. As Deaver aptly remarks: It is of value if constantly present. It is also of far greater value in the diagnosis of malignancy, if taken in conjunction with other evidence, than it is in ulcer.

A good history plus physical examination is of much greater value in arriving at a correct diagnosis of either ulcer or cancer than all other methods of investigation put together, at the present stage of our knowledge.

A few years ago it was all gastric and scarcely any duodenal ulcer. Now exactly the reverse seems to be the fad. I believe it is still an open question as to the relative frequency and will be so, for the reason that the surgeons will keep on claiming that the duodenum is the usual offender, because the cases from which their statistics are compiled are undoubtedly from the more serious cases, which come to operation, and nobody will dispute that the duodenal are more rebellious to medical treatment and hence a far greater number get to the operating table. This, however, does not by any means prove that there are more duodenal than gastric ulcers. Ulcer is not as frequent as claimed. In 108 cases gone over, not a single ulcer.

At a recent Hospital Clinical Society meeting, there was submitted by the Pathologist a report of some 60 autopsies, in order to compare the post-mortem pathological findings, with the ante-mortem clinical diagnoses.

In this series there was found no case of either gastric or duodenal ulcer. The nearest to an ulcer was one spoken of as a marked simple hypertrophy of the pylorus with stenosis.

Now, it so happened that we did not see any of these cases, else very possibly some might have been clinically diagnosed as ulcers.

With regard to the surgical indications in diseased stomach or duodenum, it should hardly be necessary to even enumerate them, as there should be no difference of opinion as to this matter.

Continued bleeding from the stomach or duodenum; intractible pain, evidence of a beginning stenosis of the pylorus, perforation, evidence of adhesions causing mechanical obstruction or unbearable pains should, of course, receive surgical attention.

Duodenal ulcer needs surgical intervention more often than gastric, in my opinion.

Owing to the voluminous glowing reports of the value of gastro-enterostomy, there can scarcely be a man doing surgery, who is not familiar with the claims which have been made for it.

There are, however, many men undertaking surgery, major as well as minor, who seldom read a medical journal, or attend a medical meeting. Now, the most able surgeons are relegating to the background the operation of simple gastro-jejunostomy for the radical cure of ulcer, because, with the pyloric canal left intact, this so-called drainage operation does not drain, as if the stomach were a paper bag, unless very marked atony be present, but after a time the food passes out the pylorus in the same old way and the new opening becomes in the gastric contractions a mere slit. (Cannon.)

Hence some harm may be done by the wholesale advocation of this operation, as it does not cure, and will continue to be practised by indiscriminate operators long after it has been discarded as a cure-all by all able surgeons.

*Another point in the surgical management of ulcer. Did you ever hear mentioned the fact that the four or five weeks' rest and proper alimentation incident upon operation played any part in the beneficial effect upon the patient? How many people receive after operation the only real, true medical ulcer treatment they have ever heard? Very many, I am sure.*

Let me cite one instance of a case in this class:

A gentleman, age 41; married; with a negative family history gave a history of stomach trouble having begun some three years before. A diagnosis of chronic appendicitis had previously been made by a gastro-enterologist whom he had seen. His story was one of pain relieved by eating, and he also gave the very pathognomonic symptom of being awakened at 1 A. M. by this pain and obtaining relief by taking almost anything into the stomach.

He volunteered the information also that he always felt better if he could belch some gas, and attributed his trouble largely to gas, a not uncommon subjective finding in these cases. I made a diagnosis of duodenal ulcer. There was no occult blood in either stomach contents or stool.

For a time he did well on medical treatment, though up and about, but as often happens the improvement was but temporary, and operation was talked of. Strangely enough he did not seem pleased at the idea, and the thing ran along for several months. Finally the usual operation with infolding of the ulcer, which was duodenal, was done. The appendix was normal.

The next I saw of the patient was in the latter part of February of the present year, some six months after the operation.

Then I got the following story: For five weeks after the operation there was perfect comfort. Then as soon as he began to move around a bit there was more or less trouble, consisting of gas and discomfort, just enough to keep patient awake nights and to distract his attention. The trouble comes on one to two hours p. c., lasting about one hour, and is still relieved by eating. Belching also relieves the pain. The pain goes to the back more for the past few days. Sometimes by drinking milk at bed time a comfortable night's rest can be gotten.

It would look as though there might still be some irritation in the neighborhood of the old ulcer.

In the current issue of one of the medical journals (*A. M. A.*), Dr. Berg (A. A.) observes:

"It is furthermore admitted that the good effects of gastro-enterostomy on ulcers in the antrum, pylorus and duodenum are not always lasting—that recurrence or recrudescence of the ulcer takes place in at least 45 per cent. of cases."

Some of us medical men may have thought this way for some time, but for a surgeon to come out in print to this effect should be pretty good proof that surgery does not do all for ulcer that some other surgeons have claimed for it.

This author also admits that with the pylorus patent, this is the channel adopted by the food, gastro-enterostomy or no gastro-enterostomy, and hence advocates an addition to the operation which seems to fill a long wanted need.

Beside the usual gastro-enterostomy a purse string ligature is passed around the stomach just proximal to the antrum, and tied snugly enough to occlude the stomach at this point, without constriction of its walls or circulation. He says that enfolding may be done instead of suture ligature, by several layers of suture and thereby exclude the antrum, pylorus and duodenum from the rest of the stomach cavity. (Done since 1901.)

Besides removing, thereby, the chance of further ulcerative activity on the old site by such a method, it seems to me that the danger of future carcinomatous degeneration would be greatly minimized, as we all know that irritation is one important factor in production of cancer, and this factor would be eliminated..

A cause of failure in gastro-enterostomy that I have not seen mentioned is the making of the opening too high up in the wall of the stomach, particularly in a large and atonic organ, which might otherwise drain fairly well. This error has occurred in one of my cases and also in another of which I know.

Many of these surgical cures do not last even as long as any one of the nine or more medical cures which have created so much mirth at medical meetings of recent years.

A laparotomy has been, is now, and always will be a serious matter to the patient, as a surgical friend of mine recently told me. He said that he believed that fully 70 per cent. of ulcer cases were amenable to proper medical treatment, and even if they should have to resort once in a while to a few weeks of treatment, they were better off than they would be to submit to an opening of the abdomen. That is the way the pendulum is now swinging. There is no doubt about it. The holder of such views as just expressed is the man who, when he does see fit to operate, gets lasting results, and it is not his cases which return after weeks or months to the medical clinics to be cured again. Furthermore, I fully believe that the average medical man is only too glad to have the advice of such surgery and to abide by the decision; but the day for simply turning this or that abdomen over to the surgical service so that there may be a "look-in" on the part of the surgeon is fast passing away. It has even been said that if a case suspected of being ulcer got well and remained so under medical treatment, it probably was not ulcer at all. This statement hardly tallies with the widely heralded one; that every case of continued severe hyperchlorhydria means ulcer (duodenal). We must either be granted the credit of an occasional cure, or else hunger pain, tenderness, etc., does not always mean ulcer.

During the past autumn I had occasion to treat a lady who displayed all the ear marks of ulcer excepting hematemesis and melena. The case did not do well upon ambulatory treatment, which is the usual treatment to which I am able to persuade my patients to submit, and I, therefore, called a surgeon to go along with me upon the case. (Patient finally consented to go to bed, where she remained four weeks. When I called him in I gave him perfect freedom to say and do whatever he might see fit, as I always do, for if there is one thing discouraging to a consultant it is to have a case handed to him with a string attached to it.) This case was severe, *i. e.*, the pain was intense, it was localized, it was relieved by food and alkalies, it produced vomiting, etc.; in short, it was a case where two out of three of our operators would have urged immediate interference, but this gentleman declined to recommend operation and the patient is now up and about and perfectly well as far as any stomach trouble goes.

I believe any sane man will admit that this case may go on without any further evidence of that ulcer.

As to the evidence proving that there is sufficient danger of carcinomatous degeneration later on; that is still in a sense a partially open question.

In Osler's series of 150 cases of stomach cancer he finds but four in which there was a possible history of previous ulcer.

It would seem that experience even at the present time teaches us that the very great majority of cases of stomach cancer occur in persons who have been particularly free from previous digestive trouble during their lives.

In one breath we are told that one of the main indications for surgical treatment of ulcer is to remove the danger of future malignant degeneration. In the next, we are instructed that duodenal ulcer occurs three times as frequently as gastric.

As we all know, duodenal ulcer takes place in the first part of the duodenum, while cancer, when it does occur, is found in the second portion. In my experience I can recall but three or four instances where the carcinoma was engrafted upon an ulcer base, and those were, of course, in the stomach and proven by operation.

In conclusion, at a conservative estimate, fully 50 per cent. of ulcer cases may be cured medically and remain cured.

We should not take it for granted that duodenal ulcer is three times as frequent as gastric, simply because operative statistics say so.

Patients about to be operated upon should have the matter clearly laid before them and should not be given promise of unqualified, permanent freedom from further digestive trouble, as is still frequently done.

Something more than gastro-enterostomy should be done for the radical cure of ulcer, and also, if the danger of future carcinomatous degeneration is anything like as great as is just now claimed, to relieve for all time the ulcer-bearing area from irritation.

Lastly, not over 40 per cent. at the outside of cases seen in the daily work done by the average internal medical man, are organic, in a surgical sense, either of the stomach or the other abdominal organs.

(For Discussion See Page 288.)

# LYMPHOCYTOSIS IN PERTUSSIS.

## By J. Horowitz, M.D.,

of Brooklyn, N. Y.

I HAVE here history records of six cases of pertussis in which I made a differential leucocyte count, and in all of which I found an increase in the number of lymphocytes.

These cases are all positive whooping cough, for in three of them I have heard the whoop in my office at the first visit, and the other three cases I was able to follow up until they reached the whooping stage.

I did not in any of them make the examination of the wet blood, as the lymphocytosis in the dry specimen implies lymphocytosis in the wet as well, and besides, to advocate an entire examination of the blood for private practice would mean that no private practitioner would go ahead and do it, for it requires more time and more difficult handling, as well as more delicate instruments to make a blood count of the red and white cells. While on the other hand, to make a smear on a slide, dry it and stain it with a standard blood stain is comparatively easy for any one who wants to do it.

The only precaution necessary in making a diagnosis in the case of pertussis by the differential count is to examine the patient well, and exclude any other causes of lymphocytosis, such as rickets, scurvy and especially hereditary syphilis and lymphatic leukemia.

To illustrate this point case number 4 will serve very well. Patient is now 5 years old, she had measles three and one-half years ago, after which she began to cough and lose flesh. The cough is mostly at night. Physical examination one and one-half years ago showed bronchial rales over the lower right lobe in midaxillary line and also in the right interscapular space. A Von Pirquet test at that time was negative.

Patient now (one and one-half years later) complains of coughing more than usual since two weeks. Two of her sisters are having pertussis since three and one-half weeks. Examination of her sputum by myself and the Board of Health on April 1, 1913, is positive. Her blood smear differs from the others in so much that her polynuclears are 20 per cent., small lymphocytes are 72 per cent., the large lymphocytes are 3 per cent., the eosinophyles are 5 per cent.

## SUMMARY.

The value of this test is at present more for the physician than for the patient, for given a case of a child who comes to the office with a cough which persists in spite of your best prescription, if you can tell the patient at the next visit that the reason the medicine did not help was because the cough was not a plain cold, but whooping cough, the mother will then not blame you for your failure, quite as much since the laity knows that, unfortunately, you can not cure pertussis with a single prescription; then there is the satisfaction of making a diagnosis.

It may in the future be useful to make an early diagnosis of pertussis in case we find a specific cure for it.

Mr. Chairman and Gentlemen, I acknowledge that these number of cases are too few to draw any scientific data, but in the course of the coming year I intend to go ahead with these blood examinations, and perhaps will be able to show more cases and thus draw more definite conclusions.

The figures of the blood counts are as follows:

Case No. 1,  3 days' duration has P. 38, S. 50, L. 12, E. 2.
"     "  2, 10   "      "      " P. 46, S. 50, L.  5.
"     "  3, 14   "      "      " P. 47, S. 17, L. 37.
"     "  4, 14   "      "      " P. 20, S. 72, L.  3, E. 5.
"     "  5,  4 weeks'  "      " P. 70, L. 30.
"     "  6,  4 ` "      "      " P. 65, L. 25, S, 10.

In which  P = Polymorphonuclears.
          S = Small lymphocytes.
          L = Large lymphocytes.
          E = Eosinophyles.

---

## TERATOMA OF THE TESTICLE.

By J. Ensor Hutcheson, M.D.,

Rockville Centre, N. Y.

and

Gertrude W. Welton, M.D.,

Pathologist, Nassau Hospital.

THE following is the history of a case of "teratoma testis." These cases are not so rare as one might suppose, as many of them lose their identity through degeneracy and are frequently diagnosed as sarcoma, carcinoma and complex growths.

Patient: J. H——. Age, 28 years. American. Consulted me on October 3rd, 1912, on account of an enlargement of his scrotum.

*Previous history:* Negative, except a possible specific urethritis four weeks previous, the discharge lasting three weeks. No history of traumatism.

Noticed one year ago a slight enlargement of right testicle. Slow growth the first six months. Rapid growth the last six months. Slight pain. More discomfort from the size.

*Examination* showed a marked enlargement of scrotum. Measurements 10 by 7 inches. Pear-shaped. Color of scrotum bluish red. Marked dilatation of scrotal veins. Tumor firm, nodular, with a central area of slight fluctuation.

Left testicle small, pushed up near the external abdominal ring. No inguinal glandular enlargement. Operation advised and patient went to Nassau Hospital.

*Diagnosis:* Sarcoma of right testicle.

*Operation:* October 12, 1912. Enucleation, high amputation of the cord. Growth partially adherent to scrotum. Scrotum very much thickened. Two-thirds excision of scrotum; enough scrotum left to form pocket for left testicle.

Patient comfortable until one week after operation, when he developed a left-sided pleural pain. A few days later the left pleural cavity was aspirated and about 70 ounces of sanguinous fluid obtained. Soon a pericarditis developed.

*Present condition:* Re-accumulation of fluid in left pleural cavity; marked enlargement of left inguinal glands. Rapid pulse. Irregular temperature. Emaciation.

*Pathological report:* The tumor was a large, firm mass, measuring 6 by 5 by 4 inches. The scrotal tissues which were adherent at the lower pole had been separated, leaving a jagged surface. Packing was in position in a pocket which had been opened the day before. The spermatic cord was seen at the upper pole, but it was impossible to identify the epididymis. The tunica albuginea was destroyed over the lower pole, the dartos greatly thickened and infiltrated with a new growth. The blood supply was abundant.

On bisection the mass was found to be a solid, vascular tumor which had apparently replaced the whole testicle.

A diagnosis of teratoma was made.

Microscopic examination showed large areas of simple necrosis, large areas of adeno-carcinoma, numerous blood spaces, with old and recent hemorrhages into the tissues, and areas where the tumor cells had lost their glandlike arrangement and were becoming diffuse.

The deeper layers of the scrotal tissues were infiltrated with adeno-carcinoma. The stratified squamous epithelium was normal.

No histological elements of testis or epididymis were seen in the twenty pieces of the growth examined.

Mesodermal structures are absent and it is a question that cannot be determined whether this great overgrowth of epithelium is of ectodermal or endodermal origin.

However this may be, it does not affect the diagnosis for, as Dr. Ewing has reported, teratomata have occurred showing very few elements of tissues derived from two of the primary germ-layers with great overgrowth from the third.

It is his opinion that a tumor of this type is to be interpreted as "a one-sided development of a teratoma, which owes its origin to a single, definite embryonic disturbance"—and that the diagnosis in this case is "embryonal carcinoma of teratomatous origin."

To those who may take further interest in this condition I refer you to an article by Dr. James Ewing, "Teratoma Testis and Its Derivatives," published in *Surgery, Gynecology and Obstetrics,* March, 1911. He concludes that teratoma testis arises from sex cells in the neighborhood of the rete. Their onset is frequently preceded by trauma.

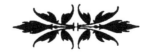

# EDITORIAL

## THE CRUX OF THE ECONOMIC CRISIS.

FROM one angle of view we, of the medical profession, seem to be living under a *quasi*-socialistic dispensation without rational economic adjustment. That is to say, we are partially socialized in spirit and in practice, and are actually giving much the same character and quantity of service to the relatively poor citizenry that we would be required to give under a socialistic government—with this difference, that we are not paid for it. Are we not as busy as we ever possibly could be attending to the sick in hospitals, dispensaries, and in other ways and places? Yet we do this work gratis when every rule of reason tells us that service should never be free. Service that is free is practically worthless and the givers are mentally defective. It is even worse than worthless; it is immoral, for the medical profession has economic obligations to others than themselves. The doctor cannot play the rôle of St. Francis and live in holy poverty, for he has dependants like everyone else, a home to keep up, culture to add to constantly, recreations to seek for his health's sake, and new medical learning and skill to acquire. We live and act as though we were above economic considerations and were unaffected by the operation of the law of supply and demand, as has been said before in these columns by another. Our altruism has seemingly increased of late, too. It would appear that whole classes of men as well as individuals may be the victims of psychoses.

What a paradox! What a grim joke upon us all! We, who are so little interested in the dry subjects of economics and sociology, who, perhaps, feel a kind of contempt for Socialism and most of its propagandists, are actually applying in practice certain socialistic principles. And the demonstration is free! No charge for admission to or participation in the most ambitious object lesson that history records. We are the advanced guard of the socialized profession that is to be. We are (involuntary) volunteers, forerunners, promoters. Men say that under Socialism there will be no incentive to work so strong as the monetary considerations that inspire us today. Behold! the medical profession works for nothing, works with zest and with terrible sincerity. Are not the reactionaries confounded?

ARTHUR C. JACOBSON.

## THE VALUE OF PUBLIC CHARITY.

THE news item in another column of the JOURNAL refers to the opening of a recently established admission bureau of the Department of Charities in connection with cases of tuberculosis. The centralization of effort thus evidenced will undoubtedly be of great help to those seeking admission to the various institutions for the care of tuberculosis patients. It is only within the last few years that any concerted effort has been made toward the systematic care of the tubercular poor; the open-air treatment was still unproven, and while individuals were convinced that early tuberculosis could be at least held in check, the general belief in its curability was yet to come. The popular acceptance of this idea seems now very general, and as a result, the requests for admission to the sanitoria at Otisville and Ray Brook far outnumber the accommodations available; nor will it be possible for many years to meet the needs of the community adequately at the public expense.

While the extremely poor have some provision made for them, and the well-to-do can find ample accommodations in sanitoria of all sorts scattered throughout the country, the provision for the self-supporting classes, whose self-respect and culture forbid their being classed with the charity cases, seems sadly lacking. Personal inquiry some two years ago emphasized this fact unmistakably. The Loomis Sanitorium, near Liberty, and the Trudeau establishment, at Saranac. offer to a limited number an opportunity for cheap accommodations, and a very few sectarian institutions provide a further, though limited, number. Obviously, with the limited accommodations at hand and the rapidly increasing number of sufferers who are seeking help through sanitorium care, the advantages of such institutions must be restricted to those who promise the most rapid and complete recovery, and as a result, it is extremely difficult to provide for any but incipient cases, and by no means all of those.

The idea of Deputy Commissioner Fogarty in establishing a central bureau to act as a clearing house for tubercular patients seems a highly commendable one, as is his choice of physicians to direct it. It also indicates a closer relation between the authorities in control of the various public institutions. It would be most desirable from the standpoint of increased efficiency and economy if there could be a centralized bureau to control all of the agencies dealing with the care of the sick. The idea of complete co-operation between the various departments of the city government and private charitable organizations is perhaps too Utopian to be practical, but it certainly would minimize expense and make for greater usefulness.

Commissioner Fogarty's new bureau will make it possible to refer the applicant for public help where he may obtain all the information that is available for his particular case, which at present is so scattered that even a careful search through the none too lucid pages of the Charity Directory leaves one in doubt as to the facilities at his command.

Extremely significant in the same direction was the recent meeting of the various private charities organizations interested in measures for public health held at the Academy of Medicine on June 4th, when, after some general discussion, a representative committee was appointed to effect active co-operation looking to the unification of effort along this line, as well as to a saving in expense by avoiding duplication. The meeting itself furnished the best evidence of the need of a concerted plan, as was emphasized in a grimly humorous manner by the divergent viewpoints of several prominent speakers. who offered each his own hobby as a fundamental groundwork from which to attack the problem.

As already remarked, there are accommodations of a sort for the extremely poor and for the well-to-do, but no adequate means seem to be at hand for the self-respecting, cultured, self-supporting people who require institutional care. For them it is a hardship to associate with the ignorant and the dirty for whom the city sanitaria are primarily intended. A bureau of self-help for such as these would be a real boon. Such a bureau might search out opportunities for those suffering with incipient tuberculosis to support themselves, wholly or in part, in some healthy country district, under proper supervision; or it might go still further and interest those who are well able to contribute to such a purpose and provide a farming and woodland tract in some favorable locality where this class of patients could contribute in service toward their care and where the changes should be only those actually incurred for board and running expenses. A workshop might be added, where with proper supply of light and air, pleasant labor, such as bookbinding or basket weaving, would produce an output of sufficient value to meet the actual running expenses of the institution. Such a plan, modified to meet the particular objections which would doubtless arise in working it out, is by no means as idealistic as it may seem at first glance, and requires only to be actively championed to become an actual fact. It is earnestly to be hoped that the real needs of this large class of patients may shortly be appreciated and met in some such way as has been suggested.

H. G. W.

## PREVENTABLE BLINDNESS.

A TIMELY article by Dr. Hiram Woods of Baltimore on "Blindness Due to Wood Alcohol," appearing in the *Journal of the American Medical Association,* again emphasizes the carelessness of the public attitude toward this dangerous drug. It is not only that purified wood alcohol is used as an adulterant in cheap liquor, as is so often reported in the newspapers, the impression being given that it is only used by an occasional unprincipled liquor dealer in the lowest of dives in order to save a few cents and increase his profits inordinately. This form is probably the least frequent abuse of methyl alcohol. It is extensively used in the trades, especially as a solvent for shellac and some other varnishes, and under the name of Columbian Spirits it is largely used as a substitute for grain alcohol, the name Columbian Spirits serving to disguise its real nature. Dr. Woods points out that its internal use varies from extreme toxicity to harmlessness, depending on the susceptibility of the victim, an experience that is quite generally noted.

It is not only the internal use of wood alcohol that may bring about poisonous effects, but its inhalation by susceptible people may, and often does, produce marked symptoms of poisoning. The investigation of the Committee on the Prevention of Blindness has brought to light several instances of extreme intoxication by inhalation. For instance: "Two men were recently killed and one blinded in New York City while varnishing beer vats because a ventilator was not attached to the vats; while another man was blinded and one killed because the necessary thirty minutes in the open air was reduced to twenty minutes." The committee has reported cases of blindness following the use of bay rum, paregoric, flavoring extracts, Jamaica ginger, and some patent medicines, all prepared by firms using rectified wood alcohol in place of the more expensive grain alcohol. As ignorance of the poisonous qualities of wood alcohol, even when inhaled, is the main reason for its extensive use, so a due appreciation of the dangers attendant upon its use will deter most people from exposing themselves to the risk of blindness. For the wretches who employ this dangerous drug to save themselves a little expense and with full knowledge of the potential harm that their cupidity exposes an innocent user of their products to, restrictive legislation of the sternest sort must be had. The more widely knowledge of the dangerous qualities of wood alcohol can be spread, the more quickly can the general public be safeguarded against its consequences.

H. G. W.

## SCHOOL HYGIENE.

POSSIBLY no general subject is attracting as much attention at present as the health of school children, at least among those who have to deal directly with educational problems. Apparently the problem is two-fold—how to pour the greatest variety of facts into the child and how to fortify the child to accommodate the facts, so to speak. Times have changed since we went to school and educational methods have changed with them. We must confess ourselves too far removed to sit in judgment upon the public school system, but to our judgment it would seem that there are too many fads and not enough thoroughness. We must confess to believe that the prime idea of general education should be to produce healthy, well rounded children, well grounded in the essentials so as to be fit for any occupation but not to be so well educated as to be too proud to work. That there is real need for the improvement in the health of school children is evidenced by the program of the Fourth National Congress on School Hygiene which will be found in detail among the Notes and News items in this number of the JOURNAL and will well repay serious consideration, as it is suggestive in a very broad way of other problems than the one of keeping school children healthy. H. G. W.

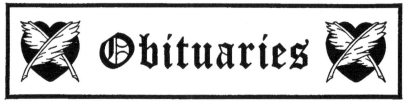

# Obituaries

DEPARTMENT UNDER THE CHARGE OF WILLIAM SCHROEDER, M.D.

## JOHN DAVIES TREZISE, M.D.

DR. TREZISE was born July 12, 1862, at Minersville Pa., and died in Brooklyn, N. Y., March 4, 1913. He was the son of John Trezise of England and Mary Rogers Davies of Wales. Educated in the public and high schools of Shenandoah, Pa., he attended medical lectures at Cornell University, receiving the degree of M.D. from the Long Island College Hospital in the class of 1901. For a number of years he was connected with the Department of Health, was a member of the Medical Society County of Kings from 1908, and the Medical Society of Greater New York. Dr. Trezise was unmarried.

W. S., SR.

## ALEXANDER MANSFIELD GOODMAN, M.D.

DR. GOODMAN was born at Saulsbúrg Mills, N. Y., May 20, 1853, and died in Brooklyn, N. Y., February 19, 1913. He was educated at the University of New York, receiving the degree of M.D. in 1876. He practiced medicine at Cornwall, N. Y., for a number of years, whence he removed to Flatbush, this city. He was a member of the Flatbush Medical Society and of the Flatbush Congregational Church. His father was Dr. Alpheus Goodman and his mother Margaret Gregg. He leaves a widow, Ruth Taylor; a son, Joseph M., and two daughters, Maud and Clara Goodman.

W. S., SR.

## EUGENE JOSEPH CAROLAN, M.D.

DR. CAROLAN was born in Brooklyn, N. Y., 1852, where he died on March 14, 1913. He received his medical education at Bellevue Hospital Medical College, where he was graduated in 1878. His medical practice was confined to the city of his birth. For a number of years he was Surgeon to the Bushwick Hospital and a member of the Brooklyn Pathological Society, and from 1880 to 1902, Medical Society County of Kings, The Associated Physicians of L. I., Hill Grove Lodge No. 540, F. & A. M., Evening Star Chapter, R. A. M., Damascus Commandery, K. T. Long Island Council, R. A. Jamaica Lodge, I. O. O. F., and Episcopal Church of St. Mary.

Dr. Carolan leaves a widow, Katherine Kellcher, two daughters, Genevieve and Virginia, three sons, Eugene, Wendell and Gallard. He was a member of the Episcopal Church of St. Mary.

W. S., SR.

## JOHN HERMAN DROGE, M.D.

Dr. Droge was born in the city of New York October 14, 1860, and died in Brooklyn, N. Y., March 15, 1913. He was the son of Fred William Droge and Eva Catharine, both of Germany. On November 3, 1886, he married Miss Amelia Vigelius. A son was born of this union, Anton William Droge.

His early education was received in the public schools and the New York College of Pharmacy. His medical education was under the direction of Dr. H. T. Swan and completed at Bellevue Hospital Medical College, where he was graduated in the class of 1884. This was followed by post-graduate study at the New York Polyclinic and Post-Graduate School, and Hoagland Laboratory.

Dr. Droge was in practice in this city during his professional life, and for a number of years held the position of Surgeon in diseases of the nose and throat at the Central Throat Hospital, Brooklyn Throat Hospital, German Hospital, St. Mary's and Jamaica Hospitals. For a time he lectured at the Metropolitan School for Nurses.

He was a member of the Medical Society County of Kings from 1886 to 1897, one of the original members of the Brooklyn Medical Society in 1894; German Medical Society, of which he was president in 1893 and in 1903-04; Associated Physicians of Long Island, 1909-13; and the New York Physicians' Mutual Aid Association. He was a Trustee of the German Hospital Society.

Dr. Droge contributed two papers: "Mastoid Abscess and Operation"; "Intubation and Tracheotomy."

W. S., Sr.

## GRANT STANLEY, B.S., M.D.

Dr. Stanley was born at Meriden, Conn., February 25, 1875, and died in Brooklyn, N. Y., on March 23, 1913. He was the son of Joseph E. and Harriet E. Stanley.

On October 23, 1907, Dr. Stanley married Bertha E. Haring, who, with one child, Nancy Martha Stanley, survives him.

The doctor's early education was received at the public and high schools of Hartford, Conn., receiving the degree of B. S. from Redfield College, class of 1900. His medical education was received at Cornell University, where he was graduated in 1904. This was followed by two years as interne at M. E. Hospital, after which he began the practice of medicine at Sea Cliff, Long Island. He was a member of the Queens-Nassau Medical Society, the Associated Physicians of Long Island from 1906, and Alumni of M. E. Hospital. Physician of Nassau Hospital and The Country Home for Convalescent Babies at Sea Cliff.

W. S., Sr.

## FRANK LITTLE, M.D.

Dr. Little was born September 30, 1856, at Ridgeway, Pa., and died in Brooklyn, N. Y., April 4, 1913. He was educated at the Western Reserve University and the Medical College of Ohio, where he was graduated in the class of 1881. He then served as interne at the Brooklyn Hospital, remaining in this city during his professional life. For a time he was Physician to the Kings County Hospital, a member of the Medical Society County of Kings from 1883, American Medical Association, Brooklyn Pathological Society, American Electro-Therapeutic Society, and from 1899 to 1902 of the Associated Physicians of Long Island.

Dr. Little in 1909 married Miss J. L. Bronson, of Geneva, N. Y. His widow and daughter, Louise Bronson Little, survive him. The funeral service was conducted at the First Presbyterian Church, the interment being at Geneva, N. Y.

W. S., Sr.

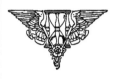 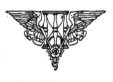

# Society Transactions

## TRANSACTIONS OF THE BROOKLYN PATHOLOGICAL SOCIETY.

*Stated Meeting, February 13, 1913.*

The President, PAUL M. PILCHER, M.D., in the Chair.

*Scientific Program.*

1. The Properties and Agglutinations of Some Non-Pathogenic Vibrios.
   By Charles V. Craster, M.D., Health Officer's Department, Quarantine Station.
2. Immunization against Typhoid Fever (with lantern-slide demonstration).
   By Major F. F. Russell, M.D., of the Medical Department of the U. S. Army, Washington, D. C.
3. Immunization against Typhoid Fever.
   By Morris Ogan, M.D., New York Department of Health.

### The Properties and Agglutinations of Some Non-Pathogenic Vibrios.

*By C. V. Craster, M.D., Quarantine Laboratory, Rosebank, New York.*

During routine examinations for cholera certain monoflagellate organisms morphologically resembling the cholera vibrio are frequently observed. These are usually obtained from persons free from disease, and are not known to cause any lesion in man. In the routine examination carried out at Quarantine in 1911, over one hundred non-cholera vibrios were found. These vibrios with few exceptions closely resemble the cholera organism in morphology and motility. In culture, slight differences were discernible in the colonies on alkaline agar plates. No typical indol reaction was obtained. They were hemolytic to a variable degree, and gelatine was readily liquefied. The action on sugars was similar to that of the cholera vibrio. Three of the strains showed pigment formation, and one was a gas former; the latter a character not usually associated with the cholera-like group. Pathogenicity tested by feeding experiments and by Pfeiffer's peritoneal inoculation test with living cultures demonstrated no pathogenicity to animals. The non-cholera vibrios agglutinated with anti-cholera serum only in very low dilutions (1/10) and not at all in high dilutions. The cholera vibrio is very sensitive to the action of anti-cholera serum, and agglutinated in serum dilutions of 1/10,000. A series of anti-sera was prepared from twenty varieties of non-cholera vibrios. The various cultures of these were agglutinated freely by the heterologous sera. The positive agglutinations were not, however, always reciprocal. The results of the tests showed the presence of certain group agglutinations, and in this way the different non-cholera vibrio cultures could be shown to be related in some degree. The rôle of the non-cholera vibrios is still uncertain. They have been regarded as "transitional" forms of the cholera vibrio by some authorities, especially Zlatogroff, who has endeavored to prove that the ability to agglutinate with anti-cholera serum may be acquired by subjecting the cholera-like vibrios to various cultural and inoculation procedures.

MAJOR F. F. RUSSELL, M.D., of the Medical Department of the United States Army, Washington, D. C., in discussion, said:—"May I ask if the water tanks were ever examined for vibrios, especially in this ship where so many vibrio carriers were found?"

DR. CHARLES V. CRASTER, answering Major Russell's question, said:—"They were examined, but no vibrios were found, doctor."

### Immunization Against Typhoid Fever.

*(See page 227.)*

*By Morris Ogan, M.D., New York Department of Health.*

DR. MORRIS OGAN, in discussion, said:—"I have nothing special to add

285

except to appeal to you to do all the missionary work you can in Brooklyn in the interest of anti-typhoid immunization.

"I have forgotten to say that in this immunity work we are ready to make the following arrangement with any physician who wants the ampules for personal or private use in his cases: If he will call us up, or write us a note, and give us the names and addresses of his cases in order that we may attend to our statistics, which are going to be valuable as you have seen, we will communicate with him and advise him where he may get his emulsion. We will ascertain from him the nearest culture station, or if he does not know it, we will look it up and tell him and the next day a carrier or messenger will deliver addressed to him an envelope or package containing the material.

"I want to speak about a little error in our circular—the circulars which were sent out to all physicians in Greater New York, some seven or eight thousand, not very long ago, in which the emulsion is there falsely characterized as a serum. I want to disclaim any personal responsibility for calling it a serum. How the name slipped into type we do not know."

### Immunization Against Typhoid Fever.

*By Major F. F. Russell, M.D., of the Medical Department of the U. S. Army, Washington, D. C. With lantern-slide demonstration.*

At the conclusion of the lantern-slide demonstration, MAJOR RUSSELL said:—

"Our present practice, I may say, is to vaccinate very man as soon as he has enlisted, on the right arm against smallpox and on the left arm against typhoid. We give three doses of typhoid vaccine, at 10-day intervals, the first dose of five hundred millions, the second dose one thousand millions and the third dose one thousand millions. If the vaccinia is severe we postpone the second dose of typhoid for a few days. We do not see many severe vaccinia cases, and very few have to be postponed.

"It is not the custom to excuse men from work to any extent after vaccination; as a rule they do their work just the same. Very few are excused from recruit duty because of typhoid vaccination and when they are excused they are taken to the hospital and put to bed, but are never kept there over one or two days.

"We have encountered no opposition, either in or out of the Army."

DR. JOSHUA M. VAN SCOTT, in opening the discussion, said:—"I would like to ask Major Russell one question and that is this: What is the theory of the 10-day interval of the inoculations, and also as to whether he has ever seen any anaphylaxis in the use of vaccines?"

DR. VICTOR A. ROBERTSON, in discussion, said:—"I should like to ask Major Russell about this age limit of 45 years; that is, as to whether anybody over that age is susceptible to typhoid. Of course, I know from my own clinical experience that they are. But I would like to know if there is any special reason why this immunization should not be done at a later age than 45 years; and, furthermore, it seems to me that I have read in the literature that in Germany they are using living attenuated live cultures, instead of dead ones, and if that is so what the possible objection might be."

DR. WILLIAM LINTZ, in discussion, said:—"The subject presented so modestly by Major Russell is certainly in great contrast to the comments that I recently heard at the Bacteriological Congress at Berlin about his work. The statistics of his recent immunization at the Mexican border were quoted again and again as the most ideal that can possibly be hoped for, and the comments of the representatives of both the British and the German armies were certainly more than a source of pride to me as an American.

"I would like to emphasize the point which Major Russell brought out relative to the susceptibility encountered by physicians and also by nurses. As a personal experience I vaccinated myself with 500,000,000 bacilli and certainly realized the truth of the statement as I had marked general symptoms, severe headaches and high temperature, so that I had to go to bed and preferred to take the second and third doses by the absent treatment. It seems to me it must undoubtedly be due to the fact that we who are constantly in contact with these typhoid patients develop a partial immunity so that when the bacilli are injected into us the ferments present break up at once and liberate endotoxins, producing instead of a slow, as in others, a marked and rapid intoxication. However, I have never seen any bad results even after severe reactions for after twenty-four or forty-eight hours there is a return to normal.

"I would like to ask Major Russell one question along with the others that have already been asked and that is this: Did I understand him to say that heating the bacteria at 54° for one hour completely sterilizes the cultures? If so, I wish to say that in my experience heating at 54 does not sterilize the cultures, but that it takes a temperature of at least 60 for an hour. However, I do not believe that even if living bacilli are present it makes any great difference for the reason that they are attenuated by the heat and are not at all harmful, and in fact, if anything, have advantages as they retain their immunizing properties to a high degree."

MAJOR F. F. RUSSELL, M.D., in closing the discussion, said:—"I am very glad to have an opportunity of answering the questions that have been asked so far as I am able to, but before doing so I would like to say something about Dr. Ogan's paper; that is, the point he has brought out, to the effect that in the Department of Health they will keep track of the immunization of contacts in typhoid fever cases so that in a short time, in a few years at most we may have some reliable statistics to guide us. This will be of the very greatest value and is the best thing I have heard in a long time. We have immunized those in contact with the disease and we believe it is the right thing to do, but we don't have much typhoid so that there is very little chance to do this now. It will need all the statistics that the Department of Health can produce to convince the average practitioner of medicine that he is doing the right thing.

"Now, the point relative to vaccinating at 7- or 10-day intervals: The reason for that is that in the military service ten days is convenient time. All of the men are on duty Sundays as well as on other days and we can spare them on the tenth as well as on the seventh day; but in civil life, with men who are employed during the week we vaccinate Saturday afternoons and they can have Sunday to themselves. Where it is more convenient to vaccinate Saturday afternoon we use the 7-day instead of the 10-day interval.

"Now, the reason covered by Dr. Van Cott's question, for the 10-day interval (the 7- to 10-day interval we might call it) is simply based upon experience with animals, as far as I know, for at the end of five, six, seven and eight days we get a good production of antibodies and the idea has always been not to give our second dose until the patient has reacted to the first dose, which they do in from five to eight days, and, therefore, we give the second dose at the tenth day. There is another possibility, an anaphylactic reaction, about the tenth, eleventh and twelfth days and the second dose is often postponed until the reacting time; and we often vaccinate on the twelfth, thirteenth and fourteenth days. When we first vaccinated people on the 14-day interval I was very much afraid of the anaphylactic reaction, but as none has been observed, it does not seem that this reaction is of any special importance. Were we using broth cultures containing more or less peptone and other things, we might obtain anaphylactic reactions, and possibly one of the reasons we do not see them is because there isn't enough peptone in our vaccine to produce a reaction. With our technic anaphylaxis does not seem to be of importance, even where we have given a second series of immunizating doses.

"I might say that we re-enlist men once in four years at the present time, and it has always been our custom to re-vaccinate against smallpox on re-enlistment and we are doing the same thing with typhoid, not because we feel the immunity has disappeared, but we do not want anything less than the maximum immunity for our men and if they are going down to Mexico they will need the maximum and not an average.

"In regard to the point relative to living vaccines: Metchnikoff and Besredka in the last few years have conducted very extensive experiments with typhoid in apes and they have found that in chimpanzees they can produce a typhoid fever by using clinical material; that is, suspension of feces containing typhoid bacilli as it comes from the patient. They found that by vaccinating them with sensitized living typhoid bacilli they were protected against these overwhelming infections, and on the strength of their experiments on 35 apes they conclude that the proper way to immunize against typhoid fever is with the living sensitized vaccine.

"Now, Metchnikoff and Besredka's work stands for itself. It is very evident that their conclusions as far as these apes are concerned are justified by the experiments, but whether you can apply it to man is a different question: whether one is justified in drawing fine conclusions on the basis of animal experimentation I do not know. Of course, you can draw general conclusions, but whether you can draw fine ones is a question. If we had only the experiments in 35 human beings to put against Metchnikoff's 35 apes we would not arrive anywhere, but we have about 200,000 human beings immunized against his 35 apes and we find that the dead vaccine *does* protect. It might not protect these 35 apes, but it protects human beings, and I do not think that for practical purposes a living sensitized vaccine will ever have any place in practical work, first, because our present vaccine is good. If it beats smallpox vaccine it is all right. If our present vaccine had failed we might have taken up Metchnikoff's, but there is no sense in dropping a good thing for something that is dangerous. Living vaccine has elements of danger in it, although it may be impossible to produce typhoid fever by injecting a living bacillus under the skin. Another thing, you cannot exclude contamination from living vaccines. You cannot sterilize living vaccine so that there would not be tetanus in it, streptococcus or staphylococcus or any other thing.

"There is for our purposes in the Army still another objection. It is more important for us to have 100 per cent. of the men immunized with dead vaccine than to have 50 per cent. immunized with living vaccine, for the time has not yet come when we can persuade cabinet officers to order every man to be vaccinated with living vaccine. They will order it if harmless, dead vaccines are used because we can assure them that no harm can come from it. That is the biggest objection. It is much better to have an army 99 per cent. immunized with dead vaccine than to have 50 per cent. immunized with live vaccine.

"These are the reasons why we have not used Metchnikoff's vaccine. We might use it on people who came to our laboratory or we might immunize ourselves and I have no doubt it will be used here and in other places by certain men competent to use it, but who would dare to put up 100,000 doses of living vaccine and send it out to every Tom, Dick and Harry to use?

"As to the reactions of physicians: It is rather curious that physicians do have bad reactions. I see it every year. In my class at the Army Medical School and at the George Washington University we get more severe reactions in physicians than among other people. People who have a bad reaction the first time might go on and take the other doses quite safely, as I have not known more than one severe reaction in any one person. We know that typhoid searches out the men who refuse the vaccine and the truth of this is astonishing. I see it all the time and get reports all the time. During the last two years that vaccination was voluntary in the Army Medical School we had one man in each class refuse to be vaccinated and he was the only man who came down with typhoid. That happened two successive years.

"Now, as to killing the vaccines: We can kill our vaccines with almost 100 per cent. regularity at 54° to 55° for one hour, but occasionally we do not kill every one and there will be a few colonies living. However, we find that tricresol when added kills those and we use the vaccine in spite of the fact that it has not been sterilized by heat. The few remaining colonies are killed by the tricresol and at the end of a few hours the vaccine is sterile. At first we did not think we could kill our vaccines at less than 60, but subsequently found we could kill them if our incubator was accurately regulated for 37°C. On the other hand, if the bacillus was grown at higher temperatures, say 38°, it took more heat to kill the cultures."

---

# BROOKLYN SOCIETY OF INTERNAL MEDICINE.

*Regular Meeting, March 28, 1913.*

The President, TASKER HOWARD, M.D., in the Chair.

### Remarks on Gastric Diseases. An Analysis of 800 Cases.

*By Dr. Harry W. Lincoln.*

*(See page 265.)*

DR. JOHN E. JENNINGS. in opening the discussion, said:—"I have listened with a great deal of interest to Dr. Cardwell's and Dr. Lincoln's papers. Dr. Cardwell's paper I am not in any way competent to discuss.

"In regard to Dr. Lincoln's discussion of the diseases of the stomach, or rather the varieties of dyspepsia, which come under the care of physicians and also sometimes under the care of surgeons: it seems proper first of all to define our field. We must, in the first place, remember that dyspepsia is somewhat different from abdominal distress in general and if we limit the discussion to dyspepsia, I think it will perhaps clarify matters a little.

"The surgeon recognizes forms of dyspepsia which originate from conditions outside of the stomach altogether; chronic appendicitis, gall-bladder disease, chronic intestinal obstruction and the two dyspepsias which originate in the stomach itself. The diagnosis of chronic appendicitis and gall stones

I shall not discuss. Those cases, when they can be diagnosed, present very fair surgical results.

"The diseases of the stomach which come under the care of the surgeon, we can also speak of in a somewhat limited way. There are a few conditions in the stomach which terminate fatally unless relieved. One of these is hemorrhage, but the surgeon no longer cares to interfere here.

"Perforation of a gastric ulcer is a surgical indication without doubt. I do not think there need be any discussion of that. When we come, however, to the true dyspepsias we begin to reach the borderline. It seems as if one could sometimes distinguish cases of almost absolute obstruction at the pylorus due to ulcer which, if unrelieved, would terminate in death. I have seen two cases at autopsy and several at the operating table in which the surgical operation brought relief, which were apparently going on to starvation. Those cases are often associated with a mass at the pylorus. They are nearly all associated with a true peristaltic wave and on opening the abdomen one finds an hyperthophied stomach wall and obstruction of the pylorus. These are the cases which are most adaptable for gastroenterostomy. In these cases I think one feels almost inclined to promise a cure. Other cases of pyloric obstruction are due to spasm which may be due to a reflex from conditions in the pelvis, kidney or intestinal tract. Some of them are due to ulceration in the duodenum; or to ulceration in the stomach itself. Certainly a very large number of cases of duodenal and gastric ulceration get well and stay well under medical treatment. Perhaps a larger number get well and have recurrent attacks. Perhaps a smaller number go on having symptoms while they develope true obstruction.

"The operation of gastroenterostomy in cases of duodenal ulcer in which relief by medical treatment has not been satisfactory, seems to promise from fifty to seventy-five per cent. of cures. In the rest of the cases operated upon recurrences will, no doubt, occur.

"In the cases of true gastric ulcer gastroenterostomy is of no particular benefit. Cases with an ulcer on the gastric side in which gastroenterostomy is done and subjected to starvation will, I think, in the main show a free period of six months or thereabouts which will be about the free period which they would get with medical care.

"In certain cases, the ulcer may be excised without undue risk. In others such an operation is attended with a heavy mortality, and it will often be wiser for the surgeon to abandon too extensive a resection rather than submit the patient to a risk that his partial disability does not warrant.

"The fact that this decision must be made during the operation should not obscure the issue."

DR. ALBERT F. R. ANDERSEN, in discussion, said:—"I have been very much interested in both papers this evening. I want to call particular attention to one point mentioned—the difficulty of making a differential diagnosis between duodenal and gastric ulcer. There are cases in which one can say 'This case is a duodenal ulcer.' This is especially true in cases with repeated attacks of melena, without hematemesis. We all see those cases occasionally, but in the majority of cases it is mighty difficult to make the diagnosis. The time of occurrence of the pain is the most spoken of point in differentiation.

"I have collected twelve cases which I saw before and after operation, of which only one was beyond the pylorus. These cases gave varying symptoms. Of the eight pyloric cases two had the pain early—less than one hour after eating, which is considered the pathognomonic symptom to differentiate gastric from duodenal ulcer. Three had the pain occurring one to two hours after eating, and in three, pain occurred two to three hours after meals. The one duodenal case had the pain coming on two hours after eating, well within the limit of the pyloric cases. Three ulcers of the fundus had pain two hours after eating.

"From the pain alone it is therefore hard to make a differential diagnosis between the duodenal and gastric cases. Some people say if the *tenderness* is a little to the right the case is a duodenal ulcer, but I do not believe that tenderness has very much to do with the location. Very often it is in the mid-epigastrium and to the left, even in the duodenal cases.

"I should like to ask Dr. Cardwell to explain the nervous mechanism of pain and tenderness in gastric and duodenal ulcers. I think that would clear up a good deal of this discussion about pain and tenderness being a differential point between gastric and duodenal ulcers. The amount of hypersecretion or hyperacidity does not have much bearing on differential diagnosis in these cases either. I did not bring this out particularly here in my summary. All of these cases were operated on for a definite indication. None were operated on just because they happened to have gastric ulcer. Four were operated on for obstruction at the pylorus. There were a few cases operated for persistent pain or persistent vomiting and they wanted to be relieved and had been under medical treatment for a long time. There were a couple which had had persistent hemorrhages which much weakened them and they were operated on between hemorrhages at their request.

Dr. Jennings brought up a point about cases with pyloric obstruction. I think, he said, we could promise a cure by doing a gastroenterostomy in those cases. Four of my cases had an obstruction at the pylorus and the three which had gastroenterostomy alone done had recurrence of all ulcer symptoms. In those which had recurrence of ulcer symptoms there must have been recurrence of the ulcer at the pylorus. Excision of the ulcer with gastrojijmostony, would seem to be the most rational operation where the patient's condition permits it."

Dr. O. A. Gordon, in discussion, said:—"I came to hear Dr. Lincoln's paper and have been very much gratified. I think there are some surgeons who are over enthusiastic and perhaps too ready to operate, and I think there are others who are too conservative. I do not think a case can be shown as a cure inside of a year. As Dr. Lincoln observed, a patient put to bed whether operated or not, and put on a restricted diet will improve. If you read the works of such men as Moynihan and the Mayos you certainly will become somewhat enthusiastic along the surgical line.

"I think there is a middle ground and that the internist should work along with the surgeon, and where there are symptoms of ulcer that are not relieved by medicine an exploratory laparotomy is much safer than to take the risk of waiting—and risking a possible perforation."

Dr. Jacob Horowitz, in discussion, said:—"I think it would be right for any medical man or gastroenterologist to decide when a person should go and be operated. Every medical man when a case of gastric disturbance presents itself should use every means to treat the case medically for a certain time and watch the progress of the case; and then if he sees in spite of medical treatment, there is no progress in the disease, the surgeon should be called in to help to relieve the patient."

---

# TRANSACTIONS OF THE BROOKLYN SURGICAL SOCIETY.

*Stated Meeting, February 6, 1913.*

The President, Richard W. Westbrook, M.D., in the Chair.

### A Case of Fracture and Dislocation of the Elbow-joint.

*Reported by Algernon T. Bristow, M.D.*

Last August this young gentleman received an injury to the elbow-joint which was a fracture of the external condyle with an outward dislocation of both bones of the forearm. The condition was not recognized at the time and I didn't see him until the end of the year, six months after the accident, when he was brought to me by his family physician.

This plate illustrates the condition of the elbow at the time. The articular surfaces were entirely separated, as you see. I have outlined here the surfaces. This is the internal condyle and both bones of the forearm were dislocated outwards and here is the external condyle which was broken off and shoved up.

The disability which he suffered from was this: The arm was fixed at a right angle and he was absolutely without the power of pronation or supination, and one feature of the case which was rather peculiar was the inability to extend the fingers, particularly the thumb and the first two fingers. The arm was practically useless.

I operated on him at St. Mary's Hospital, Jamaica, after the following manner: I saw at once that it was necessary to expose the whole lower surface of the humerus in order to thoroughly appreciate just exactly what had happened, and I did that in the following manner: I turned down a large U-shaped flap of skin, exposing the posterior surface of the arm for a considerable distance, and immediately divided the triceps muscle and turned it back and then by a little maneuvering the entire lower end of the humerus was exposed and I found that the fragment had gone right straight through the articular surfaces, filling up the olecranon fossa with callus as well as the coronoid fossa. With some difficulty I gouged away the callus in both fossæ until I had them in condition to receive the coronoid and olecranon processes respectively.

This line of callus (*indicating*) extends the tissue of the bones so that both the anterior and posterior surfaces of the articular surfaces and the cancellous tissue are without any cartilage whatever.

After some little difficulty and some further division of the soft parts I returned the dislocated structures to their place. In other words, I reduced the dislocation.

The problem which then confronted me was the prevention of ankylosis and I accomplished that, I think, by dividing a strip of the triceps muscle, leaving it attached to its tendon, and turning one piece into the coronoid fossa and another into the olecranon fossa, chiseling away the callus to restore the outline of the arm to something like normal and sewing the wound up with a drain.

A curious thing about the case was this: the very next morning on going to the hospital, the nurse said to me, "Why, doctor, he can already use his hand again!" He couldn't use it before, there being, as I said, an inability to extend the fingers.

During the course of the operation we deliberately exposed the ulnar nerve and kept it out of the way of any possible injury.

The only way in which I can explain the fact that his extensor power was limited is either that the displacement of the bones to the side stretched the posterior interosseus to such an extent that it interfered with adduction or else with the extensor muscles themselves by such a mechanical device that they were unable to act sufficiently, but the very next morning he was able to extend his fingers without difficulty.

This was done about two months ago and there is no question as far as the joint is concerned as to his getting perfectly free motion. He now has about two-thirds motion whereas owing to the absolute ankylosis he previously had no power of pronation or supination and no power of using the fingers.

The soft parts are holding the arm and we are now engaged in stretching them until we can get, as I expect, fully two-thirds motion of the arm. You may see here the scar of the original operation. If he has no more use of the arm than he has now he has an arm which is useful for all practical purposes, but my own judgment, inasmuch as there is nothing but soft tissues keeping the arm, is that in a year he will get pretty nearly free use of the arm.

I had two other cases of backward dislocation of the arm of long standing, one a case of two years' standing and the other a case of two months' standing. In these two cases I used somewhat different methods. In the first I sewed the olecranon process through and in that way managed to reduce the dislocation, and then I wired the fragments together. I have been unable to trace that case, but the last I heard of the case was that he had good use of the arm.

The other case was one of slight backward dislocation of both bones of the arm and I attacked that by two lateral incisions. This man is a night watchman and for that reason I could not get him to come here tonight. He has pretty nearly full use of the arm.

This was a very interesting and complicated fracture which fortunately came to me immediately after the accident. In this plate I show you the external condyle entirely displaced, as you see, with the ulna, and here you will see the internal condyle fractured and turned end for end. As you will see, when you examine the X-ray, it was an extremely complicated fracture. I cut down on that fragment after making an attempt to reduce it by ordinary means, and put a Lane plate on the external condyle. The internal condyle held fairly well. I do not think anything illustrates more conclusively the advantage of appreciating these injuries early and treating them early than the result which I got in this case and the result I have here. For comparison you may see that this patient has full use of the arm. She can move it up as far as the normal arm and she has full extension, whereas it is only about six weeks since the operation in the other case and you can see that he has perhaps two-thirds motion and there is absolutely smooth motion in the joint. He had no power in it before from ankylosis or filling up of either the coronoid or olecranon fossa. It is simply a matter of time when in my judgment he will get complete use of the arm.

This is a case which gave me a great deal of anxiety and much thought and certainly I think you will all agree that it was an extraordinary case.

This little lad when 3 years and 10 months old last March was run over the abdomen by one of Loeser's automobiles. I saw him about six o'clock in the evening. One of my friends had already passed a catheter and got nothing but blood. The lad was in an extremely serious condition. You could just count his pulse and no more and the question which presented itself to me was whether to abandon the case entirely or to give him whatever chance operative interference might offer, because it was perfectly evident that the only hope that could be held out for the child was in immediate operation. The situation was explained to the parents, one of them a colleague of mine, and they accepted operation with its risks. I took him to St. John's Hospital and sent for the professional anesthetist, which I think had a good deal to do with the happy outcome of the case. He anesthetized the boy and I made an immediate incision and entered a large cavity which I thought was the peritoneum, but I was surprised to find out that he had no intestines. No intestine could be seen anywhere and the cavity was filled with what appeared to be bloody fluid. I simply sponged this out and filled the bleeding area simply with hot gauze, because the problem which presented itself to me was to get him off the table alive. I opened the peritoneum above by an upper incision to make sure there was no injury to either spleen or kidney, and finding none I sutured it up and made a further exploration of the area already exposed. The bladder had been torn from its urethral attachment and with the ureters and peritoneum had been shoved up into the abdomen until the lower border of the peritoneal fold was parallel with the umbilicus. The two ureters stuck up like this (indicating) and as I looked down into the wound, confronting me was a tear into the bladder with what had once been its urethral opening.

The case was interesting from the operative standpoint, and the doctor has been kind enough to draw me a diagram of the operative procedure. The plates are numbered.

The red blood cell count was over 2,250,000 and the hemoglobin, I think, was down to 35 per cent. I therefore made no attempt whatever at repair, simply contenting myself with waiting until the red blood cell count went up to 4,000,000, which, I think, was a little over a week, and we then proceeded to the repair and the first thing I did was a perineal section. Now, you all know that in a child three and a half years of age this is rather delicate business. As soon as I made my section I found I could not get into the bladder at all, and on reopening the wound here I found the reason, which was quite simple. The bladder opening here was held and the bladder had become attached by adhesions in its false position in the pelvis. I rapidly swept my finger through and it went through the whole bladder, and recognizing the ureters, I proceeded with the operation. I found that any attempt at suturing the parts was out of the question because they were too smooth, and whatever I did in the way of repair had to be done with extreme rapidity; and this was what 1 did:

After I had my perineal section made I passed a catheter up through the urethra and passed it into the bladder in its false position, and having the ureter openings, I stitched the catheter to the bladder wound and then stitched up the bladder wound, which had extended beyond the original course of the urethral opening, and then, having the bladder, I pulled the urethra down and, turning the bladder into its appropriate position, I pulled the whole thing down until the urethral opening in the bladder was in contact with the original urethral tear and secured the bladder on each side of the ureters so as to anchor it. This, then, was the situation: here is the urethra torn through and here is the catheter in the bladder, and here is the urethral opening into the bladder with a tear which ran up this way and which was sutured. Now, I realized that that was not an altogether safe situation for the patient, and in order to get full control of the bladder opening, I then did a suprapubic cystotomy here and made an entirely independent opening through the bladder. I was dependent on the catheter with the attachment to the bladder to keep the parts in normal apposition, and it was therefore evident I should have to make an independent suprapubic opening.

The next plate illustrates the condition at the close of the operation. Here are the parts drawn together by the catheter, which was secured outside, and here is the suprapubic opening into the bladder. Fortunately, no fluid escaped. The little lad made a good recovery and here he is. He's not very big now, you see.

My policy in the future treatment of this case has been as follows: To depend largely on the increase in size of all the viscera, the bladder, urethra and so on, in order to get something like fair function finally. I am dependent on that. He accepted a No. 11 sound eight months ago; he now accepts a No. 14 without very much trouble. His present condition is as follows:

He has a small suprapubic urinary fistula about the size of a cambric needle and there is a very, curious phenomena connected with his urination which is this: this fistula has been closed for a period of eight weeks and when the fistula was closed he never urinated as well as when he has this microscopic opening the size of a cambric needle. He has passed as much as eight ounces of urine through the urethra, but less when this fistula is closed. He has two strictures, that is to say, a perineal stricture which puzzles me a little because it is entirely clean, and, of course, the typical stricture at the point of the tear in the bladder. If you will permit me, I shall read his father's memorandum:

"Present condition: Small suprapubic urinary fistula, in caliber the size of a cambric needle; stricture 3 inches posterior to the meatus. Second stricture, 5¼ inches posterior to meatus, one inch in length. In the upright position, 4 ounces residual urine; horizontal position, 1½ ounces residual urine. Expression of urine aided by suprapubic pressure performed by patient in both positions. Patient must be catheterized every alternate day to avoid pus in urine, in spite of continuous administration of 3 grains of urotropin daily."

That case still, of course, presents a very good many anxious problems to us. The first problem which presented itself was as to the nerve structures here. Was he going to have any power whatever of control of the bladder? I might add that there was no fracture of the pelvis at all. The next question was as to the other functions. I may say that we were very much gratified at finding he had bladder control and that he had sphincter power, so that so far that part of the matter is successfully ended. He has had erections, so that so far as that part of the injury is concerned it seems to be taking care of itself.

You can all see the difficult problem which still confronts us. My own solution of the problem at present is simply not to attempt any radical operation, but to trust to years. As he grows older, the bladder itself grows larger and the urethra grows larger, I think he will show marked improvement. Six or seven months ago he only accepted a No. 10 sound; he now accepts a No. 14, and as the parts grow with his years I think further operation will be unnecessary. It seemed to me that the part of wisdom is not to do any more active operation at this time, but to wait until the indications are such as to make me conclude it is possible to interfere. His father has sometimes thought he might have a hydro-ureter, because when the fistula closes he has a pain in his side. I hardly think that is possible. Of course, if he were older we could settle that very easily by cystascopy, but for the present it seems to me the wise thing to do is to let him grow up a little. Sounds are being passed once or twice a week. He is in good health apparently, lively and active, and he certainly is a credit to youth.

DR. MATHIAS FIGUEIRA opened the discussion on Dr. Bristow's case, and said:—"It seems to me that the case which Dr. Bristow presented is a case of traumatic rupture of the membranous urethra with the consequences which always follow it. You know the triangular ligament will prevent the blood and urine from going forward or backward and that is just what happened here. The blood centered and pushed them back and the bladder up, and the condition which Dr. Bristow found was the natural condition that follows in these cases and I think that the operative result would have been better in this case if the blood had been given outlet to the perineum and the bladder would have come down in place and could have been reached through the urethra."

DR. ALGERNON T. BRISTOW, in discussion, said:—"Did I understand Dr. Figueira to say that this was simply a rupture of the membranous urethra?"

DR. MATHIAS FIGUEIRA, answering Dr. Bristow's question as to whether he understood Dr. Figueira to have said that the case was one of rupture of the membranous urethra, said:—"Yes, sir."

DR. ALGERNON BRISTOW, in closing the discussion, said:—"I have seen the same thing happen once before. The bladder is torn from its urethral attachments and the perineum is shoved right up into the peritoneal cavity, stripping the perineum from the anterior abdominal wall. The same thing happened to a conductor some years ago. He was on the running-board of an open car and was struck in the side by the shaft of a business wagon and the same thing happened to him, except that he had a fracture of the pelvis, and in his case the ureters and everything, as in the case of this little lad, were stripped from their normal course. That is more than a tear of the membranous urethra. Of course, the ureters themselves were dislocated and were presented vertically on opening the wound. It was done at the time of the accident.

"I think Dr. Delatour can enlighten us on that point, as I know he has had a couple of similar cases recently."

*(Concluded in August Journal.)*

# ebical Society of the County of Kings

## MONTHLY BULLETIN TO MEMBERS

NDER the direction of the Council this Bulletin is issued every month (except July, Aug. and Sept.). It is the purpose of the Council, rough this medium, to keep the members advised all matters pertaining to the Society's work, its rious activities, its membership, and other subjects general interest.

Items of general interest to the Society and pernal notes concerning its members are invited and ould reach the Secretary not later than 4 P. M. the 20th of each month. Address all communitions to the Society's Building, 1313 Bedford Ave., rooklyn, N. Y.

## MEDICAL SOCIETY OF THE COUNTY OF KINGS.

313 Bedford Avenue, Brooklyn, New York.

Telephone: 126 Bedford.

HE Medical Society of the County of Kings (organized 1822) owns its plant, valued at $100,000, and located at 1313-1315 edford Avenue. In addition to an auditoum (seating 400) and various smaller meetg rooms, offices, etc., the greater part of the iilding is devoted to the Society's medical brary of 60,000 volumes. There are only ree larger medical libraries on this continent. the ample reading rooms over 600 current edical journals are regularly on file.

Through its public and scientific meetings, s Library, its Milk Commission, and its manild activities for the spread of medical knowlge, the promotion of scientific education, the nity of the medical profession, and the safearding of the public health, the Medical Soety of the County of Kings should enlist the tive support and co-operation of every putable physician in the county who is enged in regular practice.

## MEMBERSHIP.

*Qualifications for Membership.*—Extracts om the Constitution and By-Laws governing embership (Chapter XVI) are as follows: SEC. 1. Membership in the Society may be tained by physicians in good standing, residg in the County of Kings, and duly licensed d recorded in the office of the County Clerk Kings County, in the following manner: EC. 2. Applications for membership shall be ade on blanks furnished by the Medical Soety signed by the applicant and endorsed by o members of the County Society. Such lanks shall be sent to the Secretary, who shall resent them to the Board of Censors for investigation and report. SEC. 3. If the candi-

date be accepted the Council shall so report to the Society at a stated meeting, and after the next succeeding stated meeting the President shall declare said candidate a member. SEC. 4. Every person thus admitted resident member shall, within three months after due notification of his election, pay an initiation fee of five dollars and the assessment of the Medical Society of the State of New York for the current year, sign the By-Laws or forfeit his election."

*Blank Application Forms for Membership* may be obtained on request at the Society's Building. This form should be filled out by the applicant, signed by him, his proposer and his seconder, and returned to the Secretary.

*Dues.*—New members pay an initiation fee of $5 plus $3 (the State assessment for the current year) and are exempt from the payment of further dues until the next annual meeting after their election.

The regular annual dues are $10 plus $3 (the State assessment for the current year), payable on the first day of February. All members who have not paid on or before the first day of May shall be placed on the list of members in arrears and so reported to the Society, and shall not receive the publications, or notices of meetings, or defense for suits for malpractice until their dues are paid. All members who fail to pay their arrears on or before December 31st shall be dropped from the roll of membership (CHAPTER XV of By-Laws).

*Advantages of Membership.*—Affiliation with your confreres in the representative medical organization of your County, participation in the Society's meetings and varied activities, and proprietary interest in its property and magnificent library, membership in the Medical Society of the State of New York and the Second District Branch; monthly receipt of the *New York State Journal of Medicine* and the Society's own publications, a copy yearly of the *Medical Directory of New York, New Jersey and Connecticut;* free defense to the court of last resort of all suits for alleged malpractice; eligibility to membership in the American Medical Association.

## STATED MEETINGS.

Regular stated meetings of the Society are held in the Society's Building, 1313 Bedford Ave., at 8.30 P. M., on the third Tuesday of every month (except July, August and September). Light refreshments are served at the social hour which follows the scientific program of each meeting.

## THE LIBRARY.

The Library (60,000 vols.) of the Society is open daily (Sundays and Legal Holidays excepted), from 10 A. M. to 10 P. M. For the purposes of reference it is free to the public. Members of the Society have the privilege of borrowing books. Trained librarians are always in attendance to help and direct readers who desire such assistance.

## DIRECTORY FOR GRADUATE NURSES.

For the benefit of the profession and the general public the Society maintains a Directory for Graduate Nurses, where reliable graduate nurses (male and female), masseurs and masseuses may be procured. There is no fee for securing a nurse through the Society's Directory, which is always open, day and night. Telephone 126 Bedford.

## THE COUNCIL.

*President*—JAMES M. WINFIELD, 47 Halsey St.
*Vice-President*—J. RICHARD KEVIN.
*Secretary*—CLAUDE G. CRANE, 121 St. James Pl.
*Associate Secretary*—BURTON HARRIS.
*Treasurer*—JOHN R. STIVERS, 180 Lefferts Pl.
*Associate Treasurer*—STEPHEN H. LUTZ.
*Directing Librarian*—FREDERICK TILNEY.

### Trustees.

ONSLOW A. GORDON, *Chairman,* 71 Halsey St.
JOSHUA M. VAN COTT.     JOHN O. POLAK.
JOHN C. MACEVITT.         ELIAS H. BARTLEY.

### Censors.

JOHN A. LEE, *Senior Censor,* 23 Revere Pl.
WALTER A. SHERWOOD.     JOHN G. WILLIAMS.
CHARLES EASTMOND.         J. STURDIVANT READ.

## CHAIRMEN OF STANDING COM-MITTEES.

*Membership*—EDWARD E. CORNWALL, 1218 Pacific St.
*Directory for Nurses*—CALVIN F. BARBER, 57 So. Oxford St.
*Entertainment*—ALFRED POTTER, 491 Eighth St.
*Historical*—WILLIAM SCHROEDER, 339 President St.
*Legislative*—HENRY G. WEBSTER, 364 Washington Ave.
*Public Health*—J. M. VAN COTT, 188 Henry St.
*Visiting*—JAMES W. FLEMING, 471 Bedford Ave.
*Milk Commission*—ALFRED BELL, 37 Linden St.
*Attendance*—ALBERT M. JUDD, 375 Grand Ave.

In the conduct of the affairs of the Society the officers hope that they may have not only the frequent suggestions of members, which are heartily invited, but also their practical and loyal co-operation.

*Supt. and Librarian*—ALBERT T. HUNTINGTON.
*Counsel*—WILLIAM E. BUTLER, Esq.
*Prosecuting Attorneys*—Messrs. ALMUTH C. VAN DIVER and JOHN G. DYER. 37 Wall St., New York City.

## MINUTES OF STATED MEETI

### JUNE 17, 1913.

The President, Dr. James M. Winfie the chair.
There were about 80 present.
The meeting was called to order a P. M. and the minutes of the previous ing were read and approved.

*Report of Council.*

The Council reported favorably upo following applications for membership:

Alfred C. Beck, Long Island College Ho
Geo. F. Buttschardt, 222 St. Nicholas A
Harry Cleveland Harris, 25 Stuyvesant
Edward B. Haslam, 71 Oakland St.
Samuel Linder, 1780 St. John's Pl.
Joseph Rosenthal, 572 Fifth St.
Carl Schumann, 116 Prospect Pl.
Walter T. Slevin, 65 Eighth Ave.
Alvarez H. Smith, 382 Carlton Ave.
Purvis Alex. Spain, 911 Greene Ave.
Wm. Alfred Sprenger, 1106 Bushwick A

## ELECTION OF MEMBERS.

The following, duly proposed and ac by the Council, were declared elected to membership:

Geo. Francis Hoch, 523 Throop Ave.
John L. Madden, 262 Schermerhorn St.
Thomas Joseph Kearns, 1490 Pacific St.
Luther F. Warren, L. I. C. H.
Henry Wolfer, 678 Bedford Ave.

## APPLICATIONS FOR MEMBERS

Applications for membership were rec from the following:

David Feiner, Williamsburgh Hospital; & Bell, 1912; proposed by H. A. V seconded by E. E. Cornwall.
Louis Fisher, 318 Pennsylvania Ave.; C. H., 1911; proposed by T. Howard onded by Memb. Com.
Charles Goldman, 238 Nostrand Ave.; C. H., 1911; proposed by J. E. Jenr seconded by Memb. Com.
Frank D. Jennings, 53 Woodbine St.; P. N. Y., 1902; proposed by J. E. Gol seconded by J. G. Williams.
Henry John Kohlmann, 532 State St.; C. H., 1907; proposed by J. S. Read onded by A. L. Carroll.
Samuel Parnass, 1218 Herkimer St.; C. H., 1911; proposed by T. Howard onded by Memb. Com.
R. S. Robertson, 271 Jefferson Ave; Co 1910; proposed by J. L. Moore; seco by W. H. Lohman.

## EXECUTIVE SESSION.

The President stated that the committee on the President's address had recommended that the chair appoint a committee of 50 on Ways and Means. This committee had been appointed and had held a meeting, the report of which would appear later.

The chair requested the Society to empower him to increase the committee from time to time as occasion may arise. Granted.

## COMMITTEE ON WAYS AND MEANS.

| | |
|---|---|
| C. F. Barber. | J. P. Glynn. |
| E. H. Bartley. | R. A. Henderson. |
| S. E. Blatteis. | O. P. Humpstone. |
| A. H. Bogart. | Henry Joachim. |
| B. G. Blackmar. | J. R. Kevin. |
| W. C. Braislin. | J. C. Kennedy. |
| T. M. Brennen. | William Linder. |
| Wm. Browning. | Leon Louria. |
| S. C. Blaisdell. | E. H. Mayne. |
| Alfred Bell. | J. C. MacEvitt. |
| G. R. Butler. | T. H. MacKinnon. |
| W. F. Campbell. | J. A. McCorkle. |
| C. N. Cox | S. J. McNamara. |
| Raymond Clark. | L. S. Pilcher. |
| W. J. Cruikshank. | J. O. Polak. |
| G. J. Doyle. | J. R. Stivers. |
| H. B. Delatour. | W. A. Sherwood. |
| H. W. Dangler. | E. L. Swan. |
| W. L. Duffield. | Fred. Tilney. |
| Roger Durham. | J. M. Van Cott. |
| Cameron Duncan. | J. P. Warbasse. |
| J. W. Fleming. | J. S. Waterman. |
| R. S. Fowler. | R. W. Westbrook. |
| H. A. Fairbairn. | H. A. Wade. |
| O. A. Gordon. | J. G. Williams. |
| N. P. Geis. | J. M. Winfield. |

Dr.. Thomas Dixon stated that the Kings County Medical Society, the New York County Society and the State Society had not opposed in any way the Seeley Bill, which, he stated, was very detrimental to the welfare of the practicing physician. He moved that the Council of the Society be censured for not making active opposition to this bill. Motion not seconded.

Dr. Henry G. Webster, Chairman of the Committee on Legislation, stated that the Legislative Committees of the Kings County Medical Society, the New York County Society, The Nassau-Queens County Society and the State Society had made active opposition to the bill with the result that the bill had not been passed.

## SCIENTIFIC SESSION.

(Arranged by the Brooklyn Society of nal Medicine.)

1. Presentation of a Patient with von licz's Disease. (10 min.)
   By William Lintz, M.D.
   Discussion by E. E. Cornwall.
2. "The Interpretation of Blood P Readings." (10 min.)
   By Henry G. Webster, M.D.
   Discussion by Horace Greeley, A. Hutchinson, Bernhard A. Murette F. DeLorme.
3. "When and How to Use Nitrogl (9 min.)
   By Edward E. Cornwall, M.D.
   Discussion by Bernhard A. Fedd
4. "Strophanthin as a Last Resort." (
   By Darwin W. Waugh, M.D.
   Discussion by B. S. Antonowsky
5. "Comparative Heat Radiations wi and Cold Sponges in Typhoid." (
   By Cassius H. Watson, M.D.
   Discussion by Wm. H. Cary.
6. "Phenolsulphonephthalein Test of Sufficiency." (6 min.)
   By Henry F. Kramer, M.D.
7. General Discussion (limited to 3 min

On motion, a vote of thanks was t the Brooklyn Society of Internal N for the interesting program.

Adjourned 10.45 P. M.

CLAUDE G. CRANE, *Secr*

*The Council of the Medical Society County of Kings desires to express found sorrow in the death of Dr. Wil Dudley.*

Dr. Dudley served faithfully this and the Medical Society of the Co Kings for many years. He was a from 1903 to 1905; the Senior Cen 1908; the Chairman of the Commi Membership for the years 1901 to delegate to the Medical Society of th of New York; and a generous contrit the Society's Library.

His courteous manner, unfailing k his abnegation of self in his work Society, endeared him to all who wer nate enough to come in contact w lovable personality.

To a sorrowing family the Council Medical Society offers its heartfelt con

It is directed that this expression Council's sorrow be recorded on its N that a copy be forwarded by the Secr Dr. Dudley's bereaved family, and th resolutions be published in the LONG MEDICAL JOURNAL.

# LONG ISLAND
# MEDICAL JOURNAL

VOL. VII.        AUGUST, 1913        No. 8

## ©riginal Articles.

### THE JUNE MEETING.
### REPORT OF THE SECRETARY.
#### James Cole Hancock, M.D.,
of Brooklyn, N. Y.

THE Forty-sixth Regular Meeting of the Associated Physicians of Long Island was held at Cold Spring Harbor, June 14, 1913, and was attended by nearly one hundred guests and members. The meeting was called to order at 3 o'clock with the president, Dr. Samuel Hendrickson, in the chair. The reading of the minutes of the previous meeting was omitted as they had already been published. The president presented his address which appears in another part of this number. Dr. Winfield's motion that the chair appoint a committee of three to consider the president's address and report at the October meeting was carried and the President appointed Doctors Winfield, Browning and Delatour.

Dr. Warren L. Duffield submitted the report of the Membership Committee as follows·

*Proposed by Howard W. Neail.*

Adolph A. Auger, 215 Fulton St., Jamaica..........Buffalo, 1887
Henry Archibald Fisher, 25 Bergen Ave., Jamaica.P. & S. N. Y., 1906
Bruce Frary Halsey, 47 Union Ave., Jamaica........Louisville, 1901
T. F. McCarthy, 5 Ray St., Jamaica................Harvard, 1896

*Proposed by George F. Sammis.*

Waldemar T. Browne, 62 Rugby Road, Brooklyn...L. I. C. H., 1908

*Proposed by Russell S. Fowler.*

Leander A. Newman, 190 Main St., Port Washington..Cornell, 1908

*Proposed by Frank T. DeLano.*

Harry L. Borland, Lynbrook.....................N. Y. U., 1895

*Proposed by Alfred Bell.*

Louis Lippman Cohen, 760 Bushwick Ave., Brooklyn.L. I. C. H., 1898

*Proposed by James Cole Hancock.*

Robert F. Barber, 191 Lefferts Pl., Brooklyn.......L. I. C. H., 1908
J. Evan Shuttleworth, 427 Lincoln Ave., Richmond Hill,
                                          N. Y. Hom., 1904

*Proposed by Warren L. Duffield.*

Edward Montgomery Wellbery, 218 Sixth Ave., Brooklyn.Cornell, 1907
Howard B. Snell, 301 Clinton St., Brooklyn.......L. I. C. H., 1899
Alexander L. Anderson, 467 Ninth St., Brooklyn....L. I. C. H., 1898
Charles G. O'Connor, 980 St. Marks Ave., Brooklyn.P. & S. N. Y., 1899
Judson P. Pendleton, 91 Sixth Ave., Brooklyn....P. & S. N. Y., 1898
Paul L. Parrish, 1030 Bergen St., Brooklyn......Bell. N. Y., 1898
George H. Smith, 235 Hancock St., Brooklyn......L. I. C. H., 1898
Eugene H. Goodfellow, 5704 14th Ave., Brooklyn......Albany, 1894
John J. Masterson, 4721 Ft. Hamilton P'kway, Bklyn..L. I. C. H., 1908
Alfred Winfield White, 360 Halsey St., Brooklyn.....Cornell, 1905
David Livingston, 323 72d St., Brooklyn..........L. I. C. H., 1905
Joseph L. Moore, 175 Sixth Ave., Brooklyn.......Univ. Penna., 1908
George Armon Clark, 348A Ninth St., Brooklyn....L. I. C. H., 1898
Wesley H. Wallace, 516 Ninth St., Brooklyn....Virginia Med., 1899
Binford Throne, 2 Macon St., Brooklyn............Nashville, 1899
William V. Pascual, 691 St. Marks Ave., Brooklyn.P. & S. N. Y., 1900
Tracy E. Clark, 85 Halsey St., Brooklyn.........L. I. C. H., 1900
George W. Beatty, 204 Hancock St., Brooklyn......L. I. C. H., 1898
James G. Ditmars, 510 Ninth St., Brooklyn........L. I. C. H., 1898
Frederick J. McCammon, 139 Decatur St., Brooklyn...Queens, 1892

The Secretary was instructed to cast one vote for the above applicants.

Dr. William H. Ross made a short and favorable statement concerning the affairs of the LONG ISLAND MEDICAL JOURNAL and was followed by Dr. Edwin S. Moore who reported the finances of the Society in a most satisfactory condition. Dr. H. Beeckman Delatour reported progress from the Committee on Humanics stating instances in which consents had been given for autopsies and referring to one case in which a will had been made containing a request for an autopsy after death.

The resignations of Dr. David F. Lucas, of Brooklyn, and Dr. J. L. Bulkley, Jr., formerly of Richmond Hill, were received and accepted with regret.

Owing to the fact that the treasurer has to meet all financial obligations of the LONG ISLAND MEDICAL JOURNAL as well as to the fact that at present he is business manager of the JOURNAL the president, deeming the treasurer of much more practical importance to the Publication Committee than the secretary, gave notice that at the October meeting he would move to amend the By-Laws so that the treasurer should take the place of the secretary as a member of the Publication Committee.

Dr. Walter A. Sherwood, Chairman of the Scientific Committee opened the scientific session by introducing Dr. Cass B. Davenport of the Experimental Station of Cold Spring Harbor who gave a most interesting talk upon the subject of "The Physician as Eugenist." At the close of the address Dr. William Browning proposed that Dr. Davenport be made an honorary member of the society. This motion being seconded the president asked for a rising vote which was given with enthusiasm. There was a short discussion of the address by Dr. J. J. Kindred.

An interesting trip through the various branches of the station followed the scientific session. The guests and members were then conveyed to the site of the clam-bake which all seemed to thoroughly enjoy.

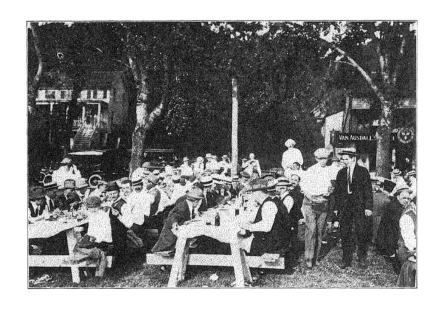

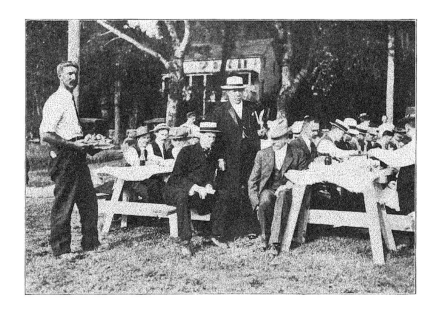

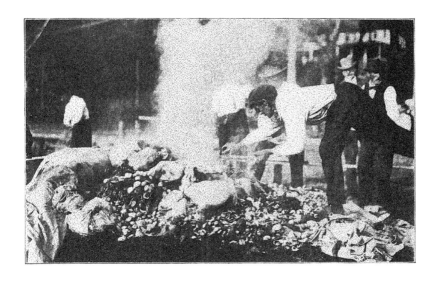

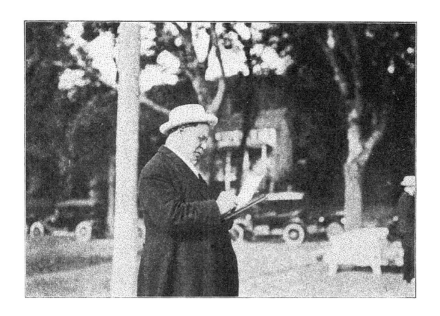

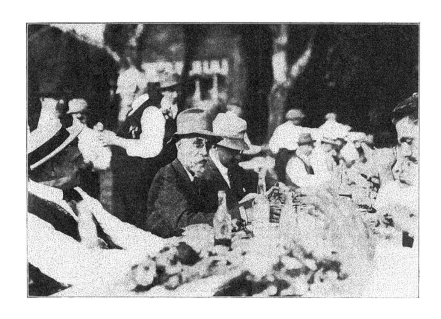

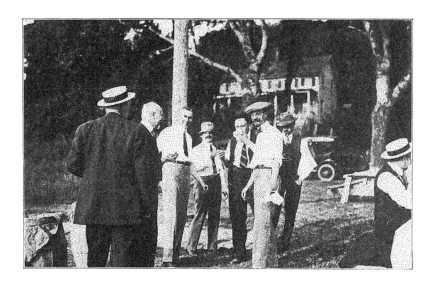

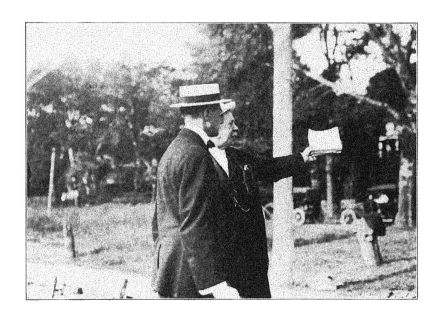

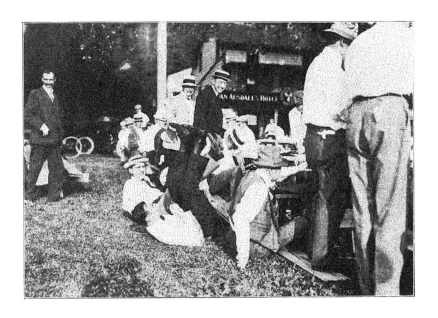

# PRESIDENT'S ADDRESS.

## Samuel Hendrickson, M.D.,

of Jamaica, N. Y.

THIS Association is in a class by itself, with just enough of the social element to stand for good fellowship. That you are a lot of good fellows is proven by the fact that during the fifteen years of its existence not a single event has occurred to mar the harmony of your organization. To know that the scientific end is not neglected you have but to refer to your scientific programs and your JOURNAL. Yours has been a steadily progressive prosperity in numbers and financially. You have as members of this Association men who will rank with the best in all this broad land. You have a medical journal which is self-supporting and second to none in the character of its articles.

All of this counts for the highest degree of success. To give proper dignity to a medical society of this magnitude and standing I would make of it an academy of medicine. You certainly meet all the requirements. You have the nucleus of a library which is bound to grow with proper care and attention in a reasonable time and if you gentlemen will remember when making your will to bequeath your medical books to this association you will help along the good work and leave a lasting memento of your kindliness, and even now if you have a book here or there for which you have no further use send them along and they will be gratefully acknowledged. You are a powerful organization capable of bringing about many needed reforms, and your opportunities are almost without limitation. One of the most pressing needs just now is a complete revolution in the existing hospital system. There are too many poorly equipped, poorly managed, and poorly financed institutions which claim and receive credit for doing a large amount of charity work that is practically all done by the physician. There should be a complete separation of the private and charity institutions. They are entirely different propositions and the combination ought never to have existed.

The care of the sick poor is an obligation which rests on every community and every municipality ought to be compelled by law to provide and maintain charity hospitals of sufficient number and proportions to properly care for all of their resident population who may be ill and too poor to employ a physician, and any physician rendering professional services to any of these institutions should be paid for his service. These institutions should be entirely removed from the domain of politics and should be governed by a board of managers selected from the various medical universities of the district.

The necessity for this is shown by the developments of recent investigation. One of the charity hospitals was called a veritable slaughter house by one of the investigators, a condition not at all creditable to a great city, nor one to call for an attitude of dignified silence on the part of the medical profession.

The private hospital on the other hand belongs to the doctor. It is a part of his general outfit and should be owned by him either individually or collectively. Any physician sending a private patient to a hospital ought to have sufficient financial interest in the institution to be able to control the situation. In this way only can the highest results be attained.

The inefficiency and lax enforcement of our immigration laws ought to receive more than passing notice. We are receiving into this country every year thousands of cases of tuberculosis, syphilis, defective mentality and insanity that never ought to be allowed to land. This is decidedly against the welfare of our race and serious injurious effects are bound to result before many years. That a chain is no stronger than its weakest link is emphasized by the fact that it is now possible for any member of an alien crew, including cabin boys and waiters, to go on shore without inspection and remain if he feel so disposed.

Thirty thousand immigrants came into this port during the last week of May. Any one conversant with methods used knows just how much individual inspection that thirty thousand received. It seems almost folly to work along preventive lines when bad conditions are increasing by leaps and bounds. This country is certainly an easy mark and it would seem as though every nation on the face of the earth was taking advantage of it. When and where will it end?

Last, but not least, I want to congratulate you on the remarkable success of your JOURNAL. Through the arduous efforts and perseverance of your publication committee it is now self-supporting and in all probability by the end of the year will show a balance in its favor and I hope that next year will see it a bi-monthly instead of a monthly publication.

---

## SOME SURGICAL SEQUELAE OF PNEUMONIA.*

### By William Francis Campbell, M.D.,
of Brooklyn, N. Y.

THE surgical sequelæ of pneumonia are manifestations of the pneumococcus infection in other tissues than the lungs.

It is well to appreciate the important fact that "the pneumococcus which in the lungs only rarely produces suppuration does so with great frequency when it attacks the serous membranes." It has also been the writer's experience that these secondary infections occur most frequently in children. Hence in these secondary infections we note the predilection of the pneumococcus for serous membranes and for young tissue.

Let me illustrate this proposition by the recital of some typical cases:

CASE I.—Boy, 7 years old, came into the hospital complaining of pain in the left chest and difficulty in breathing. For the past three weeks had been treated by a physician for pneumonia. The symptoms presented were fever, cough, difficulty in breathing, night sweats, extreme thirst, and a preference for lying on the left side. On inspection there was marked deformity in comparing the two sides of the chest. The elasticity of the child's thorax readily accommodates itself to intrathoracic pressure.

The physical signs were those of a left sided pleuritic effusion. On introducing the exploring needle a small quantity of

---

* Read before the Kings County Medical Society, April 15, 1913.

creamy pus was withdrawn which upon examination proved to be a pneumococcus infection. A subsequent resection of the rib and opening of the pleura disclosed a large quantity of thick creamy pus which was successfully drained and the boy made an uneventful recovery.

This case is typical of a group which are extremely interesting because of the frequency with which they are met, and therefore deserve special consideration. A word concerning the prognosis and treatment may not be amiss.

Remember that the metapneumonic pleuritic effusions in children are usually purulent, and that 75 per cent. of these empyemas owe their origin to the pneumococcus.

The prognosis of pneumococcus empyema is most favorable. Spontaneous cures have occured (a) by absorption of the pus; (b) by discharge into the bronchi, when it is vomited and coughed up; (c) by discharge through an external opening after perforation of the thoracic wall (empyema necessitatus).

While this spontaneous evolution of empyema in the child is not at all exceptional, it should not deter the surgeon from prompt evacuation of the pus by operative measures. A high mortality is the penalty of procrastination, or at best a crippled lung, or contraction of the chest which results in a pronounced scoliosis. Early operative intervention is the only rational procedure in order to prevent septic poisoning and secondary deformities.

In the management of these cases there are two distinct methods to be chosen, each method having its special indications. The choice of procedure requires surgical discrimination together with a proper estimate of the patient's vital index and therapeutic possibilities.

*First: Resection of the rib may be indicated.*—Resection of the rib is indicated in strong children above two years of age. The writer avoids a general anesthesia if possible. It is often superfluous and always dangerous. A local anesthesia (novocain or stovain) is sufficient for the operation which requires only a few minutes.

After removal of the rib the pleura is opened by a sharp-nosed artery clamp and enlarged to admit the index finger. The inserted finger regulates the flow of pus so that it is removed slowly.

Irrigation is not only superfluous, it is useless and often harmful.

Rubber drainage tubes are placed in the wound and securely fastened to prevent them being sucked into the pleural cavity, an accident not infrequent and always disagreeable.

The duration of the discharge varies—in the most favorable cases it ceases after a few weeks, in unfavorable cases it may exist for a long time. It is well to remember that the *earlier the resection is made, the quicker the lung expands and suppuration ceases.*

A second method of treatment is by *intermittent aspiration.* In very young children with lowered vitality the author prefers repeated aspiration with the injection of a two per cent. solution of formalin in glycerine as the safest procedure. The aspirations are repeated daily, going down one intercostal space as the pus recedes, until no more pus is found. Every third day an ounce of a two per cent. solution of formalin in glycerine is injected. This method gives excellent results in small children since it removes only a portion of the pus at a seance, and thus allows the lung to slowly expand and fill the space. On the other hand a total removal is often followed by rapid exudation and an enormous loss of serum into the empty cavity, which is a serious drain on the vital forces.

CASE 2.—Girl, 3 years old, was sent to the hospital with a painful and swollen knee. The local symptoms were those of an acute inflammatory process. Temperature 103. The history showed that four weeks previously the patient had been treated for pneumonia. The local process started 48 hours before entering the hospital. The joint was aspirated and a small quantity of milky fluid withdrawn in which the pneumococci were found. The joint was freely opened and drained, and the patient made a perfect recovery.

The writer has recently observed two cases of acute suppuration around the joint (periarthritis) which followed bronchopneumonia though the pneumococcus was not demonstrated. This is the class of cases, be it said to the chagrin of the medical profession, which not only has been, but is, being diagnosed as "rheumatism." Alas! what therapeutic crimes have been committed in the name of "rheumatism." It is responsible for more disabled joints and crippled bones and fatalities in childhood than is yet fully appreciated.

CASE 3.—Girl, 11 years old, came to the hospital complaining of severe pain in the abdomen. Her trouble began ten days previously with severe pain over the entire abdomen followed by vomiting, elevation of temperature and diarrhea. A physician was called in attendance two days later who diagnosed the complaint as appendicitis and advised operation after the pain subsided.

During the next week she was treated with vaccines which were administered four times during the week. After a few days the pain, vomiting and fever subsided, but the local abdominal conditions presented a tumefaction just below the umbilicus, and the patient became cachetic. At the end of ten days the pain again became severe, the swelling pronounced, and the mass fluctuating. Another physician was called and advised that the patient be sent to the hospital. On admission to the hospital it was learned that four weeks previous to her present trouble she suffered an attack of pneumonia from which she was apparently convalescing when the above detailed abdominal symptoms appeared.

On admission the patient's temperature was 104, pulse 135, respiration 35. The abdomen was extremely tender, and there was a well-defined ovoid tumor extending from the symphysis to the umbilicus. So much did this mass simulate an over-distended bladder that the patient was catheterized previous to operation as a preliminary precaution.

Incision into the mass showed it to be a collection of thick, creamy, odorless pus with numerous fibrin flakes. The exudate was well walled off and had no connection with the appendical region. Pneumococci were found in the pus. After a long siege of drainage the wound finally healed and the patient left the hospital at the end of ten weeks.

This was evidently a typical case of pneumococcus peritonitis and is deserving of more than passing notice. The rarity of this affection should stimulate observers to report their cases. Besides being an exceedingly rare affection, it has a special predilection for children, usually between the second and twelfth years, and is much more frequent in girls.

It is a specific infection of the peritoneum, secondary to some pre-existing pneumococcic lesion, such as a pleuro-pneumonia or an otitis media. The so-called primary form is simply the use of an illogical term to indicate that the mode of infection is obscure.

The action of the pneumococcus on serous membranes presents two peculiarities. It produces abundant suppuration and a precipitation of considerable fibrin, so that suppuration tends to become encysted. We note, therefore, that cases fall into two distinct groups, the encysted and the diffuse forms. The *encysted form* is the clinical type most frequently found in young children. The encapsulated pus is generally found beneath the anterior abdominal wall, in the median line, below the umbilicus. This pus pocket may increase so as to form an enormous cavity pushing the intestines aside and walling itself off with a whitish gray membrane.

The character of the exudate is usually thick, creamy, greenish-yellow, and odorless, and presents numerous fibrin flakes.

The *diffuse form* is rarer, more difficult to recognize and the prognosis is much more grave. Here there is no limiting membrane and the pus is scattered throughout the abdomen. It is well to keep in mind, however, that pneumococcus peritonitis is the least grave form of acute peritonitis.

*Symptoms.*—In the encapsulated form the onset is sudden, intense abdominal pain, at first diffuse, and later centering about the umbilicus; vomiting, fever and diarrhea, characterized by its fetid odor. The general train of symptoms are those of the acute abdomen. After a few days the pain, vomiting and fever abate, but the local abdominal conditions become more pronounced; the abdomen is distended, and there is distinct swelling in the umbilical region; the child appears cachetic. It is well to note, however, that there is no muscular rigidity. Aften ten or twelve days the pain begins again, there is pronounced swelling, fluctuation and occasional edema of the abdominal wall in the region of the umbilicus, and if the process is not interrupted, the skin is finally perforated and a quantity of pus is discharged. Thus the progress of the disease is in cycles, recognized by peritoneal invasion, accumulation of pus, and spontaneous rupture.

In the diffuse form, the onset is likewise sudden, abdominal pain, vomiting, diarrhea and fever; but the symptoms are all accentuated, the prostration is intense and death may occur in forty-eight hours. As Stone observes, "The picture of peritonitis develops with interesting qualifications, rigidity as a rule being far less marked than the other symptoms would seem to justify, and there is diarrhea instead of constipation." The prognosis is grave and the results fatal unless the tide is stemmed by early operation.

*Diagnosis.*—It is evident that the encysted form presents a clinical picture which simulates appendicitis and with which it may be easily confused.

Note, however, that while the onset is the same in the two affections, in pneumococcus peritonitis the pain is more diffused,

there is diarrhea rather than constipation, and the muscular rigidity of appendicitis is absent. In tuberculous peritonitis the fetid
diarrhea is rare, the swelling evolutes more slowly, the lesion is
less circumscribed, the masses are isolated and there is evidence
of ascitic fluid. In the diffused form the diagnosis is always difficult, but the indications are never obscure and no time need be
spent upon the etiology when the indications for surgical intervention are so apparent.

The treatment of either form is laparotomy and drainage.
The incision should be made in the median line below the umbilicus. The pus is gently evacuated, no irrigation, drainage tubes
are placed so as to reach the deepest possible point. In the
encysted form the prognosis is good; in the diffuse form the prognosis is always grave.

## NOTES ON THE USE OF TUBERCULIN IN THE TREATMENT OF ADVANCED PULMONARY TUBERCULOSIS.

By Wm. H. Lohman, M.D.,

of Brooklyn, N. Y.

I T is not the purpose of this short paper to discuss exhaustively
the therapeutic use of tuberculin, but rather to relate some
experiences of the writer during the last year and a half with
the use of this agent in treating advanced pulmonary tuberculosis.

Before proceding to the principal purpose of the paper, however, it might be well to review briefly a few general facts concerning the subject.

Tuberculin is a term used to designate a number of substances
differing in their method of preparation, but resembling each other
in that they are all prepared from the tubercle bacillus and the
medium on which it has grown.

It was first used by Koch, who observed that if tuberculous
guinea pigs were injected repeatedly with very small doses of a sterilized culture of tubercle bacilli, instead of death resulting, the
pigs improved, their lives were prolonged and in some cases a
cure was attained. Koch's results, which have been confirmed by
many other observers, thus show that there is an active principle
in sterilized dead cultures of tubercle bacilli which, when injected
in small doses into guinea pigs infected with tuberculosis, increases ther immunity and assists them in overcoming their infection. The many forms of tuberculin which we have to-day are
the result of the search for this active principle.

Experiments on animals have shown that the greatest degree
of immunity is attained by the use of living virulent tubercle
bacilli in small doses which the animal is able to overcome; but
heretofore it has not seemed practicable to use even cultures of
weakened virulence on human beings.

Tuberculin itself will not confer immunity on healthy animals
as it is inert except when injected in very large doses. This,
however, is not an argument against its therapeutic use, as diseased animals react very differently with much smaller doses.
Tuberculin acts first, in increasing the patient's immunity to the

tubercle bacillus and its toxins by stimulating the body cells to the production of immunizing agents, and second, by stimulating the tissue about the foci of infection by means of the local hyperemia which it produces.

There are many different forms of tuberculin. Among those most commonly used are O. T. or Old Tuberculin, Koch; B. F. or Bouillon Filtrate, Denys; T. R. or Tuberculin Residue, Koch; B. E. or Bacillen Emulsion, Koch; Watery extract of Von Ruch, and so forth. Details of these preparations may be had from any text book. Those who have had the most experience state that results may be obtained with all the forms of tuberculin, although advantages are claimed for each particular kind. Theoretically, it would seem to be desirable to use a preparation containing both the toxins given off during the growth of the bacilli (exotoxins) and the toxins formed by the breaking down of the bodies of the bacilli (endotoxins).

The form of tuberculin most used by us was the T. R., Koch. This is a watery extraction of an emulsion of living, virulent, human tubercle bacilli which have been ground in a mortar. We also used, to a lesser extent, the Bacillen Emulsion which is a glycerin emulsion of pulverized human tubercle bacilli. The initial dose used was from 1/10000 to 1/1000 mg. We used the method of gradually increasing doses recommended by Trudeau, Sahli and others, aiming always to avoid reactions. Injections were given in most cases twice a week, in some cases only once a week. The period of time during which injections were given was never less than four months. When reactions occurred, which was not very often, we usually gave the patient a rest from tuberculin medication for a week and then started again with a smaller dose than the last, increasing with caution.

Our usual method of progression was 1 - 2 - 3 - 4 - 5 - 6 - 7 - 8 - 9 - 10 - 15 - 20 - 25 - 30 - 40 - 50 etc. speaking in terms of ten thousandths of a mg. Many times patients would be continued on the same dose for some time because of minor untoward symptoms, such as poor appetite, slight pain in the chest, sleeplessness, etc. The injections were given in the back between the scapulae, care being taken to vary the location slightly with each injection so that successive injections were not given in the same spot.

Regarding the character of the cases treated it may be stated that all but two were patients in the Brooklyn Home for Consumptives. Practically 100 per cent. of the adult patients in this institution are far advanced cases; only occasionally will we get a case which is moderately advanced, according to the ordinary classification. It has been very generally held in advanced pulmonary tuberculosis, that tuberculin is useless, if not positively harmful, and our cases were selected with the idea of getting some first-hand information on the subject. They were all of the advanced sub-acute or chronic ulcerative type. Fever was not considered a bar to the treatment if the temperature did not go over 101 degrees. Several of the patients had cavities.

Eleven of the cases were started in the later months of 1911 or the early months of 1912 and have now been under observation long enough to warrant their being reported in some detail They form the basis of this paper. Our remaining cases, numbering fourteen, have been under treatment for from three to six months and I shall simply consider them in drawing my conclusions.

Attention is called to the fact that most of the cases reported had received general hygienic and dietetic treatment for varying periods before the tuberculin injections were begun. This was, of course, continued unchanged during the tuberculin treatment; hence conditions are peculiarly favorable for estimating the value of the tuberculin.

CASE I.—Male. Born in United States. 25 years of age. Conductor. Admitted, August 19, 1910.

*History.*—In October, 1909, had pneumonia and pleurisy followed by night sweats and loss of weight. Went to Riverside Hospital for 3½ months with no improvement. Came back to city for several months, then came to the Home. Now has pains between the shoulders, short of breath, cough, afternoon fever and night sweats. Appetite and digestion poor.

*Physical Examination.*—On admission: consolidation and infiltration of entire right upper lobe and upper half of left upper lobe, also partial consolidation of upper one-third of right lower lobe. Sputum positive for T. B. Pulse, 120.

*June* 9th, 1911.—Left Home improved—weight, 140½ lbs.

*July* 11th, 1911.—Returned to Hospital feeling worse, lost 8 lbs., now 132½ lbs., cough worse and pain between shoulders severe.

*November* 1st, 1911.—Improved slightly since readmission—weight, November 11th, 135 lbs. Temperature range from 96 to 99. Physical signs about the same as on first examination with additional focus in apex of left lower lobe.

Tuberculin started in December, 1911. He gained weight rapidly to 144 on January 24, 1912.

*March* 18th, 1912.—Weight, 153¾ lbs. Temperature never above normal now. Improvement in all symptoms.

During the summer the weight dropped down to about 140 lbs., although the patient felt well. Tuberculin continued until November 29th, 1912, about one year in all.

Minimum dose 1/10000 mg. Maximum dose 3/10 mg.

*November* 29th, 1912.—Very little cough—no expectoration. Physical signs show consolidation and lack of expansion over right upper lobe and upper one-third of left upper lobe. There are no rales of any kind. Signs are those of healed consolidated lesion.

*May* 15th, 1913.—Patient for last three months has been working as conductor on Manhattan Bridge three cent line. No cough or expectoration, weight 145 lbs., no temperature. Feels well.

CASE II.—Female (widow). Born in England. 53 years of age. Domestic.

*History.*—Following a pleuro-pneumonia in January, 1910, developed an empyema. Operation in Seney Hospital in April, 1910. Tubercle Bacilli found in sputum, so she was transferred to the Home for treatment.

*March*, 1911.—Empyema still discharging.

*Physical signs.*—Left sided empyema with signs of collapsed lung above. Right side shows infiltration to third rib in front, and to spine of scapula behind. Weight, 103 lbs.

Did well during summer, weight getting up to 120 lbs. in fall of 1911. All during the fall and up to March, 1912, condition remained stationary, although during this time patient was treated at Brooklyn Hospital with careful surgical dressings and mixed autogenous vaccines prepared from the sinus discharge. Surgeon reports no improvement from vaccine. March 1st, 1912, weight, 120 lbs. the same as on starting vaccine, empyema unchanged. Still signs of infiltration in upper portion of right upper lobe and many moist rales over upper portion of left chest.

Tuberculin started March 1st, 1912, and continued until about November 1st, 1912. Initial dose 1/1000 mg., maximum dose 1/10 mg. Despite periodical trouble with sinus blocking up, patient's condition improved greatly. Weight advanced to 128 lbs. Last examination about March 15th, 1913, showed right lung entirely clear; absolutely no signs could be found of disease. Left lung still collapsed but no rales heard. Sinus still discharging and diagnosis was made of lack of healing due to mechanical conditions. No active tuberculosis. Patient now in Brooklyn Hospital convalescing from an extensive Eslander operation to cure her empyema.

She stood the shock of the operation well and we are very hopeful of obtaining a complete permanent healing of her empyema.

CASE III.—Female. Born in Germany. 33 years of age. Housewife.

*History.*—First came under observation during summer of 1911. History of pleuro-pneumonia several years before while in Hamburg. Diagnosis of tuberculosis made at that time. At the time of my first examination in July, 1911, she complained of cough, pain in the left side and fever.

*Physical Examination* showed infiltration and partial consolidation of left lower lobe, also signs of acute pleurisy. Tubercle bacilli in the sputum. After several weeks rest in bed the patient's acute symptoms, that is, fever and pain, subsided, but she did not do well and gradually lost weight and strength. By January 1st, 1912, she had lost 7 lbs., weight now 107 lbs., infiltration and areas of consolidation in left lower lobe, with dulness at left apex. Tuberculin injections begun at this time and continued 4½ months to the middle of May, 1912. In all 22 injections, initial dose 1/1000 mg. maximum dose 5/1000 mg. Patient improved decidedly, gaining 6 lbs. to 113 lbs., cough and expectoration almost entirely absent. Chest signs show the rales have almost disappeared. This patient then went to the country for 4 months and continued to gain until weight was 120 lbs. On returning to the city last fall, she had no cough and no expectoration. Chest showed lack of expansion and dulness of lower part of left lung. No rales or signs of active disease. She has remained well all winter. Several weeks ago an examination showed weight 115 lbs., no cough or expectoration. Fibroid condition of left lower lobe with no signs of active disease.

CASE IV.—Female. Born in United States. 33 years of age. Clerk.

*History.*—Trouble began in 1905 or 1906 with cough and moderate hemorrhage. Examination in 1909 showed infiltration of entire right lung and upper lobe of left lung, weight 118 lbs.

In November, 1911, just prior to beginning tuberculin there were areas of consolidation scattered through right lung in addition to the infiltration, with signs about the same in left lung. Weight 114 lbs. Tuberculin was given from December, 1911 to June, 1912, in all about 50 doses. Initial dose 1/10000 mg. maximum dose 6/100 mg. Patient improved at first, gaining several pounds in first six or eight weeks, but then started to lose again and at the end of June, 1912, she weighed 110 pounds, a loss of four pounds since starting tuberculin. The physical signs in lungs showed no marked change over what they were on starting treatment. About this time patient developed signs of chronic nephritis; moderate edema of ankles, albumen and casts in urine and dyspnoea. Her pulmonary condition has remained about stationary ever since with some advance of renal trouble. In March of this year her lung condition was about the same, her weight 109 lbs. Tuberculin injections were started again in this case February first of this year, but were stopped after a few injections because it seemed useless in the face of the renal complication.

CASE V.—Male. Born in United States. 22 years of age. Electrician (single).

*History.*—Admitted to Home in July, 1911. History of illness dates back to February, 1911, when he took sick with pleurisy. Chief complaint cough, expectoration and pain in chest. Physical signs on admission showed consolidation of left upper lobe with signs of thickened pleura over left lower lobe. Patient improved gradually and examination in November, 1911, just prior to beginning tuberculin showed: weight, 150 lbs; changes in left lung more fibrous in character, with heart drawn to left so that apex was four and one-half inches to left of midsternum; also infiltration of right apex. Tuberculin administered from December 1st, 1911 to April 1st, 1912. Initial dose 1/10000 mg. maximum dose 2/1000 mg. This patient during entire time that he was an inmate of Home ran an irregular temperature which was entirely unaffected by the tuberculin treatment. He was discharged during April, 1912, for insubordination. Condition of lungs about the same as on starting. Weight 149½ lbs. Since leaving the Home this man has reported to me about once a month. He still runs a little evening temperature; cough on the whole about the same. Weight has ranged from 145 to 152 lbs. For last three months he has been doing light laboring work around a garage. The physical signs show that lesion in left lung is becoming more fibrous, the apex of heart in February, 1913, being displaced fully two inches to the left.

CASE VI.—Male. Born in Italy. 17 years of age. Bootblack.

*History.*—Admitted to the Home in July, 1911. Dates beginning of illness to 4 to 5 months previous, when he took sick with pain in the left side and cough, gradually losing weight and getting weaker.

*Physical Examination* on admission showed incomplete consolidation of left upper lobe with thickened pleura and infiltration of lower lobe. Many coarse moist râles over upper lobe, weight 95 lbs.

*November* 1st, 1911, just prior to beginning tuberculin, signs in the left lung were about the same and in addition a definite focus of disease found in the upper part of right upper lobe. Patient had gained 5 lbs. and now weighed 100 lbs. Occasional evening temperature.

Tuberculin administered for about 4 months to end of March, 1912, when his parents insisted that he go home to go to work. In all 30 injections, minimum dose 1/10000 mg. maximum dose 7/1000 mg.           ;

While taking tuberculin, weight increased to 102½ lbs.

Physical signs showed no considerable change at time of discharge. Still has occasional evening temperature rise. I last heard from this patient in December, 1912. He had been working as bootblack since leaving the institution. Still had a cough and felt about the same as on discharge.

CASE VII.—Female. Born in Norway. 30 years of age (single). Domestic.

*History.*—Admitted to the Home in July, 1910. Both parents died of tuberculosis. Patient dates beginning of her trouble three months previous to admission when she contracted a cough which did not yield to treatment. On admission there was consolidation of right upper and part of right middle lobes. Weight about 125 lbs. Patient ran considerable temperature and while weight remained stationary for a while she gradually lost ground. In July, 1911, weight 120 lbs.

*November,* 1911, prior to beginning tuberculin, still losing. Weight 114 lbs.

Physical signs then showed consolidation of right upper, part of right middle and upper one-third of right lower lobes. Also focus of disease in apex of left lower lobe.

Tuberculin given for 5 months to April, 1912, in all about 30 doses, initial dose 1/10000 mg. maximum dose 3/1000 mg. Patient continued to lose steadily and died in May, 1912.'

CASE VIII.—Male. Born in United States. 43 years of age. (Married) Stableman.

*History.*—Admitted to Home, September, 1911. Illness began in 1909 with cough, loss of weight and hoarseness. Treated at Otisville for several months about a year before admission. Chief complaint now is hoarseness, cough and shortness of breath.

*Physical Signs on Admission.*—Partial consolidation of left upper lobe and apex of right upper lobe. Signs of general bronchitis. Weight on admission 146 lbs. Temperature irregular, 100 degrees the highest.

*November* 1st, 1911, 3 months later and just before beginning tuberculin, weight 148 lbs., a gain of 2 lbs. Temperature not over 99 degrees.

Physical signs show beginning involvement of lower lobes in addition to signs noted above. Tuberculin given for 4 months, about 25 injections. Initial dose 1/1000 mg., maximum dose 7/1000 mg. Patient improved and at end of 2 months weight showed an increase of 6 lbs. At end of March, 1912, he insisted on going back to work against advice, although he promised to report every 2 weeks for examination. At this time he weighed 151 lbs. Physical signs much the same as before, except râles fewer and of dry variety. Still a little hoarse at times, cough improved. Sputum has changed from profuse mucopurulent to scant, frothy white. Dyspnoea absent, sleeps and eats well, temperature not over 99 degrees.

Patient started right in at heavy laboring work. He did not report as promised and 10 weeks later came back to the Home with high temperature and an acute lighting up of pulmonary lesions. He died about 2 months following his readmission.

CASE IX.—Female. Born in United States. 31 years of age. (Single) Saleslady.

*History.*—Admitted to Home January 5th, 1912. Illness began with a cough 9 months before which has persisted ever since. Has steadily lost weight and strength. On admission running irregular temperature 97 to 100.

*Physical signs* show consolidation of right upper lobe with infiltration of right middle lobe and apex of left lung. Weight 102 lbs. Tuberculin injections started at once and continued 7 months until the end of July, 1912, when she left the Home; in all about 60 doses. Initial dose 1/1000 mg., maximum dose 6/100 mg. Patient showed moderate improvement under treatment and gained 2 or 3 lbs., temperature coming down so that it rarely went above 99 degrees. Physical signs on discharge showed infiltration of left upper lobe in addition to lesions she had on admission. The character of the râles were very dry and disease did not seem to be active. I learn from her physician, Dr. Shookhoff, that this patient continued to improve for a few months after leaving the Hospital, but that she then grew careless and neglected her treatment. She has since been losing ground and is now in poor shape.

CASE X.—Male. Born in Denmark. 42 years of age. (Married) Machinist.

*History.*—Two severe attacks of pleurisy 10 and 3 years ago respectively. Patient dates beginning of present trouble to 3 months before admission to Home, which was in November, 1910. Complains chiefly of cough and loss of weight.

On admission patient weighed 117½ lbs. and physical examination showed consolidation of upper, middle and apex of lower lobes of right lung with a cavity in the upper lobe; and extensive infiltration of left upper lobe with consolidation of upper portion.

About 1 year later, just before beginning tuberculin treatment, examination showed subjective symptoms about the same. Chest signs about the same, except that cavity was more definite and probably larger. Weight had gradually fallen to 113 lbs. Patient has received tuberculin injection from December, 1911 to present time, in all about 90 injections. Initial dose 1/10000 mg., maximum dose 12/100 mg. For a while this patient made a decided improvement, weight getting up to 118 lbs and cough and expectoration much less. This was about 6 months after beginning tuberculin. Then he gradually lapsed into the same condition as before. He is still in the Home, his last recorded weight being 113 lbs., just what it was when starting injections about 18 months ago. His physical signs show an increasing involvement of the left lower lobe with fibrous changes in the right lung. One interesting feature of this case is the fact that while during the year before he received tuberculin he ran a very irregular temperature, since getting tuberculin it rarely goes above normal.

CASE XI.—Female. Born in United States. 22 years of age. Domestic.

*History.*—Admitted to Home, January, 1912. On admission had infiltration of left upper lobe to the 4th rib and dulness and bronchovesicular voice and breathing at right apex. Weight 99 lbs. Tuberculin started at once and patient gained consistently. Under treatment 6 months. Initial dose 1/1000 mg., maximum dose 1/10 mg.

On discharge the only physical signs were slightly impaired resonance at right apex, no active signs. Weight 106 lbs.

Patient has remained well since and is now married and keeping house.

## Conclusions.

It seems to me that from the observations made on the cases just outlined, and from the 14 cases still under treatment, which will be reported later, if the opportunity presents, the following deductions may be made:

First.—That providing reasonable care be exercised, no harm will result from using tuberculin in cases of advanced sub-acute and chronic ulcerative pulmonary tuberculosis.

Second.—That a few cases, perhaps 1 in 5, will show a very striking improvement from the use of tuberculin.

Third.—That a much larger porportion, perhaps 50 per cent., will do well while taking tuberculin and improve moderately. This may be shown by gain in weight, reduction of temperature, lessened cough and expectoration, improvement in physical signs, or disappearance of subjective symptoms; but the benefit is apt to be only temporary.

Fourth.—That the remaining cases show no improvement, the natural course of the disease being entirely unaffected by tuberculin injections.

Finally the writer agrees with Francine and Har$_{tz}$, who recently tried tuberculin in a series of chronic fibroid phthisis cases and concluded, "that in advanced chronic tuberculosis when there is fair resistance and little or no fever, tuberculin is unqualifiedly a valuable therapeutic measure."

---

## ACUTE NEPHRITIS IN INFANCY AND CHILDHOOD, WITH ILLUSTRATIVE CASE REPORTS.*

By John W. Parrish, M.D.,

of Brooklyn, N. Y.

MY reasons for choosing this subject are the frequency with which the disease occurs, the fact that its immediate or remote consequences may be disastrous and the fact that its symptoms at times are so obscure that it may be easily overlooked.

*Etiology.*—When we remember that the kidneys are the principal organs for the elimination from the blood of waste products and other poisons it is not surprising that so many and various things act as causative factors in the production of acute nephritis. Scarlet fever and diphtheria are perhaps the commonest causes, but there is probably no general infectious ailment that does not now and then lead to this disease. In practically all of these cases it is the toxin of the primary disease that produces the nephritis. There are other toxins produced in the body, in the intestines, for instance, that may cause nephritis; also toxins may be taken into the body, as in ptomain poisoning and cholera infantum, and set up this disease. Other causes are purpura and the blood diseases, pernicious anæmia, leukemia, etc., also some skin diseases and even large burns. Any one of a long list of irritant drugs may be the active agent in producing the disorder. Exposure to cold and wet frequently causes acute nephritis and finally there are cases for which no cause can be assigned.

---

* Read before the Brooklyn Medical Association, April 9, 1913.

*Symptomatology.*—Now when any of these causes have acted sufficiently certain symptoms develop with more or less regularity. There may be nausea and vomiting. There may be fever, generally slight if present, but occasionally high. In infants convulsions may occur. In older children there may be chilly sensations and pain in the back.

*Anæmia*, coming on pretty suddenly, is practically a constant symptom. It may be the first, and for a time the only thing to suggest nephritis. Whether the causative toxins directly injure the blood, or do so only through setting up inflammation of the kidney, as seems probable, the effect is a pronounced anæmia.

*Changes in the urine.*—We expect to find albuminuria. The albumen escapes largely at the malpighian tufts, but to some extent also (according to Strümpell) in the uriniferous tubules. Our ideas as to its significance have gradually undergone many changes so that we now know that it is utterly impossible to simply estimate the amount of albumen and from that deduce the gravity of the disease. Casts usually give little if any more reliable information than does albumen. Albuminuria probable always indicates some nutritional or degenerative change in the renal epithelium, but the changes are so slight as to leave little if any tendency to real inflammation of the kidney in that large group known loosely as functional cases, including the cyclic, or orthostatic, those due to unusual muscular exertion, to taking too much proteid food, to indigestion, to cold baths, to severe emotional disturbance. Osler quotes Goodhart as saying after a study of the later history of over 250 cases of this kind that "albuminuria of the adolescent has no sinister effect upon the health or duration of life." Of course in all the cases of this kind albumen is usually found in small amount only, but it may be present in considerable amount and may be accompanied by a few casts. In a much larger group, of which the ordinary febrile albuminuria is the type, including very many of the albuminurias of the infectious diseases and in which albumen may be present in small or considerable amount, there is believed to be simply cloudy swelling, or some fatty degeneration or destruction of the epithelium and aside from this no inflammation of the kidney, so that they are not, properly speaking, cases of acute nephritis.

Coming now to true acute nephritis, the abnormal elements in the urine may be present in comparatively small amounts, or in great abundance; but in neither case do they tell us whether we have to do with the exudative form or the much more serious diffuse or productive form for the obvious reason that the abnormal elements coming from the malpighian tufts and uriniferous tubules which are involved in both forms, cast no light upon what is happening in the connective tissue stroma.

In addition to this, various observers have shown that at times there may be the most marked changes in the urine, but after death from other causes very little change be found in kidney structure. On the other hand the changes in the urine may be trifling and after death very severe nephritis be discovered.

In most cases of acute nephritis urea is excreted in normal percentage, but the total amount in 24 hours is diminished.

*Edema.*—Edema was one of the cardinal symptoms of the disease as described by Bright. The old theories as to its causation, hydremia and hydremic plethora, have been discarded as inadequate and it is now believed that in certain forms of the disease, as that following scarlet fever, a poison is developed that is irritant to the walls of the capillaries and causes them to permit an increased passage of the blood serum into the tissues.

The retention of sodium chloride that often occurs in nephritis probably has a decided effect by producing an increased osmosis. It has also been suggested that certain tissue cells may develop the faculty of causing increased osmosis. The experiments of Heinecke and others in producing acute nephritis in dogs by administration of different poisons are interesting.

Chromium salts produced nephritis that was not accompanied by dropsy, whereas uranium salts produced nephritis that was accompanied by dropsy. Heinecke found that by injecting the chromium nephritis dog with serum from the uranium dog he could make the chromium dog have dropsy. In the human subject those forms in which dropsy occurs are the ones in which the malpighian tufts are prominently involved and in the young they are principally scarlet fever cases, those due to exposure and the ideopathic cases.

This theory of injury to the capillary walls by a poison is also used to explain the so-called "acute essential dropsy" which may occur without known kidney disease after scarlet fever, or after exposure to cold, or aside from either of these conditions.

*Uremia.*—This condition is often immediately preceded by a sharp drop in the quantity of urine, but it may come on without any dimination in the amount of urine. We have little positive knowledge as to the cause of uremia. Retention of excrementitious substances through failure of the kidney to functionate seems a natural explanation, but we know there may be complete retention for many days without the development of uremia.

A variety of causes have been suggested; a disordered internal secretion of the kidney, a faulty metabolism of the kidney tissue, the production of nephrolysins through the disintegration of kidney substance, and localized edema of the brain.

The milder symptoms are headaches, restlessness, sleeplessness, muscular twitching and respiratory disturbance.

These may be the only symptoms or there may be convulsions, general or local, alternating with coma or periods of great excitement. There may also be paralysis, disturbances of sensation and involvement of the special senses. Death often occurs from uremia, but it is not of necessity fatal.

*Treatment.*—This may be summed up in a few words—rest in bed, a fluid diet that does not unnecessarily increase the work of the kidney and measures to favor elimination from the skin, bowel and kidney.

For the bowels salts may be given. For increasing the activity of the skin, dry or moist heat. Pilocarpine is quite generally recommended for the latter purpose. It, however, is a very dangerous drug. I have seen death follow in fifteen minutes after the hypodermic administration of one-quarter grain to an adult.

Activity of the kidneys can be stimulated by saline enemas, colonic irrigation, Murphy drip and heat applied to the whole surface of the body. It should always be borne in mind that uremic vomiting and diarrhœa, being conservative in nature, are not to be too suddenly checked.

For convulsions we may use bromide and chloral by rectum or a hypodermic of morphine, and for immediate effect, chloroform.

With a few words in regard to some of the special types of the disease I will relate some histories that seem to me to be of interest.

*Scarlet fever nephritis.*—As is well known the nephritis usually appears any time from about the end of the second to the end of the fourth week. It is generally accompanied by dropsy, the urinary changes are usually pronounced and it is frequently of the productive type. It may end in recovery, but it is often terminated by uremia and not at all rarely it eventuates in chronic Brights. It seems to be just as common after mild cases of scarlet as after the severe ones; hence the necessity, no matter how well the child appears, of having the urine measured every day and of examining the urine carefully every day or two days.

The first case I wish to speak of presents a number of points of interest; the family history, the tendency to become chronic, the marked effect of kidney disease on the vascular system without regard to the age of the patient and the practical absence of dropsy. In June, 1898, a girl of 11 years contracted scarlet fever by sitting in private school at the side of a child who was said to have had German measles or mild scarlatina. At all events she had returned to school in less than a month. My patient developed a very severe case of scarlet fever. Now the mother of this patient had scarlet fever when a young woman, and for some months afterward was in poor health without obvious cause, so it seems fair to assume that she had kidney trouble. She married a few years later. I don't know what her condition was until the birth of her second child, but then she had severe kidney disturbance with uremic blindness for several days. Albumen and casts were present in her urine to greater or less extent for about a year. She then suffered for twenty years from a mild form of contracted kidney and died from another cause.

The daughter developed nephritis eighteen days from the beginning of the scarlet fever. The urine diminished in quantity suddenly and showed 20 per cent. by bulk of albumen, together with hyaline and granular casts, a few epithelial and blood casts, renal epithelium and some red and white blood cells. Aside from a little puffiness about the eyes there was no edema then or subsequently. The quantity of urine was quickly raised, but the percentage of albumen remained about the same for the first ten days. Then without any apparent reason the urine diminished again and the albumen jumped up to 40 per cent. by bulk. The color was smoky and there were many casts and red blood cells. The urea remained about 1 per cent. By means of saline enemas activity of the kidneys was re-established in less than 24 hours, but for the ensuing month the urine contained from 15 to 40 per cent. albumen, the total quantity of urine ranging from 2 to 6 pints daily. Then the inflammation seemed to subside somewhat and the albumen fell to 10 and 5 per cent. With the improvement in the urine she gained in flesh and strength and at the end of another month was sent to the country.

A couple of months in the country was of great benefit but the albumen did not entirely disappear. During the following winter and early spring she was housed, but got plenty of fresh air from wide open windows. Nearly a year from the beginning of her scarlet fever she was allowed to go about out of doors, and lead the semblance of a normal existance. During this year her diet had been most carefully regulated. For the next six years she lead the life of a semi-invalid, getting out regularly in any fairly good weather and really enjoying life after a fashion. From time to time headaches and digestive disturbance would cause a return to a milk diet for a month or so. During all this time a trace of albumen could always be found and at times more than a trace, but never any large amount. Gradually there had developed increased arterial tension with distinct hardening of the arteries. With this there was some cardiac hypertrophy and marked accentuation of the second sound of the heart. Finally after the disease had lasted about seven years the headaches and digestive disturbances became more frequent and severe, she lost flesh and strength, and at the end of another six months died with hemorrhagic symptoms and mild uremia. Before death she had developed as marked a case of hardened arteries as one often sees at any age.

*Diphtheria Nephritis.*—In this form the glomeruli are usually not so extensively affected and much dropsy is uncommon. The disease generally appears at the height of the diphtheria. Like that of scarlet fever it is often of the productive type.

Nephritis due to exposure to cold and wet closely resembles that of scarlet. There is apt to be dropsy and the disease is often of the productive type also.

Syphilis is said to cause a nephritis that has a tendency to become chronic. In inherited syphilis nephritis certainly isn't common. I have examined the urine in many cases and only recall one in which albumen was found, an infant of a few months who suffered also from severe malnutrition, of which it soon died.

Langstein lays much stress on nephritis due to tonsillitis and other infections of the throat and naso-pharynx and urges routine examination in these cases, despite the slight difficulty in obtaining specimens of the urine from young infants.

In October, 1910, after dining with a patient who had moved out of town, I was asked to look over his daughter of about five years. She had had a slight sore throat for a few days, but had not been confined to bed and the parents had not thought it necessary to call in a physician. The throat was somewhat red but showed no spots or patches of membrane. She had vomited that day for the first time, was decidedly anemic and very slightly puffy about the eyes, a thing the parents had not noticed. I advised examination of the urine. This was done the next day by Dr. Lanehart and albumen found. Two days later the urine became scanty and pinkish in color and her temperature ran up to over 105; she had in the meantime been put to bed on a fluid diet. I saw her the following day at her father's request in consultation with Drs. Lanehart and Keyes. No local lesion other than that of the kidneys could be made out. Dr. Lanehart had a bacteriological examination of the blood made and a pure staphylococcus culture was obtained. Before vaccines could be prepared the temperature had come down to about normal and as the kidneys were acting freely and the albumen much less in quantity the vaccines were not yet used.

She recovered completely in something more than a month and there has been no return of the disease.

I mention this case because it emphasizes the importance of paying strict attention to the apparently mild throat infections of childhood and because the bacteriological findings are suggestive in a therapeutic way.

There seems to be a marked difference of opinion as to how often the gastrointestinal diseases of infancy cause nephritis. In my opinion they rarely do so. In marantic infants from time to time we meet with edema of face, hands and feet and often at the same time an increase in weight occurs. Usually in these cases I have not found albumen in the urine, but have done so sometimes. A form of nephritis without edema I have seen occasionally in badly nourished infants.

In addition to the chronic digestive disturbances and emaciation there is a decided pallor, usually a subnormal temperature and a characteristic lifeless feeling to the skin. The skin has lost its natural elasticity and feels as if slightly infiltrated, but it does not pit on pressure. Examination of the urine reveals a small amount of albumen. High colonic irrigation at a temperature of 110 degrees I have found useful in clearing up this condition.

A remarkable form is congenital atrophic kidney. Langstein mentions that cases have been seen by Arnold, Westphal, Baginsky and Hellendall. The latter saw a brother and sister, six months and two years of age, die of contracted kidney. The mother of the children also suffered from contracted kidney.

Finally there is a type of nephritis occuring in infancy and young children without any apparent cause. Holt describes these cases carefully. Symptoms were sometimes so obscure that the disease had been overlooked. Usually in infants they began abruptly with fever, sometimes high. Vomiting and diarrhoea was present in about half the cases. Most of them were somnolent and a few had convulsions. Some had dyspnoea without lung disease. Albumen was sometimes absent at first, but casts were always found if carefully looked for. Six of twenty-four had dropsy and *all were decidely anemic.* Urine was not usually scanty until late in the disease and not always then. There was suppression of urine in a few cases and some presented a typhoid condition. Two cases seemed possibly due to highly concentrated urine, as very little fluid had been taken for a considerable period.

In March, 1896, I saw a child between nine and ten months of age who had rather suddenly become decidedly anemic. The following day a slight puffiness about the eyes suggested an examination of urine which disclosed considerable albumen with a few casts. The child had had no infectious disease of any kind nor had there been any illness in the family. Within a few days there developed general anasarca of moderate degree. The urine became somewhat pinkish in color and contained a considerable number of red blood cells in addition to hyaline and granular casts and a moderate amount of albumen. Hot packs and baths quickly started up action in the kidney and thereafter the urine was of pale color and seemingly abundant. The albumen and casts entirely disappeared in the course of six weeks and have never returned. The patient is now a healthy girl of 17 years. Her heart is easily affected by active exercise, but I can make out no hypertrophy. The sphymomanometer shows systolic blood pressure of 106- diastolic 98.

June 2, 1912, I was called to see a child of six months who had been under my care since birth. The baby had been breast fed for the first three months, then had mixed feeding for a month and after that bottle feeding alone. He had had a little indigestion all of his life, but had gained fairly regularly. I found that three days before the child had had a large vomit in the evening, a thing quite unusual with him. The mother gave no food during the night and the in the morning called in a friend of mine, in my absence from town, who ordered barley water for twenty-four hours and then food of half the usual strength if there should be no return of the vomiting. On the following day the family went to the country for the summer as the baby seemed much better, but had no more than got to their destination in New Jersey, when the child had a slight convulsion. A local doctor was called in and gave calomel and stopped all food. The following day, June 2, I saw the child and agreed with the doctor that it was a case of intoxication from milk. The child was put on a very restricted diet with the result that there was no more vomiting and the slight diarrhoea cleared up in a few days. On June 11, ten days after the convulsion, the mother telephoned that she didn't think baby was progressing as well as it should, that he was very pale and she thought a little puffy under the eyes. Instructing her to save any urine that he passed I went out to see him, taking nitric acid and test tube. On my arrival the mother had managed to save a little urine which on examination revealed considerable albumen. On the following day a larger specimen showed albumen 0.2 per cent. by weight, urea 0.4 per cent., a few hyaline and finely granular casts, a few red and white blood cells and epithelium. There was slight puffiness about the eyes. The urine could not be measured but did not seem particularly scanty. In the course of three days the urine was passing abundantly and showed 0.1 per cent. albumen, but the edema had increased in the face and showed also in the hands. There was no vomiting nor diarrhoea and temperature ranged between 99 and 100 as it had from the beginning of his illness. He was very pale, but seemed bright enough and took a fair amount of weak food. When asleep his breathing was somewhat irregular. He was given a warm bath and small enemas or large rectal irrigations every four hours during the day and for a week passed plenty of light colored urine containing about 0.1 per cent. albumen, but in spite of that the edema increased rather than diminished. Then without any apparent reason the urine became rather scanty, pinkish in color from many red blood cells, and showed 0.4 per cent. albumen with many casts. Under hot packs and the Murphy drip the urine increased in amount and continued seemingly abundant. In spite of the rather vigorous treatment the edema still increased and involved the entire body. The appetite failed but he did not vomit. He became listless and finally went into a light stupor for 24 hours and died on June 26, just four weeks from the attack of vomiting that probably was due to a commencing nephritis.

In regard to the etiolgy of the last two cases only one thing seems certain and that is that they were not due to any of the ordinary infectious diseases.

# EDITORIAL

## COLD SPRING HARBOR.

IT is a long way back to that delightful day in June when Dr. Davenport started to tell us about eugenics. The sun filtered in through the western window and we sat and wondered what those mysterious charts might mean. And then the doctor picked up the picture of a big black rooster—or was it a red one?—and the trouble began. We recall distinctly that the rooster had red hackles that were a legacy from one of his parents, and that they would have been white if his mother had been a blonde, but because of color-blindness in his father's family they were not. No, we have gone ahead too fast—the color-blindness affected a different social order, but the salient point was that we should always examine every rooster we run over with the automobile to see whether his hackles were red or white. We have followed this rule since but have not come to any definite increase in our knowledge as our kill have all been Plymouth Rocks about which Dr. Davenport said nothing. The masterly way in which the doctor handled the question of hereditary influence in the transmission of color-blindness, bringing in the maternal, then the paternal influences, and juggling them both with one hand, so to speak, dazed us quite a bit, but he came through without dropping either one and left us with the impression that mother had two chances to father's one and that somehow it wasn't quite fair. Then there was that panorama of Huntington's chorea! If Dr. Davenport had only written what he had to tell us in cold blood the editorial mind, confused by subsequent excursions into biology, where he saw asexual fungi growing luxuriantly in jars according to the rules made for them and tacked on the laboratory wall, colorless creatures pigmented by too close association with black sheep (quite according to human experience) and dear little brunette bugs blanched by being kept in a cold, dark cave,—by-the-bye, how did the genial curator keep his color so well?—would have had some hard facts to report instead these kaleidoscopic flashes, the exactness of which may be open to question. His memory of the clambake and the genial sunshine that mellowed the scene and incidentally took the backbone out of the butter and the coats off every participant except one enthusiast from Huntington is, on the other hand, clear and distinct—burnt in, possibly, by that same sunshine. The one practical point that he carried away was that the cross breeding of soft clams and incidentals with watermelon is distinctly bad from the standpoint of sound eugenics.                                                        H. G. W.

## FROM DAY TO DAY.

A S Artemas Ward once expressed it, we have removed ourselves from the busy haunts of men and are in the intimate contemplation of unpolished nature. We have laid aside our professional capacity and have announced that if we find any afflicted of disease or injured we will at once call a doctor. The telephone, accursed thing, is at the village store, too far away to break into our repose, and regarded there rather as an interesting curiosity than a thing for practical use. Its diabolic nature has not yet become manifest. The mail may be had upon request, provided we wait for the postmaster to first supply the clamor for calico and cheese that makes his life a weary grind. Two weeks ago he is reported to have mislaid the mail sack for three days. He was engaged in defending his championship in quoits against the blacksmith, but, as the mail consisted almost entirely of packages of seeds franked by the congressman to his local constituents, the delay gave them time to germinate and was rather beneficial than otherwise. We confess to a languid interest in things to eat, but fish are plentiful and cheap and canned beans may be procured without too great exertion at a moderate outlay. They are on the shelf between the calico and cheese, and are within the limits of our editorial income.

\*     \*     \*     \*

The editor of a very rural weekly once announced that when he found it too difficult to compose long vigorous editorials he would replace them with brief, caustic comments—he spelled it "costic." He further denied that the editorial "we" indicated that his wife helped in the composition. He explained that her time was too fully occupied in her domestic duties supplementing her activities in collecting delinquent subscriptions to permit of her writing editorials "for which she ain't suited anyhow, being quick tempered." We do not wish the parallel drawn too closely. "We" means our own intellectual capacity trained by the refining influence of surrounding art, as Ruskin said.

\*     \*     \*     \*

Our main concern at present is the suitable disposal of the dishonored fragments from our table. Having no Lazarus to pick up the crumbs that fall from our table, and being too æsthetic— or shall we say finikin?—to play both parts we must find some practical soul to convey to a fitting place what we no longer need. Why is it that the tender green of lettuce garnishing the golden yellow of potato salad should, when mingled with the rind of lemon in careless disarray, reverse the sensation of delight of which Lucullus so feelingly discoursed? We do not recall that the Roman epicure touched upon this darker side of the philosophy of food.

\*     \*     \*     \*

In a corner of the oak grove that shelters us from the ocean there is a Spiritualist camp, where a three week's meeting is now in progress. It seems a bit odd to find such a well attended gathering of this not over numerous sect in such an out-of-the-way corner as this, where neither the people nor the environment are suggestive of mysticism; nor are the participants themselves of the sort that one associates with the occult. Some of them are particularly plump and practical looking. But there are queer corners in almost every mind and the most prosaic are often tinctured with a thirst for the mysterious that crops up in most unexpected ways and places—tendencies that persist from generation to generation and that may have had their birth in Thebes, or Eleusis or among the plains of Chaldea. There may be here and there among these people a strain from the Indians who, long before the Anglo-Saxon invasion, in the depths of the New England forests celebrated fierce and bloody ceremonies and in their weird and awful orgies invoked the blackest and foulest of demons to their conclaves—demons that, despite the austerity of their faith, the Puritan settlers feared and in whose visible existence they held more than a passing belief. The spirits have, so far, troubled us but little, though things may be different when Mary Ann Pepper Vanderbilt and "Little Bright Eyes" arrive next week and help to make things hum.

\* \* \* \*

Speaking of oddities, we have met a character here who calls himself a "divine healer." He peddles berries and rag rugs that he weaves during the winter months, and his yellow overalls and broad brimmed straw hat look very matter of fact. But it is when one talks to the man that his inner self becomes manifest. There can be no doubt then that he believes implicitly in himself and in the destiny that is leading him to be "the greatest healer in the world." It came upon him suddenly, so he says. His had been a careless, sinful, hard-swearing life, full of hardships; the burden of which was beating him down so that he sat, partly dressed, one morning, thoroughly discouraged and bent on self destruction. At twenty minutes before seven a voice called him by name. "Ebenezer Groton, my child," it said, first in the tones of a woman, then in the deeper voice of a man. The voice went on and laid upon him an injunction of obedience and prayer and upon that first day led him to a sick boy, suffering with earache, whom he healed by "a simple prayer." Since then he has discovered that by the laying on of hands he can withdraw pain and suffering from others into himself. The nature of their maladies he divines by some inward vision that at times approaches clairvoyance.

His knowledge of Scripture is broad and fluent and his application of it apt. As he says, he has been reviled and derided, regarded now as crazy and again as a crafty pretender, but through it all he has been obedient to the voice that guides him which he firmly believes to be the voice of God.

The man is interesting from every viewpoint. His small eyes set close together, broad cheek bones, narrow jaw and forehead and flapping ears are stigmata that point to degeneracy and his obsession bespeaks abnormality of mind. But his industry—he has made and sold $4,800 worth of mats in thirteen years—his thrifty business ways and the ability he shows in his dealings with all sorts and conditions of people indicate that in the main he is sane enough. With some, indeed, he inspires something of the awe of Coleridge's Ancient Mariner, who "had strange powers of speech." When we parted with him he was discussing a sector of home-made apple pie in a manner that conveyed his complete capacity for the rational enjoyment of things that are not altogether of the spirit.

\*　　\*　　\*　　\*

Here, too, we have met the brilliant genius who first devised those fascinating little wind-mills fashioned like sailor men in blue jackets and white trousers with a diminutive vane in either hand. The first of what is now a world wide army he whittled out of odds and ends to decorate an old stump in his door yard. They were seen and coveted by a summer visitor who pestered him in person and by proxy until he grudgingly parted with them both for $5.00. She, in turn, got him orders for thirty more. The idea grew and that winter he spent his superabundant leisure in furious whittling—he makes them all with his jack knife—until today his little sailor men, a model of an old wind-mill down on the Point and a delightfully portly black rooster with a bristling red comb decorate the landscape from Cape Cod to Melbourne, Australia, and from Canada to Texas. He is genuinely proud of his work, though he speaks of it deprecatingly, as a craftsman should.

\*　　\*　　\*　　\*

Heretofore we had believed that story of how Cape Cod folk spent their winters. One old timer allowed that after the fishing was over "he set and thought, and set and thought, . . . and after a time he just set." Our closer contact convinces us that while this may be true of an isolated case in the main it vilifies a thrifty people. H. G. W.

---

## MEMORIAL TO ALGERNON THOMAS BRISTOW
## BROOKLYN, N. Y.

Be It Known by all men and especially to those nearest and dearest to him that the New York Society of Anesthetists in executive session assembled, draught this expression of respect, admiration and deep regret at the recent loss of their supporter and advocate

### ALGERNON THOMAS BRISTOW

His editorial and practical hospital support of the advancement of the Art of General Anesthesia has time and again aroused the admiration and emulation of this body of Anesthetists, and so active and influential has this work among his many followers been, that this Society wishes itself placed on record as considering it monumentally constructive and its cessation as a great loss to the surgical world.

Respectfully submitted,

W. C. Woolsey,
G. Tayloe Gwathmey,
A. F. Erdmann,
*Committee.*

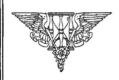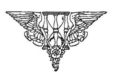

# ⚓ Society ⚓
# Transactions

## TRANSACTIONS OF THE BROOKLYN SURGICAL SOCIETY.

*(Continued from the July number of the Journal.)*

*Continuation of the Transactions of the Stated Meeting of February 6, 1913.*

DR. MATHIAS FIGUEIRA, in opening the discussion, said:—"It seems to me that the case here presented by Dr. Bristow is one of rupture of the membranous urethra caused by injury to the pelvic bones. It is evident to me from the history here given that the wheels of the car must have passed over the pelvis, compressing it and momentarily dislocating the pubic symphysis and so causing the injury to the urethra, the elasticity of the bones and ligaments springing them into place without fracture, the rupture of the urethra remaining the only evidence of the injury. Duplay, Voillemier and others give this as the sole possible explanation of similar cases met by them. I believe the hematoma in the abdominal wall was not caused by direct violence, as in that case the abdominal viscera would have been injured, but was caused by the fact that the extravasation of blood and urine caused by rupture of the urethra being confined below and in front by the triangular ligament and deep fascia, forced its way up along the abdominal planes. The bladder in children is placed high up in the pelvis, one may say in the abdominal cavity, and if torn from its urethral attachments is easily displaced into the abdomen. Surgeons doing perineal lithotomy will bear me out in this. I think also that in this class of cases besides the abdominal incision free perineal drainage is very helpful."

### Talma Operation for Cirrhosis of the Liver.

*Reported by Thomas B. Spence, M.D.*

A man, 45 years of age, began to suffer from indigestion seven months previous to operation and soon noticed enlargement of the abdomen. A diagnosis of cirrhosis of the liver was made. During the last four months paracentesis of the abdomen was done fourteen times, eighteen to twenty-three pints being drawn off at a time. The Talma operation was done on August 10, 1912, the case being a most favorable one because of the good condition of heart, kidney and lungs. The omentum was broadly sutured to the peritoneum and one portion was sutured between the peritoneum and fascia. Paracentesis of much smaller quantities than before was found to be necessary six times during the next two months, since which time (a period of four months) tapping has not been done. At the present time there is no accumulation of ascitic fluid and the patient is at work and in excellent condition.

### Operations for Gastric and Duodenal Ulcer.

*Reported by Thomas B. Spence, M.D.*

CASE 1.—For many years this patient, a woman of 39, had suffered from dyspepsia, but during the last year she was much worse than before. There were severe pain and vomiting after meals, especially at night, but never any vomiting of blood. The pain was most marked at a point to the left of the umbilicus, where tenderness could also be elicited. Blood was said to have been found in her urine before admission to hospital and renal calculus was suspected. Ureteral catheterization and X-ray examination were negative, as were gastric and fecal analyses. Exploratory laparotomy, done on February 27, 1912, disclosed a large saddle ulcer of the lesser curvature of the stomach. The ulcer was excised and because of the resulting pyloric stenosis a posterior gastro-enterostomy was performed. All the symptoms were dispelled by the operation and the patient has gained more than forty pounds in weight.

CASE 2.—This man, 30 years old, was treated for three weeks for pain in the epigastrium and vomiting. Two days before admission to the hospital he noticed tarry stools. On January 8, 1913, at 3 o'clock in the morning, he was suddenly seized with excruciating pains in the epigastrium. He suffered great shock, his whole abdomen became rigid, and all the signs of perforation developed. About thirteen hours later his abdomen was opened and a perforation was found at the base of a gastric ulcer situated close to the pylorus. There was a moderate extravasation of gastric fluid into the peritoneal cavity, but no particles of food were visible, probably because of the long fast before the perforation occurred. The ulcer was infolded by means of sutures and a posterior gastro-enterostomy was done. The patient has been rapidly gaining since leaving the hospital and is free from gastric symptoms.

CASE 3.—A male, 47 years old, suffered from symptoms referred to the stomach for four years. He had distress coming on two or three hours after meals, and a number of times he noticed black stools. He improved under medical treatment and change of diet, but had recurrences of the old trouble. A year ago his attack was accompanied by vomiting and tarry stools and he was in bed a week. Six weeks ago he had a similar attack and one week ago he fainted suddenly and has remained pale ever since, and his stools were black for a number of days. He has often been able to relieve his pain by taking bicarbonate of soda. He has lost sixty-three pounds in weight. His abdomen was opened June 16, 1912, and a duodenal ulcer was found which was buried with sutures. A posterior gastro-enterostomy was done. During the first day after operation there was some vomiting of blood. The man is now in perfect health.

The reporter has used in all cases since then three complete sutures in performing gastro-enterostomy and has not turned in the mucosa with the innermost suture, believing that in this way he can satisfactorily control hemorrhage. None of the latter cases have had any bleeding and because of that fact they have been almost free from post-operative vomiting.

CASE 4.—This patient, a man of 23, complained of indigestion for a period of five or six years. In August, 1911, he began to have severe pain in the epigastrium and to vomit, the attacks coming on some hours after meals, most frequently at night. The pain was relieved sometimes by vomiting and sometimes by taking food. In February, 1912, he began to vomit blood, this condition continuing for several weeks and causing almost complete exsanguination. Since that time the symptoms, with the exception of hemorrhage, have remained. No blood now in the stools. In October, 1912, a duodenal ulcer was found and treated as in the preceding case. Patient says he has a new interest in life and is entirely well. He has gained thirty-two pounds in weight.

CASE 5.—This man, 33 years old, has had his symptoms for four years, the attacks coming on at intervals of three or four months, and usually lasting more than a week. He has sharp pain in the epigastrium about three hours after eating, worse at night and often accompanied by vomiting. The pain is sometimes relieved by lying on his stomach but not at all by eating. The stools have sometimes been tarry and occult blood in found in the feces. On October 29, 1912, a duodenal ulcer was treated as in the other cases with the same satisfactory result.

CASE 6.—This man, 29 years of age, has had vomiting and epigastric pain for the last three years, occurring two hours after meals. Vomiting relieves the pain. He has noticed black stools and occult blood is found. His operation for duodenal ulcer was done on December 3, 1912. His stomach was greatly dilated and for a few days after getting up he suffered from vomiting caused by incomplete emptying of the stomach. He also had rather obstinate constipation. Both of these symptoms disappeared and he now claims an absolute cure.

CASE 7.—This patient, 21 years old, complained of pain in his epigastrium and back for a year and a half, the pain nearly always appearing about 4 P. M. Eating gave relief. There was some loss of weight and a moderate anæmia. Operation for duodenal ulcer, done on December 13, 1912, has relieved him of his old pain and he feels stronger, but he still has some pain in the left iliac region which he ascribes to gas. His bowels are not yet regular.

CASE 8.—This patient, 21 years old, had his vermiform appendix removed five years ago. Most of the time since then he has had attacks of pain in the epigastrium and back, coming on at 4.30 P. M. and often relieved by vomiting. He was treated in the medical service of the hospital a number of times without relief. No occult blood was found. Operation for duodenal ulcer, as described above, performed on December 17, 1912, has given complete relief from symptoms.

*Stated Meeting, March 6, 1913.*

The President, RICHARD W. WESTBROOK, M.D., in the Chair.

*Program.*

I. Report of cases.
   a. Carcinoma of the Stomach; subtotal gastrectomy. Patient. Specimen.
   b. Duodenal Ulcer. Patient.
   c. Hyperthyroidism; Anoci-Association Anæsthesia. Patient and Specimen.
   d. Prostate Case. Patient and Specimen.
   e. Multiple Post-Scarlatinal Infections. Patient. By Raymond P. Sullivan, M.D.
   Case b discussed by Dr. T. B. Spence, Dr. Mathias Figueira, Dr. H. F. Graham, Dr. Paul M. Pilcher. Discussion closed by Dr. R. P. Sullivan. Cases a, c. d and e not discussed.
II. Report of cases.
   a. Tumor of Liver.
   b. Decompression Operation.
   c. Appendicitis with Intestinal Obstruction.
   d. Exophthalmis Goitre. By A. H. Bogart, M.D.
   No discussion.
III. Paper: "Further Observations upon Angulation of the Sigmoid." By H. B. Delatour, M.D.
   Discussed by Dr. R. W. Westbrook, Dr. Mathias Figueira, Dr. R. S. Fowler, Dr. C. H. Goodrich. Discussion closed by Dr. H. B. Delatour.

### Carcinoma of the Stomach.

*Reported by R. P. Sullivan, M.D.*

Mrs. B. age 61, married, Italy, housewife.

*Family History.*—Negative

*Past History.*—Mother of three children; no miscarriages. Menopause fifteen years ago. Had a Potts' fracture of right leg three years ago; good recovery.

*Present Illness.*—About five years ago began with spells of epigastric distress—belching and occasional sour regurgitation—with pain in the pit of the stomach, coming one to two hours after meals, which was always relieved by food or alkali (vichy). Bowels very costive. Attacks at first came every six to ten weeks and last eight to ten days. This condition of affairs was the rule for three years. Then spells more often and pain more intense and relief from food or alkali of shorter duration. For the past year there has been a constant distress and dull pain in the epigastrium with increasing loss of weight and of appetite. Many spells of nausea and vomiting. Patient says that two months ago she first noticed a lump in the epigastric region, which has slowly increased in size. Lately she has had intense pain, persistent vomiting and obstipation, accompanied by a good deal of bloating and sour taste.

She was admitted to Holy Family Hospital as a case of suspected intestinal obstruction with possibility of tumor in the transverse colon. However, high enemas cleared this doubt.

On examination we found a very much emaciated woman who begged for relief from pain and vomiting. Her general examination was good. Hemoglobin was only 36 per cent. and we decided to try and build her up. The vomiting and pain decreased only moderately and she again begged for relief.

On January 3, 1913, we opened her abdomen by a median incision, and found the entire colon to be free from trouble. The stomach was in fairly good position, but contained a hard tumor, about the size of a small orange, and situated on anterior wall at about the junction of the middle and outer thirds, with extension of the growth from the greater to the lesser curve. Further exploration revealed some lymphatic enlargement along the lesser curve and in the region of the pylorus. The liver, gall-bladder and pancreas were normal. We then proceeded to do a subtotal gastrectomy after the Billroth II method, making particular effort to carry away all affected glands. To accomplish this the gastric artery was ligated close to the œsophagus and the pyloric branch of the hepatic artery ligated close to the main vessel. Then a generous portion of the lesser omentum was ligated and cut.

After ligating the epiploic vessels and the pancreatico-duodenal artery a good-sized section of the great omentum was ligated and cut.

The usual steps followed. It was rather interesting to note that the pylorus was patent and about one and one-half inches in diameter. After inverting the stump of the duodenum and removing a portion of the stomach, a Mayo posterior no-loop gastroenterostomy was done.

The patient had an excellent reaction and made an uneventful recovery. We began liquid nourishment by mouth in ten hours after operation and allowed soft diet in three days. She was out of bed on the tenth day, and on the fourteenth day was on a selected regular diet. At this point she developed a slight skin infection which cleared up in ten days. Ever since she has gained rapidly and has been entirely free from pain, distress and vomiting. The pathological report by Dr. Hulst states that the tumor is carcinoma with ulcer base. The specimen here demonstrated shows this to be true.

## Duodenal Ulcer.

### *Reported by R. P. Sullivan, M.D.*

Mr. A. M., age 40, bricklayer.

*Family History.*—Negative to tuberculosis and carcinoma.

*Past History.*—Malaria thirty years ago; denies specific history. Habits: Moderate alcohol. Excessive use of tobacco. No previous operations.

*Present Illness.*—Twenty-two years ago began having spells of gnawing pain in the pit of the stomach, coming two to three hours after meals, and always relieved by eating food. Attacks were always accompanied by nausea and epigastric distress and tenderness. Between spells was bothered with a good deal of belching and frequent heartburn. Bowels fairly regular, but loss of flesh apparent during attacks. At first attacks came about six months apart and would continue from two to six weeks. He had various treatments of highly restricted diets and absolute rest in bed. One spell of four years with little trouble and patient was able to work. He had been discharged as cured.

About eight years ago the trouble returned and the same routine of symptoms prevailed, with the addition of relief by induced vomiting. At this time he was frequently awakened at night with pain and distress. Alkali treatment and restricted diets again instituted. During the past four years relief from food or alkali lasted only an hour. Patient had become fearful of eating, thinking that this aggravated the condition, as there had been small blood-clots in the vomitus of late. Occasional tarry stool, though the color might be due to bismuth. At this time the patient complained of severe epigastric pain and obstipation and almost continuous sour stomach and has lost thirty-five pounds in the previous six weeks. Physical examination showed a man much emaciated and in a deplorable condition of mind. Abdomen presented a greatly dilated stomach and some tenderness over the region of the gall-bladder, duodenum and appendix. No palpable masses. Heart, lungs and kidneys in good condition. Gastric analysis by Dr. Hulst showed a hypersecretion, 295 c.c.; total acids, 66; free HCl, 46; combined, 8. No lactic acid; no sarcinæ, no Boas Opler.; many food remnants.

At operation (St. Marys' Hospital, March 7, 1912), the abdomen was opened by a high right rectus incision. Stomach found to be greatly dilated and many adhesions between gall-bladder and stomach. Appendix explored and found to be subacutely diseased and was removed. Adhesions dissected out and duodenum exposed. A large, thickly indurated ulcer found in the first portion of the duodenum extending up to the pylorus and down to the upper segment of the second portion of the duodenum. There were evidences of a small perforation which had been closed by adhesions. The posterior portion of the duodenum was firmly attached to the liver. Pyloric orifice was about the size of a lead pencil. A row of interrupted linen sutures infolded the anterior portion of the duodenum, thus guarding against a further perforation. Then a posterior no-loop gastroenterostomy (Mayo). The gall-bladder seemed somewhat thickened and was evidently the seat of chronic inflammation, but after being freed from adhesions it emptied easily and was, hence, not drained.

This patient made an uneventful recovery and left the hospital in two weeks, feeling like a new man. He was put on a regular diet on the tenth day and has enjoyed excellent health ever since and has gained in weight and been at work steadily since.

This case demonstrates that stomach rest is best secured by operative measures. The infolding of the ulcer has evidently closed the pylorus and hence no further passage of food will irritate the ulcer. Hence the surgical treatment of chronic duodenal ulcer is more satisfactory and complete.

## Diffuse Adenomata of Thyroid (Anoci-Association Anæsthesia).

### *Reported by R. P. Sullivan, M.D.*

Miss T. C., age 17, single, schoolgirl.

This patient was presented before this (Brooklyn Surgical) Society just one year ago. At that time we demonstrated her condition as one of tracheal pressure and dsyphagia with mild symptoms of hyperthyroidism. We removed the right lobe and isthmus and ligated the left superior thyroid artery. She had had the goitre for two years, and for eight months previous to first operation (September 19, 1911), she had had many spells of tachycardia and dysphagia and dyspnœa.

Her health was declining rapidly. The case proved to be one of diffuse adenoma, with pressure within and without the gland, thus explaining the symptoms. At operation we found the trachea dislocated laterally to the right and flattened from side to side. On releasing the enormous lobe there was a temporary collapse. Because of this we decided to defer further operation.

Her convalescence was not smooth. During the first forty-eight hours, there was difficulty in breathing and she frequently became quite cyanotic. However, from the third day there was a most satisfactory recovery. She was out of bed on the fifth day and left the hospital two weeks later, in excellent condition.

Six months later, on March 5, 1912, she reported to me and had gained eighteen pounds in weight; no tachycardia and very little nervousness, but still some difficulty in swallowing. She was able to attend to business and was in excellent spirits.

On November 10, 1912, eight months later, I saw this patient again, and she informed me that the dysphagia was more frequent; that she was again having spells of tachycardia, dyspnœa and nervousness. She had lost five pounds during the previous two weeks.

On the day of examination I found her to have a pulse of 108; respiration, 28; temperature, 98; blood pressure of 140 mm. The left lobe was about the size of an orange and very firm. By percussion we made out the gland to extend down behind the sternum to the level of the third rib.

She was admitted to Holy Family Hospital on November 12, 1912, and at a Clinical Congress Clinic we removed the gland here demonstrated. Because of the previous difficulty with breathing and because of previous tracheal collapse it was decided to follow as well as possible the anoci-association anæsthesia of Crile. The case was given morphia gr. ¼, scopolomine gr. 1/100, by hypo. fifteen minutes before operation. Then ether was administered very lightly instead of nitrous oxide.

The field of operation was entirely blocked with novocain 2 per cent. and the operation continued in the usual manner. The greater part of the gland was substernal, with the lower pole resting on the base of the heart. It was difficult to remove and tedious. However, we persisted in the novocain blocking, which proved quite satisfactory. One interesting feature in this case was the discovery of an aberrant thyroid situated in the upper angle of the neck, just beneath the mastoid process. This was removed.

During the greater part of the operation very little ether was administered and still there was absolute quiet and good muscle relaxation.

When the gland was removed and hemostasis attended to we again blocked the entire field with a 1 per cent. quinine and urea-hydroclorid solution and made the usual closure and drainage. The pulse at the finish of the operation, as reported by Dr. Ryan, was 96, showing a decrease from 102 at the beginning of the operation. There was no tracheal difficulty and the general appearance of the patient was excellent. The usual post-operative treatment, except for morphia, was instituted. Six hours later I saw the patient and found her very comfortable; pulse, 96; temperature, 99.2 (by rectum), and she had had 32 of warm water by mouth. She was delighted with her own condition and remarked that she suffered no pain or distress. Her pulse and temperature did not vary until the third day, when she was allowed out of bed for two hours. Then her pulse rose from 92 to 96; no rise in temperature. From the fifth day she was up and around all day, on regular diet and suffering no distress or pain. On the tenth day she left the hospital, having had primary union.

Two weeks ago she reported to me at my office and claimed perfect health; also she informed me of a gain of ten pounds in weight. She looked the part.

This case demonstrated to me that anoci-association anæsthesia has its place and, except for the prolongation of the operation and possibility of trouble from the quinine solution, it deserves more practice and consideration. I have used the method in several other conditions and with equally good results.

I have been amazed at some of Dr. Crile's demonstrations at the Lakeside Hospital in Cleveland and feel certain that this method of anæsthesia when used as advocated by Crile will solve many of the difficult problems of risk which are presented to the surgeons.

## Suprabupic Prostatectomy.
### *Reported by R. P. Sullivan, M.D.*

Mr. J. D., aged 60, retired, married. Examined March 2, 1912.
*Family History.*—Negative.
*Past History.*—Fifteen years had a traumatic injury to side and pelvis.
Denies specific history. Neisserian infection at twenty years. Operated upon
for hæmorrhoids nine years ago.

*Present Illness.*—About three years ago began having spells of difficulty
in starting urine. Occasionally some tenesmus, but never severe until one
year ago when there was complete retention. At this time he was treated by
a physician and secured almost complete relief for six months. Then a return
of the difficulty and tenesmus, accompanied by a good deal of backache and
cold sweats. Condition grew gradually worse and nocturnal frequency made
his rest very poor. As a result he began to lose flesh and strength and experienced loss of appetite; had a good deal of headache and constipation. One
week ago micturition became very painful and patient passed blood and sand.
Said he was never able to feel satisfied after micturition. Had backache,
intense; tenesmus, severe. Life was considered a burden. Pulse, 118; temperature, 99⅖; blood pressure 210 m.m. The physical examination showed a large,
well-developed man, but nervous and downcast. Abdominal palpation revealed
tenderness beginning at symphysis and extending up to epigastrium and some
stiffness of recti muscles. Bi-manual examination revealed a large, hard and
nodular prostate, about the size of an orange. Tenderness quite acute over
the entire gland. Blood was oozing from the external meatus.

The patient passed 300 c.c. of heavy foul urine which contained many
small blood-clots. This was very painful and difficult to start. I then passed
a No. 16 French silk woven catheter with difficulty and recovered 400 c.c. of
residual urine with a specific gravity of 1006, leaving some of the urine in the
bladder. With the residual urine there came away many small, round calculi.

Patient was put on urotropin gr. x. every four hours, and returned in
twenty-four hours, claiming to have had the best night's rest in weeks. His
bladder was again emptied and 600 c.c. of urine with a specific gravity of 1008
removed, with much less blood. This procedure was continued daily, and from
the third day we recovered on an average of 400 c.c. of residual urine. Bladder irrigations of warm boric acid solution were instituted daily, but the
specific gravity never went above 1008. The urethra became very tender and
there seemed to be no end to the small calculi. Cystoscopic examination was
attempted but was impossible because of obstruction. On March 21st, at St.
Mary's Hospital, under local anæsthesia, a suprapubic cystotomy was done and
exploration revealed a large intravesical prostate with many calculi of varying
sizes. The bladder was found to be an enormous thick-walled affair, extending
up above the level of the umbilicus.

Rubber tubing was stitched into the bladder and drainage kept up for a
period of four weeks, at which time the specific gravity of the urine came up
to 1014 and the bladder would hold only 241 c.c. of urine. The general physical
condition of the patient was much improved. Blood pressure went down to
150 mm.

On April 27, 1912, at St. Mary's Hospital, under general anæsthesia through
the suprapubic opening, we removed the entire gland, finding it very much
increased in size, a median bar about one inch square being situated at the
internal meatus. It was surprising to note the density of the bladder wall.
Incision into the capsule was possible with a scalpel. Hot packs seemed to control the hæmorrhage very well and a reflow suprapubic drainage was instituted.
The patient's reaction to operation was excellent. Gauze packing was removed
partially on the third day and completely on the fifth day. Irrigations had all
come away clear. On the morning of the eighth day I was summoned to the
hospital hurriedly and found the patient about pulseless and no drainage from
the bladder. Hot irrigations were started immediately, after introducing a soft
rubber catheter into the bladder through the urethra and continuous irrigation
of hot boric acid solution was commenced. By that night we seemed to be
getting less blood, but maintained the continuous irrigation and attended to the
shock in the usual way. The following afternoon fragments of broken calculi
were found in the fluid from the bladder and we immediately distended the
bladder under slow and low pressure and soon recovered many more calculi
fragments.

This procedure was repeated in six hours and more small calculi recovered. From this time on there was an uneventful recovery and the patient left
the hospital on May 10th with excellent bladder control and passing clear urine.

Suprapubic fistula remained open more or less until late in May, or about six weeks after second operation. The patient has enjoyed perfect health ever since; has gained in flesh and strength and has complete control, being well able to go eight or ten hours without voiding. Dr. Hulst reported the gland to be a simple hypertrophy, with an area of subacute inflammation in one lobe.

## Multiple Post-Scarlatinal Infections.
### *Reported by R. P. Sullivan, M.D.*

Mr. E. S., aged 26, single, engineer.

*Family History.*—Negative.

*Past History.*—Has always enjoyed good health up to eighteen months ago. Was then ill with scarlet fever and went through an apparently regular course. Six months later was ill with an attack of intestinal pains and was informed that it was a "congestion." Close questioning seems to show that it was either a fecal impaction or the possibility of an appendix attack. Was well again in two days.

*Present Illness.*—Two weeks previous to the date of my first visit (May 28, 1912), while at work at Mauch Chunk, Pa., was taken ill with a general feeling of malaise and headache and pains in the right hip-joint. No chills, but some fever. Bowels costive. At the time of my visit, he had been under treatment of a physician for typhoid fever for two weeks. He had had "rose-spots" on his abdomen and some tympanites in the right iliac fossa. Widal had not been taken but the Diazo had been positive. He had been having a continuous high temperature. He complained of pain in the right hip-joint and the right thigh was flexed on the abdomen and any attempt to move it was painful. His bowels were loose and watery and frequent. The abdomen was scaphoid and no masses or tender areas made out. Rectal examination negative. I advised a Widal and general blood-examination and suggested the possibility of tubercular disease of the hip-joint.

I did not see this patient for a week, but, in the meantime, Dr. Hulst reported a negative Widal, and a blood count of 16,000 W.B.C. and 84 per cent. polymorph.

During my absence the case was seen by Dr. Samuel Lambert and nothing definite made out until June 8th, when Dr. Lambert called me on the telephone and advised immediate operation for an abdominal abscess, offering the opinion that it was a retro-cæcal appendicular abscess. Rectal examination revealed a large, tender, bulging mass in the right pelvis. Six hours later I saw the case and found not only the bulging in the right pelvis, by rectal examination, but also a small, tender area, about the size of a hen's egg, presenting just at the anterior superior spine.

At the Holy Family Hospital that night we made an incision over the abdominal or inguinal mass and found an enormous retro-peritoneal abscess, about a quart of thick, creamy pus escaping.

Cultures were made and then proper drainage instituted. The patient had an excellent reaction by the next day. The temperature had come down from 104.6 degrees Farenheit to 99.6 degrees F.

The culture was reported by Dr. Hulst as staphylococcus pyogenes aureus in pure culture. The blood culture was negative. We ordered autogenous vaccines made. On the fourth day after operation we gave 150,000,000 of the autogenous vaccine and had a fairly good result. Drainage was good and the patient seemed to be making an uneventful recovery. At the time of operation we also incised a small skin infection at the level of the lower border of the second rib, near the sternum. Examination failed to show this to be anything more than a pure skin affair. For two weeks we had an easy time. Vaccines were administered in increasing doses every five days.

On the fifteenth day after operation the patient's temperature shot up to 105 degrees and there was mild delirium. Thorough examination failed to find any new focus of infection. Urine was negative; drainage was still good. However, we enlarged the opening and treated the temperature by cold baths, etc. Vaccines had not been given for six days.

The temperature varied only to 104 degrees during the next forty-eight hours. Still there was good drainage and digital exploration of the abscess cavity failed to open any new pockets. The temperature reduced gradually and by the end of the week was normal. The small wound in the chest healed completely. But still there was drainage for four weeks more from the abdominal wound. On the suggestion of Dr. Hulst we gave him a mixed vaccine during the later days.

On July 29th, the patient was allowed to go home, having had a normal temperature for six days. It seemed quite probable that the now remaining small sinus would soon close. It did so in three days.

Six days later the patient was taken with a chill and temperature rose to 106 degrees. He was delirious. He had complained of a dull ache the night previous, over the left kidney. Urine was negative; blood culture negative. On examination nothing could be made out. The following day Dr. Patterson saw the case with me and could not confirm any peri-nephritic abscess. However, six hours later, there was a tender bulging mass over the left kidney. We operated at St. Mary's Hospital the following evening and found a large perinephritic abscess. Culture showed the presence of the same staphylococcus pyogenes aureus in pure form. Mixed vaccines in large doses were instituted and continued for some time at regular intervals. On the sixteenth day after operation the patient complained of pain in the right shoulder and some difficulty in moving about in bed. Examination of the original scar from the small abscess was negative. There was no tenderness over the bones. Thirty-six hours later his temperature rose to 105 degrees and still nothing visible to account for it. The kidney wound was still draining slightly and the sinus was explored, but no pocket of pus was found. The following morning there was a tenderness over the right sterno-clavicular joint and immediate operation was done. Exposure of the joint revealed a small collection of pus. The clavicle on then being opened was found to be infected for a distance of about two inches. This was removed, leaving periosteum on the posterior aspect. Cavity swabbed with carbolic acid and alcohol and then packed with iodoform gauze.

From this time on there were no more high temperatures and vaccines were continued at regular intervals. The kidney sinus was reopened once and a small cavity drained. Tonics and general treatment had good results. The patient was discharged, cured, December 30, 1912, and is here tonight, claiming excellent health, and has gained about sixty pounds in weight.

The case demonstrates that post-scarlatinal infections are frequently slow in developing; also that persistent vaccine treatment will be a valuable aid to surgical work.

### Duodenal Ulcer. Patient.
*Reported by Raymond P. Sullivan, M.D.*

DR. T. B. SPENCE, in opening the discussion, said:—"I do not want to speak of or to discuss this particular case, but it seems to me that there is a necessity for surgeons continuing to call attention to the good results of surgical treatment for duodenal ulcer and I am certainly going to keep banging away at that subject.

"The general profession has not yet come to the conclusion that they should turn these cases over to the surgeons and the laity are not persuaded that an operation is the thing!

"I keep seeing cases that refuse operation, refuse surgical treatment because of the persuasion brought to bear upon them by others in the profession than surgeons. We hear, too, so much about the bad results of surgical cases. Frequently I hear that these cases all go bad at the end of a year. I do not know what they go bad of, but, nevertheless, I keep hearing that they go bad again; that they have all the old sypmtoms. I think we all of us believe that that is not true, but until the profession, at least in Brooklyn, is educated, they will continue to believe it and the laity are not going to subject themselves to the proper treatment for duodenal ulcer."

DR. MATHIAS FIGUEIRA, in discussion, said:—"That all of these cases do well is not so. I do not speak of my own experience, but if the doctor will read Dr. Murphy's clinical lectures of three months ago he will find there that Dr. Murphy speaks of the bad results that sometimes will follow these operations for gastric ulcer and duodenal ulcer, and he says there distinctly and plainly enough that in his experience the bad results of some of these cases cannot be explained. They do well, they go along for three weeks, for a month or for two months, and then the symptoms come back—symptoms of vomiting, symptoms of nausea, symptoms of burning after eating, symptoms of pain.

"In my own experience I have had two cases. One case was before Mayo called attention to the importance of the no-loop operation, and in that case there developed after the first month marked symptoms of vomiting. She would vomit at intervals and would have pain and distress, so much so that I reopened the abdomen and found that the loop between the pylorus and duodenum was enlarged and that the contents of the loop in place of passing on (the pylorus was not entirely closed) would go back into the stomach by way of the new opening. I did an enterostomy, joining the loop to the gut below, and the case got entirely well.

"I have since seen another case in which the loop was short and yet that patient will once in a while have distress, why I cannot say. Washing of the stomach and care in diet will relieve him, but yet he has distress."

DR H. F. GRAHAM, in discussion said:—"I had the pleasure the other evening of interrogating all the patients Dr. Spence presented at the last meeting of the Society. Of those patients (eight I think there were in all) six were entirely free from pain. The other two still complained of pain. These were recent cases, within a couple of months, and are still dieting. Their pain in the lower abdomen evidently is due to causes in the intestines and I think it will undoubtedly clear up under a carefully directed diet, *i. e.,* one leaving a greater residue for the intestines to act upon.

"Moynihan says that in his experience the only patients that have trouble after a gastro-enterostomy are physicians. I think that is entirely dependent upon their mode of living; evidently the way they eat and the conditions connected with the profession, irregular hours, etc.

"I think that there are a number of factors entering into this situation. In the first place, many of the surgeons are not yet familiar with the modes of treatment for hyperacidity which are common with the gastro-enterologist. The attending surgeon usually does not see his case more than a couple of weeks after gastro-enterostomy has been performed and many of us get through with our patients and think they are all right again and they go back to work and are not as careful to they should be, do not adopt a proper diet to neutralize hyperacidity until they have got over that tendency, so there is no reason why they should not get a second ulcer and the same symptoms all over again, only that they will get over it a good deal faster the second time under proper treatment if it is applied early.

"Another factor to consider is that most of these patients with gastric or duodenal ulcer have dilated stomachs at the time of operation and as a result they suffer from intestinal auto-intoxication for years before operation, which is a condition that undoubtedly favors the element of hyperacidity and of ulcers, and many of these cases need to have treatment directed toward their auto-intoxication after operation as well as toward their hyperacidity.

"I think that the operation of gastro-enterostomy with or without removal of the ulcer is absolutely a curative one if properly done and that these patients will not have future trouble if they will take a sufficient time to get well after operation, and if they are on a proper diet after operation, a diet that tends to neutralize hyperacidity, and are a little careful not to overwork after it."

DR. PAUL M. PILCHER, in discussion, said:—"The observations of some men, especially Lane, have shown us that in some cases at least the production of a duodenal ulcer does not depend entirely upon the secretions in the stomach or duodenum, for there will often be associated with the duodenal ulcer adhesions and bands about the intestines which produce a dilatation of the duodenum and there an ulcer may follow.

"Now, it seems to me, that some of these cases in which the symptoms recur do so because the fundamental cause has not been discovered and removed. If we make a thorough search in these cases we will often find that there are adhesions binding down the ileum and causing intestinal stasis which eventually leads to the formation of these duodenal ulcers. Lane believes this fact is so fundamental that he does not do a gastro-enterostomy in his cases, and often obtains a satisfactory result from his operations. Now, while Mr. Lane is, of course, a great enthusiast, at the same time I believe that a good many things he has observed are correct and I believe there is a good deal of basic truth in his observations, especially that intestinal stasis has a good deal to do with duodenal ulcer, and I think as a routine in those cases where the condition will allow it, that we should look in the various places he tells us to for restricting bands and adhesions."

DR. RAYMOND P. SULLIVAN, in closing the discussion, said:—"I have nothing to add except a suggestion to the surgeons that, if possible, instead of inverting these duodenal ulcers we should try and excise them. There seems to be good reason to believe that inversion does not always cure the ulcer or even guard against perforation; that if the gastro-enterostomy opening should close they have the difficulty again. I think that the problem is going to be solved along the line of excision of the duodenal ulcer if the technic can be properly developed."

## Acute Intestinal Obstruction. Appendicitis.

*Reported by Arthur H. Bogart, M.D.*

G. H., age 31 years, was taken suddenly ill thirty-six hours before I saw him in consultation with Dr. F. H. Clark. His illness began with sharp, cramp-like pains in the abdomen, nausea, vomiting and obstinate constipation. These pains continued without remission, but at no time became localized. At the same time, all efforts to move the bowels failed and Dr. Clark considered it a case of intestinal obstruction. When seen by the writer the patient had a rapid, thready pulse, a temperature of 102, and was in a condition of extreme prostration. The abdomen was distended and tender all over without any evidence of localization of the trouble. We considered the case one of general peritonitis with intestinal paresis and advised operation, but gave a very unfavorable prognosis. At the operation, which was done immediately, a general peritonitis was found which was due to a perforated appendix which was located well down in the pelvis. In addition to this, however, we found a distended loop of small intestine which had become adherent and kinked in the pelvis. Immediately upon freeing this loop, gas and fecal matter were heard to pass on and at the conclusion of the operation it was found that the patient's bowels had moved on the table. During the further course of the case the bowels responded in the usual manner to enemata and no further trouble was experienced in this respect. This patient failed to recover from his toxemia and died some five days after the operation.

Acute intestinal obstruction other than that produced by pare: ; of the intestine secondary to peritonitis, is, in our experience, a rare complication of appendicitis, perhaps sufficiently so to make it worthy of note here.

### A Case of Cerebral Tumor.
#### *Reported by Arthur H. Bogart, M.D.*

W. M., 19 years, United States, male; referred by Dr. George Barney. In October, 1911, this patient was knocked unconscious by a blow received while playing football. He had at that time a black eye, but no further after-effects until April 12th, when he began to have sick spells with vomiting and headache. These spells were severe enough at times to cause the patient to go to bed for a few days when they would pass off and he could attend to his business. In July his left eye began to trouble him with double vision and dimness of vision. During the same month he had occasional headaches and a loss of power developed in his left foot. On September 9, 1912, the patient was admitted to the Presbyterian Hospital. At this time the loss of power in the foot was considerable. He also had some flattening of the left side of the face and suffered a great deal from headache, while the eye was rapidly growing worse. After being in the hospital one week he suddenly became delirious, which condition lasted for seventy-two hours and then cleared up. He returned to his home in October, having declined operation, which was advised for the relief of his condition. He was, however, improved by medical treatment while there. Since leaving the hospital the headaches have grown progressively worse, accompanied with dizziness. He has also suffered from vomiting and hiccough. The vomiting usually occurred after the morning meal and was explosive in character, with premonition, but no nausea.

During this time his gait has been that of a drunken man and he was unable to get about without support.

*Previous History.*—Negative. Venereal disease denied.

*Family History.*—Mother died of new growth of some kind, the nature of which is unknown to the patient. His mother lost three children, all of whom died in infancy.

While at the Presbyterian Hospital a diagnosis of cerebral tumor was made by Dr. Starr and operation advised, but declined for the reason that in the absence of definite localizing symptoms the doctor was not able to promise a complete cure, but only relief from the distressing headache.

Dr. Eastman saw this case with me in consultation and while he rather inclined to the diagnosis of meningitis, recommended very strongly a decompression operation for the relief of the headache. The patient also was very anxious to have anything done which offered any hope of relief from pain.

Operation on January 24th. On this date we did a subtemporal decompression on the right side. We chose the right side because his paralysis had manifested itself on the left side, according to the history, although this was not a marked feature of the case at this time.

Immediately upon opening the dura the brain forced itself into the opening to such an extent as to make it difficult for us to close the fascia and muscle over the opening. For the first week following the operation, the pulse and temperature showed elevation and his condition was somewhat serious, but he finally straightened out and went home on the fifteenth day, the wound draining. It has since healed and on February 15th, his physician reports that the patient is sitting up and improving daily. His speech, which was very slow and deliberate immediately following the operation, is now becoming normal and the headache has been completely relieved, which was the case forty-eight hours after operation, and has not bothered him to any extent since. In view of the fact that ever since the operation he has been taking large doses of iodid, undoubtedly his general improvement is due as much to that as to the operation, which was done for the sole purpose of relieving the headache and not as a curative measure.

### A Case of New Growth in the Liver.

*Reported by Arthur H. Bogart, M.D.*

Mrs. F. K., 39 years, married. This patient was referred to me by Dr. F. H. Clark and gave the following history:

In August, 1909, the patient was seized with a sharp pain in the lumbar region. Her physician at that time diagnosed the condition as due to a floating kidney and advised operation. On August 14th, she was sent to the German Hospital, where an operation was done for that condition. Following this operation the pain in the back disappeared, but developed in the right side of the abdomen. This pain was constant, sharp and at times much worse than usual. Later she went to St. Mary's Hospital, Jamaica, where she was advised to have an operation, but declined and left the hospital unimproved. Still later she went to the New York Polyclinic, where she was again advised to be operated upon, but refused. After this she took medical treatment for about two weeks with decided improvement, both with regard to the pain and also her general health. Two years after she left the Polyclinic, March, 1912, the patient gave birth to a child, following which the pain increased. Since the Middle of December, 1912, the patient has grown progressively worse, the pain being more severe, appetite poor and bowels constipated. Occasionally while walking about or even while lying down, she has a sensation as of something moving about in the epigastrium. At times belching of gas is an annoying symptom. She constantly suffers from a severe pain in the right side of the abdomen and in the back, sometimes extending up into the thorax on the right side. She does not vomit, nor has she been jaundiced. The stools are apparently normal from her description, and there has been no loss of weight.

*Previous History.*—At the age of twelve years the patient suffered from chills and fever off and on for a period of about a year; otherwise negative. She began menstruating at fifteen years and was always regular. She has had eight children, seven of whom are living; also had two miscarriages. There is no specific history obtainable. Mother dead, cause unknown; father alive and well.

*Physical Examination.*—Well-nourished woman of middle age with no evidence of jaundice or cachexia and from her general appearance, does not seem to be suffering from malignant or other serious disease. Heart and lungs are normal. Urine examination normal. She complains of pain in the right side of the abdomen, just below the free border of the ribs. Palpation in this region reveals a tumor mass which is freely movable, somewhat tender and painful. This mass moves up and down with the respirations and from its location it might be an enlarged right kidney, a gall-bladder or an enlarged lobe of the liver. Operation was advised and accepted.

*Operation.*—Right incision as would be used for a gall-bladder. Inspection of the stomach and gall-bladder showed them to be normal. The right kidney was slightly enlarged but well fixed in a normal position. The tumor mass proved to be a very much enlarged lobe of the liver which was the seat of a tumor situated immediately beneath the capsule and apparently well defined from the normal liver substance. From its readily accessible location and freedom from infiltration, it seemed feasible to remove it. This was accomplished with very little difficulty, the tumor shelling out of its bed with very little trouble and an unusually small amount of hemorrhage, which was easily controlled with a few mattress sutures passed on a round needle. In addition to the principal mass, there was another small cystic one about the size of a walnut, situated near the large one, which was about the size of a small orange. The mattress sutures having been introduced, the capsule was closed with a running suture, a drain introduced and the abdomen closed.

This operation was done on January 27th. There has been considerable drainage from the wound, which is now rapidly clearing up, and apparently the patient is making a good recovery, though she still complains of some pain and tenderness in this region.

With the exception of secondary carcinoma and gummata, solid tumors of the liver are comparatively rare. Primary carcinoma is rare; in fact, even more so than sarcoma.

(*Continued in September* JOURNAL.)

# LONG ISLAND MEDICAL JOURNAL

## VOL. VII.    SEPTEMBER, 1913    NO. 9

## ⚙riginal Articles.

### SOME PHASES OF PELVIC INFECTION.

#### By William P. Pool, M.D.,

of Brooklyn, N. Y.

I N latter times so much has been said of infections of the pelvis, and so many rules have been laid down concerning their cause, and course, and treatment, that this subject may be considered in great measure a *res adjudicata*. But continued experience always teaches something, and the occasional unfortunate results of treatment of bacterial diseases of the pelvis would seem to indicate that there is still sometimes a lack of definite conception of the nature of these diseases and certainly a lack of unanimity as to the best methods of managing them.

Whether a case demand surgical treatment, or whether there be a possibility of a return to health with anatomic and functional restoration if it be left to nature; how to determine by the means at hand the nature of the infection; what is the proper time and preferable method of operating, if operation be necessary, are questions which we are constantly meeting, and which require not a little care in deciding.

The rational treatment of a disease must depend upon a knowledge of its natural history, and in considering the course of infections of the pelvic organs two facts must be borne in mind: 1. That many infections, whether in the uterus or parametria, or tubes, are self limited. 2. That the structures of the pelvis, particularly the mucous membranes of the uterus and tubes, are very difficult of destruction—facts which predispose to spontaneous cure—for with decrease or cessation in the virulence of the infection the second factor becomes operative, and tends to restore the tissues to their normal condition. That spontaneous cure is possible is borne out by the not infrequent occurrence of cases of puerperal or even gonorrhœal infection which present at the outset pelves filled with cellular exudate, and which after passing through an acute inflammatory stage, with or without evidences of peritoneal involvement, are gradually restored to health and comfort, the only essential treatment being rest. The exudate is absorbed and the various organs are apparently no worse anatomically for the experience. The functions of menstruation and even conception take place normally and there is freedom from pain. The effect of puerperal infections upon pelvic structures is (according to Simpson) not different from that which they produce upon tissues nearer the surface of the body, as in erysipelas, or a boil, where inflammatory exudate may be deposited and absorbed, and leave little or no trace of its existence. Gonorrhœal infection of the uterus and tubes is less likely to result in complete restoration and normal functional activity, but this also is sometimes seen even in severe cases (Simpson (*Jour. S. G. and O.,* vol. IX., page 45). Such a fortunate resolution, however, is not to be confidently expected and the end results vary with the intensity and duration of the infection. In some the organs may return to their normal condition, but, owing to an accompanying peritonitis, are left so involved in adhesions that they are a source of constant pain, and seriously interfere with health. In others there is a partial destruction of tissue, the tubes are occluded, their mucosa damaged, and their walls thickened and hardened by fibrous deposit. The ovaries have thickened tunics and are cystic, and all the organs are distorted, displaced, and massed together by adhesions of their peritoneal coats.

In still another class there is an extensive degeneration of tissue, the formation of pus foci, and the development of tubal or tuboovarian abscess, or of a true pelvic abscess in the parametrium. In all degrees and variations of the disease there is an outpouring of cellular exudate which surrounds and walls off the focus of infection, and it is due to this fact, and to its peculiarly favorable location in the most dependent portion of the trunk, that pelvic infection usually remains local. We must except those cases of puerperal origin in which the organisms advance so rapidly through the dilated blood and lymph channels leading from the cervix that the limiting exudate cannot form in time to check them. The infection passes quickly into the circulation, or peritoneal cavity, and the disease is general rather than local from the very outset. Aside from these explosive attacks, pelvic inflammations, *per se,* very rarely menace the life of the patient. The disease passes through an acute to a chronic stage, and finally she suffers from the result of the infection, not from the infection itself.

Forssner (*Archives of Gyn.,* 1907) has reported 1,555 cases of pelvic inflammations treated conservatively with eight deaths, approximately ½ of 1 per cent., and Simpson reports 465 consecutive cases of tubal origin, all conservatively treated, and then operated upon, with three deaths—7/10 of 1 per cent. Such results indicate that the life of the patient does not depend upon surgical treatment, and that during the acute period of the attack nothing is to be gained by operation. On the contrary it appears that there are excellent reasons for delaying such a measure. In the first place the patient's general state is such, at the height of an infection, that she cannot so well withstand an additional shock. The toxemia of this condition predisposes to insufficiency of the heart and kidneys and the nervous system is always more or less profoundly depressed, and to add anæsthesia and operation at this time of lowered resistence will in itself sometimes turn the scale in the wrong direction. Also the known tendency to self limitation of the virulence of infection points to conservatism until the active process has subsided.

Watkins (*S. G. and O.,* IV., page 507) has observed that inflammatory exudates furnish a protection against the spread of infection and may play an important part in the destruction of bacteria and the limitation of the absorption of toxins. "Formerly the presence of pus was considered a positive indication for immediate operation. Now it is known that pus, after a short time becomes sterile, and comparatively harmless, in the absence of a secondary infection, and that finally the bacteria and toxins entirely disappear." To destroy too soon the wall which thus seals up the infected area inevitably results in a more general mischief. A transient toxemia may be converted into a virulent bacteriemia, or extension of inflammation to the peritoneum may result.

In this connection it is desired to call attention to the enormous harm which may be done by intrauterine treatment of any kind, in puerperal infection. Instances of this abuse are too common and its invariably unfortunate results are too well established to admit any contradiction of the statement that interference with the acutely septic uterus, whether by curette or douche or even by the examining finger, is certain to be followed by a spread of the infection. It has never done the slightest good. It has frequently done serious harm. This does not refer to cases in which there is retained placental tissue which decomposes and produces foul lochia, and by reason of the absorption of the products of putrefaction causes symptoms local and general which closely stimulate those of true sepsis. It is good surgical sense to remove a sloughing mass from the uterus when that is the only cause of the trouble, but if there be present active septic organisms it is much better to leave its separation and expulsion to nature than to traumatise the uterine canal under such conditions. Another cause, though a rare one, of puerperal fever and local disturbance is the retention of lochia in a retroflexed uterus. (The writer does not recognize stenosis of the cervical outlet as a possible cause of such retention.) Here drainage is accomplished by the simple maneuvre of turning the patient on her face for a few minutes several times a day. These conditions should usually be differentiated readily. A culture from the cervical discharge may be made without injury to any pelvic structure, and this is the first step toward rational treatment, no radical measure being employed till septic organisms have been excluded beyond any question.

It has been suggested that since immediate operation is advocated in acute infections of the appendix the same rule might equally apply in like conditions in the tubes. But the circumstances are not at all analogous. The more exposed position of the appendix does not permit so complete a walling off, and the tendency to rupture is much greater. Rupture is the natural result of the great majority of purulent appendices, whereas the spontaneous rupture of a tubal abscess into the peritoneal cavity is exceedingly rare. And also limitation of the active infection is impossible in ruptured appendicitis, because of direct communication with the lumen of the bowel. A similar state of affairs exists sometimes in the pelvis when an old pus tube becomes adherent to the bowel and ruptures into it. Pus flows into the bowel and is evacuated, but colon bacilli also flow from the bowel into the tubal abscess cavity there to renew the infection and create more pus, and the process goes on indefinitely. Such a condition, wherever found, must of course be dealt with radically.

The destruction of organisms within the infected area has been accounted for in different ways: That an immunity and resistance to any specific form of infection is created in the blood by the long residence of that infection in the body, and that the infection is finally overcome by it; or, that bacteria being inclosed within a small space by the cellular exudate perish by the action of the toxins they themselves have generated. At the same time it is known that if left in a culture tube in an incubator and not in contact with, or opposed by the living organism virulent bacteria will expire in the course of time. However, the point of greatest importance clinically is that autosterilization of the focus does take place, which fact is proved by the frequency with which old accumulations of pus in the pelvis are found to be free from germ life.

In 2,973 cases of chronic pelvic suppuration (excluding tubercular) collected by Hyde (*Am. Jour. Obstet.*, 1908, LVII., page 591), bacteriologic examination showed 1,998 to be sterile, 67⅕ per cent. Andrews (*Am. Jour. Obstet.*, 1904, XLIX., page 181) has reported a series of 684 cases of which 55 per cent. were sterile.

It having been demonstrated many times by clinical and laboratory experience that the element of time is essential in the destruction of the disease organisms it is next necessary to determine the period of time required for this autosterilization, and by what means we may discover that the virulence of the attack has passed. The complexity of the question is further increased by the fact that the persistence of infection differs materially with its character. It is therefore of the first importance to differentiate the infection and to know its habit and behavior under given conditions.

All classifications show that (tubercular aside) there are two predominent forms of bacterial disease to which the pelvic organs are liable, the gonococcic and the streptococcic. Other organisms, the staphylococcus, bacillus coli communis, or the pneumococcus, may be the exciting cause in a small proportion of cases, but the number of these is so small that they may be practically regarded as negligible for clinical purposes. The two principal classes differ widely as to mode of invasion and habit, and also in persistence.

At the onset of an attack bacteriological examination is often available for differential diagnosis and an accurate knowledge of the kind of infection may be obtained, but when a case has passed into the chronic stage all external evidence of the infection has frequently disappeared, the point of primary invasion is healed and is sterile, and we must depend upon clinical evidence alone to determine with what manner of disease we have to deal.

Crossen (*S. G. and O.*, IX., 1909, page 406) has called attention to certain clinical characteristics by which a fairly accurate diagnosis may be made, viz.: 1. The apparent cause as learned from the history and examination of the lower genital organs, and 2. The location of the focus of the infection.

In the gonococcic class the deeper pelvic inflammation is preceded by external gonorrhœa, or comes on without any apparent cause, and the focus is situated in the tube. The onset is comparatively mild in the majority of cases. Fever does not run very high or remain very long, and pain and prostration are not extreme as a rule. A woman recently married, of previous good health, who presents an inflammatory mass in the pelvis, is always under suspicion of gonococcic infection, and careful questioning is necessary to discover any history of vulvitis, discharge, or burning micturition which may have occurred weeks or months before the patient is seen. In some cases there is no history of previous inflammation of the external genitals, and the infection has developed in the upper organs before the patient is aware of its presence. In such cases the germ is probably deposited directly in the cervix, and the vulvar structures escape infection to a great extent. There are often, however, signs of inflammation in or about the vulvo-vaginal glands and glands of Skene, and·the typical maculæ gonorrhœa may be seen in these localities. Frequently there is a considerable leucorrhœal discharge from the cervix, and muco-pus may be expressed from the vulvar glands and from the urethra. Although bacteriologic examination of these discharges may be negative this fact cannot rule out gonorrhœa.

Any previous examination, local treatment, or operation, must be excluded as a possible cause. The diagnosis of a gonococcic infection may be complicated by the occurrence of abortion or childbirth at which time the gonococcus, which has probably lain dormant in the lower genital tract, invades the deeper structures. The frequency with which this may take place is shown in statistics collected by Crossen, which follow: Sanger (*Vehr. d. Deutsches Gesselch. f. Gyn.*, 1886, page 177) examined the secretions of 389 pregnant women and found the gonococcus in 100. Steinbuckel (*Weiner Klin. Wochenschr.*, 1892) examined the lochia of 274 women, in whom the puerperium was normal, and found the gonococcus in 18 per cent. In Leopold's clinic (*Centralblat. f. Gyn.*, page 675) 25 per cent. of the puerperal infections were of gonorrhœal origin. But puerperal infection from this source alone is distinguished by its mild degree and short duration.

It is well understood that the gonococcus produces essentially a surface infection, and that its mode of invasion is along the mucous membranes of the cervix and uterus, whence it extends to the tubes by continuity of structure. It rarely invades the wall of the uterus or reaches the parametrium. Thus the usual lesion which results is pyosalpinx, or by extension, tubo-ovarian inflammation or abscess. Diagnosis of this may usually be made without difficulty by its location high in the pelvis or its prolapse into the cul-de-sac of Douglass. A certain amount of perisalpingitis is always present, causing induration, which, however, is readily distinguished from the hardness of parametrial infiltration.

The gonococcus is said to be the only organism which will spontaneously invade the adult pelvis, but infection by the streptococcus is almost always, if not invariably preceded by traumatism of some sort: Childbirth, miscarriage, examination, or instrumentation, cancer, or chronic inflammation. Like other organisms it may be present in the pelvic passages and fail to produce inflammation, even under conditions most favorable for its invasion. In the examination of fifty-eight puerperal women Lea and Sidebotham (*J. Obstet. and Gyn., Brit. Empire,* Jan., 1909) found hemolytic streptococci in 20 per cent., without any abnormal symptoms. But while infection does not always follow injury, the streptococcus depends upon injury to give it a point of entrance to the circulation, and careful search in the history of a chronic inflammation should be made for an element of trauma, however remote in point of time. Streptococcic inflammation is usually characterized by greater violence of onset, with higher temperature and symptoms of more profound toxemia and depression, which follow rapidly after the first entrance of the infection. Still, there are milder cases in which the onset resembles that of the gonococcic type, when differential diagnosis must depend upon other points, chief among which is the location of the lesion. This, in the streptococcic class, is in the connective tissue area of the pelvis. Streptococci entering by way of abrasions or lacerations penetrate the uterine wall and pass to the parametrium where a focus is established. From this point they may spread to the adjoining parts and no organ is immune from infection. Streptococcic salpingitis may occur, but it probably begins in all cases as a perisalpingitis and is secondary to the lesion in the broad ligament.

Therefore, in this class the disease is found lower in the pelvis and is distinguished by the extensive hardness of infiltrated connective tissue, and the massing together and immobility of the uterus and all structures on the side effected. When both sides are involved the whole pelvis may be so choked with cellular exudate that the recognition of organs is impossible. As the acute attack subsides the exudate is gradually absorbed and its site restored, or a chronic inflammatory mass remains, in the center of which is an accumulation of pus. It may be affirmed that such a lesion is never caused by the gonococcus except in rare cases of extension from the tube, and that it is nearly always the result of streptococcic infection.

Thus by a careful examination of the history of the case and by its physical characteristics a chronic inflammatory mass may usually be traced to its original source and cause. Instances of mixed infection as shown by Stone and McDonald (*S. G. and O.*, 1905, page 151) when one form is superadded to the other, no doubt exists, but the more severe and virulent type overshadows the minor, and the disease should be regarded and treated accordingly.

In respect to the persistence of virulence in these two classes, experience, sometimes regretable experience, has been the only teacher. Variations in the time necessary for autosterilization in either are no doubt due to differences in degree of virulence and to the resistance of the individual. The gonococcus, when enclosed within a limited area, is much the shorter lived. Watkins believes that its activity may pass in from one to two weeks. Simpson places the minimum time at three weeks after acute symptoms have subsided. Hartman and Morax have found that it persists from three weeks to four months, with an average of four to five weeks. Crossen (*S. G. and O.*, IX., 1909, page 411) summing up the experiences of a number of observers, concludes that sterilization of gonococcic pus confined in a tube may be expected in from six to eight weeks, but that in some cases it may remain active for a considerably longer period.

Consensus of opinion as to the streptococcus is that its duration is indefinite. It quickly disappears from the cellular tissue along with the exudate it has caused, but when enclosed in an abscess cavity shut off from all outside communication, it may remain active a very long time. Cases reported by Miller and by Martin have shown that it was found in a state of virulence six, twelve and nineteen years after the date of the original infection. The conclusion, therefore, must be that no time limit can be placed upon the longevity of this germ, and that there is no assurance of autosterilization of an abscess caused by it at any time.

The object of this review is simply to point again to the desirability of conservative treatment in pelvic infection. In those cases which have been so damaged by the disease that surgery is necessary to restore health and comfort, the time and method of operation must obviously depend, to a great extent, upon the type of infection.

In the gonococcic class the character and location of the lesion almost always require abdominal section, and while this inflammation usually runs a mild course when localized, this fact must not be presumed upon too far. The liberation of pus from a tubal abscess of this kind may be followed by severe peritonitis, or the infection of distant parts through the blood. Septic endocarditis and joint infections have been caused in this way.

To say definitely at just what point of time the virulence of any case has passed away is impossible. The amount of pain is unreliable as a sign, for after the acute period pain is often greatly relieved or may cease. Disappearance of fever indicates only that general toxemia is relieved, and does not of necessity mean sterilization of the focus. Blood examination may be entirely negative after thorough localization has taken place. The absorption of exudate is one of the most useful clinical signs, as its removal from about the point of infection indicates that local inflammation has subsided, because active infection has ceased. Therefore, when softness and flexibility have been restored to the pelvic structures, it may be concluded that abdominal operation is fairly safe. As this process occupies an average of from six to eight weeks, additional safety is secured by waiting a still longer time. A period of from three to four months from the time of original infection should ensure the sterility of practically all cases, and during this time it is surprising how many will become free from pain and improve in general health, even in the presence of an extensive anatomic lesion. A tubal abscess when situated in the cul-de-sac may be drained by vaginal incision at an earlier time, but when high in the pelvis it is not easily accessible by this route, and in reaching it so much traumatism of tissue is necessary that the patient is exposed to much the same danger as in the radical operation. Unless the exigencies of the case demand immediate evacuation it is better left till later.

As the period of activity of the streptococcus is indefinite it is never safe to expose the peritoneum to the contents of an inflammatory mass of this character, and its proper treatment is always by extraperitoneal drainage. This, fortunately, is more easily accomplished because of the lower and more accessible situation of the mass. When a parametrial abscess has formed it is, of course, useless to wait for sterilization, but it is wise to delay even a vaginal incision until the acute symptoms have passed, and complete localization has taken place. To plunge into an indurated mass in the acute stage in the hope of finding pus may be followed by serious consequences. Sometimes upward extension of inflammation causes a mass to appear above Poupart's ligament. This does not always break down, but if it does, it is best to wait until the abscess points at the skin surface, when incision and drainage may be accomplished by the shortest possible route and with the least traumatism.

With the pus focus removed sterilization of a streptococcic inflammation may proceed promptly, and secondary radical operation, if necessary, may be possible and safe.

# THE ROLE OF NEGATIVE CURRENTS IN THE GROWTH OF NEOPLASMS.

## By Martin J. Sgier, M.D.,

of Richmond Hill, N. Y.

PHYSIOLOGISTS are agreed as to the existence of currents of electricity in muscle. These currents are of two kinds, and are sufficient to cause a deflection of a galvanometric needle. They are known as (a) Currents of Rest, and (b) Currents of Action.

(A) In muscles that have been removed from the body, it has been found that for some little time, electrical currents can be demonstrated passing from point to point on their surfaces; but as soon as the whole muscle dies or enters into rigor mortis, these currents disappear. The cut ends are always *negative* to the equator. These currents are constant for some time after removal from the body, and in fact remain as long as the muscle retains its life. They are in all probability due to *chemical* changes going on in the muscle.

If the uninjured tendon be used as one end of the muscle, and the muscle be examined in situ, without removal from the body, the currents are very feeble, but they are at once much increased by injuring the muscle, as by cutting off its tendon. This appears to show that currents do not exist in uninjured muscle in situ, but that an injury, either mechanical, chemical or thermal, will render the injured part electrically negative to other points on the muscle. These currents are called either natural muscle currents, or currents of rest, accordingly as they are looked upon as always existing in muscle, or as only developed when a part of the muscle is injured. In either case, up to a certain point, it is agreed that the *strength* of the current is in *direct proportion* to the *amount of injury.*

(B) When a muscle contracts the natural muscle currents, or currents of rest, undergo a distinct diminution, which is due to the appearance in the actively contracting muscle of currents in an opposite direction to those existing in the muscle at rest. This causes a temporary deflection of the galvanometer in a direction opposite to the original current, and is called by some physiologists the negative variation of the muscle currents, and by others a current of action.

It has been shown by Hermann that in an entirely uninjured, resting muscle there are no differences in electrical tension. If the skin be removed carefully from the gastrocnemius of a frog, no current at all, or only the very weakest one, is obtained when the muscle is connected with the galvanometer. If, on the other hand, the muscle be injured in any way in the neighborhood of one electrode, a strong current appears. (The current does not appear in its full strength immediately, but develops gradually.) Herrmann's theory is that the cause of the difference in electrical potential in the resting muscle lies in the injury which it receives. In a partially injured muscle, every point of the injured portion is negative to every point of the uninjured part. The facts may be expressed in the following general proposition: In every injured muscle fibre the demarkation surface between the living and the dead contents of the fibre is the seat of an electromotive force, directed toward the living part.

Tigerstedt sums up the question in the following statement: In muscle and in nerve, every active or injured part maintains a negative electrical relation toward every other part which is at that time at rest or uninjured.

Biedermann observes that one cannot draw a sharp line of separation between current of rest and current of action in epithelial and glandular cells for the reason that the differences of tension met with are always the expression of differences in the chemical relations of the neighboring parts.

In reading the foregoing, it occurred to me that the negative variation, or electric current in the contracting muscle might also be due (as in the case of the muscle at rest) to *chemical changes* going on in the muscle, this time because of the formation of a new chemical substance or compound (the product of its metabolism) which was *positive* to the muscle and consequently reversed the polarity of the current. Immediately the whole question of chemico-physical science as applied to electricity was brought up, and I concluded that these currents were due to the chemical dissociation of molecules and atoms into negative and positive ions and electrons, whenever the equilibrium of a resting part was disturbed, whether by injury or by action; anabolism causing a positive electrical phenomenon and katabolism, a negative condition of the part.

It is only possible for a current of electricity to exist between two points when there is a difference in potential between the two points: the greater the difference, the stronger the current, and vice versa. In the case of any healthy inactive muscle, I believe that it is ISOELECTRIC because the electric equilibrium is complete, and hence no currents are demonstrable; but any cause that will upset the equilibrium will cause a current, *i. e.,* any influence (mechanical, chemical or thermal) which will lower the vitality or even in the slightest degree alter the metabolism of any part of the muscle, creates a difference of potential with reference to the uninjured part, and it becomes negative to the latter. In the case of currents of action, I believe that the products of the metabolism of the contracting muscle alter the equilibrium and in this way cause a current.

The problem therefore resolves itself into a question of metabolism: whether it be a current caused by the perverted and consequently lowered vitality (potential) of an injured or dying part, as compared with a healthy part, or one caused by the active metabolism and higher potential of an active part, as compared with one that is at rest. The currents will continue to flow until the equilibrium is restored, in every case.

Inasmuch as the question is now one of metabolism, I think that it is logical to argue that electric currents occur in all organs and tissues, for although none have yet been detected,* it is reasonable to suppose that they must exist because of the vital changes (metabolism) which take place and the consequent differences in potential which must be caused by them. But if *metabolism* will by *chemical activity,* liberate or create negative and

* Recently currents have been shown in the heart and all internal organs, when in a state of activity.

positive ions, and thereby cause electric currents which will flow until a state of equilibrium is reached, what determines the equilibrium?

We are told that it is certain that "the cells of most adult tissues retain the power of multiplication. This is not manifest under normal conditions, possibly because the blood-supply that is received by the tissues is only sufficient to maintain the status quo, while the resistances opposing growth (such as pressure within the tissues) are equal to the force with which they tend to multiply; but if the intercellular pressure be loosened by wound or by destruction of tissue, absorption of the damaged elements and multiplication of the cells around about will begin." The foregoing extract from "Green's Morbid Anatomy" may be perfectly in accord with the latest scientific teaching, but somehow I cannot help imagining a direct connection between the so-called Vis Medicatrix Naturæ and the currents of metabolism. When a structure is diseased, as in the case of a granulating wound or ulcer, is it not possible that the Vis Medicatrix is simply the electric current generated by the difference in potential between the healthy and the injured part, which will cease when the gap is filled up, or in other words, when the equilibrium is restored?

Applying the foregoing to cancer and other tumors, the deduction would lead to the following conclusion or theory. A traumatism (mechanical, chemical or thermal) exerted on a part of an organ or a tissue, devitalizes the tissue affected, lowering its vitality (altering its metabolism) and consequently generating, because of the difference in potential, an electric current or vis conservatrix. This electrical stimulation causes an increased growth of cells, which by their very presence further lower the vitality (by the added pressure which they exert on the blood-supply, etc.) and thereby increase the electrical discrepancy (and consequently, the strength of the current) and augment or hasten the metabolism of the growth.

It is a well known fact that cancer flourishes only after forty years of age, when the vitality is beginning to wane, and when the recuperative powers are no longer far in excess of the injury, so that the part of lowered metabolism has a chance to start (and thus add its weight to the metabolic discrepancy) at a time when any organ or tissue that has recently or even remotely been injured or devitalized in any way (whether directly by traumatism or irritation, or indirectly, by interference with its nutrition or blood-supply) has a poorer chance of a restitutio ad integrum than in early life, because of the general senile changes in blood vessels and tissues. Is it not possible that these *senile changes* may be reduced to *a chemical basis,* whereby new chemical combinations (ions and electrons) are formed, producing a state of metabolic equilibrium which is more readily altered or destroyed, and hence creating a condition in which these electric currents are more easily generated, and counteracted or destroyed with great difficulty, if at all?

Between benign and malignant growths, I do not think there is any difference in growth and development. It is a well known fact that the more normal tissue (adult tissue) in a tumor, the less malignant it will be; in other words, the more tissue that is in electrical equilibrium, the less electrical stimulation and hence the slower growth. If, perchance, the metabolism of a benign tumor should by any interference with its vital conditions (blood-supply, etc.) increase the discrepancy of electrical potential, and hence cause a stronger current, and thus increase stimulation of cell growth, a rapid growth would supervene and we would say that the benign tumor had become malignant; and in proportion as the emunctories were unable to eliminate the products of its accelerated metabolism, toxæmia or cachexia would ensue.

Metastasis and metastatic growth I regard simply as a process of auto-inoculation, by which a portion of the metabolic products of the primary growth is taken up by the lymphatics and carried to a point or points separate and apart from the original tumor, where it lodges, altering chemically the tissues with which it comes in contact, and producing a katabolic phase in their metabolism. This condition of lowered vitality results in their becoming negative to the surrounding healthy tissue, a current is generated which by its stimulation causes cell proliferation and a new (secondary) tumor appears at the site of inoculation.

With regard to the morphology of cancer, I believe that the cancer cells are atypical simply because of their atypical and unrestrained growth. In embryonic and pre-adult tissue (to which all malignant tumors tend to revert) I believe there is a greater difference in electrical potential, causing by this constant stimulation, an increased and proportionately more rapid growth than in the adult tissues, in which the equilibrium is more constant.

The recently discovered fact, that the products of carcinomatous growth are acid, and those of sarcomata, alkaline, is simply corroborative of the foregoing, inasmuch as the result of chemical action in carcinoma would naturally be some combination or derivative of sarcolactic acid, and in connective tissue or bone (sarcoma) alkaline, because of the alkaline elements (calcium, sodium, potassium, etc.) involved. I think the proposed treatment, as outlined, of neutralizing acid by the use of alkalies and vice versa, is simply treating effects or results and not causes.

Cancer is at present a surgical disease, and from present indications will continue to be one for a long time to come. This is simply for the reason that there are no nerves in neoplasms, and consequently they cause no pain or discomfort until by pressure or interference with some tissue or organ, they make their presence felt. The only hope then lies in recourse to surgical methods. If the surgeon accepts any or all of the premises named in the foregoing hypothesis, his technique will include, in addition to the regular routine, two propositions, as follows:

1. Cut in tissues that have the lowest available vitality, so that there will be the least discrepancy between the normal and the resulting scar-tissue.

2. Cut in such a manner that the minimum scar will result, keeping in mind always, loss of vitality and of nutrition, due to altered blood-supply.

While surgical treatment is at present the only treatment for cancer, it is admitted that 65 per cent. recurs in one year, 20 per cent. in two years, 5 per cent. in three years and after that it is of rare occurrence. Cures have been reported of epitheliomata and superficial carcinomata by means of the Roentgen ray.

I believe, in accordance with the foregoing hypothesis, that every case of recurrence of cancer (unless some of the original growth has actually been left behind) is not a recurrence at all, but a *primary new growth* caused by undue and unrestrained electrical stimulation, which is generated by a *difference in potential* between healthy tissue and one devitalized by injury caused by mechanical or surgical means; and I am further strengthened in my belief in this by the statistics mentioned under the question of recurrences. The fact that they decrease in such enormous ratio (25%) each year, seems to me to indicate the degree of success that was attained in complying with the two propositions mentioned above . . . the cases of least number and longest immunity being in all probability those in which the ideal circumstance (where it was possible to cut in tissues whose vitality (metabolism) was very little, if at all higher in grade than the resulting scar, and hence the difference in potential and consequent stimulation was practically nil) was attained . . . and that the greater percentages and quicker recurrences were in direct proportion to the metabolic discrepancy whch existed between the healthy and the incised tissue at the close of the operation . . . for a current will flow, as stated above, until the equilibrium is restored, and is in direct proportion to the injury.

Mayo estimates that 50 per cent. of cancers of the stomach are engrafted on the scar of an old ulcer; and Moynihan says that 72 per cent of all the cases of carcinoma of the stomach operated upon by him had been preceded by a gastric ulcer.

Electricity in some form, by fulguration or some other means, seems to me to be the logical method of treatment, in an effort to neutralize or destroy these currents of injury, but I believe surgery will be required in every case. Much has already been done in electro-therapeutics by way of experiment, and many cures reported. A copy of a recent article in the *Medical Record,* by Dr. William Seaman Bainbridge, on this subject, which I had the opportunity of reading through the courtesy of the author, and in which he describes the DeKeating-Hart Method of Fulguration and Thermo-radiotherapy was very interesting and instructive. This treatment is at present being tried at the New York Skin and Cancer Hospital, with great success. One of the statements that impressed me most forcibly was the announcement, attributed by Dr. Bainbridge to DeKeating-Hart, in which he says that the spark acts

"not upon the cancer itself, but upon the soil upon which the cancer develops."

This seems to be in perfect accord with the foregoing hypothesis, inasmuch as it is only another way of saying that it is the surrounding healthy tissue which stimulates the growth . . . and I believe that the stimulation is electrical, . . . and that it is carried on by means of the above mentioned Currents of Rest . . . Currents of Injury . . . Demarkation Currents . . . as they have been variously designated, and if the foregoing has any foundation in fact, the problem confronting us is merely the addition, subtraction, transposition or substitution of one or more molecules or radicals (simple or compound) whereby the chemical nature of the devitalized part is altered and becomes negative to the unaltered tissue, thus generating a current in precisely the same way that any two electrodes of different potential do when brought into contact under suitable conditions; and I believe that the very many attempts that have been made to devise a method for the cure of this dreaded disease (enzymes, serum, fulguration, X-ray, radium, etc.) have all been more or less successful, accordingly as they were able or unable to readjust the original chemical molecule; and the converse of this may be presumed to exist in the instances in which cancer has been successfully inoculated.

In recapitulation, I desire to say briefly, that according to the foregoing hypothesis

1. Healthy, inactive tissue is isoelectric, because the equilibrium is perfect and complete.

2. Whenever the vitality of a part is lowered, or its metabolism altered even in the slightest degree, by injury or action, a current is generated.

3. These currents are due to chemical changes, taking place in the area of altered metabolism, whereby it becomes negative to the healthy part.

4. These currents cause tissue metamorphosis. (Cell proliferation, etc.)

5. The chemical constitution of the human body is altered gradually as the individual grows older, and eventually becomes such that the equilibrium is very easily destroyed and very difficult to restore, hence the prevalence of cancer after middle life.

6. Cancer is neither infectious nor contagious; nor do I believe that heredity has any part in the causation, excepting possibly the influence of certain inherited peculiarities on the metabolism and chemical composition of the individual, relative to the above mentioned senile changes.

7. Treatment of this most terrible and fatal of human diseases should be directed to overcoming these currents (neutralizing or destroying them by X-ray, fulguration, violet ray, radium, etc.) or in an attempt (by means of enzymes, sera, etc.) to alter the chemical composition of the negative pole.

In conclusion, I wish to say simply, that I earnestly hope the foregoing may be the means, even indirectly, of lessening the misery of some poor sufferer. Every one of us has experienced that feeling of desire to do something to assuage the pains of a fellow mortal,—and has also experienced the opposite feeling of sorrow, regret and utter helplessness, when he has not known the right thing to do; and if the foregoing pages be the means of affording a clue, or stimulating to profitable research and investigation those who have the facilities, the experience and the ability which I have not at my command; and if their efforts be the means of relieving even one poor human being, I shall consider that I have been well repaid for whatever time and labor I have given to the theory submitted in the foregoing pages.

# A CASE OF BANTI'S DISEASE.*

## By L. Albert Thunig, M.D.,

### of Brooklyn, N. Y.

PATIENT.—January 13, 1913. Mr. B., age 25, Italian, in the United States for 14 years, and driver of milk wagon by occupation.

Family History.—Father, mother, two sisters and one brother are all alive and well. No tuberculosis. No carcinoma. Patient's wife is well, and though five years married, has never been pregnant.

Personal History.—When seven or eight years old suffered with some enlargement of his spleen; this gradually disappeared. When nine years old had diphtheria. The patient has no knowledge of ever having had malaria or any prolonged intermittent fever. From the age of nine was well until present illness.

Venereal.—Gonorrhea at seventeen years of age. Denies sore of any kind.

Habits.—Has used imported Italian wines moderately at meal time. Never intoxicated.

Present Illness.—Following a day of horseback riding, October 11, 1911, patient felt ill and had loss of appetite. He was examined and a large spleen found. He then had fever and chills for a few days and felt weak. Upon two occasions he passed a moderate amount of blood (per rectum).

In December, 1911, he commenced to have noticeable ascites, which became very great, but subsided spontaneously in March, 1912. This condition remained until August, 1912, when the ascites again became enormous and paracentesis was necessary about August 15, 1912. Since then this operation has been performed about every two weeks. During his entire illness he has felt quite well except for local discomfort from the weight and size of the ascites and the dragging weight of his spleen after paracentesis. Appetite always excellent, no vomiting or nausea. Bowels move well until ascites becomes very great, then a temporary constipation takes place. Patient has never had any local symptoms of hæmorrhoids. Has lost weight and flesh. No night sweats and no cough. Slight dyspnœa on exertion and slight œdema of ankles when the ascites is at its maximum. At other times both of these symptoms are absent.

*Physical Examination.*—Before Paracentesis.—Thin adult with marked ascutes. Slight flush of cheeks during examination. Color of lips good in comparison to surrounding skin, which is very white. No superficial lymph node involvement on inspection and palpation. Large dilated veins on abdominal wall.

Eyes, Throat.—Negative.

Thorax, Lungs.—Negative.

Heart.—Transmission of apex impulse to abdomen over fluid; otherwise negative.

Abdomen.—Tense and greatly enlarged with all signs of ascites present. Liver not palpable, area of dulness diminished from above. Spleen palpable and movable, but not easily definable.

Rectum and Anus.—Normal, no hæmorrhoids, internal or external (ascites at its height).

*Physical Examination.*—After Paracentesis.—A large ventral her-

---

* Read before the Brooklyn Pathological Society, March 14, 1913.

nia is at once discernible and when the patient is in the dorsal position the relaxed skin and parietes fall over the enormous spleen and its anterior edge can be seen to form an elevated ridge about two inches in height extending from the free border of the ribs almost into the pelvis.

Thorax.—Same as before with exception of loss of transmission of apex impulse.

Abdomen.—Liver cannot be felt, evidently small.

Spleen.—Greatly enlarged, dislocated downward and towards the median line, it being impossible to get the finger beneath the lower pole owing to its position in the pelvis.

In other respects the *physical examination* is the same as during ascites.

· *Pathological Examination.*—Urine.—Negative.

Blood.—Wassermann negative.

| Date | I<br>Jan. 13, '13 | II<br>Feb. 11 | III<br>Feb. 14 | IV<br>Mar. 9 | V<br>Mar. 12 |
|---|---|---|---|---|---|
| Hæmoglobin | ? | ? | ? | ? | 40% Dare |
| Red Cells | 4,960,000 | 2,148,000 | 1,852,000 | 2,400.000 | 3,440,000 |
| Pòikylocytes | Few | Not | Few | ........ | Many |
| Macrocytes | ........ | ........ | ........ | ........ | Many |
| Microcytes | ........ | ........ | ........ | ........ | Few |
| Skeletal Cells | ........ | ........ | ........ | ........ | Many |
| Normoblasts | None | None | None | None | None |
| Other Abnormal Reds | None | None | None | None | None |
| White | 5,200 | 9,600 | 7,400 | ........ | 7,200 |
| Polynuclears | 64% | 55% | 70% | ........ | 75% |
| Mono-Nuclears and | 20% | All Lymph | 20% | ........ | 13% |
| Large Lymph | ........ | 45% | ........ | ........ | ........ |
| Small Lymph | 16% | ........ | 10% | ........ | 12% |
| Eosinophiles | ........ | ........ | ........ | ........ | ........ |
| Basophiles | ........ | ........ | ........ | ........ | ........ |
| Abnormal Leucocytes | None | None | None | None | None |
| Parasites | None | None | None | None | None |

The above blood examinations show a rather marked variation, being made by two internes and myself. The first and last were made by myself and I paid special attention to the character of the cells, at least a two hours' search having been made in quest of abnormal red and white cells. As shown none were found.

*Progress of the Case.*—I sent the patient to St. John's Hospital on January 24th and the following is a brief report of his case:

His general condition is really excellent, being up and about with the exception of a day or two before paracentesis; then owing to the weight of the ascites he remains in bed. His appetite at all times is excellent. His temperature has ranged between 97.2 and 100. His pulse between 80 and 128, always regular and of good quality. Of more importance is the following table showing the frequency of recurrence of the ascites and the amount of fluid withdrawn at each occasion.

Jan. 25................2 gal. and 6 pts. (probable error, as
                      there were almost two pails of fluid.)

Feb. 6................6 gal. 4 oz.

Feb. 19................4 gal. 6 oz.

Mar. 4................5 gal. 4 oz.

Mar. 14...............Paracentesis performed at the meeting
                      of the Brooklyn Pathological Society. One large 16-quart pail and one-half of a large specimen jar full of fluid was obtained.

On February 19th patient had two severe nose bleeds which came on at night without any apparent cause.

On February 24th he had moderately severe hemorrhages from the bowel, some bright red blood and some tarry material.

*Treatment.*—The treatment has consisted of X-ray exposures which have been given by Dr. Search every week; also iron, arsenic, and nux vomica. The iron and arsenic had been given by mouth but are now being given by hypodermic.

*Present Condition.*—The general condition shows little change, if any. The blood is in worse condition although there is certainly a very marked diminution in the size of the spleen, it being now possible to get the fingers well underneath lower pole.

*Diagnosis.*—In view of a primary splenomegaly, an anemia of the secondary type, an atrophic liver, a severe and rapidly recurring ascites and the presence of hemorrhages, I feel that I can safely call the foregoing a typical case of Banti's Disease. The differential diagnosis will be given in the following discussion of splenic anemia and Banti's Disease.

*Splenic Anemia Including Banti's Disease.*—Splenic anemia is an anemia of the chlorotic or secondary type associated with a primary splenomegaly. Banti's Disease is that form of splenic anemia associated with cirrhosis of the liver.

Osler, in reviewing fifteen cases of splenic anemia, gives the following as the chief symptoms: I. Primary splenomegaly. II. Hemorhages, which are common, sometimes profuse or even fatal. Sometimes the hemorrhages are the chief source of trouble. III. Ascites. This is not necessarily due to a cirrhosis but may be due to the enlarged spleen or to the anemia. IV. Absence of enlargement of the superficial or deep lymph nodes. V. Anemia may vary from a mild chlortic type to a severe progressive pernicious type. The red cells averaged 3,336,567 in his cases and the hemoglobin was very low, but no average was taken. He found poikylocytes in five cases and degeneration of the red cells in two cases.

Cabot reports one case with the red cells as low as 384,000.

Einhorn, of New York, considers the following the typical symptom complex of Banti's disease: Splenomegaly, anemia, cirrhosis of the liver and ascites. He has found the red cell count low and the hemoglobin very low. In his experience the ascites has always been severe, recurring very rapidly after paracentesis. The liver was often atrophic. The skin sometimes pigmented. The hemorrhage was sometimes severe or fatal. He describes three forms:

I. *Primary.*—Splenomegaly, anemia, cirrhosis, ascites.

II. *Hemorrhagic Type.*—Primary type plus hemorrhages.

III. *Last Type.*—Splenomegaly, large liver, severe gastric symptoms and anemia.

*Pathology.*—Dr. Clark, in an excellent paper, reports a case in the Bristol *Med. and Chir. Journal,* 1903, with autopsy. In this case the red cells were as low as 1,171,000 and the hemoglobin 12 per cent., leucocytes 7,200 and the disease had been in progress about four years. The patient had many attacks of severe epistaxis. The temperature ranged between 99 and 100. Under iron, arsenic and digitalis the blood improved remarkably and the spleen decreased in size. The patient had an attack of diarrhœa and in the course of five days the temperature rose from 100 to 105 without any physical signs to account for it. It suddenly subsided and three days later the patient died of hemorrhage from the stomach, losing five pints of blood. Dr. Clark goes very minutely into the pathological findings and I would refer you to his article for the details. In brief, the changes were those of a sclerosis of the spleen with decrease of the malpighian corpuscles. The vessels of the spleen showed a proliferative process of the endothelium. The liver showed a cirrhosis. Slight change in the vessels of the glomeruli of the kidneys was present. The hemorrhage had evidently taken place from a small abrasion near the cardiac end of the stomach close to œsophageal varices. No gastric ulcer was found.

*Theory of the Pathological Cause.*—Moynihan believes that the increase in the size of the spleen is due to the absorption of toxines, probably from the intestine. These toxines are in turn given off from the spleen and carried to the liver by the portal vein, producing the cirrhosis.

Barr believes that the condition is due to a vasomotor paralysis of the splanchnic area due to disturbance of the sympathetic ganglions. This produces engorgement of the abdominal viscera, especially the liver and spleen. This in turn causes a change in the red cells and an increased hæmolysis. Owing to the chronic congestion of the liver and spleen an interstitial change finally takes place.

The latter theory supports Banti's findings in two cases of the disease in which he found post-mortem a lymphoid infiltration of the solar plexus and semi-lunar ganglion.

*Differential Diagnosis.*—Banti's Disease must be differentiated, according to Osler, from the following:

Pernicious Anemia.—In pernicious anemia abnormal red cells are always found and the spleen is usually not enlarged.

Splenic Leukæmia.—Ordinarily there is no difficulty whatever owing to the large leucocyte count and abnormal cells. Splenic anemia must at times be differentiated from those cases of leukæmia in which a temporary decrease in the leucocytosis has taken place. In these cases the change is only temporary and abnormal white cells are always found.

Hodgkin's Disease.—In this disease the superficial lymph nodes are always enlarged.

Cirrhosis of the Liver with a Large Spleen.—In these cases we can usually get an alcoholic or syphilitic history. The liver is the organ primarily involved and the blood changes are not marked.

*Prognosis.*—The prognosis is grave. Nearly all the cases grow progressively worse and die of gradual exhaustion or hemorrhage.

*Duration.*—No definite knowledge as to the duration of the disease is at hand. The duration has been quoted as three years. Osler reports a case of twelve years' duration.

*Treatment.*—Some cases have been cured by splenectomy. Moynihan states that it is impossible to give any accurate information as to the results of splenectomy, either immediate or remote, as many cases of simple hypertrophy of the spleen have been called early Banti's disease and many cases of cirrhosis with a secondarily enlarged spleen and ruptured œsophageal varices have been called late Banti's disease. Splenectomy, in his opinion, should be done before change in the liver is marked. Tansini and Rafferty, however, report cases of cure when splenectomy had been performed after the appearance of the ascites.

*Medical Treatment.*—The usual drugs, iron and arsenic and other tonics are advised. The X-ray has been beneficial in some cases.

NOTE.—The author does not claim any originality for the latter part of his paper. His statements are based upon papers and articles by Osler, Einhorn, Moynihan and Clark.

*(For discussion see page 374.)*

# A REPORT OF A CASE OF TRICHINOSIS.

## By Henry Joachim, M.D.,

of Brooklyn, N. Y.

DURING the past year the opportunity presented itself of observing seven cases of trichinosis. During this era of rigid meat inspection there is a tendency to convey the impression that the incidence of trichinosis is practically nil and its existence extinct and only of historic interest. In addition to these seven cases, Drs. Van Cott and Lintz reported the occurrence of three others to me, making a total of ten cases. This series would tend to controvert our sense of security in the efficiency of meat inspection in the extermination of trichinosis. It may be that its existence often remains unrecognized, as its clinical picture often simulates that of nephritis or muscular rheumatism. In the absence of a routine blood examination, which in all our cases revealed an eosinophilia, this error might well occur, for in one of our unsuspected cases it was this fact which aroused our suspicion as to the true diagnosis.

Nine of our ten cases occurred in Italians, two of whom succumbed to respiratory paralysis, thus giving us a lethality of 20 per cent in our series. With a few preliminary remarks on trichinosis in general, I shall report one of our cases somewhat in detail, as it serves as a type for the remainder which ran a somewhat similar course.

The importance of trichinosis was first recognized by Zenker in 1860. In that year a young girl was admitted to the hospital in Dresden, supposedly suffering from typhoid fever. Throughout her illness Zenker was impressed by the predominance of muscle pains. The girl succumbed and at the necropsy he removed a section of muscle which, upon microscopical examination, revealed the presence of the trichinella spiralis, which had been previously described by Owen and Paget in 1833. Previously to Zenker's discovery no particular significance was attached to the trichinella, and its presence was considered merely accidental. Zenker, however, associated its presence with the symptoms in his case, and attributed the malady to their presence. His findings were confirmed by Virchow and Leukhardt. Since Zenker's original case a great many epidemics have been reported, particularly in Germany, and all ascribed to the ingestion of raw or insufficiently cooked pork which harbored the larvæ of the trichinella.

The symptoms are usually grouped into three stages:

1. Intestinal irritation or period of ingression, in which the ingested encysted larvæ are liberated in the gastro-intestinal tract.

2. Myositis and fever, or digressive stage, characterized by the migration of the embryos into the muscles.

3. Subsidence or regression, in which œdema predominates.

The initial symptom is usually vomiting and a profuse diarrhœa with colicky abdominal pains suggestive of cholera. These symptoms usually appear a few hours subsequent to infection. The severity of these symptoms varies directly as the number of ingested trichinæ. Curiously enough, the severer the initial vomiting and purging, the better the prognosis and the greater the likelihood of the case eventuating in recovery. This apparent paradox might be explained on the assumption that a greater number of parasites are eliminated by the excessive vomiting and purging, and thus less are likely to enter the lymph and muscles. During this stage there is often a transitory initial œdema, usually appearing on the eighth day and persisting for from two to five days.

On the tenth day the second stage is ushered in by the appearance of muscle pains (myositis), which marks the invasion of the muscles by the young embryos. The muscles become tumid, hard and tender. Fever ranges between 102 deg. and 103 deg. The flexor muscles, rectus, masseters, diaphragm, intercostals and oculars usually show the greatest involvement. The patient assumes a posture of flexion suggestive of meningitis, but the knee-jerks as a rule are wanting.

About the third week the characteristic œdema appears involving chiefly the head and eyelids, hence the old name of "big head disease" of the Germans. There is also slight general œdema, but the genitals are usually spared. The œdema occurs in about 90 per cent. of the cases. During this stage the patient is bathed in a profuse perspiration which may be accompanied by sudamina, a roseola or desquamation. If the outcome is to be fatal, the typhoid state with its concomitant signs of dry tongue, frequent pulse rate, prostration and delirium intervenes.

It is during this stage that pneumonia may occur from involvement of the intercostals which makes expulsion of accumulated secretions impossible on account of muscular paralysis or pain provoked by coughing. If the case is to recover, convalescence begins about the fifth or sixth week. The lethality of 14,820 German cases compiled by Stiles was 5.6 per cent. Death usually occurs from asphyxia, pneumonia, excessive purging, marasmus or entorrhagia.

*Diagnosis.*—1. The most constant and characteristic finding is a leukocytosis with a marked increase of eosinphiles, first described by Brown of Johns Hopkins in 1897. This was a constant feature in all of our cases, reaching as high as 83 per cent. in one of them.

2. The demonstration of the trichinella in the fæces. This must be undertaken early in the disease before the parasite passes into the muscles. In none of our cases in which the search was instituted, could we demonstrate the parasite as most of them were seen in the second or third stage of the disease.

3. Lately, Janeway and Herrick have demonstrated the presence of the trichina in the circulating blood.

4. The occurrence of several cases in the same family, or other participants in a feast of pork should arouse the suspicion of trichinosis, and should lead to an examination of the blood for cosinophilia and the stools for the trichina.

5. The presence of a painful non-inflammatory œdema involving chiefly the head, sparing the genitals, and unaccounted for by a cardiac or renal lesion, should indicate the excision of a piece of the biceps for the microscopical demonstration of the encysted embryo.

Differentially, the following diseases must be taken into diagnostic consideration: typhoid, meningitis, muscular rheumatism, neuritis, beriberi, neuralgias, diaphragmatic paralysis, nephritis, etc.

*Prophylaxis.*—The key word to prophylaxis is abstention from raw or improperly prepared pork. The rat has been demonstrated to be the natural host of the trichinella. These or their excrement are ingested by the swine in whose muscles the parasites lodge. Rat extermination would therefore abolish the occurrence of trichinosis.

*Treatment.*—If seen in the first stage, which rarely happens except in epidemics, calomel and intestinal antiseptics, such as thymol, beta-napthol and glycerine, are indicated. The latter is advocated because it is supposed to destroy the parasite by extracting water from it. The rest of the treatment is purely symptomatic and supporative. Dr. Lintz will tell you of the salvarsan treatment of two cases.

The following case was one of our typical ones:

An Italian barber, age 35, was seen by Dr. Lintz and referred to the Jewish Hospital on December 19, 1912. His previous and family history were negative except for the existence of a right otitis media purulenta of eighteen years' duration. On Thanksgiving Day, 1912, he and his family partook of some veal and pork sausage prepared in the following manner: The bought skins were filled with a finely minced mixture of raw pork and veal. The mixture was then boiled for a few minutes. The day following the consumption of this delicacy the patient was taken with severe abdominal cramps followed by sixteen loose watery bowel movements. He then complained of nausea, vomiting, anorexia and severe prostration which necessitated his taking to his bed. On the eleventh day he noticed that his eyes and face were swollen and he felt very tired and drowsy. On the thirteenth day he experienced pain and stiffness in all his muscles and joints and consulted Dr. Lintz who advised hospital treatment. His wife and three children had similar but milder symptoms.

The physical examination was as follows:

Marked œdema of the face and eyelids with moderate swelling of the hands. Purulent discharge from the right ear, slight rigidity of the neck with some tenderness and stiffness of the sternomastoid muscle. There was also tenderness of the biceps and rigidity of the masseters which made it impossible for the patient to open his mouth widely. The knee-jerks were absent and there was a slight Kernig.

On admission the blood examination was as follows:

There was a leukocytosis of 22,750 with 45 per cent. polynuclears and 42 per cent. eosinophiles. Four days later the white count was 25,750 with 73 per cent. eosinophiles. The red count was 5,800,000 with 90 per cent. hæmoglobin. On discharge the count was 17,000 with 16 per cent. eosinophiles. The Widal reaction was negative.

The urine showed a faint trace of albumin, a few red blood cells but no casts. Three examinations of the fæces were negative. His temperature on admission (December 19) was 104 degrees and gradually dropped by lysis on January 8, 1913.

The treatment was purely symptomatic, with the exception of a salvarsan injection, about which Dr. Lintz will have something to say. On discharge the patient had completely recovered from his trichinosis as far as the subjective symptoms went.

# OBSERVATIONS ON THE USE OF PHENOSULPHO-NEPTHALEIN AS A FUNCTIONAL RENAL TEST.

## By Henry F. Kramer, M.D,.

of Brooklyn, N. Y.

THE data here presented on the use of phenosulphonepthalein as a test of renal function have been obtained from forty-eight cases, normal and abnormal, occurring in the services of Drs. Butler and Roberts at the Brooklyn Hospital.

Phenolsulphonepthalein as originally prepared by Dr. Ira Remsen was first used as a test of kidney function by Geraghty and Rowntree in July, 1910. The technique as recommended by them has been closely followed, except in the estimation of the percentage of dye excreted. The patient's bladder being empty, he is given two glasses of water. One c.c. (6 mg.) of phenosulpho-nepthalein is injected with a long needle into the lumbar muscles. The urine is gathered hourly thereafter for three hours in separate receptacles. Only a few cases had to be catheterized to obtain the specimen at the proper time. Some cases complained of pain at the site of injection the next day, but no other untoward effects were noted. To each specimen is now added 10 c.c. of a 10 per cent. solution of NaOH and the whole diluted with water up to 250 or 500 c.c. depending upon the concentration of the dye. Instead of using the modified Helige Hæmoglobinometer, as recommended by the originators to estimate the percentage, the Fleischl-Miescher Hæmoglobinometer was used in the majority of the cases. This was done on account of the tendency of the solution employed in the former to fade, this error being obviated by the crimson glass wedge of the latter instrument. By reflected artificial light the shades of the dye and glass are identical. The scale was first tested against successive dilutions from 10 per cent. to 100 per cent. of a 1-1000 sol. of phenosulphonepthalein plus 10 c.c. of 10 per cent. NaOH. The readings tallied exactly with the dilutions from 10 per cent. to 70 per cent. No single reading in the series following was above 47 per cent.

### NORMAL CASES

The excretion in a series of four individuals whose kidneys appeared to be normal averaged 37 per cent. of the drug for the first hour and 57.3 per cent. for the first two hours. During the third hour we have an average of 6.9 per cent.

### TABLE 1.

| Case. | Albumen. | Casts. | 1st Hr. | 2d Hr. | 3d Hr. | Total. |
|-------|----------|--------|---------|--------|--------|--------|
| I.    | 0        | 0      | 40      | 17     | 5.5    | 62.5   |
| II.   | 0        | 0      | 30      | 21     | 9      | 60     |
| III.  | 0        | 0      | 38      | 20     | 0      | 58     |
| IV.   | 0        | 0      | 42      | 23.5   | 6.4    | 71.9   |
| Average | | | 37 | 20.3 | 6.9 | 63.7 |

### FATAL CASES.

In nine cases which were fatal the average excretion for three hours was 7.3 per cent. Only one case with a percentage less than this was able to leave the hospital and he was removed in a mori-bund condition. Two cases showing no trace of the dye in three hours died of uremia in less than 24 hours. One case survived for three months after having a three hour excretion of only 5 per cent. These figures are raised somewhat by one case in which the excretion was 27 per cent in three hours, the real cause of death being a cardiac lesion.

TABLE 2.

| | 1st hr. | 2d hr. | 3d hr. | Total. | Special Symptoms. |
|---|---|---|---|---|---|
| I. | 0 | 0 | 1 | 1 | Albuminuric retinitis. Uremia, Sys. Bl. Press, 180. |
| II. | 3.9 | 1 | 2.3 | 7.2 | Partial heart block. Myocarditis. |
| III. | 0 | 0 | 0 | 0 | Uremia with convulsions and coma. Mitral regurg. |
| IV. | 0 | 0 | 0 | 0 | Myocarditis Sys. B. P. 170. |
| V. | 4.4 | 2.8 | 1 | 8.2 | Chr. nephritis. |
| VI. | 10 | 0 | 0 | 10 | Edema, hydrothorax. |
| VII. | Tr. | 4 | 4 | 8 | Dyspnea, anuria—aortic and mitral regurg. |
| VIII. | 2 | 11 | 14 | 27 | Endocarditis. Died of ac. cardiac dilatation. |
| IX. | 2 | 3 | 0 | 5 | Pulmonary edema. |
| | Average............... 7.3% | | | | |

ACUTE NEPHRITIS.

In three cases of acute nephritis occurring in young persons the average excretion at the apparent height of the inflammation was 38.2 per cent. It was possible to demonstrate in two of these that with the disappearance of albumen and casts the excretion of the dye rose to over 59 per cent. in three hours.

TABLE 3.

| | Date. | Alb. | Casts. | Total Excretion. |
|---|---|---|---|---|
| I. | Mar. 10 | ++ | Hyaline and Granular Casts R. B. C. and W. B. C.......... | 26.5 |
| | Mar. 26 | 0 | 0 | 30.8 |
| II. | May 7 | ++ | Epithelial and Granular Casts. Blood cells. | 50. |
| III. | Mar. 10 | Tr. | Few Haline and Granular Casts ........ | 13.7 in 40 min. |
| | Apr. 10 | 0 | 0 | 52. in 3 hrs. |
| | | | | 33% in 1st hr. |

It is very difficult to classify clinically the affections of the kidney. It seems of value to reproduce the facts as established by Austin and Eisenbrey in the hope that they may serve as a guide in the classification of the cases of chronic nephritis.

These investigators (*Jour. Exper. Med.*, Feb., 1911) have shown in their studies of experimental nephritis that the pathological result varied with the irritant used. Thus cantharidin caused chiefly glomerular congestion and swelling of Bowman's capsule with granular degeneration of the epithelium of the convoluted tubules. In nephritis caused by uranium nitrate or potassium chromate the glomeruli appeared normal while the epithelium of the convoluted tubules showed granular degeneration and fat vacuoles. The medullary loops contained granular casts, the tubules being totally occluded in some places. In further experiments (*Jour. Exper. Med.,* Nov., 1911) phenosulphonephthalein was used to test the excretion powers of animals with these various forms of experimental nephritis. Animals with cantharidin or glomerular nephritis showed an average excretion of 69.7 per cent. as compared with 51.1 per cent. in uranium nitrate (delayed) or tubular nephritis and 8.6 per cent. in acute insufficiency produced by a stronger solution of uranium nitrate.

The following table is adapted from data of Austin and Eisenbrey:

TABLE 4.

|  | Cantharidin. | .0075 gms. Uranium Nitrate. | .015 gms. Uran. Nitrate. |
|---|---|---|---|
| I. | 78.9 | 78.8 | 25.3 |
| II. | 62.9 | 68.6 | 4.1 |
| III. | 67.4 | 44.4 | 3.5 |
| IV. |  | 12.8 | 1.8 |
| Average.. | 69.7 | 51.1 | 8.6 |

The obvious deduction is that phenosulphonepthalein is excreted chiefly through the tubules, a very small proportion going through the glomeruli.

Returning to our series, cases of chronic nephritis can be divided into two groups: I. Those showing a three hour excretion of more than 35 per cent. and, II. less than 35 per cent. In the first group there are nine cases whose urine showed no casts and no albumen, or only a faint trace at times. These correspond to the glomerular types as produced by cantharidin experimentally in animals.

In the second group of 23 cases showing less than 35 per cent. excretion, eighteen showed considerable albumen and casts. These might be classed as cases of tubular nephritis. Half of these cases died in from a few hours to a few months after the test was used. In these cases the average excretion was 14 per cent. Of the five cases without more than a trace of albumen and a few or no casts the average excretion was 26.9 per cent. Only one of these five has died and this is the one previously mentioned as having died of cardiac lesions. Of the 18 cases all obviously presented the clinical picture of nephritis. Of the group of five cases only one showed such a picture and in this one the percentage excretion was 5 per cent., although there was no albumen and casts on repeated examination.

TABLE 5.

CASES WITH A THREE HOUR EXCRETION OVER 35 PER CENT.

| | Albumen | Casts | Excretion | Diagnosis | Special Symptoms |
|---|---|---|---|---|---|
| 1. | Trace | 0 | 40. | Hysteria | Systolic Blood press. 150. |
| 2. | 0 | 0 | 52. | Intestinal parasite | 45% Eosinophiles. Areas of analgesia. Blood press. 120. |
| 3. | Faint Trace | 0 | 46.5 | Tonsillitis | None. |
| 4. | Trace | 0 | 42. | Myocarditis | Obesity—Edema of legs— Dyspnea—Acne rosacea. |

| | Albumen | Casts | Excretion | Diagnosis | Special Symptoms |
|---|---|---|---|---|---|
| 5. | 0 | 0 | 45.5 | ? | None. |
| 6. | 0 | 0 | 35. | Hepatic cirrhosis | Hemetemesis. Dyspnea. Secondary anemia. |
| 7. | Trace | 0 | 45. | Chronic nephritis | Edema. |
| 8. | Trace | 0 | 52. | Chronic nephritis | Anemia. |
| 9. | 0 | 0 | 50.5 | Acute articular rheumatism | Pericarditis with effusion. |

TABLE 6.

CASES WITH A THREE HOUR EXCRETION UNDER 35 PER CENT.

| | Albumen | Casts | Excretion | Diagnosis | Special Symptoms |
|---|---|---|---|---|---|
| 1. | ++ | Hyaline, Granular | 1. | Chr. Nephritis | Album. retinitis. Bl. press. 180. Uremia—Death. |
| 2. | ++ | Hyaline, Granular | 1.8 | Chr. Endocarditis and Nephritis | Edema Scrotum. Aortic regurg. Bl. press. 270. Album. Retinitis—Death. |
| 3. | ++ | Hyaline, Granular | 0 | Myocarditis and Nephritis | Partial heart block. Edema. Bl. press. 170—Death. |
| 4. | + | Hyaline, Granular | 16. | Myocard. and Nephritis | None. |
| 5. | ++ | Hyaline, Granular | 8. | Chr. Endocard. and Nephritis | Mitral regurg. Anuria. Bl. press. 118—Death. |
| 6. | + | Few Hy. | 31.4 | Chr. Nephritis | ................... |
| 7. | + | Few Hy. | 34. | Chr. Nephritis | ................... |
| 8. | ++ | Hy. and Gran. | 12.7 | Myocard. and Nephritis | Vincent's angina. Edema of lids. Pulmonary Edema. |
| 9. | ++ | Hy. and Gran. | 5. | Myocard. and Nephritis | Pulmonary Edema—Death. |
| 10. | +++ | All casts Bl. cells | 0 | Endocarditis and Nephritis | Anuria. Uremia—Death. |
| 11. | ++ | Hy. and Gran. | 10. | Myocard. and Nephritis | Hydrothorax. Anuria—Death. |
| 12. | + | Gran. | 7.2 | Myocard. and Nephritis | Partial heart block—Death. |
| 13. | Trace | Few Hy. and Gran. | 8.2 | Chr. Nephritis | Edema general—Death. |
| 14. | Trace | Hy. and Gran. | 27. | Chr. Endocarditis | Aortic and Mitral regurg. Edema scrotum—Death. |
| 15. | 0 | 0 | 5. | Chr. Nephritis | Anemia. Dyspnea. |
| 16. | Tr. | .. | 24.8 | Chr. Nephritis | Sys. Press. 185, Diastolic 125. |

|  | Albumen | Casts | Excretion | Diagnosis | Special Symptoms |
|---|---|---|---|---|---|
| 17. | Tr. | Few Hy. | 31.4 | Chr. Nephritis | .................... |
| 18. | + | Few Hy. | 34. | Chr. Nephritis | .................... |
| 19. | + | Hy. and Gran. | 30.2 | Chr. Nephritis | Pneumoconiosis. |
| 20. | Tr. | Hy. and Gran. | 19.5 | Chr. Nephritis | Bl. press. 225 Sys. 140 Diast. Hemiplegia. |
| 21. | Tr. | .. | 33. | Ac. Artic Rheum | .................... |
| 22. | Tr. | .. | 24. | Mitral and Arotic Regurg. | Dyspnea. |
| 23. | Tr. | Few Hy. and Gran. | 23.2 | Chr. Nephritis | Intestinal obstructions. |

Two cases of diabetes with polyuria seemed to show that the amount of dye excreted does not run parallel with the urine excretion.

### TABLE 7.

|  | 1 hr. | 2d hr. | 3d hr. | Total excretion. | Sugar. | Recent Total Urine. |
|---|---|---|---|---|---|---|
| I. | 31 — | 5 — | 4 — | 40. | 7.2% | 5 qts. |
| II. | 10. | 20. | 8.7 | 38.7 | | 3 qts. |

In conclusion:

I.   Normal cases excrete over 60 per cent. of this dye in three hours.

II.   In acute nephritis the excretion increases synchronously with the improvement of urinary symptoms.

III.   It is possible to indicate the degree of functional impairment of the kidney in cases of other than renal origin and without renal or urinary symptoms.

IV.   It may be possible to designate a nephritic case as being glomerular, or tubular, or both.

V.   A more definite prognosis is possible in cases where dissolution is more or less imminent.

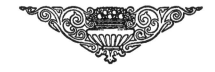

# EDITORIAL

## A NEWSPAPER HEADLINE AND A WORD TO THE WISE.

"Guests of Bride-to-be Ill—Five of Twelve Who Attended Linen Shower Are Stricken with Typhoid."

WE have noted in the billboard advertisements that an enterprising undertaker will furnish a "Complete Casket Funeral for $65.00." This is consoling and may possibly mark a decided advance over a hitherto extravagant if not barbarous custom, but starting with the proposition that a funeral cannot be more economically conducted, we estimate the cost of 1,128 ceremonies—and there were 1,128 deaths from typhoid fever in the State of New York in 1912—at $73,320. Truly a small sum for so much splendor and yet one cannot suppress the thought that practically all of those 1,128 victims might have been immunized against that hideous malady for less than one per cent. of the estimated cost of burial.

Were we a better disciple of Euclid we might attempt to compute the magnitude loss which the State has sustained in those 1,128 preventable deaths—a loss incalculably great for the reason that the majority of the victims were vigorous, wage-earning adults or the mothers of young children.

In view of such facts the continued apathy of the profession is quite incomprehensible. Surely apathy is not an immoderate word when, in *the immediate families* of Brooklyn physicians, there have been several deaths from typhoid fever during the past twelve months!

BURTON HARRIS.

## SHORT CUTS.

EARN $3,000 to $5,000 a Year as a Doctor of Chiropractic." "More Scientific, More Simple, Easier to Learn Than Osteopathy." "Easily Learned in Spare Time at Home." These few extracts from the advertisement of a "School of Chiropractic" situate in a western city famed for its enterprise, whet one's curiosity to learn more of this enticing "Science." One has but to turn to the advertising pages of a certain reputable monthly to read for himself the advantages that the art affords. There it is, among dozens of other advertisements of correspondence courses of all sorts: how to become a successful chicken farmer—how to write display ads—how to succeed in real estate—how to become an expert accountant—how to learn plumbing and bricklaying; all taught by the "university extension" method that requires no previous education, no manual training, no brains, only a few dollars, a few months of reading in spare time and sure graduation into the class of skilled workmen, with a handsome diploma and a title to "put the gilded dome on the horror"! Did the founders of the Chautauqua and University Extension courses ever foresee how useful their system would become to the ever increasing class that includes on the one hand a crew of clever charlatans with schemes to peddle, and on the other a horde of potentially dishonest incompetents who crave the craftsman's wage, but shirk the drudgery of his apprenticeship?

But to return to our advertisement: The dignified, scientific looking gent whose picture adorns the upper left hand corner and who points so convincingly to the compound convoluted spine held as the virtuoso grasps a violoncello in his left hand, we judge to be a sample chiropractor. His looks should place him in the $5,500 class at least. But read the following excerpts and then know what envy is!

> "There are twenty-three million people in this country who believe in drugless healing, and the number is constantly increasing. They are to be found in every community. Splendid openings for Chiropractors everywhere. It's a profession that is far from over-crowded. Immensely lucrative. Dr. W., a graduate, made $500 the third month after starting. R. M. J. added over $3,000 a year to his income. V. S. makes $40 a day. We taught these men by mail and in class. You can do as well or even better. Treat members of your own family free—earn handsome fees for treating others.
>
> Our simplified home study course, profusely illustrated, and with 14 big free charts and a spinal column, makes it easy to acquire a thorough, practical knowledge of this dignified, profitable profession in a surprisingly short time. A common school education is all you need—our absorbing, easy-to-learn-lessons will do the rest. It means financial independence, social position—a profession that is looked up to, for you.
>
> Free sample lesson sheets, big illustrated book, also names and addresses of successful students mailed free on request. Write today—a lucrative practice awaits you."

This is an insidious appeal to the cupidity rather than the ambition of the man who is seeking a near cut to a competence. "Easier than Osteopathy"! Here is the gist of the whole matter; not how good a craftsman one may become, but how he may most cheaply and most speedily place himself in a position to gain dollars. It is the old cry that Charles Dickens heard when in 1846 he recognized the same unworthy spirit and held it up to ridicule in the pages of Martin Chuzzlewit. Then, as now, there flourished the same brotherhood of schemers whose one thought was riches before honor. Now, as then, it is the desire to substitute tinsel for the pure metal. There is no royal road to learning, and therefore every effort to better the art of healing, every limitation that is placed upon the aspirant for the right to practice medicine—a right that carries with it graver responsibilities than any other human calling, save only the call to the priesthood, with which it is in no small measure linked—is met by a fresh outcrop of just such schemes as this. It is hard to believe that our national life turns only upon worldly gain. It is hard to think that the American motive is money only, and yet it is to be feared that the leaven of unselfishness, of honest effort, and of high ideals, has but a sorry loaf in which to germinate. It is not the healing art only that is compelled to struggle against incompetence and lust for mere gain, for in almost every occupation we see the same tendency to produce, not better goods, but cheaper ones at increased profits.

The responsibility that is laid upon the physicians of this country is a great one. We have in our keeping the flame that Prometheus got from Olympus, and it is laid upon us to see that it shall burn bright and clear. The need for loyalty to our ideals of honor, unselfishness and public service was never greater than today. Small jealousies, narrow-mindedness and dogmatism must have no part in the struggle that we are called upon to make against the besetting sin of the time if we are to prove to a great people the folly of permitting lust for gain to interfere with the march of scientific truth.

H. G. W.

## DOCTORS AND THE "SUCKER LIST."

A RECENT news item recalls vividly enough some two or more years ago the receipt of a series of pamphlets most entertainingly written, signed by a name of high honor in American literature but composed with one end in view—the sale of mining stock. That the talented author is now confined in a Federal jail is a sort of poetic justice, but the flood of similar, if less artistic, appeals to doctors as investors flows steadily on. Sometimes it is gold, sometimes silver, sometimes copper. Again a sure road to rapid wealth is offered through the stocks of industrial corporations, but always the appeal is the same—the rapid transmutation of meager savings into comfortable fortunes, and always it is physicians who are approached. Again and again the news columns chronicle the downfall and apprehension of "promoters" whose pluckings from credulous victims total not hundreds, but hundreds of thousands of dollars. The classified lists of prospective purchasers—the "sucker lists"—contain a separate pigeon hole for doctors. Are doctors really easy victims? Are we, as a class, particularly gullable? Is cupidity one of our failings? If not, then why is the bait so often dangled before us? Our dealings with individuals are most often characterized by a true estimate of the personality of the patient, otherwise we would fail more often than we do. Perhaps the very frankness with which the average patient opens himself to our approach—the confidential attitude that so many readily assume toward the physician— engenders a false estimate of one's ability to read character. In matters of ordinary business we are not qualified, as a class. Our profession prevents it. Our training has taken no account of it. We are flattered to think that we should be chosen, that we should have the opportunity for investment that is denied the professional financier; and the reason is always the same. "We prefer," says the plausible solicitor, "to have our stock held by the small, intelligent investor, whose interests are our own, for we find that the capitalists (who are clamoring for our stock) demand too large a share in our management, and we are anxious that the control be kept out of such selfish hands." How many of us stop to wonder why, if the investment is so enticing and the returns so sure, it was ever allowed to be offered outside the immediate circle of the promoter's friends? But we rely on our ability to read character, and are tickled by the flattery of the specious appeal, and make a dash with our sprats to capture such a whale—and are sucked in.

H. G. W.

## OCTOBER MEETING

The President, Dr. Samuel Hendrickson, announces that he has planned a visit of inspection to Blackwell's and Randall's Islands for the October Meeting, which will be held on Saturday, October 4, 1913.

The present plan contemplates a trip by boat from some convenient pier in Brooklyn, with stops for inspection first at Blackwell's Island and then at Randall's Island, where opportunities will be afforded to view the various institutions under the control of the Department of Charities. There is much of unusual interest to be seen at both places; the number and variety of the activities under the Charities Department is surprisingly large and so varied that it is doubtful whether many physicians have any adequate appreciation of what the Charities Department controls and conducts. Those who recall our delightful voyage of inspection to Quarantine a year ago will do well to set this date aside. Details will be announced by the Secretary through the usual folder, when the full plans for the meeting have been perfected.

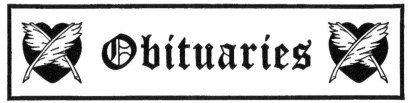

# Obituaries

DEPARTMENT UNDER THE CHARGE OF WILLIAM SCHROEDER, M.D.

## WILLIAM H. McLENATHAN, M.D.

DR. McLENATHAN was born at Jay, N. Y., and died at Willsboro, N. Y., July 30, 1913. He was graduated from the New York Homeopathic Medical College in 1878, and practiced for many years in this city. He was a member of the Kings County Homeopathic Medical Society. He leaves two sons, Harrison W. and Paul.

W. S., Sr.

## OVID ALLEN HYDE, M.D.

DR. HYDE was born in Brooklyn, N. Y., August 6, 1852, and died at Queens, L. I., August 5, 1913. He was graduated from the New York Eclectic Medical College in 1884, in which college he was professor of anatomy. He leaves a widow, Mary Crawford Murray, and a son, Chester Ovid.

W. S., Sr.

## WILLIAM P. MANATON, M.D.

DR. MANATON was born in New York City in 1865 and died at Greenport, L. I., August 6, 1913. He was graduated from New York Homeopathic Medical College. Dr. Manaton was a member of Peconic Lodge, No. 349, F. & A. M. His widow survives him.

W. S., Sr.

## JAMES LEWIS WATT, M.D.

DR. WATT was born in New York City, October 17, 1871, and died at Dunkirk, N. Y., June 24, 1913. He was the son of George Watt, of Scotland, and Elizabeth F. Kidderminster, of England. Dr. Watt was educated at the public and high schools of this city; his medical education was under the direction of James Watt, M.D., graduating M.D. from the Long Island College Hospital in the class of 1893.

Dr. Watt practiced medicine in this city for a number of years and about fifteen years ago went West to take charge of a hospital at Circle City, Alaska. He was for a few years physician to St. Gile's Home for Crippled Children and the Contagious Disease Hospital. He leaves a widow, Mary E. Marshall, and three children. During the years 1895-96 he was a member of the Kings County Medical Society.

W. S., Sr.

## EDWARD WILLIAM CARHART, M.D.

Dr. Carhart was born at Clinton Hollow, New York, September 23, 1856, and died in Brooklyn, N. Y., May 15, 1913.

He was graduated from the Albany Medical College in 1878. He practiced medicine in Dutchess County for a number of years and came to Brooklyn in 1894. He was a member of the Dutchess County Medical Society, and in 1895-96 of the Kings County Medical Society; Merchant's Lodge, No. 709, F. & A. M. He leaves a widow, Amelia Woolsey, and a son. W. S., Sr.

## JAMES LESTER CARNEY, M.D.

Dr. Carney was born in Dublin, Ireland, in 1850 and died in Brooklyn, N. Y., April 22, 1913. He was educated at the public schools and Harvard University; his medical education was received at the Long Island College Hospital, where he was graduated in 1888.

Dr. Carney was in practice in this city during his professional life and was a member of the Kings County Medical Society from 1888 to 1911.

His wife Elizabeth, to whom he was married in 1883, and daughter Lillian Alice, survive him. The funeral services were conducted by the pastor of the Hanson Place M. E. Church.

W. S., Sr.

## JESSE WILLIAMS HENRY, M.D.

Dr. Henry was a native of Brookfield, Mass., where he was born May 8, 1830, and died in Brooklyn, N. Y., May 16, 1913. His father was Charles Henry, and his uncle was James Harvey Henry, M.D., President of the Kings County Medical Society in 1850.

During the war Dr. Henry was private in the Twenty-seventh Connecticut Volunteers. After the war he was connected with the War Department at Washington, D. C., attending medical lectures at the Georgetown Medical College, where he received his degree of M.D. in 1866. From 1872 to 1908 he was a member of the Kings County Medical Society; for thirty years physician to the Home for Aged and Orphans, and for more than fifty years a member of Wooster Lodge, No. 79, F. & A. M., of New Haven, Conn.

He is survived by his widow, a daughter and two sons.

W. S., Sr.

## WILLIAM HENRY CLOWMINZER, M.D.

Dr. Clowminzer was born in New York Mills, Oneida County, N. Y., on January 28, 1867, and died in Brooklyn, N. Y., June 21, 1913. He was the son of William Clowminzer and Sarah Hepworth, both of New York. His early education was received in the public and high schools of this city. His medical education was under the direction of W. E. Wetmore, M.D., receiving the degree of M.D. from the Long Island College Hospital in the class of 1891. During the years 1892-93 he was instructor in obstetrics in the same institution, and for a number of years was physician to the Bedford Dispensary and Home for Epileptics. He was a member of the Kings County Medical Society from 1891-95 and the Long Island Medical Society, of which he was president in 1897.

He was married on June 21, 1892, to Annie Forsyth McKeachie, who survives him. **W. S., Sr.**

---

## BERNARD ALOYSIUS DUHIGG, M.D.

DR. DUHIGG was born on April 15, 1870, in Brooklyn, N. Y., and died at St. James, L. I., July 29, 1913. He was the son of Bryan Duhigg and Anna T. Cummings, both of Ireland.

He was educated at St. Leonard's Academy and St. John's College. His medical education was under the direction of James C. Kennedy, M.D., graduating from the Long Island College Hospital in 1894; this was followed by a term as interne in St. Catherine's Hospital. He practiced medicine at Bath Beach, L. I. From 1901 he was a member of the Brooklyn Medical Society.

**W. S., Sr.**

---

## GEORGE RANSOM WESTBROOK, M.D.

DR. WESTBROOK was a native of St. Louis, Mo., where he was born February 1, 1847. He died at Benson, Vermont, July 19, 1913. He was the son of George W. Westbrook, of New York, and Harriet Ransom, of Vermont. His early education was received in the Free Academy of New York; his medical education was under the direction of his brother, the late Benjamin F. Westbrook, M.D., receiving the degree of M.D. from the Long Island College Hospital in 1878. During his professional life he was surgeon to the L. I. C. H. Dispensary; from 1879 to 1884 St. Mary's Hospital; from 1860 to 1890 a member of the Kings County Medical Society; from 1879 to 1913 of the Brooklyn Pathological Society.

Dr. Westbrook was married on June 3, 1874, to Ida Blanche Wilmshurst. His second wife was Jessie Kellogg, of Benson, Vt., who, with a grandson, Frank Westbrook, survive him.

**W. S., Sr.**

---

## MATTHEW JOHN LELAND, M.D., LL.D.

DR. LELAND was born in Dublin, Ireland, and died on May 29, 1913, in Brooklyn, N. Y. He was graduated from Trinity College. His medical education was received at the University of New York, where he received the degree of M.D. in the class of 1883. In 1893 St. John's College conferred the degree of LL.D. upon him.

His time was devoted in a large degree to teaching at St. John's College, St. Francis College and Manhattan College, where for a number of years he was professor of sciences and languages.

He was a member of the Kings County Medical Society from 1884-90; Fulton Council, No. 299, R. A.

He served as interne at St. Mary's Hospital from 1883-85 and for a number of years was physician to the hospital.

On June 6, 1888, he was married to Annie F. A. Kleider, of Brooklyn, N. Y. **W. S., Sr.**

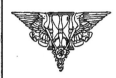 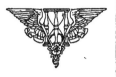
# TRANSACTIONS OF THE BROOKLYN SOCIETY OF INTERNAL MEDICINE.

*Stated Meeting, April 25, 1913.*

The President, TASKER HOWARD, M.D., in the Chair.

### Lung Changes in Asthma.

#### By Dr. Luther F. Warren.

DR. LOUIS C. AGER, in opening the discussion, said:—"I would like to ask whether the heart in this case, during the considerable degree of distension, showed any murmurs, whether the valves were thrown out of gear by this change in the heart shape?"

### Second Infections in Pulmonary Tuberculosis, Etc.

#### By Dr. Avary.

DR. LOUIS C. AGER, in discussion, said:—"I am sorry that Dr. Avary has not emphasized one interesting fact in connection with his work, that is, that with the same technic and the same culture medium, he was getting positive cultures in pneumonia. These findings are certainly very different from those reported by other observers and they have a very practical bearing on the treatment of pulmonary tuberculosis. If Dr. Avary is correct pulmonary tuberculosis, even in the later stages, is a local and not a systemic infection. It has been very generally taught in the past that the so-called septic symptoms are due to secondary infections with pyogenic organisms. If this is true and if Dr. Avary has shown that the infection is entirely local, we have a condition in which the mixed vaccines ought to be successful. For this reason I tried out a mixed vaccine on a series of ten children at the Brooklyn Home for Consumptives with the unexpected result of getting no reaction in any of them. This would appear to be a strong argument in favor of the theory that the tubercle bacillus itself is responsible for the septic symptoms usually attributed to the pus organisms."

### Notes on Tuberculin Treatment in Advanced Pulmonary Tuberculosis.

#### By Dr. William H. Lohman.

(See page 308.)

DR. LOUIS C. AGER, in discussion, said:—"I think the most important thing to be learned from this paper of Dr. Lohman's is the fact that to get any benefit from tuberculin in pulmonary tuberculosis there has got to be thorough co-operation on the part of the patient and there has got to be the utmost patience and care on the part of the physician. There is absolutely no use in trying to use a treatment of this kind unless we are prepared to carry it out continuously with the same careful technic. I want to emphasize that fact, because I have repeatedly seen childish attempts in the use of tuberculin on the part of physicians without any realization of what they must expect to do if they are going to get any results, or even know whether the use of tuberculin is going to be of any use in the particular case under treatment."

DR. BENJAMIN WHITE, in opening the discussion, said:—"In the use of tuberculin there is a point of importance which is not always appreciated and that is the great variation which is found in different preparations of tuberculin. Some of the commercial preparations of old tuberculin are absolutely inactive and it is difficult to obtain two lots of tuberculin of equal potency.

"We have used a method at the Hoagland Laboratory which is always employed at Saranac Lake for testing new lots of tuberculin. Each lot of tuberculin before use is tested out on the skin of an individual who is known to show marked skin sensitiveness to tuberculin. By using tuberculin in 100 per cent., 50, 25, 10, 1 and 0.1 per cent. dilutions by the von Pirquet method, it is possible to compare the reaction obtained with a maximum reaction obtained by any previous lot. The tests are made on the forearm with the first scarification of the weakest tuberculin nearest the wrist, placing the other scarifications in order on the arm, about 30 millimeters apart. This is a very simple method and produces no disagreeable or harmful symptoms in the person on whom this is tried. By carrying out all tests on various individuals with the same lot of tested tuberculin it is possible to obtain a more accurate measure of their sensitiveness by this method.

"In determining the therapeutic dose of tuberculin in any patient, we have been using a modification of the method described by Dr. White, of Pittsburg. We give intradermic injections of old tuberculin in the following amounts: 0.000000001, 0.00000001, 0.0000001, 0.000001, 0.00001 gram in 1/10 cubic centimeter. The smallest amount giving a zone of reaction 5 millimeters in diameter is considered as the minimum reacting dose. Then the initial therapeutic dose is 1/10 to 1/100 of the minimum test dose on the skin giving a reaction of 5 millimeters. By this method it is possible to give a dose which will not produce general reactions, while in other individuals it is possible to give them a much larger dose than would be possible when the original method of beginning tuberculin administration is used. The method seems accurate for most individuals but numerous variations have been observed in children under five years of age.

"It is highly desirable to obtain some accurate method for determining the proper dosage in tuberculin treatment, and the above described procedure seems to me to constitute an important step in placing this therapy upon a more systematic and accurate basis."

DR. EDWARD E. CORNWALL, in discussion, said:—"When Robert Koch discovered tuberculin, I think it was in 1890 or 1891, I was an interne in a hospital in New York City. This particular hospital was one of the first in this country to get a supply of the wonderful lymph. As I remember, we tried it on three cases, one of lupus and two of pulmonary tuberculosis. The lupus case was not improved; one of the phthisis cases had a severe reaction after the injection and was apparently made worse; the other phthisis case left the hospital before any observations could be made on it. Since that time, over twenty years ago, I have given no serious consideration to the use of tuberculin in tuberculosis for therapeutic purposes, and, of course, from such a very slight experience with the remedy, I have no right to hold any opinion regarding its merits.

"I was interested in Dr. Lohman's report of his cases, which show painstaking observation, which is the basis of clinical achievement. It may be that there is some good in this treatment. But Dr. Lohman's results were not particularly conclusive in its favor; certainly temporary improvement in 50 per cent. of the cases was not more than could be expected from other well-established methods of treatment, notably the hygienic method.

"Dr. Lohman mentioned the fact that the patients felt better after the injections. Could it be that suggestion had something to do with that?

"An impression which I have received regarding tuberculosis is, that it is one of the diseases which are not easily affected by vaccine treatment: if the patient has not been able to acquire immunity by natural methods after months or years of stimulation with the toxin of the disease, it seems difficult to understand how injection of more of the toxin can stimulate the development of that immunity. But the subject is one of which I have no practical knowledge."

DR. TASKER HOWARD, in discussion, said:—"It seems to me that it is difficult to judge, as a rule, how much good you are getting from the use of tuberculin in any one case, and it is only from a consideration of a large number of cases that fair conclusions may be drawn as to its value. Dr. Lohman's experience with advanced cases, getting such good results in as large a proportion as he did, is very encouraging because we know how hard it is to get results in this stage of the disease.

"Dr. Lawrison Brown published a paper only a few years ago in the *American Journal of Medical Sciences* in which one would rather gather from the introduction that after using it for many years there was still some doubt in his mind as to its value. He analyzed the end results obtained in patients treated with tuberculin and compared them with the end results in patients who had not been treated with tuberculin. The series included all the discharged patients from Trudeau who could be traced and he found that the end results were distinctly more favorable in the cases treated with tuberculin than in those who were not."

DR. JAMES P. BECKER, in discussion, said:—"I want to report two cases in which tuberculin was used. My cases have all been seen in private practice. As Dr. Ager has said, one of the most difficult things to accomplish is to have patients submit to tuberculin treatment and to induce them to carry on the treatment long enough to get any permanent results therefrom. In these two cases the patients are the only ones I have succeeded in getting to carry on the treatment long enough. It is now over a year since stopping the treatment and both patients are apparently cured. One of them was a graduate nurse who contracted tuberculosis when she left Brooklyn and went to Nova Scotia and got married. She had something like fifteen or seventeen hemorrhages— very profuse ones. When she came to Brooklyn she had not had a hemorrhage for a month or so, but did have several later on. At that time she weighed about 122 pounds. I speak of this case particularly because I saw her this morning for the first time in nearly a year, and she now weighs 145 pounds and has not had a hemorrhage in about eighteen months.

"The other patient had signs of incipient tuberculosis. She had them for sometime and they had not advanced possibly because she had been taking a certain amount of treatment most of the time. She was carrying a temperature is high as 102 at times and had a long course of tuberculin treatment lasting nearly a year. It is now about sixteen months since stopping the treatment and while her weight has not increased much (she is not of the type to put on a great deal of weight), she apparently has been well now for sixteen months or more. She is apparently cured. In fact, both of these cases are apparently cured."

DR. WILLIAM H. LOHMAN, in closing the discussion, said:—"I was interested in the method described by Dr. White for determining the dose. It would be very nice if we could have some scientific way for determining the dose beforehand so as to know it without depending upon clinical reactions. My experience is not in accord with this. It may be because, as Dr. White suggested, the preparations of tuberculin vary. At times a patient, who was apparently going along smoothly on a given dose, would suddenly get up a reaction and we would have to drop down a number of notches. Later we could double the dose on the course of a few weeks without trouble. In other words, the tolerance or point of reaction does not appear to be stationary. It may be a good means for determining the initial dose, but it seems rather elaborate. That was the criticism made upon the method of determining the dosage by means of the opsonic index; that it was not very accurate and not as practical as the clinical method.

"It has been remarked that suggestion was accountable for the results in our cases; that it may have had something to do with their improvement. I admit that it may and I am not at all convinced that it doesn't have much to do with the improvement of these patients.

"One advantage of the treatment, especially in private practice, is that it enables a man to keep his patient under control. You stick a hypodermic needle into him and it undoubtedly gives the patient a little psychic stimulus. You see the patient at certain intervals weekly or twice a week, and in this way you are able to use a little suggestion on him. The whole secret of the treatment of the tuberculous is in keeping everlastingly at it, and, of course, this weekly or periodical injection helps in the effect that the doctor's personality has on the patient.

"On the other hand, we have one rather interesting case—the one of empyema. This patient received vaccines for a number of months prior to tuberculin. In other words, she was getting a mental stimulus before that time once or twice a week and we simply changed the character of the material we were injecting. She did not improve with vaccines, but did improve with tuberculin. This was one case which convinced me that the benefit was not due entirely to suggestion.

"The point brought out by Dr. Ager that prolonged treatment is necessary is undoubtedly a very good one. A short course of treatment is useless. I do not believe that less than four months is worth bothering with, although sometimes patients seem to improve considerably. It was very striking to note that all of our cases in the first few weeks gained three or four pounds and said they felt better (although some were growing worse) simply because they were getting the treatment.

"Regarding the small number of cases, no doubt a large number of cases is very much better. But I believe that the character of the observations counts for something. With a prolonged period of observation before and after treatment, I think more may be proved with a small number of cases than with a large number, where the preliminary observations are not taken or where the subsequent observations are more or less of an indefinite nature.

"I did not expect to have to defend the tuberculin treatment as a whole. I thought that it was pretty well established as a valuable treatment, especially in the earlier cases. Even such an observer as Brown, after saying that he does not think it much good, turns around and cites may cases that have improved after injections.

"I do not recall any person who has had an extensive experience with tuberculin who is not at least a moderate advocate of it. If they did not see benefit from its use some would certainly be frank enough to say so. The only men condemning it, I think, are the men who have not had very much experience with it."

---

## BROOKLYN SURGICAL SOCIETY.

### Stated Meeting of March 6, 1913.

### (Continued from August Journal)

#### "Further Observations Upon Angulation of the Sigmoid."

#### By H. B. Delatour, M.D.

Remarks of Dr. Delatour at the conclusion of the reading of his paper:— "I have had one other case under observation. A Murphy button was used in that case and the patient suffered from some gas on the day following the operation and the interne ordered a two-quart enema without knowing the point at which anastomosis was done. The patient suffered immediate severe pelvic pain and had a rise of temperature following it. I believe in that case some of the fluid must have forced out the button, which was only a few inches from the anus, and the two quarts of fluid introduced there must have produced considerable pressure. There was apparentaly a localized peritonitis from which she has recovered all right, but it gave me some anxiety for the first day or two.

"I will draw a rough diagram of the condition which you find and you will find it in many, many cases, the colon going down to the brim of the pelvis around the loop, the sigmoid coming back to the upper end of the rectum and passing down to the rectum. You will find this portion of the sigmoid distended and the wall of the gut much thickened and enlarged, showing the same condition that you find in the portion of the large intestine immediately behind the band or stricture of any sort. That portion of the intestine has been working hard to overcome the stricture there and the musculature of that portion of the intestine becomes very much thickened and in these cases of ptosis of the sigmoid with angulation we find exactly that same condition existing in the sigmoid.

"Now, these people all suffer from obstinate constipation; they have the greatest difficulty in getting the bowels to move and, as I said in the paper, sacral backache is a very prominent symptom.

"Now, the problem of treatment is to obtain a direct line for the fecal current from the colon to the rectum and that is done either by a direct suturing anastomosis between the colon and rectum or the placing of a button there. When that is placed apparently this section of the sigmoid very soon is taken out of the fecal current.

"All five of these cases which have been done recently have ceased the use of cathartics which they had been in the habit of using constantly before.

"I think in this whole question of disease and conditions due to bands and adhesions we have to bear in mind all the points at which this trouble can occur. There is no question in my mind as to the existence of the so-called Jackson's veil or bands and the method with which they produce constriction of the ascending colon. You can demonstrate that in many cases, and when we open the abdomen for these conditions it is well to bear in mind all the conditions that can occur, and I present this subject again tonight to emphasize the fact that in many cases this is the more important point of the trouble."

Dr. R. W. Westbrook, in opening the discussion, said:—"What has been the age of these patients for the most part?"

Dr. H. B. Delatour, answering Dr. Westbrook's question, said:—"The cases presented in my early paper were all people advanced in years and, as I said at that time, I considered it a condition of the age, but in the recent cases two were as young as 30, the other three, I think, were between 40 and 50, and one of them was 60 years of age. The 60-year old case was that of a lady who came to me with symptoms of distress in the left iliac region and a tumor could be distinctly felt there and it was a question as to whether it was an enlarged kidney which had slipped down. She was very stout and it was very difficult to determine as to this. In that case a cystoscopic examination was made and an attempt to catheterize the ureters by the gentleman who had the case in charge by the use of the Kelly cystoscope by direct vision putting the patient in the knee-chest position. The attempt at catheterization was unsuccessful, but as soon as the patient was put back in bed she had a movement of the bowels and said she felt much more comfortable than for a long time. There was a very copious discharge from the bowels and the tumor mass entirely disappeared which practically cleared up the point that it was a simple loading up of the descending colon. In that case I operated and found a loop at least eighteen inches long.

DR. MATHIAS FIGUEIRA, in discussion, said:—"Could you make out the distended loop of intestine by vaginal examination in women?"

DR. H. B. DELATOUR, answering Dr. Figueira's question, said:—"No; you could feel the resisting mass in this particular case in the pelvis. It felt as though she might have an ovarian cyst. You could feel a mass which we suspected might be an ovarian cyst. There was a resisting mass in the pelvis, which in all probability was the distended colon."

DR. MATHIAS FIGUEIRA, in discussion, said:—"I mean by examining through the vagina you could not satisfy yourself that there was a distended loop of intestine?"

DR. H. B. DELATOUR, answering the further question of Dr. Figueira, said:—"No."

DR. RUSSELL S. FOWLER, in discussion, said:—"There was one point on which Dr. Delatour has not laid sufficient stress and that is anastomosis in the right direction between these various loops of intestine, an anastomosis to carry out the continuity of the intestine in the proper direction, as he has done in these cases. He showed some cases at the Norwegian Hospital the other evening in which there had been prolapse of the transverse of the colon, in which the same idea was also carried out. I think that is the secret of success in cases of both resection and anastomosis."

DR. R. W. WESTBROOK, in discussion, said:—"I would like to ask Dr. Delatour whether anything short of an anastomosis would be sufficient to cure the symptoms in these cases, such as suturing the sigmoid to the abdominal wall?"

DR. H. B. DELATOUR, answering Dr. Westbrook's question, said:—"I did that in two cases where there was not a very long loop, both males, and the primary result was satisfactory, but they were both hospital cases and I could not follow them for any length of time. I brought up the loop of intestine from the pelvis and sutured it in the iliac fossa, but it is very difficult to get a straight line of intestine in doing that. I do not believe it would be satisfactory permanently."

DR. C. H. GOODRICH, in discussion and answering the question put by Dr. Westbrook, said:—"I can speak of one experience along the line of which you ask. About two years ago I diagnosed such a case and had it proven by the X-ray. I opened the abdomen and found an apparently short loop and sutured it and for about six months that man had comparative relief and then there was a return of his pain in the left side of the abdomen which he referred to the region of the spleen. I reopened the abdomen and very promptly found a considerable sized enterolith in the loop of intestine corresponding to the splenic flexure, which I removed, believing that it accounted for his pain, and he was again relieved for the period in which I followed him (about three months), but I do not feel certain that he continued to have relief, because I have since heard of a number of reports where the suturing has not been satisfactory remotely. It may be satisfactory at once, but not in the remote results. I have been trying to locate this patient during the past month, but have not succeeded in so doing."

DR. H. B. DELATOUR, in closing the discussion, said:—"I feel the point Dr. Fowler spoke of is well worth speaking of further; that is, not only in this condition, but in all these cases of intestinal trouble where we make an anastomosis or try to correct the deformities to be sure of our point of anastomosis giving us a straight and direct current for the intestinal contents.

"I will just make a diagram of the case Dr. Fowler referred to. It will show that a little better than any of the cases we have shown here. This was a child, seven years old, who suffered from most obstinate constipation. Every time the bowels were forced to move by the use of enemata he had a convulsion and he had been through all sorts of treatment without relief. Now, in that case the transverse colon dipped away down toward the pelvis and then you had another ascending colon practically and then the descending colon and sigmoid. In that case the question was as to where to make your anastomosis. It will do you no good to make a short circuit there because you will still have this loop in which the fecal current can travel. Make your anastomosis between the lowermost point of that loop and the sigmoid; get your direct point there and tie off that loop so that none of the intestinal contents can travel around and you have a direct current into the sigmoid. This loop is still open so that whatever secretion may come from that portion of the intestine will travel on down. You then make a direct current between the lowermost portion of that trap so you can completely and absolutely drain that trap. In making our anastomosis we must be careful to see that we do not leave a chance for that same trouble to continue. This boy I operated three years ago by making a good-sized anastomosis between the lowermost portion of the loop in the transverse colon and the sigmoid and he is perfectly well today, takes no cathartics and has had no more of his convulsions. That is why in these cases, in certain cases you should get your anastomosis at the brim of the pelvis where you get your most direct flow. Occasionally it is more satisfactory to use the Murphy button than suture because you cannot get your clamps well in and it is very difficult to keep them clean because it is almost impossible to thoroughly empty out the bowel of fecal matter. I do not recall a single one of these cases which I have done in which the intestine was thoroughly emptied of feces. This loop prevents the complete emptying of the bowel and in every one of these cases which I did recently there was a good deal of fecal matter still in the intestine, notwithstanding persistent efforts to try and empty it."

---

## TRANSACTIONS OF THE BROOKLYN PATHOLOGICAL SOCIETY.

*Stated Meeting, March* 13, 1913.

The President, PAUL M. PILCHER, M.D., in the Chair.

*Scientific Program.*

I. A Case of Banti's Disease. Presentation of Patient. By Albert Thunig, M.D.

II. a. Ulcers of the Stomach and Duodenum Co-existing with Obstruction at the Ileo-Cecal Junction. Demonstration of Specimens Removed at Autopsy.

  b. Stomach of a Case of Achlorhydria Hemorrhagica Gastrica. Demonstration of Gross Specimen and Photo-Micrographs. By James T. Pilcher, M.D.

III. A Report of Two Cases of Colon Bacteraemia. By Arthur Holzman, M.D.

IV. A Report of Five Cases of Diplococcus Rheumaticus Recovered from the Blood. By Benjamin Koven, M.D.

V. Trichinosis. A Report of Two Cases, with Lantern Demonstration. By Joshua M. Van Cott, M.D.

### A Case of Banti's Disease.

*Reported by Albert Thunig, M.D.*

(See page 350.)

DR. HENRY A. FAIRBAIRN, in opening the discussion, said:—"Dr. Thunig has gone into this case and presented one of the best detailed histories from beginning to end I think I have ever heard. He has covered every point and has arrived at a diagnosis of Banti's disease, but the question, I think, that is uppermost in the minds of us all is, Is there any such entity, pathologically, as Banti describes? Is it worthy of a separate division in pathology? The French school, I suppose, would say yes. I would like to ask what they would put down as the basis of Banti's condition. What is the cause of it? Dr. Thunig informs us that the removal of the spleen has cured some of these cases. Now, if that is so, we do not know any other condition of that kind that it will cure. Where you get cirrhosis of the liver and involvement of the spleen, to remove the spleen and have the cirrhosis of the liver recover is remarkable and makes me think cirrhosis of the liver was dependent upon the condition of the spleen, but still, as I have said before and as I have always felt, I am a little skeptical about the pathological entity called Banti's disease."

DR. JOSEPH SAMENFELD, in discussion, said:—"I would like to tell you about a case which occurred in Dr. Fuhs' service in St. Catherine's Hospital of a girl who had the same enlargement of the spleen seen in this patient, with a slight enlargement of the liver, leukopenia and the usual anemia which these patients have, and which was diagnosed by Dr. Fuhs as Banti's disease and operation performed, spleen removed and patient recovered. She came back to the hospital a few months later with a severe attack of typhoid fever, had five or six severe hemorrhages, and recovered. She again came back a short time after with appendicitis, had the appendix removed and one of the kidneys, all of which goes to show that probably the patient was able to use her liver to a certain extent in order to aid in the formation of anti-bodies to overcome the toxins of the various diseases which superseded Banti's disease. The patient is now in good health. It also showed that the blood itself was able to maintain a normal equilibrium as to chemical and physical properties without the aid of the spleen."

DR. ARTHUR H. BOGART, in discussion, said:—"I have had but little experience in this disease, as I have had but one case, and in that particular case I advised operation but gave a rather poor prognosis, so I did not operate. If, however, this man has a blood count of perhaps 3,000,000 and a hemoglobin of 40 per cent., and his kidneys are all right and he is in fairly good condition, as he seems to be, he is a proper case for splenectomy."

DR. SIMON R. BLATTEIS, in discussion, said:—"Banti's disease is essentially a primary cirrhosis of the spleen. The theory of its production seems to be that of a toxin circulating in the blood, attacking the connective tissue first of the follicles of the spleen, and then of the pulp. These changes are continued into the liver along the course of the portal vessels, producing an hypertrophic cirrhosis of the liver and later an atrophy with ascites.

"Removal of the spleen seems to diminish the amount of toxin produced; these not entering the system any longer, at least not to the extent as before, results in some improvement in the general clinical condition.

"The histological changes in the spleen are quite different from the changes observed in sections of splenomegaly of the Gaucher type which I showed; there isn't that characteristic proliferation of hyaline, seemingly swollen endothelial cells; there is here a general sclerosis.

"Changes in organs other than the spleen and liver, I think, have not been mentioned to be at all characteristic; those changes that are noted are consequent to a secondary anemia of varying grade."

DR. ALBERT THUNIG, in closing the discussion, said:—"There have been many points of advice given for which I want to thank you, but I feel that the point for discussion which remains is the point Dr. Fairbairn brought up, and that is as to whether or not this condition deserves a special name. Apparently some men, from what I have read, seem to have that undecided feeling about the condition and tend to call it simply splenic anemia. It is only in just that small group of cases of splenic anemia in which you have cirrhosis that the term Banti's disease should be given. On the other hand, if we take the broad term of splenic anemia, it has been shown that there are many cases classified under this name which are not truly splenic anemia. Many cases of simple hypertrophy of the spleen due to other causes, associated with anemia, have been classified under this condition; I do not see that I can give any definite ideas as to whether it should be given a special name or not."

## Demonstration of Ulcers of the Stomach and Duodenum Co-existing with Obstruction at Ileo-Cecal Junction.

### *Reported by James T. Pilcher, M.D.*

The specimen presented was obtained from a man 69 years of age, who gave a history that for thirty years he had suffered from recurrent spells of chronic indigestion which were characterized by pain coming on three or four hours after meals, always being relieved by the ingestion of alkalies or food, and from the fact that he had been repeatedly awakened at a stated time at night by pain. He had lately been under the treatment of lavage by his physician and seemed to be in his usual health after supper on the evening of the catastrophe to be reported. At half-past eleven in the evening he was seized with sharp, persistent pain in the upper abdomen, accompanied by vomiting of large quantities of grumous material. Opiates failed to relieve the pain, although given in fairly large doses. He was seen by the speaker in consultation with his physician, Dr. Thayer, two hours after the inception of the attack, at which time he was suffering intense pain, with a board-like abdomen of stony resistance over the upper right rectus. The liver dullness had been obliterated by encroaching tympanites and he was in a pronounced condition of shock. The case was considered one of perforated ulcer near the pyloric outlet and he was operated upon within the hour under gas oxygen anesthesia. On opening the abdomen there rushed out a quantity of free, odorless gas and several quarts of grumous material similar to that which had been vomited. A blown out ulcer the size of a dime was found in the neighborhood of the pylorus, which was reefed and inverted, and the abdomen closed, with adequate drainage. After return to his bed he suffered from a marked degree of acapnia and died in six hours without fully regaining consciousness.

At the restricted autopsy which was allowed this specimen was removed in conjunction with the accompanying portion of the gut which represents the cecum and terminal ileum and appendix. The speaker primarily called attention to the ease with which the stomach and duodenum could be recognized at post-mortem, as the duodenal mucosa up to the pyloric vein was invariably stained with bile, while that of the pyloric antrum was always unstained, and demonstrated this fact very clearly in the specimen presented, in which the pylorus was seen to be contracted to a diameter of one-quarter of an inch, just proximal to which obstruction on the inferior posterior aspect of the pyloric antrum was to be seen a perfectly healed, very definite round ulcer, while on the anterior superior surface was the blown out perforation which caused the death of the individual.

Of further interest was the presence of an extensive ulceration of the duodenum punched out in character and which had perforated deeply into the pancreas. It gave evidence that it was an old process and was probably not causing the patient any particular discomfort.

Dr. Pilcher then called attention to the observations of Mr. Lane, of London, who has been calling our attention lately to the fact that various conditions of the upper abdomen, including obstruction of the duodenojejunal angle, ulcers of the stomach and duodenum, gall bladder conditions of various kinds, or adhesive processes in that region, were in many instances due to a distal obstruction of the intestine which is most usually found at the ileo-cecal junction. This phenomenon was shown very definitely in the specimen presented in this case, the cecum being covered over by thick, membranous films. The appendix, which was in a state of complete obliteration and was fastened to the right iliac wall, was dragged taut. The very greatly enlarged mesoappendix, which instead of running posteriorly to the ileum, crossed the ileo-cecal junction anteriorly, and owing to traction of it by the appendix directly kinked and compressed the terminal ileum, proximal to which compression the ileum was very greatly dilated.

### Stomach of Case of Achlorhydria Hemorrhagica Gastrica, with Demonstration of Gross Specimen and Photo-Micrographs.

*Reported by James T. Pilcher, M.D.*

The specimen was obtained from a case dying post-operatively, who had a marked grade of acute pancreatitis, diabetes and many gall stones. Preoperatively, it had been found to present the symptom of achlorhydria hemorrhagica gastrica, which the speaker wished to be considered as indicative of an advanced condition of chronic gastritis; from the test meal findings in which cases it had been inferred that there must be some erosions of the stomach mucosa present. The specimen demonstrated that this was, in fact, the condition. The micro-photographs, of which bromide enlargements had been prepared, showed that there was a marked destruction of the mucous membrane and a very evident round-celled infiltration of the submucosa, which illustrations the speaker believed to be the earliest formation of confluent ulcer of which any record could be found in which definite pathologic and microscopic examination had been made. He believed, further, that this condition was due solely to the presence in these stomachs of great numbers of pathogenic bacteria, which are invariably present in patients presenting this symptom.

### Two Cases of Colon Bacteraemia.

*Reported by Arthur Holzman, M.D.*

Within the past three months two cases of colon septicæmia have been studied in the laboratory of the Jewish Hospital. The occurrence of this organism in the blood stream, producing its own peculiar type of septicæmic symptoms, makes it well worth the while for presenting these two cases of bacteræmia.

*Case* 1.—J. V. G., age 64, male, white; admitted to the Jewish Hospital in the service of Dr. Linder on December 25, 1912.

Family and previous history negative. Has had a left-sided hernia for the past fifteen years, but for the last three years has worn a truss. The hernia was never painful. Its size was that of about two fists and it was partially reducible.

On the day before admission the patient became extremely nauseated, did not vomit, was unable to urinate, and had to be catheterized. It was deemed advisable that an operation be done and a Bassini operation was performed on the day after admission to the hospital. Upon opening the sac the sigmoid flexure was found.

For the next nine days the patient ran the usual post-operative course, being troubled only with distention and inability to void urine.

On the tenth day, at 8 P. M., the patient suddenly developed a chill and temperature jumped to 103, pulse 124, respirations 36, at which time there was only a slight degree of distention and involuntary defecation.

Ten hours later the patient had another chill; temperature again rose to 103; the involuntary defecation became more frequent; vomited twice a large quantity of a very sour, watery fluid. On this, the eleventh day, the sutures were removed, the wound looking good.

On the twelfth day the patient had another chill; temperature this time rose to 104.8, pulse 140, respiration 40.

For the next six days the patient felt rather comfortable; temperature ranged between 100 and 103; there was but little distention, and no difficulty upon urination or defecation. At times the patient complained of abdominal cramps, which were relieved by enemas. Repeated examinations of the urine at this time showed only slight traces of albumin and the blood a slight leukocytosis. The general condition of the patient, however, was growing gradually worse; the temperature assumed the septic curve and the patient the septic facies.

On the nineteenth day there was another chill, the temperature rising to 102.8, pulse 144, respirations 42. On this day a blood culture was taken and a Gram-negative, slightly motile bacillus was isolated in pure culture, which proved to have all the cultural characteristics of the colon bacillus. The patient's condition became rapidly worse and the next day (twentieth) expired. No autopsy.

*Case* 2.—I. S., 34, white, female; admitted to the Jewish Hospital in the service of Dr. Polak on January 15, 1913.

Ten days before admission the patient suddenly developed a uterine hemorrhage and fainted; had sensations of heat and cold; curetted at home. Two hours after the currettement she was seized with chills and pains in the lower part of her abdomen.

Upon admission to the hospital, examination showed a lacerated pelvic floor, lacerated cervix and a hard, tender mass in the posterior cul-de-sac, with infiltration extending into both fornices. Post-vaginal section was performed and a large amount of pus evacuated. Bacteriological examination showed the streptococcus.

Within twenty-four hours the temperature dropped and for the next two days the patient felt fairly comfortable.

On the third day, post-operative, the temperature rose to 102.8, pulse 126, respirations 24. She was restless, noisy and somewhat distended. Under treatment the distention gradually disappeared, but the temperature assumed the septic curve and the patient a septic condition.

On the ninth day the condition of the patient was of a septic nature, temperature 103.2, pulse 132, respirations 28; somewhat noisy and irrational.

On the tenth day, post-operative, a blood culture was taken and a Gram-negative, motile bacillus was isolated. At this time she was delirious; distention was much relieved, and involuntary defecation was present, and on the eleventh day, post-operative, patient expired.

In this case we were fortunate enough to obtain an autopsy, and upon opening the peritoneal cavity encountered free pus. The smears of this pus shows a streptococcus longus and a Gram-negative bacillus; the cultures secured showed only a colon bacillus. A rat was injected intra-peritoneally with a saline emulsion of the organism and died two hours after inoculation. The colon bacillus was isolated from the liver and the heart's blood, and a second rat was injected with an emulsion of the organism obtained from the first rat. The dilution used this time was much weaker. This rat died in about six hours, and again the colon bacillus was isolated from the liver and heart's blood. This organism still maintained all the cultural characteristics of the colon bacillus and proved that not only was it pathogenic, but extremely virulent.

As far back as 1894 Hanot found colon bacilli in the blood of acute icterus gravis and maintained that changes in the liver were due to the presence of these organisms in the blood. In 1906, Gibson and Douglass, in the *Lancet,* reported a case that they called microbic cyanosis. Patient was a woman 36 years of age who, for a few years, was troubled with headache, dizziness, persistent diarrhea and cyanosis. After various examinations a bacteriological examination was made of the blood and the colon bacillus isolated. Their interpretation of the case was as follows: that the bacillus had gained entrance into the blood-stream through the intestinal tract, its presence there had caused the formation of nitrites and that the nitrites held the oxygen of the blood in such firm combination with the hæmoglobin so as to form methæmaglobin, thereby producing cyanosis.

In 1909, Jacob, in the Klinik of Strassburg, collected 26 cases, to which he added 13 of his own. He divides his cases into three groups:

1. Those running a course somewhat resembling typhoid fever.
2. Cases with secondary abscesses.
3. Cases of terminal infection in which the organism is removed from the blood a short time before death.

The most common point of entrance into the blood-stream is from the intestines, caused by any break in the mucosa. The biliary passages, urinary tract, female genital organs are next in order of occurrence.

The symptomatology of colon septicæmia is marked by a high temperature with rapid fluctuations with pulse in proportion. A constant feature is the presence of chills, sometimes occurring twice daily, most often daily. A high leukocyte count is always present. Small hemorrhages in the skin often take place, as is manifested by the disease in infants a few days old, namely, Winckel's disease.

The prognosis is, as a rule, bad, and depends upon:

1. Whether or no another organism is present with the colon bacillus.
2. Lessened resistance due to other disease.
3. Altered cultural characteristics of the intestinal tract.

Treatment—Symptomatic; vaccines.

The conclusions which may be drawn are as follows:

1. Colon septicæmia is more frequent than was formerly supposed.
2. It must be considered as a terminal infection.
3. Must always be borne in mind after an operation, especially laparotomy.
4. Prognosis is bad.
5. Diagnosis can be made early by blood cultures.
6. In the two cases studied by us the leukocyte count was not high.

# LONG ISLAND MEDICAL JOURNAL

| VOL. VII. | OCTOBER, 1913 | NO. 10 |

## 𝔒riginal 𝔄rticles.

### THE DIAGNOSIS OF CARDIAC DISEASE.*

By Richard C. Cabot, M.D.,

of Boston, Mass.

I HAVE chosen a very well worn subject rather than trying to give you the latest discoveries and researches, first, because I have not made any discoveries and researches; secondly, because if I had, they would not interest you.

When I meet another physician what I want to know from him is what his experience is with the common things we meet every day. I want to know his personal reaction to the matters that are sure to fall in my own sphere. I took, therefore, when asked to address this society the subject of cardiac diagnosis. I shall speak also of some points of treatment of cardiac disease.

I though it would be worth while to get a fresh start in the study of this very ancient and honorable subject by going over the last thousand cases I had seen in the Massachusetts General Hospital, in reference to the commoner types of cardiac disease and what is the relative frequency in a general way.

The figures of 1,144 cases of cardiac disease as studied at the Massachusetts General Hospital divide themselves roughly into two groups, first, those diseases affecting the heart itself primarily, and, second, those diseases in which something outside of the heart has brought about disease within the heart. In the first place, cardiac disease arising within the heart itself belongs in two groups, the rheumatic group and the syphilitic group. In the rheumatic group is, of course, the familiar rheumatic heart affection affecting the valves and the myocardium and pericardium and in children especially affecting all three. I have lumped together the cases of chronic diffuse pericarditis with cases of acute endocarditis and of chronic valvular disease.

When one thinks of heart disease ordinarily one thinks especially of that group and I was rather struck in going over these figures to find that that group made up only about one-third of the total number of heart cases; that is, the number of cases in which the valves were deformed made up only about one-third of all the cases of heart disease. Out of 1,144 cases, there were 425 in the rheumatic group affecting the valves, mostly, of course, the mitral and aortic valves, then the syphilitic group of 59 cases, a much smaller number, to be sure, but still I think about 59 more cases that I should have recognized myself five years ago. I want to emphasize that a little later as being one of

---

* Presented before the Brooklyn Society of Internal Medicine, May 14, 1913.

the newer points to me certainly in relation to heart disease—rheumatic cases, 425; syphilitic cases, 59; and then outside of the heart, 655, a good deal more than those inside the heart. Among those arising outside the heart arteriosclerosis with secondary effects upon the heart, is the chief cause; 328 cases. What we call the kidney heart, that is, the weakening of the heart secondary to kidney disease comes next, with 280; and then the goitre heart, the heart secondary to exophthalmic goitre, 47. Now, if you leave out the goitre-heart and the negligible item of congenital heart cases (only 5 cases out of those 1,144), the cases fall into four groups, the rheumatic group, the syphilitic group, the arteriosclerotic group and the kidney hearts. The last two together make up more than any other type of case that I see. I am speaking now of cases of failing compensation which turn up at the hospital or at your office with dropsy, dyspnea and cough and the ordinary symptoms of a failing heart. I will take those up in the order in which I have given them.

In the first place, the rheumatic group, affecting the valves and also the myocardium and pericardium.

## 1.

I will speak first of mitral regurgitation. I noticed in looking over the catalogs of hospitals a great number of diagnoses of mitral regurgitation and a very considerable number of diagnoses of death due to mitral regurgitation. I think if you take the trouble to look over the rather uninteresting statistics in the hospital reports you will generally find a large number of deaths put down to mitral regurgitation.

In the study of 3,000 autopsies at the Massachusetts General Hospital there was one solitary case where in our belief death was due to mitral regurgitation. I think that death due to mitral regurgitation is very rare. On the other hand, there were 81 cases of death due to mitral stenosis in that same series. As a cause of death mitral regurgitation is not a common disease. Where mitral regurgitation occurs and the patient dies there is generally something else more responsible, for example, arteriosclerotic conditions. The mitral regurgitation is only one item in the group of processes which finally produce death. In the same way, chronic interstitial nephritis—then hypertrophy of the heart, dilatation of the mitral orifice, mitral regurgitation, death; but the patient really died of chronic interstitial nephritis.

Now, as to the diagnosis of mitral regurgitation: I am very much in the habit of saying to medical students that it is like a three-legged stool; that is, it rests on three legs, but take away any one of those legs and it will fall. Three things are characteristic, the murmur at the apex, enlargement of the heart and accentuation of the pulmonary second sound. In the presence of those three facts one is very seldom wrong, but with less, with only the murmur of the apex, one is very often wrong and I have been very often wrong. I am not in the least shy about criticising my confrères, because I am wrong so often that I imagine others are, too.

In children I have made a number of wrong diagnoses of mitral regurgitation. Children very frequently show systolic murmurs and loud systolic murmurs at the apex, but there is no incurable change in the heart at all in those cases for the child grows up and gets well and nothing remains of your diagnosis. Never make a diagnosis of regurgitation because there is a systolic murmur, however loud, at the apex and however widely transmitted or you will make as I have made, many mistakes. But if you make a diagnosis on those three items then you will not make that mistake nearly as often as I did.

## 2.

Mitral stenosis, as I have said, is a very different article with reference to the production of death. In the series of 3,000 autopsies which I have analyzed, 81 deaths were due to mitral stenosis primarily and only one to mitral regurgitation. Among the cases of mitral stenosis the great majority can be diagnosed correctly during life. It is one of the easier lesions to diagnose provided you see the case sometime before death. But if you see the case the first time only forty-eight hours or so before death, diagnosis is generally impossible. In a moment I will speak at greater length as to why that is so. Imagine you are more fortunate and see the case some weeks or months before death. The series of events is classical and pretty nearly characteristic. In the first place, the quality of the impulse felt with the hand on the chest wall. I have often said to medical students that we can make a diagnosis of mitral stenosis merely by feeling the chest wall in a great many cases. What one feels is, of course, the well known crescendo presystolic roll which sounds like a galloping horse because it ends in the first sharp sound. When you have heard it a few times there is nothing easier to recognize. The difficulty of it is that it is not always there; when it is there a diagnosis is simple, but the roll has a habit of falling out and getting lost, which is unequaled by any other murmur.

When the heart weakens with the approach of death it is often impossible to hear any murmur whatever. The left auricle does not contract hard enough or push the blood down through the orifice fast enough to produce a murmur and therefore there isn't any murmur to that class of cases; hence diagnosis, as I have said, is usually impossible.

There is, however, one point even in these advanced cases, what we call the third-stage cases near death—one point that sometimes helps us; that is the quality of the first sound. I tried a moment ago to symbolize this murmur, this presystolic murmur, by tapping my fingers on the table. By the final sound I intended to represent the first sound of the heart. That tapping first sound is one of the characteristic things remaining even when the murmur itself disappears near death and by noticing that point you can sometimes make a diagnosis of mitral stenosis even when there is no murmur present.

Then, as in mitral regurgitation, you have enlargement of the heart and accentuation of the pulmonary second sound, but there is also another point which helps you and that is the doubling of the pulmonary second sound; in about nine-tenths of all cases of mitral stenosis the doubled second sound is heard. It is not heard in any other lesion with anything like that frequency.

Another point of value in the doubtful cases is the absence of the second sound at the apex of the heart. In normal cases we hear two sounds at the apex, the first and second sound. In mitral stenosis we generally hear only one and that is the first sound. The reason is that the second sound at the apex is the transmitted aortic second and the aortic second sound is so feeble in advanced mitral stenosis that it is not transmitted to the apex.

One of the great things in auscultation of the heart is to get used to noticing the absence as well as the presence of things, the absence of the second sound at the apex, for example.

Mitral stenosis has been said in the text-books for a great many years to be commoner in women and I have repeated that statement to my students many times. I have often been asked by students and by physicians, Why is mitral stenosis commoner in women than in men? but I have not known the answer to that question until this year. Now I think I do. I began to analyze this same series of 3,000 autopsies in reference to this point and in nearly 150 autopsies on mitral stenosis of the adult at the Boston City Hospital and the Massachusetts General, I looked up this question of sex and I found that the sexes are exactly equal. So the answer to the question, Why is mitral stenosis commoner in women? is that it isn't. That is one of those characteristic mistakes transmitted from text-book to text-book. I do not believe that you can find a text-book that does not contain that. I know my text-book does. The reason for it is simple; no one has yet taken the trouble to go to the autopsy table to settle this point.

Another characteristic point about mitral stenosis is the occurrence of hemiplegia—of paralysis of one side of the body in connection with it. That happens much more frequently in connection with mitral stenosis than in any other form of heart disease. The reason for it seems to be this: In mitral stenosis the blood circulates very slowly through the left auricle and in the left auricle there are places where the blood clots so that intracardiac thrombosis in the left auricle is very common. A little bit breaks off and goes down through the mitral and up to the brain; similar emboli go to other parts of the body and do no harm, to the kidney and spleen, for instance, but when emboli of the same size are being thrown off in showers and some go to the brain, the brain being more sensitive and some of its arteries being terminal, we get hemiplegia. If in a doubtful case of heart disease hemiplegia occurs, that is in itself a good reason for believing that you are dealing with mitral stenosis, whatever you hear.

### 3.

Now, as to aortic regurgitation: I would say the same thing for that as for mitral regurgitation. It is very seldom the cause of death, because nearly 90 per cent. of the cases of primary aortic regurgitation are due to syphilis, and has been so proven. Syphilitic arteritis, syphilis of the arch of the aorta, including the valves, is the cause of 90 per cent. of all cases of primary aortic regurgitation, and if it is there it is, of course, elsewhere throughout the body. The patient dies of syphilis and not of aortic regurgitation, one part of that syphilis.

One of the things which we have been recently following in the hospital is the condition of the central nervous system in syphilitic heart disease. In these cases of aortic regurgitation as they come into us for hospital care for their heart trouble, shortness of breath, swelling of the feet and all the ordinary heart symptoms, we often find, on testing the blood, the Wassermann reaction to be positive. If it is and even if it is not we tap the spinal cord in these cases and we find very often an excess of mononuclear cells in the spinal fluid, showing a low grade inflammation of precisely the same kind that leads to tabes and to general paralysis of the insane. In other words, you may have the opportunity of stopping by treatment the development of tabes or general paralysis which you discover by tapping the spinal cord, to which you are led by finding the Wassermann reaction in the blood, to which again you are led by finding aortic regurgitation. Given aortic regurgitation, try for syphilis in the blood. If not in the blood, try and see what the spinal cord shows. If you find an excess of cells; that is, over fifteen cells to the cubic centimeter, · counted in the ordinary way as blood is counted, you have an excess of cells and should treat the patient as for syphilis and especially by the methods recently introduced here at the Rockefeller Institute. Dr. Swift there gives salvarsan intravenously and then bleeds the patient and puts the salvarsanized serum into the spinal cord. You cannot put salvarsan into the spinal canal; it is too dangerous, but you can put the salvarsanized serum from the patient into the spinal cord and in that way you can apparently check tabes and general paralysis in this way at times.

Aortic regurgitation is one of the easiest of all diseases to diagnose and in my records there have been fewer mistakes in this than in any other type of valve lesion when we come to post mortem. As a rule the murmur is easily heard and easily recognized; moreover, we have the peripheral phenomena in the peripheral arteries, the jumping of the arteries, the Corrigan pulse, a group of facts making the diagnosis much stronger. In aortic cases, as in mitral regurgitation, you should never make the diagnosis from the murmur alone; but if you have the murmur and jumping of the arteries you get a diagnosis that will stand. Practically all these cases have a very high systolic blood pressure, with a low diastolic blood pressure.

Aortic stenosis is one of the hardest of valve lesions to recognize. It is the one in which we have made more mistakes at the Massachusetts General Hospital than in any other lesion, as shown post mortem. It is generally a mistake in the direction of saying that stenosis is there when it isn't, rather than of saying it isn't there when it is. A diagnosis of aortic stenosis made by some men simply because they hear a systolic murmur in the second right space. This murmur is very common without any stenosis in the aortic valve, very common with slight arteriosclerosis of the aortic arch; the blood makes a rough noise going over the arch. It is not uncommon to find functional murmurs heard best there; so that you can never make a diagnosis on the murmur alone. We need at least four things for this diagnosis. I have spoken of the three-legged stool for mitral regurgitation. I think we have a four-legged stool here. We need all four legs before we can make a diagnosis of aortic stenosis; first, the murmur, secondly, the palpable thrill, in or near the second right interspace, systolic in time; thirdly, diminution or absence of the second sound, the sound produced by the shutting of the valve, which cannot shut because it is stiff; fourthly, the characteristic pulse which is best defined as being the opposite of the Corrigan pulse; it is sometimes called the plateau pulse. With those four things you can generally make a diagnosis, but it is hard to get all those four things.

As I have said, these valvular lesions make up in my experience the minority of cardiac cases in the stage of failing compensation mainly; the majority is made up by cases of kidney trouble and cases of arteriosclerosis leading to hypertrophy and then to failure of the heart. It is in these two diseases, of course, that the heart undergoes degenerative changes or wears out by chronic fatigue, and it is on these two diseases in the last few years that my attention has been specially centered.

I do not suppose I need express to an audience like this the strength of my feeling about the value of blood pressure measures. I will say, however, that in this series of 3,000 autopsies, to which I have referred, wherein we compared our diagnoses made before death with the actual facts after death, there has been no single method of examination which has stood the test on confrontation with the facts as well as blood pressure measurement. Compared with percussion, with auscultation, with urinary examination, with blood examination, with anything you can mention, there has been no test that has stood up against the facts as well as blood pressure measurement. When the blood pressure has said there ought to be a big heart there has been a big heart practically every time. It is an easy test to make. You can make it about as well the first time as the thousandth time. Then the quickness of it. Very few tests have anything like the same value that we can do as quickly as blood pressure.

I will say a word about the instruments. I believe strongly in employing the mercury column and not the smaller types of instruments which look more or less like a watch. They are very tempting because they are small, but check them up against mercury and you will find that in time they will play you false. Now as to the mercury instruments, some of them are portable and cheap, which is a consideration. The best type I know of can be had for $12. It is one that can be easily put into an ordinary doctor's bag without any trouble. If there is anybody here who does not make routine blood pressure examinations on his patients at the bedside and at his office I would strongly advise him to try it and see if it does not prove itself more valuable in his own experience than the cost. It helps, especially in the early diagnosis of arteriosclerosis and chronic nephritis. Those are two of the commonest diseases we meet with in general practice and I do not think there is any doubt but that we can make a diagnosis of those two diseases earlier by means of blood pressure measures than we can in any other way. I have noticed the change in our hospital statistics—a change in the increasing frequency of diagnoses of kidney disease and arteriosclerosis. That change began coincidently with the greater use of blood pressure instruments.

(Here Dr. Cabot took up the question of pain in the heart, stating that pain may be serious or of no importance; that in this relation blood pressure measures were of very great use; and that pain may be organic or functional.)

Continuing, Dr. Cabot said:

Given a case where there are no murmurs, no enlargement, irregularity of the pulse and of the apex beat, there are two things which seem to me positively of value: First, make the patient walk up and down your office as fast as he can go four or five times. If the trouble is functional the heart will act more regularly; if organic it will act more irregularly. I have very seldom known that test to fail. Putting it in more modern terms: if the irregularities are due to premature contractions those are usually banished or nearly banished by exercise; if the irregularities are due to auricular fibrillation they will be made worse by exercise.

Blood pressure in this field also helps us. The great majority of irregular hearts due to organic disease have a high blood pressure.

(I am speaking of cases without murmurs), and the great majority of functional irregularities have a normal blood pressure.

One of the greatest helps that come from blood pressure measurements is in chronic nephritis and cardiac diseases secondary thereto, in that they enable us to make a diagnosis of organic disease when the urine shows little or no albumin and no casts. Every one who has had much to do with chronic nephritis knows that there are such cases, knows also that cases which this week show albumin and casts may show none next week and the week after will show them again. If you happen to see the case the first time, perhaps the only time in that intermediate week you will get no albumin and casts; it is then that blood pressure is our only guide to the presence of nephritis. Blood pressure is just as high in cases without casts and albumin as in cases with them and if you can exclude arteriosclerosis, as in many cases you can, and if there is a high blood pressure and no other obvious cause for it, you can say with almost complete certainty that you are dealing with chronic nephritis.

I will give some slight limitations and exceptions to that statement. If you have a high blood pressure and can exclude arteriosclerosis, you can almost say that it is due to chronic nephritis, the chief exceptions being, in the first place, goitre hearts, the heart secondarily enlarged as the result of exophthalmic goitre, which also have a high blood pressure, and the rarer cases of brain tumor or other intracranial disease with high blood pressure.

The question is often asked, Aren't there people who have a high blood pressure from idiosyncrasy without any disease? It is impossible to make an absolutely positive statement on such a point, but I can say I have never seen a case of that kind and I do not yet see reason to believe that there are such. The cases of so-called idiosyncrasy that I have seen turn out when carefully studied to be one of the things I mentioned, usually nephritis or arteriosclerosis.

In all doubtful cases it is well to test the apex impulse with the patient lying on the left side. Many of us, in examining patients in the office or at home, examine them lying down on the back and sitting up. That is all right, but there are cases in which the presence of an apex beat in the sixth interspace, a space below where it should be, is demonstrable only with the patient on the left side. The chest arches forward in such a way, or the thickness of the chest wall may be such that you do not get the apex beat with the hand in the ordinary sitting or lying position. But put the patient on the left side and if you feel the apex beat in the sixth space, you have valuable evidence of an enlarged heart; this is sometimes the best clue you have of the presence of kidney trouble.

In relation to this class of doubtful cases of kidney disease. I would like to pass on to you one rule which I have been using for a good many years without seeing any reason for changing it. I have already spoken of the presence and absence of albumin and casts as not being a deciding factor. One of the things I have learned from this same series of autopsies is how frequently we have albumin and casts in the urine in normal kidneys post mortem. When you are confronted with that situation and you are not sure you have kidney disease or not, I would commend to your experience this course of reasoning:

If you have kidney disease it is either acute or chronic. If it is acute it will usually show in the urine by obvious evidences. If it is chronic, it practically always leads to hypertrophy of the heart and so to high blood pressure. If you have not an hypertrophied heart and high blood pressure you probably have not got chronic nephritis. If there are no obvious evidences of acute nephritis and no cardiac hypertrophy there is usually no nephritis at all—no matter *what* the urine.

Now, as to arteriosclerosis and its effect upon the heart: I remember some years ago seeing a case in consultation with a physician in which I made a diagnosis of arteriosclerosis and he was a good deal surprised at my diagnosis. He said, "I did not know arteriosclerosis was a diagnosis. I thought it was just a symptom. I thought that arteriosclerosis meant that the arteries were tortuous, rough and stiff. Isn't it a symptom like the arcus senilis." I do not think that that is now a common view. I think most of us know it is a common disease and, more than that, the commonest of all diseases in adult life.

1. It can affect the heart by narrowing the tubes into which it has to pump and stiffening them, so as to increase the work of the heart and induce hypertrophy. 2. It can affect the heart by narrowing the coronary arteries, diminishing the blood supply of the heart and so producing interstitial myocarditis or scars in the heart wall, which scars again may stretch and produce aneurysm, not of the aorta, but of the heart itself and so at last actual rupture of the heart, the broken heart, which occurs not only in novels but in real life, although in a very different class of cases! 3. Arteriosclerosis can affect the heart by roughening the inside of the aorta and then crawling down from the aorta on to the aortic valves so as to stiffen and contract them and produce aortic regurgitation. I spoke a few minutes ago of aortic regurgitation as being usually due to syphilis and I do not mean to take that back, but about 10 per cent. of the cases of primary aortic regurgitation are due to arteriosclerosis extending back from the aorta in this way on to the heart.

Those are the most important ways in which arteriosclerosis affects the heart; when it does not produce these effects the diagnosis of arteriosclerosis is not a simple one. In many cases I have felt hard, tortuous, roughened arteries at the wrist, perhaps also in the temple, but when I came to post-mortem it has turned out that none of the internal arteries had arteriosclerosis. It was confined practically to the arteries of the arms and wasn't, therefore, of very great importance. Thus we may be very seriously misled. On the other hand, in many autopsies on patients whose arteries were felt in life soft and straight and smooth at the wrist, there is, post-mortem, a most extensive arteriosclerosis in the internal arteries. If that is true, and I am sure you can convince yourself it is, palpation of the arteries, our ordinary method, misleads us often, and in both directions. Hence we need especially any method that will minimize the number of such mistakes. Such a method is blood pressure measurement.

That brings me to the differential diagnosis between chronic nephritis with high blood pressure and arteriosclerosis with high blood pressure. It is a very frequent and difficult problem.

I will give you such points as in my own experience I have found to work. On the average arteriosclerosis is seen in older patients and nephritis in younger patients; nephritis may last a long time, but does not ordinarily last as long as or begin as late as arteriosclerosis. Hence, other things being equal, the younger the patient who has high blood pressure the more likely it is to be nephritis, while the older the patient the more likely it is to be arteriosclerosis. Secondly: As to anemia and uremia. Both are commoner in high blood pressure cases due to nephritis than in high blood pressure due to arteriosclerosis.

In spite of those points you will make a mistake every now and then, but it is not a mistake of any great importance, I mean in the cases you would be likely to be mistaken in. In the cases where there is not much albumin or many casts, not much edema, not much uremia, the diagnosis between nephritis and arteriosclerosis does not make much difference because the treatment is essentially the same in both.

Lastly, I want to speak about two drugs. Most of you know more about the treatment of disease than I do. I do not know much about the treatment of any disease, but there are two or three things which I would like to say. First, I would like to emphasize the value of the drug diuretin, which you can get much cheaper if you call it the sodio-salicylate of theobromin. It takes longer to say, but it saves money. If you buy it under its trade name of diuretin it is more expensive. Sodio-salicylate of theobromin is, I think, the most valuable of all the cardiac drugs in the treatment of cases of "kidney hearts," "arteriosclerosic hearts" and "goiter hearts," the whole group I have been speaking of. Diuretin certainly acts upon the heart as well as on the kidneys, and while it does not act always favorably (of course, there is no drug that does), I know of no drug that helps as many times, not only in dropsical cases, but in cardiac failure without much dropsy.

Let me advise you in dropsical cases of heart disease to begin with diuretin and purgation, say, with magnesium sulphate, and keep that up for five days before you give any digitalis at all. If you will begin in the dropsical cases with diuretin and sulphate of magnesia and keep that up for five days before using digitalis, you will do a great deal more good with your digitalis than if you start it at the beginning when your patient is water-logged and often has a very bad stomach.

Another point: I know of no drug oftener misused than morphin, but in the one disease I see it used too little is heart disease. Morphin is a heart stimulant, not a heart depressant; yet I meet many men who are afraid to use it for fear of depressing the heart. It never depresses the heart, in my experience. It supports the heart. It is valuable at the beginning and at the end of our treatment in cardiac stasis. I have seen cases live on it that couldn't get along on digitalis. In the first twenty-four hours of your treatment of cardiac failure with dropsical disease it is of very great value. The patient is generally sleepless and if you can give him one good night's sleep it will give the heart a rest (the heart needs a rest just as well as you do). After that relief the heart will pick itself up and take hold of its job in a different way. Use morphin as a heart stimulant in the first twenty-four or forty-eight hours in the treatment of acute cardiac failure; after that diruetin and magnesium sulphate and after this digitalis.

In regard to the digitalis preparations: I suppose every one has his own favorite brand. As to the tincture of digitalis preparations: All of you who use the tincture method know that you get one tincture which will be splendid and another one that is no good. I advise you to use digipuratum, because it is reliable. The only thing against it is its expense, but you, no doubt, all have some patients to whom the expense of a drug is rather a recommendation than otherwise.

# THE RATIONAL TREATMENT OF GASTRIC AND DUODENAL ULCER.

## By Henry F. Graham, M.D.,

of Brooklyn, N. Y.

THE rational treatment of digestive disorders must be based upon a knowledge of the physiology of digestion and nutrition in man as modified by the pathological conditions present.

The facts of especial interest in the therapy of gastric and duodenal ulcer are those concerned with the secretion of gastric juice and the motility of the stomach.

They may be briefly stated as follows:

When hunger is present the sight and smell of appetizing food cause a profuse flow of a powerful gastric juice and the mere acts of tasting and chewing such food are quickly followed by an active secretion from the gastric glands, even though nothing is allowed to enter the stomach. The more pleasant the taste the stronger the juice is.

The response to different kinds of food varies in the properties, rate, duration and quantity of the secretion, and there is almost an exact proportional relationship between the quantity of gastric juice and the amount of food taken.

The acidity is greatest with meat and meat extracts. It is lowest with bread. Flesh also calls forth the greatest quantity, while milk is followed by no "appetite juice" and the least quantity, a low acidity, and a slow secretion which is neutralized as formed. Bread and the white of egg introduced directly into the stomach do not excite the flow of gastric juice.

Water produces a small quantity of very weak secretion. Olive oil, cream, and all kinds of animal and vegetable fats inhibit the secretion of gastric juice, although they stimulate the flow of bile and pancreatic juice. When put into the stomach half an hour before meat, olive oil lessened the gastric juice to half the quantity usually secreted, and prolonged the digestive process. Carbohydrates seem to have little influence in the stomach.

As a diet is maintained for a long period of time, more and more the digestive juices conform to the digestive requirements of the food eaten.

What conditions influence the motility of the stomach?

Carbohydrates commence to leave it normally in fifteen minutes, and are all gone in three hours. Fats of the same quantity and consistency are only one-half gone at the end of six hours.

Proteids require six hours to reach the intestine in their entirety, although egg white or soft-boiled egg escapes quickly into the duodenum, and fully 50 per cent. of the milk ingested reaches the cæcum in two hours.

When hard particles are present in the food they cause pyloric closing and delay the exit of the softer food, so that it may take even three times as long.

Absence of stomach movements may occur as a result of excitement, anger or anxiety, causing stagnation of food; and respiratory distress may cause antiperistalsis.[5]

Periodic propulsive movements occur in the empty stomachs of fasting animals about every two hours, lasting about twenty minutes.

There may be five to fifteen waves, the contraction taking one-half to one and one-half minutes and the pause one to one and one-half minutes.

It is evident that this may have an important relationship to the "hunger pain" of duodenal ulcer.

What is the influence of drugs?.

We will mention only two: A ½ per cent. solution of sodium bicarbonate at intervals over a period of time diminishes hypersecretion and lessens the excitability of the glands, thus giving the stomach a rest.

Atropine experimentally destroyed the irritability of the vagus nerve and inhibited secretion.

Now, a word in regard to the pathological conditions that we find present in ulcer—hypersecretion, hyperacidity, pylorospasm, gastric dilatation, and marked constipation are the most prominent of these and are the ones toward which our treatment must be most often directed. Perforation, peritonitis and hæmorrhage will not be considered except to say that the latter condition will usually be best met by treatment of the underlying cause—the ulcer.

As our main reliance must always be upon diet we must briefly consider what is necessary to keep a normal individual in good health.

Chittenden's studies have been so exhaustive and his conclusions seem so well proven that they are worthy of acceptance. (Chittenden, Low Protein Standard.)[2]

The average individual weighing 150 pounds requires while leading a moderately active life about 2,200 calories or food units per day, and of these 225 should be in the form of protein—three times that amount in fat (700) and six times that amount carbohydrate (1,200).

In treating diseased conditions it is often necessary to throw added strain upon one or more organs that are not diseased, and depart from normal standards. In ulcer of the stomach and duodenum we are forced, in combating the hyperacidity and dilatation, to use excessive amounts of proteid and fats, but we must always bear the normal in mind and get back to it as soon as possible.

How, then, shall we handle these cases? The first requisite when possible is rest in bed. Physical rest, mental rest, freedom from worry and excitement in a cool, pleasant room with plenty of sunshine—far removed from any odors that may suggest enjoyable food.

The food should be simply served and, even later, when the patient is up and about, he should not eat at the the table with others where the sight and smell of food that he cannot enjoy will only excite a greater amount of "appetite juice" to do harm. The food at first should be entirely liquid or in the form of a puree or gruel to eliminate chewing and lessen pylorospasm. The food, like a suit of clothes, must be fitted to the individual, but most cases will probably do well to start with a milk and egg diet below their permanent requirements, such as four tablespoonfuls of ice-cold milk every half hour from 7 A. M. to 9 P. M., and one egg at midnight, another at 3 A. M. After a time the quantity can be doubled and the interval increased to one hour.

If improvement is taking place, at the end of ten days or two weeks it will be possible to get nearly up to a normal standard by the following diet, which furnishes 308 calories of protein, 842 of fat and 836 of carbohydrate. Total, 1,986 calories.

```
 7 A. M.    Glass milk, 6 ounces, with oatmeal and sugar, 1 ounce;
 9 A. M.      "      "       "
11 A. M.      "      "       "      "   pea or bean puree, 1 cup;
 1 P. M.      "      "       "      "   baked potato and 2 ounces cream;
 3 P. M.      "      "       "      "
 5 P. M.      "      "       "      "
 7 P. M.      "      "       "      "   rice and sugar, 1 ounce;
 9 P. M.      "      "       "      "   2 ounces cream;
12 Midnight.  One egg beaten up;
 3 A. M.       "    "     "    ".   Total, 1½ quarts of milk.
```

The protein and fat are still somewhat above the normal. The milk should be cold and should be slowly sipped, or, better, taken from a teaspoon.

Someone will say, How does this differ from the Lenhartz treatment for ulcer?

Here is the tenth day of a Lenhartz cure as applied in one of our New York hospitals.[4]

Eight eggs, 1 quart of milk, 50 grams of chicken, 70 grams of beef, 20 grams of butter, 200 grams of rice, 40 grams of sugar, 40 grams of zwiebach. Total, 450 calories of protein, 1,225 calories of fat and 675 calories of carbohydrate.

It does not seem necessary to use such excessive amounts of protein and fat with their ever-present danger of an intestinal upset, and it surely is illogical to use beef and chicken, which excite a stronger gastric juice than any other food stuff and which are slow in leaving the stomach, when we can use milk, which is more digestible and absorbable than any other proteid and excites a minimum amount of acidity, which it promptly neutralizes. Eggs act in a similar way, but are much more likely to cause the familiar "bilious attack."

Because of the large amount of fat which they contain they are valuable for use at night, when longer intervals are necessary between feedings.

A constant watch must be kept for evidences of colitis, hepatic disturbance or renal irritation. This is not an imaginary danger, for I have seen it occur.

In the long run, it is poor policy to rob Peter to pay Paul, and little gratitude is expressed when the gnawing, burning pain of an ulcer has been converted into the colic and diarrhœa of an acute colitis or the constipation, pain and toxæmia of a chronic one. It is too much like Mark Twain's horse doctor who was called to see a man with acute indigestion and gave him medicine which changed it into blind staggers.

Later on the milk and eggs may be gradually reduced, the night feeding eliminated and vegetables, such as squash, carrots, peas, beans, spinach, etc., added. The variety of cereals may be increased, and fruit, such as baked apples, apple sauce, muskmelon, pears, prunes and oranges added. All food of this kind, of course, should be carefully chewed and the frequency and size of the meals adjusted to the size of the stomach in inverse proportion to the amount of dilatation. The ravenous appetite must be kept in check by a reminder that most indigestion comes from an attempt to "fit a square meal into a round stomach" and that a "gastronomic debauch" will inevitably be followed by a relapse. Meat should be avoided for a long time, perhaps better forever, as the intestinal flora are much more toxic in carnivorous animals.

A daily enema will be necessary for a time, and later Russian white oil may be given in one-ounce doses at bedtime. Most cases can be handled with very few drugs.

If alkalies are necessary it is better to give them with the meals to inhibit gastric secretion, rather than an hour or two later to neutralize it.

. Atropine inhibits secretion. Clinically, sodium bromide gives splendid results in lessening pain.

Experiments should be made to determine whether a pure mineral oil, such as a white liquid petroleum oil, will inhibit the secretion of gastric juice as animal and vegetable fats do. If it does it should be valuable, because it does not split up into irritating acids in the intestine.

The bacillus bulgaricus seems to aid in combating intestinal toxæmia, which we know will of itself cause hyperacidity. It is best given in the form of a liquid culture and not as the lactic acid milk. I have known the latter to cause severe pain when an ulcer was present. Bismuth subnitrate in large doses has been warmly advocated.

The dietetic and medicinal treatment is recommended for acute ulcers, relapsing ulcer when the relapses have not been frequent and the free intervals have been long ones, in acute hæmorrhage from an ulcer, and in cases presenting a contraindication to surgery.

. As to the surgical treatment: No one who has seen many of these cases on the operating table will doubt that surgery is the only means of cure for some of them. They have tried palliative means and cures again and again. Others are too shiftless to carry out any prolonged treatment, or, from economic reasons, cannot afford the time and expense. They must get back to work as soon as possilbe.

Still others insist upon operation and will not consent to try diet and medicine first.

Perforation—often like a bolt from the blue—forces to the operating table one who has been timid and reluctant before.

The operative technique for these cases is now established on a firm basis and it may be stated with much emphasis that nearly every case of gastric or duodenal ulcer properly operated upon and receiving the proper after care will be cured and stay cured. This means that we must try in every case to discover the conditions originally responsible for causing the ulcer and remove them.

The diet after operation for a considerable period of time may well be one for diminishing acidity and restoring tone to an atonic and dilated stomach. The administration of broths, as is often done, has no rational basis.

The phrase, "We operate and God completes the cure," has been overworked. We must help God out. He works through human instrumentality.

A prominent New York surgeon recently went out of town, resected two-thirds of a stomach and did a gastroenterostomy for carcinoma. The condition of the patient was so critical he was afraid to telephone and inquire about her. One week after operation he met her doctor and asked, "When did she die?" The reply was, "Oh, she's eating some strawberries today."

Let us watch these patients; keep them from work if we can until they are up to their normal weight and strength—several months at least. Keep them on an ulcer diet until all tendency to hyperacidity has subsided, and on soft, well-chewed food in moderate amounts until gastric motility is normal.

After a gastroenterostomy there is a tendency for food to reach the colon more quickly than before, so large quantities of milk are not advisable. A quart a day should be sufficient. Meat is better omitted.

These measures, with avoidance of overwork and worry as far as possible, and ordinary dietetic and general hygiene, will avoid future digestive disorders.

### BIBLIOGRAPHY.

1. Pavlov: "The Digestive Juices."
2. Chittenden: "The Nutrition of Man."
3. J. H. Kellogg: "Diet List."
4. S. W. Lambert: "The Lenhartz Treatment of Gastric Ulcer." *Amer. Jour. Med. Sc.,* January, 1908.
5. Cannon. *Amer. Jour. of Physiology,* 1898.

## "VACCINATION AND ANTIVACCINATION."*

### By Jay Frank Schamberg, M.D.,

of Philadelphia, Pa.

Member of the Pennsylvania State Vaccination Commission.

IT would appear an act of supererogation to address a medical body in support of the efficacy of vaccination as a safeguard against smallpox. I shall, with your permission, advert to certain historical, statistical and clinical aspects of the subject, and then address myself to some of the arguments of the opponents of vaccination. It is a rather remarkable fact that despite conclusive proof of the efficacy of vaccination, opposition to this prophylactic measure has for over a century been manifested by small but active bands of individuals.

In order to appreciate the value of vaccination, one must comprehend the extent to which smallpox prevailed in the pre-vaccination era. Admiral Berkeley, Chairman of the Committee of the House of Commons in 1802, to whom Jenner's petition for a parliamentary grant was referred, stated that 45,000 persons died annually of smallpox in Great Britain.

Upon the screen, you will note a statistical table showing the actual number of smallpox deaths in London from 1647 to 1800. It is seen that smallpox was not only continuously present in the English metropolis during this period, but the yearly smallpox mortality was enormous, averaging for the century 1700 to 1800, about 2,000 deaths annually; this would indicate about 10,000 cases a year. Smallpox caused about one-twelfth of all deaths during this century in London.

To demonstrate that this mortality was not peculiar to the English capitol, one may cite the smallpox record of several small English towns.

Haygarth gives an account of an epidemic of smallpox in Chester, England, in 1744, at which time, of a population of 14,713 there were 1,202 persons who took smallpox, of whom 209 died. At the termination of the epidemic, there was only about 7 per

---

* Address delivered before the Medical Society of the County of Kings, March 18, 1913, with lantern demonstrations.

cent. of the population who had never had smallpox. Thus 93 per cent. of the people had suffered an attack of this fell disease.

In the small town of Ware, England, in 1722, in a population of 2,515 souls, 2,213 had had smallpox; 302 persons were referred to in the record as yet "to have the smallpox." Eighty-eight per cent. of the people had already had smallpox.

In our country great epidemics were not unknown. The case of Boston is most striking. In 1752 Boston had a severe epidemic of smallpox. The population of Boston at that time was 15,634; of this number, 5,545 persons contracted the disease in the usual manner, and 2,124 took it by inoculation. Over 5,000 people had previously gone through an attack of smallpox. Eighteen hundred and forty-three (1,843) persons escaped from the town to avoid the danger of infection. There were, therefore, left in the city, but 174 people who had never had smallpox. The population at the end of the epidemic practically consisted of persons who had survived an attack of this great scourge.

As you all know, the discovery of vaccination was made known to the world in a modest brochure, which was published by Jenner in 1798. Within a few years, a remarkable decline in the morbidity and mortality of smallpox became apparent in most of the countries of the civilized world. The opponents of vaccination allege that this decline was not due to the introduction of vaccination, but to the cessation of smallpox inoculation. Without entering into detail upon this contention, let me state that the conclusion of the Royal Commission on Vaccination was that inoculation exerted a favorable influence by saving the lives of thousands of persons who would otherwise have succumbed to natural smallpox, but likewise exerted an unfavorable influence in tending to perpetuate the disease; that there was no appreciable influence upon smallpox mortality, as the two influences neutralized each other. Even before the introduction of inoculation into England in 1721, smallpox was a constant and ever present scourge that decimated the population. If the introduction of vaccination in 1798 was not the cause of the decline in smallpox deaths that set in at the beginning of the 19th century, then this must be regarded as one of the most remarkable coincidences in the history of mankind.

Within recent years, striking statistical evidence of the efficacy of vaccination has been available. Prior to the American occupation of Porto Rico "smallpox existed in all directions and was a constant menace to the people and to the material interests of the Island." A general vaccination of the people was ordered by the United States authorities in 1899. After this, there were no smallpox deaths in Porto Rico up to 1910, the date of the Government report, a period of over ten years.

A similar eradication of smallpox from Cuba has resulted from the general vaccination carried out by the United States authorities in 1898.

But the most remarkable achievement was that brought about in the Philippine Islands. In certain provinces contiguous to Manila, where there had annually been from time immemorial a loss of 6,000 lives from smallpox, there has not been since 1907, when systematic vaccination was carried out, a single death in a successfully vaccinated person, and only a few scattered cases have occurred.

An incident exhibiting in a striking way the efficacy of vaccination, occurred in Cuba, in 1898. An epidemic of smallpox was raging in Holguin; two battalions of United States Volunteers under Major Woodson were sent into this intensely infected district, where they came into intimate contact with the people. Although the sanitary conditions were execrable, more than 700 soldiers, protected alone by vaccination, remained on duty for six months, without a single case of smallpox developing among them.

The opponents of vaccination allege that vaccination failed to protect the American soldiers in the Philippines in 1898 and 1899. As a matter of fact over 99 per cent. of the soldiers were protected although living in a country which was a hot-bed of smallpox infection. The surgeon-general of the army remarks that at the time the army was rapidly recruited from 28,000 to 280,000.

Great difficulty was experienced with the preservation of vaccine lymph in the hot moist climate of the tropics. This necessitated the appointment of a Commission to devise ways and means of preserving the virus en route. Vaccine virus is now transmitted in thermos bottles and then placed in refrigerators.

Some of the smallpox in the army was due to purposeful frustration of the vaccination by subsequent removal of the vaccine lymph. Surgeon-General Torney publishes instances of confessions of several men in this connection. Col. Kean said that he knew of three volunteer officers who had lost their lives as a result of their unwillingness to be vaccinated.

The opponents of vaccination likewise refer to the smallpox mortality in Japan in 1898 as evidence of the inefficiency of vaccination. Japan has a compulsory vaccination and revaccination law, but the number of vaccinal failures runs into the millions, so that there is always ample susceptible material for the smallpox infection that is so frequently introduced from China, Korea and Manchuria. The Japanese government, with a depleted treasury, has recently spent enormous sums of money in vaccinating the people of Korea. The English and American Antivaccinists may tell us that vaccination in Japan is a failure, but it is quite possible that the Japanese government, which is convinced of the value of vaccination, has a more intimate knowledge of the results of vaccination in its own country.

The most convincing statistical proof, on a large scale, of the efficacy of vaccination, is observed in the smallpox history of Germany, in the past 37 years. In 1875, the new Imperial compulsory vaccination and revaccination law went into effect. Since that time, smallpox has been stamped out as an epidemic disease. During the past 22 years (from 1889 to 1910) the average number of deaths in the entire German empire has been only 53 per year. No other great country of the world can boast of such low mortality. These remarkable figures are all the more significant when we consider that Austria, one of Germany's neighbors had, for the 20 years following 1874, an almost thirty times higher smallpox mortality than Germany. During this period, 239,800 persons perished in Austria from smallpox.

The smallpox mortality in Russia, another neighbor of Germany, has been much higher than that of Austria. From 1901 to 1908, Russia lost on an average, by smallpox, 38,833 persons per year in but 60 to 70 million of her population.

Despite England's insular isolation, she has for the past 30 years, suffered infinitely more from smallpox than has Germany. From 1875 to 1905, England has had 31,642 deaths from smallpox. For the 20 years from 1889 to 1908, England and Wales had, proportionate to the population, over thirteen times as great a smallpox mortality as did Germany. England had no legal provision for revaccination.

Germany leads the world in the thoroughness with which her excellent vaccination laws are administered.

### The Arguments of the Opponents of Vaccination.

The arguments generally set forth by the opponents of vaccination are as follows:

First, that vaccination does not protect against smallpox.

Second, that cowpox and smallpox are unrelated diseases, and therefore, inoculation with the one could not possibly protect against the other.

Third, that vaccination may, and in fact does at times, induce smallpox, and

Fourth, that vaccination is injurious.

In view of what has already been said, it is unnecessary to refute the first argument. The efficacy of vaccination has been proven beyond the peradventure of a doubt. The antivaccinists close their eyes to the facts and consequently do not see them.

The question of the unity or duality of cowpox and smallpox is an academic one and is not vital to the discussion of the efficacy of vaccination. Human experience has proven the prophylactic power of vaccination, and even if the duality of vaccinia and smallpox were established, this fact could not controvert the almost universal experience of medical men. As a matter of fact, however, it is almost conclusively proven that smallpox and cowpox, or vaccinia, are related in the closest manner. The virus of smallpox may be converted into that of cowpox by the inoculation of a successive series of calves. Furthermore, monkeys may be protected against smallpox by vaccination, and may in large part be protected against vaccination by smallpox inoculation. Finally, Guarnieri bodies are found in sections of the skin in smallpox and in vaccinia and in no other condition. Vaccine virus is a benign, modified smallpox virus which has been robbed of its contagious properties.

The third proposition that vaccination may produce smallpox is advanced only by the radical and totally unscientific opponents of vaccination. The argument cannot be supported by an iota of real evidence. Germany, which employs more vaccine virus of variolous ancestry—so-called variol-avaccine—than any other country, has less smallpox than any great country of the world.

Variolous material must be passed, however, through at least two generations of the bovine species, in order that one may be sure that it is completely deprived of its variolous properties. The argument above referred to is a gratuitous assumption without any basis in fact.

Now, in answer to the contention which receives and should receive the most important consideration, namely, that vaccination is injurious, we may say that there is no human act which is entirely devoid of risk. If one rides in an elevator, in a railroad car, in a pleasure vehicle, if one travels upon the seas or engages in sports, one takes a certain risk which may be mathematically calculated. This risk is a minute one, although the aggregate of accidents and deaths from these various causes is considerable; but the risk is so minute that we disregard it. So it is with vaccination; considering the enormous number of vaccinations performed, millions upon millions, the risk of serious accident or death after vaccination is so small that it may be disregarded.

Vaccination is safer today than at any time since its discovery. According to the Federal Law of 1902, the Secretary of the Treasury is empowered to license vaccine farms doing an interstate business. An official is constantly busy at Washington making bacteriological experiments of vaccine virus. This virus is purchased in the open market without the knowledge of the firms who make it. There are stringent regulations of the Government which require that every vaccine propagator shall make certain tests on laboratory animals before placing the virus upon the market. In addition animal tests are made in the laboratory at Washington.

Of the various infections following vaccination tetanus is one of the most serious. Dr. Anderson, Director of the Hygienic Laboratory at Washington, recently stated that 100,000 tubes of vaccine virus had been examined within recent years without the tetanus organism being once found. Furthermore, most important experiments were conducted by Dr. Anderson in which it was attempted to introduce tetanus into suitable animals by vaccination; vaccine virus purposely contaminated in the laboratory with countless numbers of tetanus organisms was thoroughly rubbed into scarifications made upon monkeys and guinea pigs: it was found impossible to produce tetanus in this manner. Dr. Anderson concluded from these crucial experiments that it was practically impossible to convey tetanus to an individual or suitable animal by the mere act of vaccination.

The explanation of the cases of tetanus following vaccination is to be sought in secondary infection; a study of the incubation period of tetanus and of the mortality of vaccinal tetanus confirms this view.

Mr. Higgins, the treasurer of the Antivaccination League of America, recently published a brochure in which is contained the remarkable statement that "vaccination now actually produces more deaths than smallpox." He made a similar statement before the Pennsylvania State Vaccination Commission. In support of this general statement, he selected English statistics from the year 1906 to 1910, a period when England happened to be almost free of smallpox; and the gentleman carefully selected the year 1906 to begin with, when England had but 21 smallpox deaths. From 1900 to 1905 there were 4,291 deaths from smallpox in England, but this was not a favorable period for the gentleman's argument.

He then compares the death rate *per million vaccinated* from 1900 to 1910 in England, and finds that it is greater than the smallpox death rate *per million of population*. The absurdity of such statistics is patent to all. By this astounding sort of figuring, 10 deaths among approximate 300,000 vaccinations carried out yearly in England, would represent a higher rate than 1,000 annual smallpox deaths in England.

The actual deaths from smallpox and from vaccination for

the decade are not given in the antivaccination pamphlet for they would render the sophistry of the statistical argument too evident. In 1902, for instance, when there was an epidemic of smallpox in England, there were 2,464 deaths from smallpox and 22 deaths following vaccination.

Mr. Higgins also stated that smallpox nowadays was a disease the mortality of which was relatively and absolutely insignificant. In 1901-1904 there were over 5,000 cases of smallpox in Philadelphia, with 890 deaths. In Pennsylvania, from 1898 to 1904, there were 21,727 cases of smallpox with 1,613 deaths. From 1900 to 1903, 5,177 persons died from smallpox in the United States. In a little over one-half of Russia, 38,000 persons die annually of the smallpox at the present time. Figures might be given showing the great mortality in Italy, Austria, Hungary and other countries in recent times. They suffice to show that smallpox is still a dread disease.

The opponents of vaccination charge vaccination with being the cause of many chronic, insidious diseases. The increase of cancer, and of degenerative diseases of the heart and kidneys is attributed by these gentlemen to vaccination. There is no evidence worthy of the name that can be adduced in support of this proposition, but the assertion is grist to the mill of the antivaccinationist. We might say with the British Royal Commission on Vaccination that if vaccination is to be charged with the increase of mortality in those diseases which have a higher death rate than formerly, it ought likewise to be credited with the decrease of mortality in those diseases whose death rates have declined. The whole proposition is, of course, absurd.

In the Philippines in 1907 and 1908, according to the report of the Sanitary Director of the Philippine Islands and the Secretary of the Interior, over 2,000,000 persons were vaccinated by the United States authorities without a single death and without a serious complication.

The opponents of vaccination pay no heed to these statistics and brush them aside by casting doubt upon their accuracy. There is one point of importance to which I wish to advert. I think the vast majority of accidents and complications are the result of neglect and maltreatment of the vaccinal wound, and we as physicians are not entirely free of culpability in this matter. We do not take sufficient pains to instruct the patient with regard to the subsequent care of the wound. A vaccination wound is subject to the same infections to which any wound of the skin is liable. My belief, from evidence introduced before the Pennsylvania State Vaccination Commission, is that vaccination shields should not be employed, as they are likely to do harm. A perforated linen shield may be allowed to remain on the arm for a few hours until the vaccination abrasion is dry; after that it should be discarded and the vaccinal area protected by sterile gauze. I think that some of the accidents and complications of vaccination are due to the peripheral pressure made by a shield which causes not only congestion but rupture of the vaccine vesicle; an opportunity is thus created for secondary infection of the wound. Care of the arm after vaccination is a matter which deserves the serious consideration of physicians; I am sorry to say it does not always receive the attention which its importance demands.

One might speak at much greater length on this subject. I fear I have already trespassed too long on your time; permit me, however, to mention one other point. The opponents of vaccination claim that the decline in smallpox during the past century has been due not to vaccination but to improvement in sanitary conditions. We all know this is not true. We know that specific diseases requires specific measures for their prevention. Typhoid fever and cholera are largely water-borne and the protection of the water supply is the dominant factor in the prevention of these diseases. We know that malaria and yellow fever are to be prevented by the destruction of the intermediate hosts—the mosquitoes which carry these infections. We all know that another group of highly contagious diseases including smallpox, measles, chickenpox, whooping cough, etc., are probably due to an air-borne infection, and do not depend upon general vices of sanitation, but rather upon personal susceptibility. Measles and smallpox are among the most contagious of all diseases.

The opponents of vaccination point to the history of Leicester in England, as an instance of protection against smallpox by sanitation. While Leicester has enjoyed considerable immunity against smallpox it did not escape an epidemic of the disease in 1892 and a smaller outbreak in 1902. A certain city in this country, Cleveland, in 1902, attempted to follow the same procedure, *i. e.*, to protect the community by sanitary measures without vaccination. Dr. Friedrich, health officer of that city, testified before the Vaccination Commission of Pennsylvania, that at the end of 1901 he thought he had stamped out smallpox by disinfection, and he published an article in the *Cleveland Medical Journal* to that effect. In 1902, smallpox again appeared; the people believed the health officer that sanitation would suffice and they refused to accept vaccination, even when he later urged it upon them. The epidemic spread until 1,240 cases of smallpox had developed, resulting in a loss of 224 lives.

The city of Buffalo then threatened to quarantine against Cleveland, and the physicians of Cleveland held a mass meeting and protested against the unnecessary loss of life. Vaccination was then begun; in three months 200,000 people were vaccinated and the epidemic was stamped out.

Thomas Jefferson in a letter written to Jenner in 1802, a letter no less remarkable for its phraseology than for its broad humanitarianism, said "you have erased from the calendar of human afflictions one of its greatest; mankind can never forget that you have lived and future nations will know by history only that the dreaded smallpox has existed and by you has been extirpated;" this prediction has failed of becoming a prophecy only because vaccination and revaccination have not been carried out among the nations of the earth.

### Discussion.

DR. TRAVERSE R. MAXFIELD, in discussion, said:—"I have very little to say in regard to this subject except that during the past year we have vaccinated in the Borough office, in the Borough of Brooklyn, 14,280 odd children who have been brought to us for vaccination by their mothers or fathers or guardians, 80 per cent. under the age of 10 years, and not one death has occurred from any of those vaccinations of which I have any official knowledge."

Dr. Jay Frank Schamberg, in closing the discussion said:—
"I desire briefly to advert to the statements made by Mr. Higgins.
It is said by him that smallpox inoculation was a medical blunder
and has now been abandoned. Let me state that it was abandoned
because it was superseded by vaccination, which possessed distinct
advantages over inoculation. Inoculation saved the lives of thousands of persons who would otherwise have succumbed to natural
smallpox; inoculated smallpox was, however, contagious, and it
tended therefore to perpetuate the infection.

The British Royal Commission on Vaccination, composed of
distinguished scientists and headed by Baron Herschell, Lord
Chancellor of England, sat for seven years. The Royal Commission concluded that smallpox inoculation had a two-fold influence
and that these two influences neutralized each other as far as any
effect on smallpox mortality was concerned.

I must admire the complacency with which Mr. Higgins dis-
credits the figures which I have quoted of smallpox mortality in
London in the prevaccination era. These figures, which were
based on the London Bills of Mortality, were carefully studied by
the British Royal Commission; they are regarded as the most
reliable data in existence concerning smallpox mortality prior to
1800. It was only in a certain period prior to 1700, that measles
and smallpox deaths were not differentiated; Mr. Higgins' statement to the contrary is erroneous.

Mr. Higgins' statement published in a widely distributed
pamphlet that "vaccination now produces more deaths than smallpox" is indefensible. As a general statement it is unqualifiedly
false. To attempt to demonstrate its truth by circumscribing the
proof to a single county for a brief period when that county was
remarkably free from smallpox, serves to exhibit the extremities
to which the antivaccinists are driven.

The opponents of vaccination are sincere and zealous, but
woefully misguided. Their ranks are made up largely of laymen
who are not qualified by technical training or education to pass
judgment upon a medical subject; there is also a sprinkling of
physicians who have lost their scientific sense of proportion.
When Dr. Charles Creighton of England, appeared before the
Pennsylvania State Vaccination Commission, he was asked
whether he could name one professor of medicine or pathology in
any reputable university of Germany, England or the United
States who was an opponent of vaccination; he replied that he
could; he was then challenged to do so, but he remained silent.
There is no medical scientist of real standing who is not an enthusiastic advocate of vaccination. Mr. Higgins has stated that vaccination is a dangerous procedure. We all know that this statement
is untrue. I am sure that in this audience few, if any practitioners
of medicine have ever encountered a death from vaccination.

**EDITORIAL**

## COMMMENDABLE ACTIVITIES.

FROM time to time the United States Department of Agriculture issues bulletins of its various work of investigation, which covers a field surprisingly wide and including subjects wonderfully diverse. Some of these are reports on water supply and drainage, some on food impurities, while others range from diseases of cattle to the ravages of insects and the food value of codfish. Unfortunately they are like the seed in the parable: some fall upon stony ground, some by the wayside, and a very few in fertile soil, where they bear fruit worthy of the care and patience that has produced them. A recent communication from the department is a warning to the general public in regard to so-called radioactive waters. It has long been considered a recognized fact that the benefit derived from drinking various mineral waters at the Spas is far greater to the patient than the consumption of the same when bottled and shipped to a distance, although chemically the mineral water is identical. Since the discovery and exploitation of radium, it has been proved that considerable number of natural mineral waters are radioactive, a property that is probably highly advantageous to the consumer. Investigation by the Bureau of Chemistry of the Department of Agriculture, supplementing investigation by other chemists, has definitely shown that this radioactive property is evanescent, lasting at the most but a few weeks and disappearing to the extent of 50 per cent. four days after bottling and 90 per cent. twelve days after. This is probably due to the fact that the waters do not contain any radioactive substance, but are active by reason of radium emanation, possibly from their passage through radium-containing earth.

The exploitation of radium cures in the public press, the known value of radium treatment and the fabulous properties attributed to the substance in the public mind have already been reflected in the exploitation to the public of so-called radioactive bottled waters, and a considerable industry has already sprung up in their advertising and sale. That the department has taken steps to prevent any extensive fraud upon the public is evidenced by the following passage quoted from their latest report:

"The department is now investigating a number of the so-called radioactive waters with the object of securing evidence that can be made a basis of prosecution for misbranding. In the past, before the Food and Drugs Act was enacted, a number of mineral waters made claim to curative properties which they did not possess and succeeded in creating a misplaced confidence on the part of the consumers. This was particularly true of a number of imported waters which were sold extensively in the United States with a statement on the bottle that they were wonderful or magical cures for all sorts of incurable or chronic ailments. The Treasury Department, acting in co-operation with the Department of Agriculture, now refuses admission to the country of foreign waters labeled so as to mislead consumers as to their real or curative properties. The department fears that unless the public is warned that the fraudulent trade in so-called radioactive waters will develop, just as the fraudulent trade in other mineral waters was developed to the point where people with strong imaginations will supply their bottlers with all sorts of testimonials asserting that these supposed radioactive waters have effected wonderful cures."

Such commendable activity should be met on the part of the profession by an effort to keep in touch with and spread abroad as far as possible the work of the Department of Agriculture, a work to which the JOURNAL is glad to contribute in every way in its power.

H. G. W.

## HOBBIES.

THE line that separates the man with a hobby from the harmless crank is often so faint as to be well-nigh imperceptible; and on the other side there is often little to distinguish the man of a single idea, shrewd, hardheaded, intent upon business, from the hobby-rider, if you view him from the right angle; for the man of a single idea concentrated upon the acquisition of dollars, having but the one idea, may, and often does develop a concentration that amounts to obsession. He becomes a monomaniac with but a single hobby, and his very singularity makes him a monotonous person to associate with. Diversity of interests, variety of thought, if guided by a reasonable purpose, constitute the most companiable aspects of the average man. That man soon palls as a comrade who can only talk about the delights of soliciting life insurance and who desecrates the sacred hour reserved for the worship of Dea Nicotiana by purely mundane discussion of the business which occupies his whole time. Such a man is devoid of imagination; his mind for social purposes is a monotonous waste studded with sordid facts as the Mojave Desert is with prickly pears and is just about as capable of giving pleasure and refreshment to the hungry and thirsty. Facts have their uses and so have prickly pears—fondle one and see—but too close application to either leaves a tingling pain or an aching head. Followed to its logical conclusion, this train of thought leads one to the conclusion that hobbies should be avoided, but it is with hobbies as with the prickly pear aforesaid. Treat it in the right way, apply to it the methods of a Burbank and it loses its spines and becomes not merely a harmless vegetable but a valuable article of food. Too close application to a single occupation, be it study, politics or the acquisition of wealth, surely tends by its very monotony to exhaustion of the brain cells, made and provided that there is no compensatory physical effort to give them rest. Applied to physicians this principle means that sooner or later the doctor who bends all his energies to practice alone becomes a monotone, capable only of talking "shop" and as time goes by his tired brain loses its capacities for new ideas and the man is apt to prematurely lose his diagnostic and therapeutic ability. To counteract such a tendency there is nothing better than to cultivate a hobby that will be so different as to make it impossible when pursuing it to think of his ordinary avocation. For such a purpose nothing can

equal a purely mechanical pursuit, for mechanical exactness precludes speculative thought. The eye, mind and hand must act
together to accomplish mechanical nicety. If any one doubts this
let him try to drive a nail while his mind wanders in pursuit of
the abstract—if he doesn't hammer his thumb he possesses a true
dual personality worthy of study. Wherefore, buy a set of golf
sticks, or a horse if you can afford them, or rig up a carpenter's
bench in the cellar if you can't, and give your friends and patients
the advantages of a mind keen on its professional and diverse upon
its social side.                                              H. G. W.

## JOHN R. STIVERS, M.D.

THE death of Dr. Stivers has come as an unexpected blow to
his many friends, of whom the greater number were ignorant
of his illness. His active participation in the work of various
medical bodies of Brooklyn and the services which he has rendered
in the positions or responsibility that he has held have made
him a well-known figure among Brooklyn physicians. Dr. Stivers'
ability, his faithful services and sterling character contribute to
make his untimely death a loss which will be keenly felt.
                                                             H. G. W.

## THE CONVENTION OF DISEASES.

WE attended one of the great national gatherings of the profession recently and took in all the sessions that we could. So
surfeited did we become with the interminable talk that one
afternoon, as some estimable gentleman proclaimed the virtues and
defects of salvarsan in somnifacient monotone, we slipped down a
plane or two from the conscious, and suddenly found ourselves in a
convention of diseases.

Here, strange to say, we found the usual conditions completely
reversed. The diseases were discussing the medical profession, its
aims and methods and results, as well as the possibilities held by the
future both for physicians and diseases.

The convention hall was crowded with diseases and bacterial
proxies. Most of the diseases gave a venerable impression, but here
and there flashy young diseases, like pellagra and the sleeping sickness,
were to be seen. Tuberculosis presided, with cancer occupying a place
of honor on the dais. Flitting about the hall we observed many Cohn-
heim cells with metastasis licenses conspicuously displayed. Syphilis
wore a curiously designed robe, which upon close inspection we saw
bore side-chain figures, woven out of amboceptors and complements.
Acting as a kind of chief usher, or master of ceremonies, was Alcoholism, who seemed to be popular with everybody. The greetings
between Alcoholism and Arteriosclerosis were particularly effusive.

Proceedings opened with an address by Tuberculosis. In the
course of the address Tuberculosis expressed somewhat optimistic
views. Despite the feverish activities of the crusaders there was much
to be thankful for. Thus the phthisiophobia which had been engendered through an overreaching campaign had led to much inhumanity
on the part of fear-inspired relatives toward the victims, and Tuberculosis was glad to say that while the mortality had perhaps been lessened

there had been compensations. Then, again, there was still much congestion of population in the big cities, and certain interests could be counted upon to perpetuate this state of affairs. An instance was cited where the head of a great corporation directly interested in crowding three thousand people into each acre of its city property was the president of the charity organization society. These things were most encouraging and it could almost be hoped that the disease would gain its old ascendency once more. There were many things about the existing social order and the capitalistic exploitation of the industrial classes which also gave ground for future hope. Upon the whole, Tuberculosis saw but little reason for pessimism.

Typhoid Fever, speaking for the whole class of preventable diseases, thought the immediate outlook fairly good but sounded a note of warning for the future. Much was to be feared from the constantly growing enlightenment of the people and the persistent efforts of medical educators. Much encouragement was to be derived from the activities of such bodies as the League for Medical Freedom, the anti-vivisectionists and the anti-vaccinationists. A National Department of Health was the thing mostly to be feared, and Typhoid Fever confessed that its foundation seemed inevitable. It would probably be a wise plan for the preventable diseases, instead of working far afield, to concentrate their energies toward "getting" such enemies as the A. M. A. propagandists, particularly the public lecturers.

Acute Rheumatism spoke in a rather cheerful vein. The damp and insanitary houses and working quarters of the poor were supplying a plethora of victims, as always. These people, after discharge from the hospitals, were perforce obliged to resume their old habits of life, and could usually be depended upon to suffer recurrences. Nor had any great advance been made in the therapy of the disease. It was true that cardiac complications were perhaps not so common, owing to the enforcement of prolonged rest, or even fixation, as in children, but still there was no end to the mischief worked in the hearts of the victims. This, after all, was Rheumatism's chief aim, and by it must its usefulness be judged.

The Venereal Diseases were perhaps the merriest among all the attendants of the Convention. Gonorrhea, their spokesman, could see no immediate likelihood of the passing of prostitution, public or clandestine, nor any probability of society putting its economic and moral house in order for some time to come. The age at which young girls seemed to be falling out of the impossible industrial struggle into the ranks of the courtesans was constantly lessening, until now mere children were on the streets in increasing numbers. The value of prophylactic measures was understood by few physicians, seemingly, though the Philippine army surgeons had tried them out with great success. The boards of health could be trusted not to educate the public along such lines, for reasons too obvious for discussion. Incredible as it might seem, many general practitioners neglected prophylaxis against ophthalmia neonatorum. The therapy of gonorrhea could hardly be said to have been signalized by any great advance, though the spokesman confessed to considerable discomfiture upon the few occasions when it had been compelled to try conclusions with hot water irrigations after the Harrison-Houghton method, as described by them in the *Journal of the Royal Army Medical Corps* for February.

Diabetes reported, grumpily, some recent disagreeable experiences with massive doses of *Bacillus lacticus bulgaricus.* This treatment had caused it more concern, to say the least, than any it had yet encountered. Aside from this there was but little cause for complaint; indeed, the disease was distinctly on the increase among certain classes of citizens.

The many diseases due to the colon bacillus all tried to talk at once against the pernicious activities of certain physicians who had waged successful war against them with hexamethylenamin and sodium benzoate in combination. Thus they had been obliged to retire from the gall-bladder, the kidney, the blood, the urinary bladder, the ureter, the ovary and Fallopian tube, the lung and the cervix uteri. Even Urinary Incontinence in Children had a sad story to tell.

Pneumonia was sorry to say that since the more or less useless ammonium salts, used with fatuous faith by the profession for so many years, had been replaced by calcium chloride it was having greatly increased difficulty in effecting the demise of patients.

The Poisonings were too busy to be present but sent a report to be read by the secretary in which they reported a hitherto unsuspected recruit in the shape of Magnesium Sulphate, which Boos, of the Massachusetts General Hospital (October, 1911, *Publications*), had shown the profession to be really toxic. Still, the laity could be depended upon to keep on using the stuff.

Appendicitis was feeling very happy and prosperous, thank you. The high operative mortality at the Massachusetts General Hospital was cause for felicitation. Conservative medical treatment of colitis, Appendicitis was glad to say, was growing less and less popular, despite the repeated warnings of Beverley Robinson and other reactionaries, and the appendix would continue to be removed more and more. The surgical progressives had the inside track and the whip hand and there was little to be feared from the ultraconservatives. The devil and the gods of disease were to be sincerely thanked for keeping up the heresy hunt against these reactionaries.

The Diseases of Childhood, represented by Malnutrition, seemed to be obsessed by fears proceeding not so much from the direct activities of the medical profession, tremendous though they were, as from those of the social reformers, agitators like Ellen Key and the advocates of small families, and the constantly growing army of enlightened mothers and restless, if not fully emancipated, women who were beginning to see what their proper relations and responsibilities in the social scheme should be.

At this point we began to look around the hall to see if our old friend, "A Complication of Diseases," was in attendance. But the meeting suddenly broke up in confusion, due to the unexpected appearance of a body of shoo-fly cops, made up of opsonins and antitoxins. We awoke just in time to catch the last words of the lecturer on salvarsan. So the menu which we had read on the Convention's programme was not partaken of, to wit:

Ptomain Cocktails

Serum, Plain

Muscæ Volitantes        Small Round Cells

Bundle of His, Vitreous Sauce

Pineal Croquettes        Cilia

Phagocyte Punch

Agar-Agar Pudding, Albumin Sauce      Opsonic Ices, all Strains

Lady Fingers        Casein Nodes

Caffein Cordial

A. C. JACOBSON.

# Correspondence

## WHY ARE SO MANY NERVOUS AND MENTAL PATIENTS SENT OUT OF OUR STATE FOR TREATMENT?

THIS circular is written with the purpose of informing the physicians and laymen of the State of New York of the laws governing the licensed sanatoriums of this state.

Not so many years ago, the laws regulating the treatment of those suffering from nervous and mental diseases were so unwieldy that many legal difficulties beset the way of those who wished to place their relatives in sanatoriums, and it became a practice with New York physicians to send their patients to institutions in other states where a less complicated legal process existed. Today New York State has a statute governing its *"Licensed Private Houses and Sanatoriums"* as liberal as that of any other state, and clearly framed for the protection of its nervous and mental patients. The old law set up difficulties in the way of receiving voluntary patients, and it is this class of patients that the later statutes especially benefit.

New York has more than twenty licensed institutions known as *"Licensed Private Houses and Sanatoriums."*

The requirements of the law governing these institutions are these:

1st. The physician in charge must have had five years' actual experience in an institution for the care and treatment of the insane.

2d. There must be a qualified medical assistant.

3d. There must be a graduate nurse.

4th. The premises, which are examined at frequent intervals by state officials, must be up to standard in hygienic conditions, have proper fire protection and provisions for the comfort of the patients.

5th. The number of patients which any such institution is allowed to take is limited by the state authorities.

Such "Licensed Private Houses and Sanatoriums" are permitted to take both "voluntary patients" and those "committed."

It was the lack of a statute allowing licensed institutions to take voluntary patients which originally drove so many patients of this class to patronize sanatoriums outside of the state, and it is believed that a large percentage of such patients from the State of New York who are today receiving treatment in institutions in other states would be in New York institutions if the facts as they exist today were understood.

One provision of the New York statute is that every patient in a licensed sanatorium is seen and examined by a state alienist, and this gives added protection to a class of patients unable to protect themselves.

The form of application which a voluntary patient is required to sign on admission to a sanatorium in this state is as follows:

### VOLUNTARY APPLICATION.

*To the Physician in Charge:*

I desire to be received as a voluntary patient for care and treatment in .........................., and promise, if my request is granted, to obey all its rules and regulations, and to give ten days' notice, in writing, before leaving without your permission.

..............................

Witness:

..............................

When persons of intelligence neglect advantages which are at their very door to search for those which are both dubious and remote, it must be because they are uninformed or misinformed. The fact that a large percentage of the residents of New York who require treatment for mental or nervous diseases are sent to institutions outside of this state comes to be remarkable when it is realized that there is absolutely no reason for this discrimination against home sanatoriums.

It is curious that the pride in his home institutions, supposed to be so characteristic of the New Yorker, should be absolutely wanting in the case of the sanatoriums, and yet a very slight investigation of the facts will demonstrate the unquestionable advantages which he would derive by patronizing one of them when the occasion required. Convenience, economy and efficiency alike appeal for the New York sanatorium.

The foregoing refers, of course, expressly and specifically to *Licensed Private Houses and Sanatoriums* only.

D. A. HARRISON, M.D.

Whitestone, L. I., N. Y.

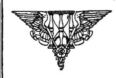 **Society** 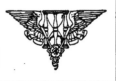 **Transactions**

## TRANSACTIONS OF THE BROOKLYN GYNECOLOGICAL SOCIETY.

*Stated Meeting, February 7, 1913.*

The President, DR. CARROLL CHASE, in the Chair.

### Presentation of Specimens.

DR. POMEROY: The first specimen which I present does not show very much in its present condition. The drawing submitted was made by Dr. Dickinson from the fresh specimen. This patient was sent into the hospital by one of our graduates with a diagnosis of recurrent appendicitis. She was 32 years of age; had not had a child for some years. She had a temperature of 100, with a pain on the right side, no vomiting, but a general tenderness of the lower abdomen; some fixation of the uterus. After three days' rest there was a subsidence of all symptoms. After waiting three or four days longer the patient began to grow indignant that nothing was being done for her, and I told her if she wished it we would operate. The interesting thing about the case was that the appendix was found to be innocent. Both tubes were edematous and inflamed but not closed; on the left side the ovary was found slightly adherent and considerably enlarged, about 1¼ to 1½ inches in diameter. In freeing adhesions the ovary ruptured and everted a clot about ¾ inch in diameter. There was free fluid but no blood in the peritoneal cavity. Suspecting a tubercular process, I removed both tubes, the affected ovary and the innocent appendix. The patient showed a temperature of 101 to 102 for several days. We had the ovary examined by Dr. Hulst, who reported that he found very distinct chorionic villi.

The second specimen was removed from a woman 43 years of age who had been sent in by Dr. J. H. Andrew. She had been advised by Dr. George McNaughton some years previously to have operation for fibroids. I saw her last summer when she had acute peritonitis involving the lower abdomen mainly on the left side, but she was then in such a serious condition as to preclude operation at the time. She recovered from that condition and was operated on by me ten days ago. She appeared to have a large fibroid uterus reaching nearly to the umbilicus and projecting in the lower abdomen when she was recumbent. The bulk of the mass consisted of a large left side tubo-ovarian cyst containing more than a pint of foul pus, and after a great deal of care it was separated from the densely adherent gut. It was necessary to tap the cyst to get at the posterior adhesions; the tapping was effected without soiling. The cyst and uterus are here shown. The interesting point was that the other tube looked entirely innocent. After removing the cyst, the uterus and the other tube, on opening the uterine cavity was found to contain a small amount of foul smelling pus. The mid-section of the apparently innocent tube was found blocked, it being impossible to pass a probe through, and for this reason presumably no inflammatory process was formed around that tube. The condition must have started as an endometritis, with defective drainage because of distortion of the uterine cavity by the fibroid. The patient has made a good recovery. Culture from the pus showed streptococcus pyogenes.

The President announced that the cases were open for discussion; a case of true ovarian pregnancy should certainly be discussed.

DR. JUDD: The first specimen which I wish to present tonight is that of a uterus which I removed per vaginum four week ago for a complete prolapse. This operation followed one for prolapse which I did on this woman three years ago, when I dilated, curetted and made an amputation of the cervix. I put the patent back to bed and three weeks later removed both tubes and ovaries. Understand that this cervix had been amputated previously. The operation I did four weeks ago was after the method of Goffe. The convalescence of this patient was interesting. She suffered a great deal from pain and required large doses of morphine. On the eleventh day she vomited a large quantity of fluid in the morning and in the afternoon, and began to go into a sleepy, semi-comatose condition. The next day I asked Dr. Polak to see the case and he said at once that it was a case of acetonuria. I had had the patient's urine examined previously but not for acetone. A specimen was sent to Dr. Murray who found large quantities of acetone. The patient was treated with carbohydrates and peppermint candy, and the convalescence was so rapid that I have since been looking for acetone in all of my cases.

The second specimen was from an emergency case upon which I operated last Saturday at the Jewish Hospital. She had had her last period two months previous to admission to the hospital. Eleven days previous to admission on rising in the morning was seized with sudden acute pain in lower abdomen and was treated by a doctor for several days. On the third day after the seizure she had severe genital bleeding, which ceased in the morning. On the day of admission she had another attack of acute pain and was brought into the hospital. We diagnosed ruptured tubal pregnancy. I operated under spinal anæsthesia, as the patient had practically bled out. The method is interestinng to me as I had not done many operations with this form of anæsthesia. I found a tubal pregnancy but was not able to find the attachment of the tube to the uterine cornua. I found that less than one-half inch from the uterus it had ruptured at the site of the pregnancy in the tube. The special points are the method of finding the rupture and the form of anæsthesia.

The third specimen is an X-ray picture of a patient of mine taken at the Kings County Hospital. Dr. Pfeiffer was the first to call my attention to the fact that it was a twin pregnancy. We could hear fœtal heart practically all over the abdomen. We could not find two heads nor two buttocks, but plenty of small parts. I asked Dr. Charles Eastmond to take the picture at the hospital, though the X-ray machine there is not very powerful—110-volt current. The doctor took three exposures, one directly antero-posterior, the second from side to side, and the third was made slantingly, with a lateral exposure from the right side downwards and backwards towards the table. That exposure gave us this plate and from this I have attempted to have some prints made. Many men of many climes have used the X-ray for diagnosis of fibroids, for pregnancy and other conditions, but this is the first case of diagnosis of twin pregnancy that I have found in print in English. Both of the fœtal heads were found in the upper abdomen. This woman was delivered one week later and one child presented transverse and the second normally. One child weighed 6 pounds, the second 6¼ pounds.

DR. BEACH: I should like to ask Dr. Judd what he considers the fault in the technic in his operation and what was the cause of the recurrence of the procidentia. I had a similar case upon which I operated about a year ago, where I did very much the same thing, and this woman returned in four months with a recurrence of the procidentia, which was a very extensive and complete one. The fault in that case was that the uterus was entirely too large and should never have been left. I finally cured the case by amputating the uterus, leaving the cervix and fixing the vagina to the broad ligaments.

DR. JUDD: The fault was in my technic. I depended too much upon the mucous membrane and did not get enough fascia.

DR. CARY asked if the urine in Dr. Judd's case had been examined for anything besides acetone, and what were the conditions of blood pressure?

DR. JUDD: There was also diacetic acid in that case. The blood pressure was low. The condition of acetonuria is usually due to some debility, and can be brought about by starvation, with diminishing of the amount of carbohydrates ingested. This woman had been given broths but no carbohydrates.

DR. POLAK: I wish to put on record the results of four cases which were recently reoperated on, who had had a previous Webster-Baldy operation. As you know, in this procedure the round ligaments are brought through the broad ligaments and underneath the utero-ovarians and stretched behind the uterus and sewn to its posterior wall. We are just beginning to have our patients, on whom this operation had been performed, come back to us with complaints of persistent pain, and I wish to call attention to a pathological condition through which some of these troubles are brought about. Through the weakness of the varied ligaments in some cases where they are called upon to support a large anteverted uterus (particularly if the cervix is not lying well back toward the sacrum), the uterus will sag. This brings the ovaries up through the supporting loop made by the round ligament and throws them toward the median line and they become adherent to each other and to the transposed ligament behind the uterus. In these four cases we had persistent pain in the hypogestium. The uterine mass was enlarged and sensitive posteriorly. This has been a constant symptom in this pathological condition. We may have placed the round ligaments too high and thus raised the utero-ovarians so that the ovaries fell inward as the uterus sinks, yet we have been careful to avoid just this possibility. Lately we have used the Webster-Baldy in small movable uteri. In these cases the posterior surface of the uterus is found on examination to be exquisitely sensitive. I report these cases for the lesson it has been to me.

DR. CARY: I am very happy to hear Dr. Polak speak of this condition. In the dispensary of the Brooklyn Hospital, where we have opportunity to watch these cases post-operative, we have found very bad results in a very few cases, possibly two, from that operation, and I thought the trouble to be due to the fact that the round ligaments had been brought through the broad ligaments when some subacute inflammation of the tubes existed and a subsequent feritonitis occurred with exudate adhesions. We have one woman who has been coming for two years with this trouble. This woman has a mass posterior to the uterus that is exquisitely tender, and the pain is almost constant. It is certainly not a pleasant result. I thought it some inflammatory condition lighted up by the trauma of the operation.

DR. JUDD: The condition Dr. Polak speaks of I have not seen myself, but there is another result of the Webster-Baldy operation in several cases, and that is adhesions of the small intestines when the round ligaments are brought through the broad ligaments. I have seen it produce annoying and nagging pains.

DR. POLAK then read the paper of the evening, "Observations from Foreign Clinics During the Recent Trip of the American Gynæcological Club."

DR. PILCHER:. It is very rare that we have an opportunity to listen to a man who has seen the inside of the clinics of Europe. During my last trip I did not visit the gynæcological clinics but I had an opportunity of working in Wertheim's clinic in the pathological department, and I learned cystoscopy in his clinic. I was impressed, as Dr. Polak was, by the fact that we are doing as well as Wertheim did or ever will do, and we get as good results. He has taught us one thing, and that is the safeguarding of the ureters. At the time I was at his clinic I had an opportunity of catheterizing the ureters in a number of cases, and all of his cases were catheterized. I do not believe in his statistics, the character of the cases, as Dr. Polak says, are often of the hopeless type, and they do not list all of the cases. Schauta is, I believe, a remarkable operator. It was he who demonstrated that in doing a Cæsarian section it is not necessary for an assistant virtually to climb into the abdomen of the patient to put a rubber band about the uterus. He turns the uterus out onto the abdomen, almost. It is very true, in some of the clinics that they do not observe the technic of asepsis as we do, but in many of the clinics, surgical particularly, which I visited on my last trip, they were very careful. The things they do which we do not do here is they make almost post-mortem incisions; they do seem to care for the patient. They care more for the technic and the demonstration of the operation. They are slow in taking anything from America, and if they can find anything in their literature that has a similar bearing they will credit the innovation to one of their own men. The way Dr. Polak saw the clinics is the proper way. If one goes as a student one is not apt to gain very much. If a young man starts out on a trip to Europe to pick up what he can, he knows that he is going to certain cities and to see certain men, but if he is not properly introduced he will sit among the students and not learn much. If you want to see work and get at the basis of subjects you will not do much unless you go with a prearranged plan. It is better to go to study the work of one man, and to study that one man well, than to go to all of the principal places. If a student is going to Berlin or Vienna it is better to go to the American Medical Club. In Vienna they have formed practically a medical trust, because the Americans control the teaching clinics there, and you cannot get anything unless you get it through them. When I was over I saw Germans and Austrians visiting the club to get assistance in securing admission to the clinics. In order to get the best you have got to be introduced. Copenhagen has one of the most beautiful hospitals in the world. It is organized on the latest plan and they do some of the finest work that is done anywhere. If a man wants to learn gynæcology he can do better in Brooklyn and New York than he can anywhere else.

DR. CARY: It seems hardly proper to discuss such a delightful informal paper as that presented by Dr. Polak this evening. I am sure we have all, especially those who have not had an opportunity to see the work on the other side, enjoyed this splendid paper. The impressions of Dr. Wertheim have been very interesting. In reference to extraperitoneal Cæsarian section, I have not had an opportunity to see the operation. but I have some personal ideas on the subject. I know that Dr. Küstner in sixty cases has injured the bladder in six, and has had a fœtal mortality of 5 per cent. Other operators have had a maternal mortality of 5½ and 5 per cent. respectively, which is certainly not better than the other methods. One indication for the extraperitoneal operation, according to its advocates, is when infection is suspected to exist. In doing some study of infections of the parametrium and adjacent tissues, I have been impressed by the abundance of soft areolar tissue, the freedom of the blood and lymphatic circulation in the space of Retzius, and I recall vividly some infections in the tissues back of the symphysis where the trouble has started after operations upon the prostate, and have seen the condition kill the patient. I am inclined to think that the peritoneal tissue is more suited to resist the attack of infection than the tissues posterior to the symphysis pubes. This operation is also more difficult, and any operation that has this objection, unless it offers some good reason for its use, must soon fall into the background. Momberg's method of pressure for postpartum hemorrhage I have not used, but I should hate to wait for the application of the apparatus. The method that Davis reported some time ago—I am not sure that he is the originator of it—of putting the hand up into the uterus and making pressure on the aorta through the posterior wall of that organ, seems to me to be more practical. I have had opportunity to watch a few of the "twilight sleep" cases. I know that this method of relieving patients has come into disrepute because of the additional doses of morphine and its bad effect upon the child. The method has these objections: (a) It is hard to know just what the right dose is that is suited to the different patients. (b) It is not always possible to estimate when the woman will deliver herself, therefore morphine may be given too near delivery. (c) It is very difficult to control the patient when she is under this form of narcosis. I believe this method will be limited to selected cases. It seems adapted to the highly neurotic type where the labor is held back by the nervous tension of the patient.

DR. BEACH: I had an opportunity a few years ago to make observations in the German clinics. In regard to the conditions of operative technique, I was very much disappointed, except at the clinic at Dresden, Leopold's clinic, in 1905. I did not see anybody do as clean work as we do here, especially in the surgical clinics. The great operation then was pubiotomy. They made enormous tears of the tissues in some of the cases at the time of operation, due mainly to the lack of any preliminary dilatation of the soft parts. I saw two or three cases where the laceration extended through the skin and mons veneris, and through the vagina. There was no question at that time but that there was going to be a reaction from that operation, and I believe they do not do it now so frequently.

With regard to the vaginal Cæsarian section which they were doing, and doing well, the secret was in the type of anterior retractor which they were using to hold the bladder back.

The question was asked, "What was the length of time used by Wertheim and other operators in their interposition operations?"

DR. POLAK, in closing the discussion, said: "Three points have been brought up which are of interest. 1st, The matter of un-Americanism was very pointedly brought out in Schauta's clinic. On one of our visits to Schauta's clinic they had a patient who was about to be operated upon for retroversion. Prof. Schauta said: 'We will now show you an operation for retroversion which I devised about three years ago,'" and he then proceeded to do a Gilliam operation. Dr. McMurtry, of Louisville, watched him for awhile and then remarked that the same operation had been done and published in monograph and textbook on this side of the Atlantic by Gilliam over fifteen years ago. Everybody in Germany uses the Bozeman needle forceps. When Wiebel was over here he could not operate till they sent down to Kny Scherer's and got a Bozeman forceps, and he does not know yet that the instrument was invented by Bozeman, a New Yorker. No credit is given to anything American. Dr. Cary has brought the weak point in the extraperitoneal Cæsarian section, *i. e.*, the incision goes through the least resisting area and one that is supplied with the greatest number of lymphatic vessels. With regard to the interposition operation the results depend a great deal upon who operates. Most of the German operators are slow in their work, they have a profound fear of hemorrhage and clamp and tie the smallest twig; they pay little or no attention to the condition of the cervix, simply interpose the uterus and do a split flap perineorrhaphy, which takes from thirty to forty minutes. Regarding the teaching facilities, they are best in the smaller towns, and not so good in Munich, Vienna and Berlin. I would certainly advise a student to go to Frieberg or Tubingen. The material at the foreign clinics is certainly immense in amount, but not better than that which we have for study on this side of the Atlantic."

## Stated Meeting of March 7, 1913.

### The President, DR. CARROLL CHASE, in the Chair.

#### Naration of Cases.

DR. BEACH: I should like briefly to report a case of pregnancy complicated by cardiac disease. Mrs. A., primagravida, aged 18 years. Previous history of rheumatism followed by cardiac disease, there being one break in compensation before marriage. At the time of admission she was five months pregnant. She had vomiting, edema, and dyspnœa. Physical examination disclosed rales in the lungs, with fluid at the bases. There was a double mitral lesion, with enlargement of the right side. The edema of the lungs was the cause of a constant cough. She was in the hospital five or six days, during which time the symptoms were practically the same, and we decided to empty the uterus. There was some thought given to the type of anæsthesia, as ether was out of the question on account of the condition of the lungs, and chloroform was contraindicated on account of the mitral lesion. We decided to empty the uterus under spinal anæsthesia. The injection was given by Dr. Chrystal, and my assistant, Dr. Blum, did an anterior hysterotomy. The patient was conscious during the operation and toward the end complained of pain, probably more on account of the position of the limbs than from the operation. There were no untoward symptoms after the operation, the pulse was good and strong, and the convalescence ran an uninterrupted course. I do not know how many cases of this character have been done under spinal anæsthesia, but it seems to be safe. One point in the technic was that the last suture in the cervix was taken with silk-worm gut instead of catgut. Very often there will remain a notch in the cervix at the juncture of the two edges due to the suture. In this case the suture ends were allowed to remain long so as to be found easily. The result was perfect. I can recommend spinal anæsthesia in such condition, and it seems to be indicated in gynæcological work.

DR. CHASE, SR.: Incidentally this case and the results which Dr. Beach got from spinal anæsthesia recall very vividly a paper by Dr. Crile regarding the ushe of local anæsthesia to block the nerve transmission and thereby save the nervous system from shock. This paper was published last fall in the *Journal of the American Medical Association,* and is not altogether new. I should like to ask Dr. Beach if he does not think the blocking of the nerve transmission in this case by the spinal anæsthesia may have been the reason why the woman did not suffer from shock?

DR. BEACH: There is no doubt that what Dr. Chase says is true. The woman had no shock and there was no transmission of impulse from the lower abdomen.

DR. HUMPSTONE: I wish to report a case of dystocia from ventral fixation and amputation of the cervix. A woman, 38 years of age, who had had three children. She had suffered from procidentia and was operated on in New York by ventral fixation and a fairly high amputation of the cervix. She went through her pregnancy without pain or other symptoms until labor commenced. At the time of labor there was no advance, and after being in labor for six hours the head was in the pelvis and was boring its way through the anterior wall of the uterus. The os was of pinhole size. It seemed to be a case for operation if ever a case of dystocia required such assistance, and I did a vaginal hysterotomy and with forceps delivered an eight-pound baby. The cervical canal was left of sufficient size for drainage, and the result was satisfactory.

DR. POMEROY: About six weeks ago, at the Methodist Hospital, there was sent in from Bay Ridge a patient with a history of amputation a year before, but with no ventral fixation. The report from the doctor was that she had been in labor for twenty-four hours without any dilatation of the cervix. The condition found was something like that mentioned by Dr. Humpstone. The head was in the pelvis and there was only a one-finger dilatation. Careful study of the condition showed that there had been a complete amputation of the cervix, and it indicated that the head was obstructed by the inverted vagina. There was no cervix and the dilatation was in the vault of the vagina. It seemed impossible for the woman to deliver herself, and I did an anterior hysterotomy and an anteroposterior colpotomy and delivered the child by forceps, restitching the incision in the vagina. I noted that after delivery the contracted uterus was entirely separated from the inverted vagina. The mechanics of the condition was that in doing the circular amputation of the cervix the vault of the vagina was stitched to the level of the internal os. Except for this circular attachment there was no connection between the uterus and the vagina and in

4

the dilatation the vagina was inverted and pulled over the head of the child. That is my understanding of the reason for the failure of the parts to dilate.

DR. HOLDEN: About four years ago there was a case at the Methodist Hospital wherein a woman had been in labor for two days and the pains had ceased. In the vagina was felt a smooth cervix with a pinhole opening. The fœtus was dead. An anterior hysterotomy was performed and the child delivered piecemeal and macerated.

DR. BEACH: I saw a case in Bum's clinic in 1905 which seems to me explains some of the mechanics in question. She had an old type of dystocia where the cervical opening was thrown way high up posteriorly five or six inches. It had been a neglected case and there was a temperature which made an abdominal operation out of the question. In this case Professor Bum took a curved scalpel in his fingers and did an anterior hysterectomy and anterior colpotomy through which opening the child was delivered. He did not injure the bladder, as I think the bladder in such a condition is drawn well up out of the way.

DR. POMEROY: I wish again to emphasize the fact that if there has been an actual amputation of the cervix that when the head is in the pelvis there is no tissue on which to do a colpotomy. There is nothing but vagina. The bladder goes up with the os and the incision extends from that os wherever it may be.

DR. HUMPSTONE: I have a very high regard for Dr. Pomeroy's observations, but in this case I do not see how the uterus is going to separate from the vagina. What was lacking in my case was the shelf of the cervix. If I had done as Professor Bum did I should have cut into the bladder. The anterior wall of the uterus boring down into the pelvis. In this case those mechanics did not apply.

DR. POMEROY: I was referring to my own case only.

DR. RALPH H. POMEROY then read the paper of the evening on: 1. The Medical, Legal, and Sociological Status of Obstetrics. 2. Rotary Version in Posterior Positions. 3. Contraction Ring Dystocia. 4. The Third Stage Management of Postpartum Hemorrhage.

Dr. HUMPSTONE: Dr. Pomeroy's philosophy is one of the most interesting features of my professional life. I always enjoy him when he is discussing a philosophical topic and certainly tonight his remarks have been of the first water. There are just a few points which I should like to speak of, though in most of what he says we agree with him fully, particularly in the matter of the legal status of obstetrics. It is news to me that there is no legal status of that branch of practice. The midwife problem, it seems to me, in the centers of culture, is one that we will not have much trouble with, but in the lower classes what we will have to do is to get into touch with the people and to get them to understand that it is to their interest to have educated assistance in their confinements. I believe in that way we are going to solve this problem. Regarding the problem of Cæsarian section, Dr. Pomeroy has always been very conservative. In Boston they are very radical, about every third woman is operated on and anything is an excuse for it. It is a question whether in cases of dystocia we have really anything that will show a better general average than this operation. The problem of long drawn-out labors with the occiput in the posterior position is a matter that jeopardizes the patient and the child. I have been instructed by what Dr. Pomeroy has said, but it is not easy. When the head has moulded and the uterus has retracted it becomes exceedingly difficult. Dr. Pomeroy can do it where others would not be able to accomplish it. That problem of long drawn-out labor from posterior positions I think will be recognized before many years as a justifiable cause for Cæsarian section. The problem of why the occiput posterior is a little different when there is a retraction ring is that we have a great big hump in the way, and whether the position is in the diagonal or not the hump is in the way and that is the reason the head does not come down. I think in comparison with the use of forceps above the brim, which is so dangerous, Dr. Pomeroy's procedure is much to be preferred. As regards the treatment of postpartum hemorrhage, I must disagree with the doctor a little. I think it is best to let the uterus alone unless the placenta is partially separated. If it is not partially separated then we do not have postpartum hemorrhage. If there is hemorrhage then it must be controlled by manipulation or by removing the placenta, but there will be no hemorrhage unless the placenta is partially detached.

DR. BEACH: It seems like an anticlimax for two such authorities to differ. I have a few ideas on the subjects mentioned in the paper. Dr. Pomeroy brought forth the thought that the general practitioner is to blame in cases where the consultant is not called in early enough. Labor is considered to be a physiological process and the practitioner feels that he is depreciating himself when he asks for assistance and so puts it off as long as possible, hoping that things will right themselves, as they often do. Regarding the moulding of the uterus, that condition does occur, as is shown by frozen specimens. With regard to rotary version, I should like to question the nomenclature. Is it really a version when the position of the head is changed from an anterior to a posterior position? I do not think so. Whether the procedure should be undertaken or not is a matter of judgment. It is very dangerous both to the tissues and from the danger of infection. Many cases will rotate themselves and come down anteriorly if left alone. We are not patient enough. The judicious use of morphine will often be valuable in gaining time. In turning it is sometimes easier to turn toward the larger than the smaller part of the circle. As to management of the third stage, it seems to me that in the cases in the hospital the large majority of the cases are caused by over-manipulation on the part of the internes. In the cases which I witnessed during a month at the Charité, the patients were delivered on the table and were immediately put to bed and no effort made to express the placenta. I saw over three hundred and fifty cases and in only three were there any hemorrhages. Manipulation will tend to separate the placenta partially and thus produce the hemorrhage.

DR. POOL: In regard to persistent occipitoposterior positions, I have not thought that the retraction or moulding of the uterus was the cause. I believe it is due to the substituting of the larger for the smaller diameters that makes the trouble. It is without question that this retraction resulting in moulding of the uterus does occur. The rotation of the head above the brim which I have practiced differs slightly from that advocated by Dr. Pomeroy. It is useless to rotate the head without rotating the trunk. If the position is the right occipitoposterior I introduce the right hand and grasp the posterior shoulder which is opposite the palm of the hand and push it toward the right of the mother, rotating over the mother's front and use the opposite hand externally. This all sounds very easy, but when you have the uterus moulded around the fœtus it is difficult. You can turn the fœtus but you also turn the uterus sometimes, and the position is the same as soon as you let go; it returns to its old position. I think in many of these cases internal version is the wise solution. If we have such a case it is not wise to let it get into such a position. We then get a thinned out lower segment of the uterus, and it is better before we get a really dry labor to complete the delivery by some other means. In this procedure of internal version the head must be flexed and shoved into the pelvis until the uterus can force it further down. I think this is more simple and certainly a minor procedure and is to be commended in preference to Cæsarian section.

DR. POLAK: I regret that Dr. Pomeroy did not present his able paper before a larger society, for it is worthy of it. Most of the points he has instructed me in and I have followed them to a limited extent and have had some success. The question of rotation of the occiput has been gone over very thoroughly, but it is a more difficult procedure than one would get the impression of from his description, as I have found in the cases that we have seen in counsel together, and that because of the neglect we were frequently unable to do it and compelled to use the podalic version. The presence of a retraction ring has been apparent to me, but I did not know what it was until a few years ago. I had found it in cases where I had used Voorhees' bag, but thought it had something to do with a tired uterus and dystocia. The question of post-partum hemorrhage is most interesting to me because I had not supposed it was so frequent. Recently I have had several experiences with the house staff. I have followed the plan of never interfering with the uterus unless the placenta was partially separated, or unless it was injured. I have been on the side with Dr. Beach and never bother with the placenta if the women are in good condition, and simply watch and let them deliver themselves. Some physicians seem to have got in the habit of hurrying the condition, as though they had to be making a living and had no time to spare. I agree with Dr. Pomeroy and believe in raising the uterus, as Dr. Dickinson has suggested. Frankly speaking, I have not had a case of hemorrhage in ten or eleven years until the recent ones. I think the douche is a most useless procedure. There is nothing that wastes so much time as the preparation of a douche. The whole principle of the Momberg pressure on the abdomen is based on the raising of the uterus. The whole subject has been so thoroughly and so well discussed that I feel that all that I can do is to express my deep appreciation for the points brought out by Dr. Pomeroy and to thank him for what he has taught me in the last ten or fifteen years. They have been of great value to me.

DR. POMEROY, in closing the discussion, said: "The most impressive thing about the discussion to myself is the conviction that I have not succeeded in getting close to you on some subjects. One point I have not succeeded in getting to you is the proposition that the rotating of the posterior position is not intended for doubtful cases, but for those where the head has sunk into the pelvis and has shown no disposition to advance and hours have passed without any dilatation of the os. There you are dealing with a scant liquor amnii. This procedure is not to be compared to the operation of last resort. My idea is to rotate early and to get the head into a good position and let the woman deliver herself. The matter of postpartum hemorrhage also shows some little defects in my efforts to convey the differentiation between the postpartum that may be suspected and the cases which will deliver themselves if left alone. The complete emptying of the uterus does not add to the risk of postpartum hemorrhage. I speak of tampering with the fundus that is done by hospital internes. My belief is that immediate emptying of the uterus does not add to the danger. I do not know of any argument that proves that the empty uterus is more likely to bleed, and I am hopelessly at a loss to be able to detect a whole or a partially detached uterus. It may be detached immediately on the expulsion of the child, or before."

## BROOKLYN SURGICAL SOCIETY.

### Stated Meeting, April 3, 1913.

WALTER A. SHERWOOD, M.D., President, pro tem., in the Chair.

#### Program.

I. Presentation of Clinical Cases:
    1. "Bone Transplantation for Spinal Disease." Patients. By Dr. Walter Truslow.
    Discussed by Dr. C. D. Napier, Dr. J. S. Wight and Dr. Walter Truslow.
    2. (a) "Adeno-Carcinoma of the Rectum." Specimen.
    (b) "Hystero-Myomectomy." Patient. By Dr. F. W. Wunderlich.
    No discussion.
    3. (a) "Fracture of the Lower End of the Humerus, with Displacement." Patient. X-ray plates.
    (b) "Tubercular Disease of the Red Marrow." Patient. X-ray plates. By Dr. J. Sherman Wight.
    Case "a" discussed by Dr. J. B. Bogart.
II. Paper of the Evening:
    "Review of 150 Cases Observed at the Mayo Clinics." By Dr. John A. Lee.
    Discussed by Dr. Mathias Figueira, Dr. R. P. Sullivan, Dr. Walter Truslow, Dr. J. B. Bogart, Dr. L. W. Pearson; closed by Dr. J. B. Bogart.

#### Bone Transplantation for Spinal Disease. Patients.

##### By Dr. Walter Truslow.

This must of necessity be preliminary reporting. I think we cannot feel that as yet this procedure is an assured thing. I feel that the cases I am to report—two of these which I have done—I can present to-night. In their cases it appears to be, so far, absolutely an assured thing, but time only will tell the final results. Just a very brief review of the history of the condition and of the procedure.

Of course, Pott's disease of the spine, tubercular spine, is no new thing. Percival Pott was the first to describe it with any great accuracy, but it was not until somewhat later, in the early part of the last century, that some Frenchman seemed to be able to tell us the pathology of it with any degree of accuracy, and since that time the treatment has tended very largely in the direction in which it still tends; that is to say, tuberculosis here is as tuberculosis elsewhere to the extent that good hygiene is a very important factor, and then the localized fixation of the part to relieve strain on the diseased bone, the disease taking place practically always in the body of the vertebræ. The method of treatment up to this time has been largely that of fixation and the use of plaster jackets and of spinal braces. Probably an efficient means has been the Bradford frame or, as Whitman has modified it, to let the child lie recumbent.

Now, as far as I know, Langer, of Berlin, a few years ago suggested something similar to the Lane plate to go from spinous process to spinous process. This effects an internal fixation of the spine, as he called it, and he presented it to the American Orthopedic Association several years ago, but it did not seem to meet with much favor. It is not unlike the Albee operation, which is to be reported to-night and which consists in cutting the bone across and placing it between the spinous processes of one or two vertebræ—sometimes three—thus getting internal fixation.

The theory seems to be that here the weight of the entire frame rests largely upon the body, centrum above centrum, which is the function of that portion of the vertebræ. Shifting the weight a little more to the articular processes and holding it there by this fixation from behind seems, mechanically, a very good procedure.

The question of bone transplantation I shall not go into, except to recall to you Dr. Murphy's principles. You recall he made the statement that grafts taken between species, from one species of animal to another, practically never take, and grafts between individuals of the same species much more rarely take, if we may use the expression, but with grafts from the same individual there is much more frequently a final union.

The method of regeneration seems to differ according to different writers. Albee maintains that the graft itself remains intact, and that in any piece of bone that is transferred the blood vessels will enter and form an actually new bony structure. Murphy, I believe, maintains that it acts only as a nidus long enough for other bone to gradually take its place, but it seems to me to make but little difference what is the method as long as in either case it remains long enough to get a final fixation there.

The first case that I tried this on was that of a boy who had been under my care for a number of years—this boy. He is fifteen years of age, had disease in the dorsal region, much deformity, and a duration as long as twelve years.

Previous treatment included jackets off and on for about five years, and braces for about seven years. In July of last year operation was performed by bridging seven spinous processes. The graft was not as well obtained as later experience showed me how, there being some splitting of the graft.

In my cases the graft has been taken entirely from the crest of the tibia, a splinter of bone more or less.

I will tell you why he is in a partial plaster jacket now. The incision in this case and the next was made directly over the spinous processes, a bit of technic which was improved upon in the later cases. The bones of the lower end of the graft became loose within a week or so and a little portion of the lower end of the graft was finally removed through a little opening in the splint, but a great deal remained, enough, in my judgment, to be a good strong bridge.

There was a little post-operative temperature, probably due to that portion which sloughed away, healing by granulation at the lower end of the wound.

The second case was that of a child five years of age, mid-dorsal region, much deformity, duration a number of months. In a few of these cases I have not been giving previous treatment. This case was mostly on a frame. Operation in October, 1912, bridging of four verterbræ, incision over the spinous processes. I can show you an X-ray taken before operation. A good deal of deformity in the mid-dorsal region, some post-operative temperature, but healing per primam. There was pyuria for two weeks, for which we could not account.

I want to say of that second case that I have heard within two weeks through Dr. Taylor, of the Hospital for the Ruptured and Crippled, that the boy was later brought there. The doctor wrote to me that he was in bad condition and that the father reported this operation had been done by me, and he therefore wanted to know the facts, and I told him. In a second letter he told me that an X-ray showed absolutely no sign of the graft. This is one of the reasons why I say this is still in the experimental stage—one example of the possibility of absorption. In this case apparently there has been absorption and the child is going around, as we have done in all of the cases, without support, except as I shall tell you in this case.

The third case is that of a boy eight years of age; disease in the dorsal region, with a great deal of deformity. You will notice how very small and very short the spinous processes were, the disease involving the bodies of several of the vertebræ, and it seemed to me something of a qustion whether we could get much bridging. He had been on a frame for three months. All these cases had been in the Kings County Hospital. In this case, operation at the end of last October, bridging of seven spinous processes, some slight sloughing at the lower end.

I think all of the cases in which the incision was over the spinous processes healed with some difficulty, but this second case shows no such trouble.

This child, the fourth case, is seven years of age and I had seen her for some years. There was a good deal of deformity in the mid-dorsal region; previous treatment, Bradford frame, plaster jackets and braces; operation in January, 1913, bridging of seven spinous processes, graft about three inches long; the first case with the crescent incision; no post-operative temperature, and healing per primam. That child, the mother tells me, is playing around without any support and is robust and never complains of the slightest pain anywhere, but this is a comparatively recent case. As you see, there is deformity, but I feel the results are better with the crescent incision; there is better nourishment of the bone.

Now, the fifth case was a low dorsal, a little girl of four years, not much deformity, duration over two years; most of first year on a Bradford frame and a few months' neglect. About sixteen months ago, before operation, one month before admission to the Kings County Hospital, abscess in the right groin and right side of the back, spontaneous rupture; for fifteen months on a frame; operation decided on, though sinuses not healed. We here followed Albee's idea of operating, though sinuses are not healed. If you can keep the wound clear of the sinus discharges, and that was done, you are all right, and it has been entirely successful as far as that is concerned. In the operation on January 15, 1913, bridging of eight processes, graft about four inches long. That is the only one I am able to show with the graft in. I think you will appreciate how in some hospital services the X-ray machine goes out of order just when you would like to have it most in order to show our cases. This was in the lumbar region. That shows the graft in place there, about four inches, crescent incision, practically no post-operative temperature, healing per primam.

This is the last of the six cases I have to show. The seventh one I do not care to include, as the child is older and still in bed in the hospital.

The sixth case is a high dorsal. I want to say in passing that I think that is an unusually good X-ray picture, for it is difficult to get a lateral X-ray in that region, cervical dorsal, practically at the junction of the two regions. Duration in this case about three years. Patient could not hold the head up. Had worn head and back brace six months before coming to the hospital. On admission, sinuses in the neck, front and back, and left side. In hospital on frame ten months. Operation decided on. On January 29th bridging of six processes, graft about three and one-half inches long, crescent incision, no post-operative temperature, and healing per primam.

Now, the question is, What about the future of these cases? The seventh case is in bed, and I do not know about its future. Both girls are in the hospital and both are healing. Heads are a little bit in rotation, but if it interferes with motion, one can go down and clip the bones between those processes in these high regions and chisel away enough to correct the deformity.

I want to speak a little of this boy's condition here, and the reason for operating. This is the first case. There was a very great deal of deformity. I believe that we should be accurate in what we say as to whether a case has improved or not. I have followed him more carefully, as I have had the better opportunity to do. The tracings of the spine I am reducing to figures which I call the ratio deformity as a record to tell later whether it is increasing or decreasing. Now, that was taken about a month or so afterwards and the ratio deformity there, we will say, was perhaps 28¼ per cent. and is here reduced to about 25½ per cent. Now, is that a fictitious reduction or is it real? I think one can feel only that it is or is not, if one does it one's self both times.

Now, what about this boy? I found that he was reducing his main trouble, but how about the compensatory deformity? He had been used to a support for years. His compensatory deformity was increasing, and increasing to a considerable degree, and it seemed to me a question of anteroposterior balance. He had so much of his body weight backward that he was tending backward. We tried exercise to strengthen the abdominal muscles to tend to drawing in and for a little while he seemed to improve, but this thing was going on to a considerable increase and pain was increasing. For about three or four weeks he has had this thing on. I thought I would leave it on on purpose. Since this has been on he has been relieved of pain. He had pain in the compensatory region and I have not decided what we should do, whether we should have a light support here which he can discard slowly. I at least wanted to get the stoop different from what it was. It was backward, and I believe we have accomplished that to a certain extent.

I have that apparatus. That is a modification of a Philadelphia one (Elkington). Elkington worked out these parallel points on the upright and you place them one after another. With a thumb-screw you fix it and can transfer it to this and trace it out.

Before I sit down I would like to speak of the operation. It consists in this: A crescent incision and getting as much extension as the present condition will allow; then cutting down and chiseling one after another right through the number of spinous processes you decide to use, not very deeply. I do not know whether I have gone deeply enough. Albee, I think, goes a little deeper than I have, represented by that picture, and takes a little broader graft, chiseling and cutting through the spinous processes until you have a wedge-shaped bit. I have not yet broken any of those bones. I do not think it is a thing which would happen unless one went more deeply. There is a little matter of technic. Instead of having to turn over, the leg is simply drawn up and an assistant holds it sharply against the thigh. At first we simply measure with a probe the length of the graft we want to use before cutting into the front of the leg, and just chisel out the necessary splinter of bone. That is where Albee's technic is fine, in that he uses a motor saw. I think he does it much quicker than we have been able to do at the hospital. Dr. Napier has recently gotten a circular saw and taken it out there and has used it on some of his cases. To my mind, that is an important part of the operation.

Now, suppose the graft is a curved one; the graft is simply arranged as a carpenter would a piece of wood when he wants to make a curved piece of wood. If he wants to get that curved he turns it on its base on the side, and makes a few sawings. You can bend the graft into whatever shape you wish. An assistant must saw that up for you and then fit it nicely. Thumb pressure, I found, brought it in best to fit it into the groove. The point is to sew the graft, sewing over the superior spinous and interspinous ligaments; get it completely imbedded. I think that the protrusion in the first case was owing to the fact that I did not use strong enough sutures.

The after-treatment: In bed, and keeping the spine in a fairly extended position. We generally in the cervical region keep the head slung upon the portion there so as to see that they do not move.

I feel, gentlemen, that it is simply an interesting possibility of reducing what is admittedly a two to three years', or even longer, treatment, to possibly a two to three months' treatment, but I feel we should not consider this thoroughly settled as to its final utility.

Dr. C. D. NAPIER, in opening the discussion, said: "From what I have seen of other cases operated, Dr. Albee's and Dr. Truslow's, in addition to my own, I am very much in favor of this operation. I also think it is a very big advance over what we have done.

"I want to speak of what I think the special indications for the operation. In the upper and mid-dorsal disease I find that many cases present an increase of deformity in spite of long recumbency on the Bradford frame, followed by plaster and braces, and the after-treatment of exercise of the muscles. I do feel now that the operation is decidedly indicated in upper and mid-dorsal disease. Probably it should be done early. However, in other cases, the lumbar and cervical variety, if we can get the cases early enough, we can undoubtedly, without operative procedure, by long recumbency and fresh-air treatment, get a return to the normal bone. If we follow, as I have in some cases, with the X-ray at intervals of six months or a year, we find that the bone returns to the normal, so we have a normal bone and normal joint and perfect motion in the spine—a perfect cure. If we can get that, we certainly do not want to fix four or five, or even six vertebræ, as we have to at times, entirely ankylose them by this bone-grafting operation. In the lumbar Pott's, and lower dorsal and cervical, the spine, especially in a child, can be thoroughly fixed on the Bradford frame and later with plaster jackets. In the mid and upper dorsal they are very difficult to fix, and we may get increase of the deformity,—very likely partially due to the respiratory movements. I think it is also indicated rather decidedly in adults, particularly in workingmen.

"I saw today at the Kings County Hospital an Italian whom I operated eight weeks ago, now walking around the wards. When he was sent in he had had the preceding recumbency, long recumbency in bed, followed by plaster jackets, and going out working in his jacket, became worse and came back. He had a family to support and readily consented to operation. Now, after eight weeks in the hospital, he is going home, not, I hope, to work yet, but certainly to get back to a supporting position very much quicker than he could by any other means; so that in these adult cases men, and probably women as well, this new procedure certainly affords very great hopes of putting them on their feet and getting them back to their work very much quicker. I feel about the Albee operation that it is probably a little better than the Hibbs method, brought out about the same time. This latter operation appealed to us at first for some reasons, that by turning down the spinous processes one against the other, in that way we reduced the kyphos and did not introduce any foreign bone, even from the leg of the same patient. I think if that could succeed it might be better, because it would form the same bridge of bone that the Albee operation does between the vertebræ. It seems to me more difficult. Where there is considerable kyphos it is hard to make one spinous process come down and reach the point where you want on the next vertebra, and the bones in children are exceedingly soft and easily break off and are hard to hold in place; and this does not give us the firm, solid spine which we have in the Albee. In the latter, the piece of bone from the tibia at once splints the spine, which the Hibbs operation does not do until the spinous processes grow together.

"It does seem to me that it is a very great advance in our work, but I do feel like saying that it is not the only advance in the treatment of Pott's disease in the last fifty years, as one of the Western surgeons I heard speak here in Brooklyn not very long ago said, for the Bradford frame and improved plaster jackets have enabled us to give complete cure to cases which was not obtained fifty years ago."

DR. J. S. WIGHT, in discussion, said: "I want to take issue with one statement made by Dr. Napier, and that is, that the placing of a solid piece of bone in position will act immediately to reinforce as a splint. Of course, it will, compared with the lack of that general support from the turning down in the Hibbs operation if it was fastened in there rigidly enough or firmly enough so as to give splinting or reinforcement immediately, but it should not be relied on, as the pressure will become less through the establishment of an equilibrium on the part of Nature. Just as soon as there is pressure on the bone there is a tendency to produce equilibrium; it will loosen up in a very short time.

"There is a collateral matter coming up here of importance to all the men doing this work; that is, the men cutting into the tibia or other bones to get grafts may have a claim made against them on the basis of malpractice which may be successfully pressed. From what has transpired in a recent case a man has not protection against what is termed an assault. The case I refer to is that of a gentleman from New York who operated on a case and did some bone grafting, removed a fragment from the tibia and had a consultation with his associates on the staff in the presence of this woman who sued him. He brought them to court to establish the fact that she had knowledge of what was going to be done, but the lack of consent was sufficient to bring in a verdict against the doctor, showing the necessity of getting not a verbal consent, but a form of consent signed by the patient before a witness, in order to protect ourselves against such actions."

DR. WALTER TRUSLOW, in closing the discussion, said: "I would merely agree with Dr. Napier.

"Now, my judgment so far is that the operation is mostly indicated in the upper and mid-dorsal regions. It is very much easier to bring about artificial support in the lumbar region, and yet I rather hope that it may be a procedure for the cervical region, it is so difficult to get artificial external support for that region. We can do it, of course, with a chin cage or jury mast, but both of these are considered by patients as being very unsightly and are much objected to, although, of course, I agree that that objection must be overruled if it is an essential.

"That question about immediate splinting does interest me somewhat. I feel my early cases, especially that boy that was shown right here, were due to the insufficient size of the graft taken; that is to say, I did not splint it well enough. The immediate splinting is the object I would make, that it does occur and the graft sewing in was a very important point in the later cases.

"If I might just add another phase to the whole subject. Albee claims that more than this point for which we originally operated, namely, quick recovery from disease—more than that, we get in a child still within growing age a decrease in the deformity, and he says that it is because he will make the curvature of the graft just less than the best curvature obtainable in the child's back and he will let that act as a kind of spring, a bony spring to hold it, to draw back the two segments in the body segments. Personally, I cannot feel quite so sure that this point is correct. It is a point in favor of immediate splinting."

*(Continued in November.)*

# LONG ISLAND
# MEDICAL JOURNAL

| VOL. VII. | NOVEMBER, 1913 | No. 11 |

## ®riginal Articles.

### INDICATIONS FOR COMPLETE AND PARTIAL OOPHO-RECTOMY CONTRASTING CLINICAL AND HISTOLOGICAL CRITERIA.*

### By Robert T. Frank, M.D.,

of Manhattan, N. Y.

THIS is the first opportunity I have had of seeing the program, and I find that some of the things which I intended to speak of really fall in the province of other speakers. Therefore if I should encroach upon their field, I beg to apologize in advance.

Your chairman struck the right note when he said that frequent complaints are still met with that ovaries are unnecessarily removed. The practicing gynecologist, the operator, is at a disadvantage. He finds these ovaries at operation. Frequently he has a number of technical difficulties to overcome and hence his attention is divided. Furthermore, when an ovary is, for instance, fixed in the pelvis, he is not as well able to judge the conditions as exactly as the pathologist, who has an opportunity to examine them at his leisure in the laboratory and if any doubt remains is in a position to satisfy himself as to the difference and kind of condition by microscopical verification. The condition the operator meets with, as I have hinted, is entirely different; and, therefore, as I myself operate, I appreciate this, and feel that it is wise to refrain from unjust criticism. At the same time certain facts should be known to the gynecologist, particularly if he is an operator, and he ought to possess certain basic pathological knowledge as part of his armamentarium.

The first point to be discussed is the primary indication for operation. Before a society of this character I need not dwell at any length upon these criteria. At the same time it is wise at least to touch upon these points. In most instances the patient consults the physician because of pain. Most commonly, pain is produced by inflammatory conditions, in acute cases more intense; in chronic perhaps not as intense, but wearing, as it lasts for so long a period of time. Acute or chronic ovarian pain, as such, is extremely rare. In almost every instance it is combined with tubal disease and we are, offhand, unable to determine whether the pain is due to the tubal or ovarian inflammation. But probably it is caused more often by the tubal disease than by the ovarian inflammation. Pain is also caused by pressure as in the case of large

---

* Read before the Brooklyn Pathological Society, April 10, 1913.

tumors or tumors pressing on the bladder; and occasionally in malignant disease if there are adhesions and obstruction.

Hemorrhage into a tumor or unaltered ovary may furnish a locus minoris resistentia for infection. In ovarian tumors infection is rather rare, but I have seen a case of gonorrhea and a typhoid infection of an ovarian cyst. Tubercular infections have also been reported.

The second symptom which causes the patient to seek advice is the increase in size of the abdomen. This may be due to the growth of the tumor itself; the size of the tumor attracting the patient's attention; or to the concomitant ascites. Ascites in ovarian tumors is apparently more common than I thought it was until I looked up the statistics. It is known to occur in one-quarter of all tumors of the ovary and in fibromata (which in themselves are absolutely benign tumors) it occurs in three-fourths of all cases, while in malignant tumors it occurs in over sixty per cent.

Occasionally uterine disturbances call the patient's attention to the ovarian condition. This may be due to functional ovarian conditions such as overaction of the ovaries, or it may be due to organic lesions, such as inflammation, or, in rare instances, to tumors, usually intraligamentary tumors, where the metrorrhagia probably arises from the mechanical pressure exerted upon the pelvic veins.

One other cause for advising operation is the sometimes accidental finding of a tumor which has caused no symptoms.

The second heading I had in mind dealt with conditions met with at operation, but I am afraid if I go into that to any extent I will encroach upon Doctor Pool's field, so on the whole, I will practically skip this paragraph. Let me, in passing emphasize that I am unwilling to recognize ovaritis as a distinct disease. It is true that diseases of the ovary are encountered with tubal inflammation; the other varieties, uncomplicated by tubal inflammation, occur only in general infectious diseases. Therefore, I come to what really is the main part of my theme, and that is the pathological criteria.

As I said at the outset, every gynecologist ought to be well equipped with certain fundamental pathological knowledge, otherwise he will be greatly handicapped at the operating table. He is called upon at a moment's notice to decide upon radical or conservative measures, and unless he is very familiar, at least with gross pathology, he will frequently err.

As far as the inflammatory conditions are concerned, we find again the acute and chronic conditions. Personally, I rarely encounter acute conditions at the operating table because I try to avoid operating in the acute stage. Acute conditions are recognized at once by the surroundings, as much as by actual disease in the tube or ovary. Exudation in the broad ligament, recent adhesions, serous cysts found in the pelvic cavity, that is, encysted serous fluid, which ruptures while the intestinal adhesions are freed, or actual purulent collections in the pelvis, are characteristic of this condition.

Under those circumstances, at the operating table, it is impossible to judge just what portion of the tube or ovary is healthy.

In the chronic conditions, the purulent process has usually stopped. If we find pus, it is usually shut off in the tube. The cultures are then most often sterile. Ovaries may be cystic or may be buried in adhesions. They may have the appearance of being intraligamentary. They may be in direct communication with a hydrosalpinx. So we encounter tubo-ovarian cysts, the different variations of which are innumerable.

As the actual operative conditions and method of treatment will be discussed by other speakers, I shall not dwell upon them.

Now, turning to tumors. The most important thing when you encounter a tumor in the pelvis, a tumor of the ovary, is, in the first place, to determine its nature; in the second place to decide whether it is safe to leave an apparently healthy ovary on the other side. These things are not easy to determine at the operating table. They are sometimes not even easy to determine after microscopical sections have been made, and hence many errors, some of omission, some of commission, occur. Not only have we to decide upon the just mentioned facts, but we are, soon after the operation, asked by relatives as to the prognosis; and, as you know, the future of a patient depends largely upon the nature of the neoplasm removed. We have local recurrences, if we have been unable to remove the tumor radically. We have in some instances recurrences in the incision, whether vaginal or abdominal, that is, scar recurrences; we have lymphatic gland recurrence; we have general metastases, either in the peritoneal cavity itself or in distant organs.

Now, turning to the varieties of tumors we meet with. The most innocent is the so-called simple cyst of the ovary which rarely attains large size, which is readily recognized by its thin wall, and by its clear contents. We sometimes meet with simple cysts of the ovary which have slight and localized papilliferous portions but yet are not malignant. These cysts, of course, are entirely harmless and do not recur.

Probably the most common is the rapidly growing multilocular ovarian cyst, or pseudomucin cyst, which may attain a very large size. It is of interest to note that it is frequently, although not so very often (in 17 per cent.) bilateral. When one encounters a pseudomucinous cyst it is easily recognized. It is wise to remove the affected ovary or ovaries entirely unless there are very special indications, usually social, that contraindicate the inducing of sterility, and warrant the assumption of the additional risk resulting from resection. It is wiser to remove the entire ovary because the condition verges on the border line of malignant disease. These cysts ought not to be punctured as pseudomyxoma of the peritoneum may follow.

Serous papilliferous tumors are more malignant. They are often bilateral and recur in 75 per cent. In other words, when we encounter one of these serous papilliferous cysts, it must be treated as a serious condition which requires thorough and complete surgical interference. They are recognized by the papilliferous contents and by the fact that the fluid portion is thin and serous.

Then we come to the more solid types of tumors which merge from the cystic into the solid. Sometimes macroscopically it is impossible to distinguish between the two. They occur more often in older people and recur with even greater frequency than the preceding form, and are more often bilateral; in fact, most statistics say they are bilateral in 90 per cent., and by bilateral in this case is meant that the opposite ovary may be absolutely normal to macroscopical appearance, but already show microscopical involvement. I make a habit of removing both ovaries when I encounter a condition of this kind, and have always subjected them to microscopical examination, and almost regularly found minute foci showing malignant changes. When we find them already macroscopically bilateral at operation, the indication for doing a complete double oophorectomy is absolute. Solid carcinoma falls under the same heading and requires the same treatment.

Sarcoma is only bilateral in one-third of the cases. It is very malignant; particularly the soft varieties. Sarcomata have a yellowish to reddish color, are meaty and have a great tendency to disintegrate or tear in the hands of the operator during removal. Such an accident, of course, greatly increases the danger of recurrence.

Teratomata, those mixed tumors in which we see almost all the tissues that can be found in the fetus, are easily recognized. They are solid tumors containing numerous minute cysts, or sometimes larger cysts. They are very malignant and I have never seen a patient recover in whom a teratoma was removed unless it was a simple struma ovarii (thyroid tissue). Sometimes as many as four or five years may pass before these patients die of metastases.

There are a few other things which I would like to call to your attention, especially metastatic tumors in the ovary. The gynecologist and general surgeon should be aware of this condition and be able to diagnose it in some instances. For example, if a sarcoma is limited to a portion of the ovary, that is, if it does not involve the entire ovary, it is practically in every instance metastatic, and if a primary tumor cannot be found and removed no benefit will accrue from oophorectomy. Certain colloid carcinomata of the ovary are absolutely characteristic of metastatic involvement. The primary growths are found in the intestines; (stomach tumors) the breast and most frequently in the uterus. When I see such a tumor in the ovary which is colloid, and yet differs macroscopically from the ordinary more solid primary colloidal carcinoma of the ovary, I am sure it is a metastasis.

There is only one other point I would like to dwell upon, and that was mentioned by Dr. Pilcher; that is multiple simple cysts of the ovary, or polycystic ovary. I can best illustrate what I think about the polycystic ovary by referring to certain analogous conditions in animals. I have examined many hundreds of ovaries of sows and a much smaller number of cows' ovaries. In rabbits and guinea pigs, the same thing practically holds true, but the sow is the best instance of this condition. When a sow is in rut, the ovary enlarges enormously. The normal ovary in the sow is a little smaller than the human ovary. After rut, it assumes proportions five times as large, of which perhaps only a quarter is due to the corpora lutea. I feel confident for many reasons that the human ovary undergoes similar functional changes. I have clinically followed this out in patients whom I have been able to examine repeatedly for long periods of time. I have made repeated vaginal examinations and watched the ovaries. I feel confident that I can usually determine the side in which the corpus luteum develops and it is about time we took this more generally into consideration when speaking of minor enlargements of the ovary.

If you have occasion to operate a patient and find a polycystic ovary, leave it alone. If for any other reason you re-operate that patient, you will find in most cases this same ovary normal in appearance, if you strike the right period in the menstrual cycle. Resection, unless very special conditions are present, which I do not care to discuss here, is entirely unnecessary, and unless we are forced to perform oophorectomy, on account of persistent pain, which we feel sure can be ascribed only to the ovary, we are much wiser to leave such organs entirely alone.

(*For discussion see p.* 456 *et seq.*)

## PELVIC CONDITIONS REVEALED ON THE OPERATING TABLE WHICH CALL FOR REMOVAL OF THE OVARY.*

### By William P. Pool, M.D.,

of Brooklyn, N. Y.

CONDITIONS as found at the time of operation sometimes make the decision to remove or leave an ovary very difficult, since it must be made purely upon a clinical basis and must be made upon the spot.

Briefly, diseases of the pelvis which may require removal of the ovary wholly or in part may be divided into two classes; those outside the ovaries, and those which affect the ovaries themselves.

In the first class I believe there is only one absolute and unvarying indication for the radical and complete removal of all ovarian tissue, and that is malignant disease. Hysterectomy for fibroid or fibrosis, or for chronic inflammatory disease need not include the ovaries, nor is it always necessary to disturb them when operating for disease of the tubes. The rule is well established that under such conditions, as much ovarian tissue as possible be conserved—both, or one, or at least a part of one. But in the presence of cancer, the wide dissection, and complete removal of all glandular tissue from the pelvis which is necessary, must include the ovaries along with other organs extirpated.

In other forms of disease outside of the ovaries the indication for their removal will depend upon the extent of the secondary involvment of ovarian tissue itself.

Diseases of the ovary which require ablation, partial or complete, may be classified as tumors, inflammations, and certain trophic disorders.

Dr. Frank has already spoken so fully of the tumors that there is no need of my saying more, except to emphasize the necessity of differentiating clinically between those that are benign and purely local, and therefore harmless, and those that are malignant. In the former class we may place fibroids, retention cysts and pseudomucinous cysts. These are undoubtedly benign and require excision simply of the local disease. If they be unilateral the other ovary should be left undisturbed. If bilateral, a cure requires that the entire disease be removed, but it is usually possible to leave a part of one or both ovaries and highly desirable to do so.

Dermoid cysts are in a class by themselves. These tumors, while they are local and non-malignant, contain a very infectious material and great care must be used to make a complete excision

---

* Read before the Brooklyn Pathological Society, April 10, 1913.

of the tumor, and at the same time to avoid puncturing it. This not infrequently requires entire extirpation of the ovary. When bilateral, which is comparatively rare, both ovaries may have ·to be sacrificed, if the disease be so intimately blended with the remnant of ovarian tissue as to make dissection dangerous.

Pseudomucinous cysts, which are probably the most common of all ovarian tumors, are not difficult to recognize. The possibility of malignant development in such a tumor has been considered, but while malignancy has occasionally been found in these cysts, it cannot be considered in any way a characteristic of the growth, and should not affect its classification as benign. The removal of the disease from one ovary may be followed at a longer or shorter time by its appearance in the other, but there is nothing to show that this occasional secondary involvement is by extension, or that it is at all dependent upon the disease in the first ovary. Therefore a unilateral pseudomucinous cyst is not an indication for the removal of both ovaries.

Papillary cysts were formerly classified as malignant, and they certainly do present some characteristics of malignancy, but investigations by Pfannelstiel and others have shown that they do not entirely fulfill the definition of a malignant growth. While it is possible that they may be implanted upon the peritoneum by a rupture of the cyst or a perforation of its wall, they are not metastatic in the sense that they are carried by the blood and lymph to distant parts. The removal of the focus of the growth will sometimes be followed by a disappearance of the secondary growths which may have been started in various parts of the peritoneum. Still they must be regarded as upon the border line of malignancy, and are dangerous because of the extensive local damage they do in·the pelvis and peritoneal cavity, and also the injurious effect they produce upon the general health of the patient. They recur in some cases, though it is believed that when found growing again upon the pedicle from which the original tumor was removed, it is due to an imperfect removal in the first instance. At the same time, they are very prone to develop in the opposite ovary after a brief space. With these facts in mind, I believe it is wise to regard these tumors as malignant and to remove both ovaries with as much of their pedicles as possible. Panhysterectomy even, may be the best operation and give the most favorable and permanent results.

In ovarian tumors of unquestioned malignancy, even though only one organ is the seat of disease, and the other entirely normal, the most rational procedure is the same that we would follow in operable malignant disease of the uterus; the complete extirpation of all the pelvic viscera possible. Recurrence is the rule and the chances of success are slender in any case, but a permanent cure is sometimes possible by such radical treatment, if early. This is rather in opposition to the conclusion of Hofmeier, who has held that in the case of malignancy of one ovary, it is not always necessary to remove the one that is apparently sound. He cites cases in which sarcomata and carcinomata of large size have been excised from one side, the other side being left alone, and which have resulted in complete recovery, the patients remaining in good health, the pelvic functions being performed normally, even conception and childbirth having occurred. But I believe that these cases must be looked upon as exceptional, and that unless radical removal is practiced, other adjacent structures will become involved by direct extension, in the great majority of cases.

Since ovarian inflammations are for the most part secondary to inflammations of other organs in the vicinity, they frequently do not deeply invade or completely destroy the tissue of the ovary, and hence do not necessarily require its entire removal. In many cases the inflammation is quite superficial. This is notably true in gonorrheal infection of the tubes with secondary involvment of the ovaries. In such a case the ovary may be found buried in an inflammatory mass, and densely bound by adhesions. There are evidences of inflammatory change upon its surface, but further examination shows that its parenchyma has escaped serious damage, and when it has been freed from its entanglement and restored to its proper position, it is capable of regeneration and normal function. The gonococcus rarely reaches the inside of the ovary, unless in the case of tubo-ovarian abscess when the whole organ is converted into a pus sac.

The streptococcus usually strikes more deeply and causes extensive destruction of tissue by forming numerous pus foci which enlarge and coalesce, and finally result in a general abscess. Such advanced conditions, of course, demand ablation of the affected organ.

In the superficial variety of infection the treatment must depend upon the extent of involvement of the tunica and the chronicity of the inflammation, for while restoration is possible in some, in others the thickness and cirrhosis of the tunica prevent ovulation, retention cysts form, and as they multiply they crowd upon and destroy the normal follicles, and the ultimate result is a mass of small cysts inclosed in a thick and rigid shell. Such an ovary is painful, particularly at the menstrual period and is absolutely useless. If this condition be unilateral it is well to remove the ovary entirely, leaving the sound one. If both are diseased in the same way it is desirable to excise such portions of both as seem to be the worst affected, and to leave a small fragment of at least one. It is a fact that a mere shaving of ovarian tissue if it bear follicles, will functionate and prevent the distressing symptoms of the artificial menopause. It is therefore necessary to examine both ovaries carefully at operation before attempting any surgical procedure upon either one.

Another class of cases is that in which there is no history of preceding inflammation and no evidence in the pelvis of inflammatory change, except possibly a few slight adhesions. But the pain which the patient suffers is unquestionably traced to the ovaries. They are found to be enlarged and often prolapsed into the cul de sac, and may be moderately adherent. They are studded with unruptured and degenerated follicles, the pressure of which has resulted in the atrophy and practical disappearance of the stroma, and much of the normal parenchyma, and the organs are almost functionless and cause extreme pain. The chronic suffering is greatly exacerbated by the premenstrual afflux of blood to the part, and by futile efforts at ovulation, and patients so afflicted manifest many phases of the so-called reflex neuroses.

What has started this process is often difficult to determine. Whether it be due to simple trophic change induced by displacement, or kinking of blood vessels with interference with the return circulation, or whether it be the result of some remote inflammatory attack, which is undiscovered, may not be known. But it is certain that in its advanced stages the changes in the ovary are permanent and are likely to be progressive. The treatment of these conditions is one of the most perplexing things we have to deal with in ovarian surgery. To remove the ovaries means a bad time for the patient; to leave them means, in many cases, continued pain and invalidism, in spite of puncture, or excision of tissue, or suspension. Puncture is of no value and gives only temporary relief, if any. Excision of tissue removes only a part of the disease, which promptly recurs in however small a fragment that is left. Suspension, which theoretically straightens out the vessels, improves the circulation, and relieves congestion, often results in a vicious adhesion which seems to add to the trouble rather than allay it. The bad results of so-called conservative surgery in this kind of ovarian disease are so common as to be familiar to all, and with these facts in mind, I believe that it is fair to conclude that there is a certain small class of cases of this character, in which total ablation of the ovaries is justifiable and desirable. For unfortunate as the effect of this may be, it is less distressing than the continued pain, the neuroses, and even the psychoses from which the patient will suffer if any ovarian tissue be allowed to remain.

It is, of course, necessary to make a careful clinical study of cases before and after operation; to note the relation between the symptoms and the findings upon the operating table; and to note the modification of symptoms as the result of operation. It is only by much accurate observation and large clinical experience that one may hope to attain success in solving such problems at the time of operation.

(*For discussion see p. 456 et seq.*)

## THE IMPORTANCE OF CONSERVING A PORTION OF THE OVARY.*

### By Lewis S. Pilcher, M.D.,
#### of Brooklyn, N. Y.

THE phrasing of the title expresses very well the scope of the remarks which I wish to make, "The Importance of Conserving a Portion of the Ovary." That hinges entirely upon the importance in the economy which the ovary itself may play. One who is familiar with the surgery of the past thirty or thirty-five years might very readily come to the conclusion that from a surgical standpoint the ovary had no rights that any surgeon need respect. That that condition has continued up to the present time would seem to be the case from the remarks which have been made by the chairman of the evening in introducing the subject for our consideration tonight.

Is there any real reason why the ovary should be conserved?

We have been in the habit of looking upon the ovary very largely as important chiefly in its relations to the perpetuation of the species, as the organ in which the ovum is formed and matured sufficiently for its final expulsion that it may become impregnated and that pregnancy and child-bearing may result. The importance of its preservation from that standpoint depends entirely upon how desirable it may be that children should be multiplied, or, in

* Read before the Brooklyn Pathological Society, April 10, 1913.

particular, that the particular strain, which is represented by the woman in question might be perpetuated. In many instances, of course, we are quite ready to believe that sterility in a particular strain would be a good thing, and that the quicker we bring it to pass and the more easily and safely we accomplish it the better for the human race. That would seem to be the state of mind, apparently, with which many have performed these operations; that is to say here was a case in which the further perpetuation of this particular strain was undesirable and a good opportunity was presented to benefit the human race by stopping this particular strain in it.

Is this, however, the most important view from which to consider the ovary? The surgical relations of the ovary have commanded my interest from the beginning of the time that ovarian surgery was introduced and more especially from the time when that Georgian surgeon introduced to consideration the removal of ovaries which were practically normal because of the supposed possibility thereby to control certain psychoses which the bearers of the ovaries had manifested. The demonstration that by the removal of a normal ovary, the patient would possibly be benefited in some respects by the loss, was the beginning of a most extensive development of ovarian surgery, which has continued to the present time.

During all this time, however, not enough attention, I think, has been paid by surgeons to the importance in the economy of the ovary as an organ aside from its relations to the process of ovulation. More recently attention, however, has been more directed to other functions of this organ as one which has to do with development, with the production of an internal secretion, which internal secretion may have an important bearing upon the general metabolism of the body and particularly that portion of it which involves the questions of sex.

Is it not true, in the light of our present knowledge, both of histology and of physiology, that the ovary is a complex organ; that ovulation is but one of its functions; that in a special degree it is the source and center, especially of those influences which make for what I would call femininity, not that an individual is a woman because she has an ovary, the fact being indeed that she has an ovary because she is a woman, but in the later development of the woman it is this organ which becomes endowed with a special influence over those traits of body and mind which especially characterize the feminine species? Just as the testes dominate the quality of virility in the male, so it is with the ovary in the female, it influences the quality of femininity in the female.

No such tests on a large scale as in man, where there has been an early removal of the testes, have been made in woman as to the effects of the removal of the ovaries in early childhood, but what we are more familiar with is the result of the removal of the ovaries in persons reaching adolescence, and more especially in those who have reached adult age.

Notwithstanding the absence of any experiments in woman as to the influence of the removal of the ovaries in very early childhood upon later development, I think we are justified in the conclusion that the ovary is:

*First.*—A special gland presiding over the peculiar sexual characteristics of woman, and,

*Second.*—That while it is the special gland presiding over the sexual characteristics in the female, it is not exclusively so. It is this which perhaps is the key to the very great differences in individuals which have been noted as resulting from the removal of the ovaries in different women.

That the ovary is but one of a chain of ductless glands which have profound influence over the metabolism of the body is well worthy of our consideration. We have but recently learned somewhat, though as yet faintly, of the influence of the pituitary body over the genital functions and sex characteristics. We have longer and more full knowledge of the close relations of the thyroid and parathyroids over this phase of the bodily changes. Added to these also, as members of this chain which act and react upon each other and upon the body as a whole, we must take the thymus gland, the adrenals, the spleen and possibly, the marrow of the bones, all of which belong to this inter-related and correlated chain.

If we examine the ovary in its histology, we find that there are entering the composition of the ovary, as possible sources of an internal secretion:

First and most important, the lutein cells which form a portion of the corpus luteum, and second, in addition to that and possibly in many cases even more important, the interstitial cells of the stroma. From all these sources there may be, and I am convinced is being continually formed a secretion which is being absorbed and which by its stimulating or activating effect upon the other members of this chain of glands or upon the general other changes throughout the body, has an important relation to the development and maintenance of the nutrition and welfare of the body as a whole exercised by the ovary.

That is the first point which I would make in my reasoning as to the importance of preserving this organ.

In this reasoning there must be at once thrown out all those more important conditions which have been so well developed in the remarks of the previous speakers in which it is a question as to whether, whatever relation this organ may have to the body, its preservation does not entail imminent danger to the body as a whole if it be allowed to remain. If the local condition is such as makes the presence of the ovary one of danger to the whole body it must be taken away ruthlessly without question, but in the greater proportion of cases coming to surgeons for treatment and for decision as to what should be done this is not the case. The great mass of the cases of ovarian trouble are of a much simpler kind. They are the painful ovaries. It is because they are painful, because they are the source of suffering month by month and often day by day, continual suffering to our patients, that they are brought to us and not that they are a source of peril to life or the seat of malignant disease, but they are the seat of pain and the question is as to what should be done to them and if it is proper to remove them *in toto.* Now, when an ovary is removed both local and general effects follow. The immediate effect of the removal of the ovaries is the atrophy of the uterine muscular tissue. In former days when immense myomatous tumors of the uterus often presented themselves for treatment, and the removal of these tumors was attended with extreme, immediate danger of life; many times we contented ourselves with the removal of the ovaries for when the ovaries were removed, the tumors in many cases shrunk and ceased to be of further trouble. Such an effect upon the uterine tissue was a main and immediate local result of the removal of the ovaries.

We know from experimental sources when an ovary is removed that the calcium output in the urine is diminished 50 per cent. The effect, then, of the ovary upon the general metabolism is demonstrated by its relation to this one element alone, the excretion of calcium salts. Further also it has been demonstrated that when the ovaries are removed the phosphorus secretion is very much increased.

Aside from these more manifest results which we can determine by our test tubes and can see with our eyes, after oophorectomy we know that many patients become the subject of all manner of psychoses and neuroses, while, on the other side, others suffer very little. As I have already suggested in a previous paragraph, the difference in this effect upon the different individuals may be due to the varying ability in individuals of the other ductless glands which are related to it to supplement, or take over, the work of the ovary. All of the other ductless glands are roused to increased activity by total ovarian insufficiency, so much so that it is a well-established clinical fact that the thyroid may be so stimulated by the removal of the ovaries that a condition of extreme hyperthyroidism is produced.

My conclusion, then, as the result of these considerations, is that the internal secretion of the ovary is a subject of the highest importance. A natural corollary is that we may have also a condition of hyperovarianism produced from an excessive production of this internal secretion just as in the condition of the thyroid we have an hyperthyroidism where there is an excessive production of thyroid secretion. We know practically and clinically what the symptoms of this hyperovarianism are. We are familiar' with them—that exaggeration of the special sex characteristics, that morbid introspection which seems to attend it, that peculiar mental activity, that exaggerated emotional temperament, that highly excitable nervous tendency which is characteristic of these patients who come to us with their painful ovaries and which it seems not unreasonable to refer to an excessive production of this internal ovarian secretion.

Now, this excessive production of the ovarian secretion, this hyperovarianism, is attended locally with pain, pain referred to the ovary. This pain is exaggerated by the normal ovarian congestion of the menstrual period. Tenderness upon pressure exists, the organ is swollen, tends to prolapse, and when prolapsed further congestions arise and are perpetuated. As to the changes in the ovarian tunic and its contained stroma in the condition referred to, these bear every mark of a chronic inflammatory origin, and the term *microcystic ovaritis* is quite appropriate.

As to the etiology. May it not be—is it not true that there is a possibility of a superficial infection early in life in many of these cases which has caused the thickening of the tunic of the ovary, just as in the testes we have a thickening of the tunica as the result of a mumps or of a scarlet fever or similar infectious disease? May it not be through the tonsils there are infectious materials carried in, which conveyed by the blood-stream, and arrested in the superficial tunica of the ovary so irritate it as to cause this thickening which has interfered with its development and, more particularly, with the proper bursting of the graafian follicles when they are matured and the time for their rupture has come? May not this be the cause of the cysts, these retention cysts, which I am quite sure in many cases are not a temporary thing that come and go with varying conditions of congestion in the ovary, but are a positive entity, a durable affair and that in many cases go on to larger and larger development? Many, many times have we as surgeons when we have uncovered these ovaries seen the stroma of the organ nearly destroyed by the pressure of multiple cysts varying in size, some of them as large as a good-sized marble. And in other cases have we not seen such cysts which have developed to become real tumors attached to or a part of the ovary, the ultimate development of these cystic elements which I am now striving to describe?

Multiple microcystic degeneration, then, I am not as yet convinced is not a disease. It is an accompaniment of much of this condition of ovarian change associated with the symptoms that I have endeavored to describe and which may and does call for treatment.

Then the question is, What is the proper treatment? Shall we when this condition of the ovary is presented to us simply make a pedicle below the ovary and sweep it off? Ofttimes both ovaries are equally affected. Shall we do it on both sides and unsex the patient at once? Too often this has been done. Thereby a surgeon may secure immediate results, but is it the best and proper thing for the surgeon to do in the cases now under consideration? If the ovary is simply—mainly—for the purpose of ovulation in very many cases it would be a great deal better thing if its total removal were done, because of the undesirability of prolonging a peculiar psychical or neurotic strain in the community, but I take it that this is not for surgeons to decide. Our duty is to the particular patient. What is the best for that particular patient?

One point I would make and which I desire to emphasize and to place deeply upon the conscience of all is that total ablation of even such ovaries as have been described is rarely necessary to secure the best results in an individual case as far as the relief of the symptoms suffered by them, while such loss is certainly a very great detriment to the individual as a whole. Partial resection even if there is only a sliver of the ovary left behind, would seem to be far more rational, far more desirable and defensible a procedure. Preservation of some of the ovarian tissue whenever possible certainly should be the aim of the surgeon, and thereby the preservation to the individual of a ductless gland which has important relations to the highest qualities of the woman.

(*For discussion see p.* 456 *et seq.*)

## HYDROTHERAPY AND MASSAGE IN THE TREATMENT OF NERVOUS DISEASES.

### By Henrik N. Hulander,
#### of Brooklyn, N. Y.

PEOPLE have always taken baths in some form, and it appears that the ancients had an instinct for bathing although perhaps they were not able to give a scientific reason for their belief. In Sweden, Finland and Russia are still to be found on some old farmsteads small log houses built exclusively for bathing purposes, and the old folks will tell the visitor that such steam bath cabins were formerly considered a necessity on every farm, and that invariably every Saturday afternoon the members of the family would gather in this "bastun," so called.

In the northern parts of these countries the country people are still in the habit of taking a weekly steam bath in such cabins, and the guest is, as a matter of course, invited to take part. On entering through the low door he gradually distinguishes in the center of the room a great pile of rocks which are being heated by a log fire. Water is occasionally thrown on the stones, which causes a sudden formation of steam, and before long the heat becomes so intense that the visitor—unused to such hot treatment—heartily wishes to escape; but outside are large drifts of snow and he is advised to cool himself in them. Each bather is provided with twigs of birch, and one and all generally succeed in arousing the circulation by lashing himself and the others. The grandfather, 70 or 80 years old, but still strong and active, having taken these baths regularly during his whole life, is generally able to endure the extreme temperature better than the others, which gives him occasion to express his contempt for the younger generation and to utter regretful remarks on the decline and disuse of his favorite bath.

This is apparently water treatment for robust individuals.

The employment of hydrotherapy in disease, however, requires thorough knowledge and good judgment, and many physicians, therefore, not knowing nurses or other persons qualified to carry out their prescriptions, and not having the time to administer the treatments themselves, use these measures little or not at all. Including hydrotherapy as a subject in training schools for nurses somewhat relieves the difficulty, but post-graduate courses in standard schools for these particular subjects are greatly needed.

Peripheral nervous diseases—neuritis, etc.—are extensively treated by massage and hydrotherapy, the best results being accomplished in cases of rheumatic and other origin, when infiltrations around the affected nerve and in the surrounding tissue exist without actual degeneration of the nerve.

The massage treatment in such cases consists of firm, small, circular frictions on and around the nerve, in order to disintegrate the abnormal formations, followed and alternated by effleurage (sweeping frictions) on a large area, for the purpose of bringing out into the circulation the dislodged substances.

In sciatica the nerve and surrounding tissue are thus treated, but the nerve is generally also stretched by raising the leg as far as the pain permits. This is accomplished by first placing the patient's lower leg on the operator's shoulder, then the leg is slowly elevated while the hands clasp the knee in order to prevent the same from bending.

The diabetic, alcoholic and gouty varieties with degenerative changes in the affected nerves give less rapid and satisfactory results, but are nevertheless benefited by general gentle massage. Even peripheral neuralgia of central origin is treated by effleurage and vibrations, since experiments and observation have shown that the treatment of peripheral nerves favorably affects the corresponding nerve center.

Gentle effleurage is the only form of massage used in acute

inflammations, but various hydropathic measures then offer considerable relief. Very hot fomentations applied on a large area over an inflamed nerve are capable of congesting the surface blood-vessels, thereby lessening the congestion of the interior blood vessels vascularly connected, and thus removing the undue pressure and relieving the pain. The application over a painful nerve superficially situated must be short and more often repeated because prolonged heat readily elevates the temperature of the superficial tissues, thereby increasing the pain.

The atonic reaction from heat is prevented by finishing the hot treatment with a short and cold application, or by frequent changes from heat to cold (revulsive), but in these cases the cold should merely absorb the surplus heat in order to produce a pure circulatory effect without a thermic reaction, since the latter, by increasing vital activity, is likely to increase the pain. ‾

Scotch douches, incandescent and arc light, hot air and steam, may be similarly employed, but are less convenient when the patient is confined to bed.

Eliminative treatments are generally prescribed in acute, as well as chronic cases to combat toxemia and for that purpose sweating baths followed by the neutral bath, Scotch douches, or other suitable measures are employed.

In central nervous diseases massage and medical movements, as well as hydrotherapy, often constitute a valuable adjunct to the medicinal and other measures.

The Fraenkel movements and ordinary resistive and medical movements are, as is well known, capable of improving the power of co-ordination in cases of locomotor ataxia. This system is equipped with complicated and expensive apparatus as in La Salpetriere, Paris, but fortunately these movements can be and are given effectively with very simple and inexpensive means. The exercises are performed slowly so as to be controlled by the antagonistic muscles and may be taken in lying, sitting, or standing positions. Overexertion must be guarded against, since the patient himself has more or less lost his sense of fatigue.

However excellent these movements are, they should not be allowed to wholly take the place of massage which was employed with remarkable results even before the Fraenkel movements.

In hysteria, neurasthenia, melancholia, and in the various degrees of nervous exhaustion, general tonic measures that involve a stimulation of vital activities without undue taxation of nervous energy are commonly employed, although sedative and analgesic measures often are indicated and necessary when irritability and pain exist.

General tonic massage is employed since it gives the benefit of exercise at small expense of energy, but the dose must be carefully graduated so as not to cause fatigue. This cannot be too strongly emphasized. Very carefully graduated cold and alternating hot and cold applications, cold friction, revulsive compresses to back and abdomen, Scotch douches, salt rubs, half baths, sitz baths, etc., provide means of stimulating the vital functions without tiring the patient.

The insomnia in these disorders may be relieved by one of the following means given before retiring—the neutral bath, the neutral wet sheet pack, general gentle massage with particular attention to back, neck and feet and the neutral head compress. All these measures lessen the excitability of the cerebral cells and equalize the circulation, but if the head is much congested, special derivative treatments, as hot and cold foot, leg, half or sitz bath with cold compress or ice bags on head and neck, may be employed. The heating abdominal girdle or compress worn over night is capable of drawing large quantities of blood into the abdominal blood vessels, thereby lessening the congestion of the brain.

Insomnia, headache, giddiness and other symptoms resulting from anemia of the brain may naturally require measures that increase the circulation of that organ. Vibration on the head has been tried with good results. Fomentations and revulsive compresses to the head, not only draw more blood to the brain, but cause it to flow at a more rapid rate. A heating head compress effects a continuous increase of circulation in the brain. Moderate heat around the neck dilates the carotids, thereby inducing a more abundant flow to the head. Massage on head and neck is very frequently prescribed in these cases.

Congestive headache requires clearly opposite procedures. Revulsive and derivative measures to the extremities draw the blood mechanically downward, while cold to the neck and head constrict the cerebral blood vessels. Ice bags to neck (back and front) and top of head, with hot fomentations over face, often help when other measures fail.

Irritability of the solar plexus and umbilical ganglia, with accompanying symptoms are often greatly relieved by fomentations or revulsive compresses to the abdomen, as well as by the heating abdominal compress with or without a hot water bag over the stomach.

Muscular activity, although capable of promoting sleep in health, exerts a stimulating influence on the nervous system, which in neurasthenic cases almost invariably causes wakefulness if taken immediately before retiring. Vigorous hand massage, medical movements and general exercises, therefore, are, in these cases, best taken in the forenoon or early afternoon.

The hot water bags and radiators, although convenient, do not constitute the best means of warming the feet, and, if habitually used, not only make the feet more anemic and sensitive to cold, but exert the debilitating effect of heat on the whole body. The alternative hot and cold foot or leg bath, on the other hand, may be repeated not only without harm, but with decided benefit to the whole system, as often as desired.

Nervous and feeble persons are generally enervated by prolonged and repeated heating procedures, but when in such cases an occasional sweat bath is indicated, it is best taken in the form of the electric light bath which induces perspiration at the lowest temperature, and therefore is less weakening than the steam or Turkish bath.

In the treatment of many forms of paralysis a system of exercises and movements calculated to restore and facilitate the normal transmission of motor impulses is successfully employed.

In hemiphlegia, for example, the motion of the affected side is greatly facilitated by letting both sides execute the desired movements simultaneously. The movements are often first demonstrated to the patient, then performed passively, and finally the patient himself makes an effort. Many exercises are more easily performed when the body reclines in water and are therefore, often given in a neutral bath.

Massage prevents the muscles from degenerating and acts indirectly on the nerve centers and is therefore generally employed together with the exercises. Experience has also proven that the most satisfactory results in these cases are accomplished by alternating the two measures, first a few minutes effleurage and kneading of the whole of the disabled affected limb, with particular attention to the affected muscle groups, then a few exercises are given which are followed by more massage, and so on.

The neutral bath and partial tonic applications (cold friction, salt rubs, revulsive compresses, etc.) with the brain well protected by suitable cold applications to head and neck, are the only hydropathic measures that may be given safely in these cases.

To what extent massage is capable of restoring motion in infantile paralysis is not fully known, but the subsequently developing joint deformities (abnormal angles) are certainly checked by systematic employment of that means. When discontinued, however, the deformities gradually develop.

Surgery has won triumphs in these cases by establishing an equilibrium of the muscle arrangements while massage and medical movements have proven their efficiency as an indispensable after-treatment. A mutual and perfect understanding between the surgeon and the masseur becomes, in such cases, necessary, since the latter, by not fully understanding the anatomical changes, may treat the wrong muscles, thereby increasing the difficulty.

In writers' cramp, massage and general tonic hydropathic applications are employed together with the rest of the affected parts.

The usual procedure in severe cases of acute chorea is first massage in conjunction with immobilization for a short time, followed by simple and carefully graduated, self-controlled, and resistive movements, which are most easily controlled by the will, while free-standing exercises are employed only in cases the recovery of which has considerably progressed.

## SOME PHASES OF INHERITED SYPHILIS.

### By Paul L. Parrish, M.D.,

of Brooklyn, N. Y.

SYPHILIS is not a disease of recent discovery but is always of interest, as it is always present with us and its vicious influence is so far reaching.

It is a question of interest whether it is increasing in frequency among the population. I believe it is. There were 1,029 deaths reported due to this cause in the registration area of the U. S. in 1900; in 1909 there were 2,858. The ratio per 100,000 was 3.4 in 1900; in 1909 it had reached 5.6. New York City rose from 4.3 to 7.8 and the rural districts from .9 to 3.1. It is doubtful if the reported cases represent more than one in fifty of the deaths actually due directly or indirectly to this disease. In the year 1909, in which 2,858 deaths were reported, there were but 655 deaths reported caused by smallpox.

A question which has long been discussed is, which parent transmits the disease. It was for long contended that the mother alone could transmit the disease to her child; that the sperm could not carry it. This has been disproven by recent cases in which infection has occurred from contact with the semen. Also it is sometimes possible to cause the birth of healthy children following the birth of syphilitic children by curing the father of his disease. There have been cases where a woman impregnated by a syphilitic man has given syphilitic children without contracting the disease and later given healthy children when impregnated by a healthy man. On the other hand syphilitic mothers usually give syphilitic children, the severity of the infection in the child frequently seems to depend on the recency or age of the infection in the mother, and the more recently the disease has been acquired by the parent the more severe the disease in the child.

Along this line Colles' law is of interest. His theorem as laid down was that a woman acquires immunity by carrying a syphilitic child; also Profeta's law, that a recently infected woman may give birth to a healthy child which is immune to the disease. These laws have fallen into disrepute of recent years since the discovery of the Wassermann test, the modern theory being that they have latent syphilis. But why may not both laws be founded on fact? If the child be infected by the sperm why may not the placenta act as a filter or modifier of the toxic organism so as to allow the mother, or the child in the case where the mother is syphilitic, to be vaccinated by the modified substance passing the placenta? They should then by the formation of immune bodies react positively to the Wassermann test just as the person who has been vaccinated against typhoid reacts to the Widal test.

If the mother contracts the disease while pregnant the child may or may not be syphilitic; if the child is infected there is probably involvement of the placenta allowing the organism to pass through.

What is the mortality of children born of syphilitic parents?

It is very high. Fournier states that in investigating 18 families where there was syphilis, of 161 births there were 137 still-births or 85 per cent. J. N. Hyde reports 916 deaths in the first year out of 1,121 births. In the foundling home in Moscow out of 2,000 cases 70 per cent. died in the first six months. Out of the last 45 cases that I have studied at St. Christopher's Hospital, 28, or 62 per cent. +, died; 16 were improved greatly and one was so greatly improved as to be called cured. As a rule the earlier the child shows signs the more fatal is the case.

The gross pathology of a case of moderate severity is not characteristic except that the child is usually wasted, there is moderate general glandular enlargement, and nearly always there is some increase in size of the liver, spleen, or both. There may be scars around the anus, or mouth, or both. There may be malformations of the cranium or of the long bones.

Microscopically there are always found extensive areas of small round cell infiltration in the affected organs and the blood vessels. The spirocheta may be obtained from the blood, or more easily from the serum of blebs, or the discharge from moist surfaces, and is usually very abundant in the parenchymatous organs and especially the lungs. Two of the cases that are included in this paper had an interesting condition post mortem, the so-called white pneumonia, which is due to a desquamation of the alveolar epithelium in such quantities as to blot out the alveoli. The lung is massive and airless and looks somewhat like Swiss cheese. Children with this condition are usually born dead or die soon after birth, although one of our cases was a year old at the time of his death. All the middle and lower lobe was solid in this case.

The symptoms of inherited syphilis do not differ greatly from those in the adult except there is no division into primary, secondary, and tertiary stages. The condition in inherited syphilis is from the beginning a general infection involving the whole organism, but having a predilection for the viscera and other parts freely supplied with blood, as the growing ends of bones and the blood vessels.

It is of interest to know the symptoms which usually appear first. In children who are born with well marked symptoms there are usually present enlarged liver and spleen; coyza; there may be pemphigus or other skin lesion; and the child is weak and under weight. A child which at birth is weak and much underweight and with enlarged liver and spleen is usually syphilitic; if in addition it has the pecular scars around the mouth the diagnosis is confirmed.

When the symptoms develop after the birth of the child most authorities lay stress on snuffles as the most frequent first symptom. If the discharge is bloody or irritating it is very suggestive. In 16 of the 45 cases on which this paper is based it was the first symptom elicited. Cutaneous rash was the first symptom but once. Failure to thrive without any patent cause is commonly an early symptom and if close search is made confirmatory signs can frequently be made out.

In these cases on admission the liver was enlarged alone in 8 cases, the spleen alone in 4 cases and both in 12 cases.

The peculiar scars which are found around the mouth and nose or the rectum were present in 8 cases.

There were skin lesions in 37 of the 45 cases at some time while under observation.

There is a symptom which as far as I have been able to discover was first mentioned by Dr. J. W. Parrish, which is very suggestive of inherited syphilis. It is a bright red, smooth erythema of the soles of the feet, which may slightly overlap the plantar surfaces. It was the first symptom present in 5 of this series. It has not been observed by us in other pathological conditions.

A condition known as pseudofurunculosis is mentioned by some authors as a pathognomonic symptom of inherited syphilis. It occurs frequently in syphilitic children, but I have frequently seen it in weak hospital babies who did not have syphilis. It is manifested by an eruption of numerous pustules or abscesses which are flaccid and not inflamed.

Hochsinger says that the roseola of adults is never seen in the inherited disease. One of our cases showed as beautiful a roseola as I have ever seen in an adult.

Paronychia is an interesting symptom and is frequently seen. It may be dry or ulcerating. When present with other signs it strongly confirms the diagnosis.

Otitis was not more frequent in this series of cases than in other feeble children.

General glandular enlargement is sometimes a helpful guide to a diagnosis, but by itself I believe it of little value; as in a recent examination of 300 hospital children I found well marked enlargement of two or more groups of glands in more than 66 per cent. of the children. Eighty-two per cent. of the syphilitic children had enlargement of two or more groups of glands. The epitrochlear glands showed palpable enlargement in less than one-half the cases. Enlargement of the epitrochlear, or of a gland on the side of the chest in the 4th or 5th intercostal space has considerable diagnostic significance.

Many of the hæmorrhagic cases in new born infants are caused by a combination of syphilis and a septic condition.

The changes in the skull are sometimes characteristic.

Where the squamous bones are soft, with open sutures and large fontanels, the change may be due either to syphilis or rickets.

Abnormal protuberance of the eminences with hard bony sutures may cause the hot cross bun appearance, which is usually of syphilitic origin.

Periosteal swellings, or rarefaction of the bone in small areas, are usually caused by syphilis.

Syphilitic hydrocephalus may· be caused by an inflammation starting in the inner periosteum of the skull. This is a curable condition.

Continued fever is a symptom rarely mentioned in the books, but during any stage of the disease it may be present, without any other cause than the disease being present. It usually runs an irregular course, but there may be a regular rise and fall. It may last a week or two or may run for several weeks.

There has been much discussion of para-syphilitic conditions in children. Some authors contend that atrophic conditions, failures of proper development, nervous disorders like dementia paralytica, hydrocephalus, and the cerebral birth palsies of children when occurring in children who have not the usual manifestations of syphilis are caused by the depraved generative cell of syphilitic parents. This contention has not been proven. We only know that such conditions are more common in the offspring of parents who are affected with syphilis, alcoholism and lead poisoning than in the offspring of healthly parents.

In studying this series of cases what seems to me the most interesting fact brought out is that while collecting these cases over 11 per cent. of the cases admitted to St. Christopher's Hospital were syphilitic. When one considers that in no sense have we a foundling institution it seems to show a startling incidence of the disease among the poor of this borough. The racial order of frequency was first Italians, second Russian Jews and third Irish.

Of the 45 cases 65 per cent. died, the rest were improved. Over 40 per cent. of the infants died before reaching the age of 6 months.

### Treatment.

In hospital practice I believe the most satisfactory method in infants is by the hypodermic injection of some preparation of mercury. It is safe in a young infant to begin with a dose of one-eighth grain of mercury salicylate once a week and this can be increased to one-fourth grain once a week or even twice a week. Almost every man has some favorite means of treatment. I have found the most difficult part of the treatment is to keep the child alive after relieving the active symptoms of the disease. Every means should be employed to keep the child as well nourished as possible. In combatting the intense anemia which is usually present I have had most success with the

Zambeletti preparations of iron and arsenic by hypodermic injections every two or three days.

The one thing of greatest importance is the prophylactic treatment. In a way it is fortunate that most of these children die, or we might be overwhelmed by a race of defectives.

The last century was one most wonderful in inventions for the improvement of mankind and the relief of his ills, but what in the last century has been done for the suppression of syphilis? Nothing, except that it is probably more successfully treated than formerly.

The ideal of government in this country is one which interferes to the least extent with the personal liberty of our people. But how about the personal liberty of the infant born without any desire on his part to suffer and die, or to live a life limited by disease? The public must be educated to understand the ravages of this disease in innocent children. It is for children a terrible inherited curse. I believe the time will soon come when a syphilitic commercial traveler will not freely be allowed in his travels to infect small hamlets all over a continent with this preventable disease.

What can be done?

1st. The disease should be made reportable as a communicable disease like typhoid or tuberculosis.

2d. The prostitutes found to have it in a transmissible form should be prevented from plying their trade by being confined in an institution until cured, or until they do not show evidences of the disease to a contagious degree. To do this it will be necessary to register them and have them frequently examined.

3d. To protect innocent women and unborn children, both men and women contemplating matrimony should be compelled to show a clean bill of health in this regard, not after an examination by a family physician, but after examination by an impartial physician who is competent to diagnose the disease. In some of the western states there is now a medical examination required.

4th. A concealed syphilis contracted before marriage should be *prima facie* cause for an annulment or a divorce.

5th. The birth of syphilitic children should be reported to the department of health and supervision kept over the infant and its parents till the disease is cured. This should be done by the attending physician if he can keep them under his control; if not, then by the department physicians. In this way accurate statistics could be collected which would give an idea of the actual incidence of the disease which we do not now possess.

6th. As the public becomes educated every case must be reported and kept under supervision as the contagious diseases are now supervised by the department of health. It is said that if you report the cases the patients will not come for treatment and the cases will be concealed and allowed to grow worse without treatment. This may be so for a time, but now every case is concealed from the innocent victims and it is allowed free spread. Most of the victims now take inefficient treatment and go on spreading the disease as their desire pleases them.

This may seem like a dream of Utopia but some such measures must be adopted to control the disease and they will only be allowed after the public is awakened to the seriousness of the present conditions.

## THE OCTOBER MEETING—MINUTES.

THE Forty-seventh Regular Meeting of the Associated Physicians of Long Island was held at Blackwell's Island Saturday October 4, 1913. President Samuel Hendrickson of Jamaica presided and there were about eighty members and guests in attendance. Dr. Charles B. Bacon, our former Treasurer, representing the Hon. Michael J. Drummond, Commissioner of Public Charities of the City of New York, whose guests we were to be, met those who were to go at the foot of Dock Street, Brooklyn, and welcomed them aboard a special boat of the Charities Department. After a pleasant sail we were landed at Blackwell's Island and were received by the Commissioner and his Deputies, and were conducted to the dining hall of the nurses' home where a most enjoyable luncheon awaited us. This was followed by a brief business meeting during which Dr. William B. Brinsmade proposed that our host the Hon. Michael J. Drummond be elected an honorary member of our Society. This motion was seconded and carried by an unanimous rising vote. The Commissioner accepted membership with a few well chosen words.

As the minutes of the previous meeting had been published the reading was omitted by general consent. The Membership Committee through the Chairman Dr. Warren L. Duffield reported the following applications for membership and it was voted to add these names to the roster:

Tasker Howard, 383 Clinton Street, Brooklyn, Univ. Pa., 1903; proposed by Warren L. Duffield.

Frank S. Child, Port Jefferson, L. I., P. & S. N. Y., 1909; proposed by Frank Overton.

Rollin Hills, 216 77th Street, Brooklyn, Cornell, 1905; proposed by Charles M. Fisher.

Drs. Sgier and Freitag have failed to qualify.

Under unfinished business Dr. Elias H. Bartley, by request, read the report of the Committee appointed to report upon the President's address presented at the June Meeting. The report follows:

The Committee on the President's address appointed at the June Meeting reports as follows:

*First.*—Regarding the establishing of an Academy of Medicine on Long Island, your Committee thinks the idea an excellent one and is of the opinion that such an organization will be established on Long Island in the future.

*Second.*—The giving of books and whole medical libraries to the Associated Physicians of Long Island is heartily endorsed.

*Third.*—"A complete revolution in the hospital system.' While the Committee is in accord with the President, it believes that this is a matter that must be brought about according to circumstances and not one that requires any formal action.

*Fourth.*—"Any physician rendering professional services to any of these (charitable) institutions should be paid for his services." This fact is already recognized by the management of many municipal and county institutions and it is probable that some action will be taken, at no distant period, to bring about this reform.

*Fifth.*—"The inefficiency and lax enforcement of our immigration laws." As this matter is in close correlation with the question of National Health, and as active interest is at present being directed toward the establishment of a National Department of Health, the Committee recommend that the Associated Physicians of Long Island do all in its power to further that measure, and the Committee would also suggest that the Associated Physicians of Long Island do its share in seeing that when such a department be added to the National Government, that the Secretary of that bureau be selected from the professional civilian class rather than from the medical ranks that are already receiving pay from the government.

(Signed)    JAMES M. WINFIELD,
WILLIAM BROWNING,
H. BEECKMAN DELATOUR.

The following resignations were received and accepted.

Dr. Leo J. J. Commiskey.
Dr. John F. Fitzgerald.
Dr. Harris Moak.
Dr. Edward F. Marsh.

The following Nominating Committee was appointed by the President to report at the January Meeting: Dr. William B. Brinsmade, Brooklyn, Chairman, Dr. Frank Overton, Patchogue and Dr. Frank T. De Lano, Rockville Centre.

At the close of the business session we had the pleasure of listening to an address by the Hon. Michael J. Drummond who, after saying a few words of welcome, explained the work that had been done by his department in the way of bettering conditions on Blackwell's Island with regard to the care of the sick poor. Mr. Drummond urged the members of our Society to make other visits to the Island and to fully inform ourselves with regard to the work being done there. At the close of the address we were divided into parties, each party in charge of a medical officer, and with the Commissioner in the lead we started a most interesting inspection of the Island institutions, beginning with the City Hospital, from which we went to the well appointed home of the medical internes, then by boat to the hospital for the treatment of tubercular cases, then to the Metropolitan Hospital with its splendid nurses' home and internes' home and finally to the pathological department. We had a most enjoyable and satisfactory visit due to the greatly appreciated courtesy of all whom we met and who did everything possible to make us feel that we were welcome.

The special boat landed us at the point of departure at dusk and we then went to the Hamilton Club, where an excellent dinner was prepared and fully appreciated by the seventy-six members who attended. During the dinner Dr. Sylvester J. McNamara with a very neat speech referred to the success of the meeting and moved that a vote of thanks be tendered Dr. Charles B. Bacon, who had done so much to make it successful. The motion was seconded and carried with a will.

JAMES COLE HANCOCK, *Secretary.*

# CASE REPORT.

## TUBERCULOUS PERICARDITIS WITH COMPLETE OBLITERATION OF THE PERICARDIAL SAC.

### By Louis C. Ager, M.D.,

of Brooklyn, N. Y.

JENNIE M., 14 years, Italian parentage, was admitted to the children's ward of the Home for Consumptives on September 19, 1911. Her father and two children had died, cause unascertained. Mother and several children normal.

The patient had had some minor ailments and had been ill and coughing for about one year.

At the time of admission she was a tall thin girl, flabby, icteroid color; mucous membranes pale; round shouldered with protruding abdomen; tongue coated; hands cold and damp. Her temperature was 101.2; pulse 98; respiration 22. Von Pirquet test positive. Urine, trace of albumin, few hyaline casts.

*Chest Examination.*—Dullness at both apices, more pronounced on the right. Marked dullness over lower half of right chest posteriorly, extending round to the midaxillary line. (Thickened pleura.) Prolonged expiration and subcrepitant rales at right apex. Expiratory sounds almost lost over lower right base at area of dullness. Tactile and vocal fremitus increased at apices, lost at right base. Heart sounds rather faint, otherwise negative.

During her stay in the hospital the temperature (rectal) ranged from 98 to 100, the respiration ranged from 22 to 28 and the pulse from 90 to 105.

The weight rose slowly at first from 74 pounds; later more rapidly but the increase was due to fluid in the abdomen. The question of tubercular peritonitis was discussed and Dr. Jennings was called in. By that time there was considerable edema of the legs and the heart was showing more definite signs of weakness and the conclusion was reached that the fluid was due to cardiac failure and not to abdominal tuberculosis. On November 22d 3,750 c.c. of clear yellow fluid were drawn from the abdomen. This fluid had a low specific gravity, contained very few cells and no tubercle bacilli were found; apparently a true transudate. The patient showed the usual temporary improvement but the abdomen filled up rapidly and on December 19th 5,250 c.c. of fluid were drawn. Temporary improvement again occurred, but the patient died on December 30th, at 6 A. M., of heart failure.

Autopsy, 10.45 A. M., December 30th.

Abdomen distended, walls very edematous, edema extending into the neck. Veins over thorax very prominent. Fair amount of adipose tissue in abdominal wall. Abdomen full of pale straw colored fluid. Omentum small, drawn up, dusky red, old adhesions to intestines. Stomach distended, thin. Old adhesions between the colon and liver. Meso-appendix thickened. Adhesions between stomach and transverse colon. Many old cheesy tubercular glands in mesentery.

Spleen adherent on all sides, many superficial cheesy tubercular areas.

Kidneys normal in size, capsule slightly adherent, kidney tissue dark and congested.

Liver firmly adherent to diaphragm, greatly enlarged and shows amyloid degeneration.

*Thoracic Cavity.* Left lung, recent adhesions to pleura more marked at base posteriorly and to diaphragm. Right lung, old adhesions over most of its surface, particularly at base. Both lungs edematous with patches of consolidation but almost entirely free from tubercles except at apices, particularly the right where there were old tubercular foci with contractions. Tracheo-bronchial glands tubercular, moderately enlarged, some calcified. The pericardial sac completely obliterated; heart removed by cutting out the entire section of the pleura with some lung tissue attached. Cross section under the microscope shows numerous giant cells in both layers of the pericardium with a layer of firmly organized connective tissue, from one to two millimeters in thickness, lying between.

For some unknown reason, in this particular case the inflammatory processes were confined almost entirely to the serous membranes throughout the body, although the point of entrance of the tubercle bacilli was apparently the usual one—the thoracic glands. Either the lungs had some peculiar power of resistance, or the infecting organism had a peculiar affinity for serous surfaces.

There is not very much literature on this subject. Wall, of Georgetown University, had a short paper with bibliography at the Sixth International Congress.* According to him about one-fourth of all cases of pericarditis are tubercular. This statement, however, is very misleading as the conclusion is based on the fact that in a very large percentage of cases of tuberculosis almost all the organs of the body will show infection in the terminal stages. As seen clinically pericarditis in children is in most cases either of rheumatic or influenzal origin.

---

* "Tuberculosis of the Pericardium in Children." J. S. Wall, Sixth International Congress on Tuberculosis, Vol. II, p. 464.

# THE ANNUAL MEETING

## OF THE

# Associated Physicians of Long Island

### WILL BE HELD ON

## SATURDAY, JANUARY 31, 1914

# EDITORIAL

## THE INCOME TAX.

THE following brief resume of the new Income Tax has been received by the JOURNAL from the Treasury Department, with a request that it be published for general information.

"Every citizen of the United States, whether residing at home or abroad, and every person residing in the United States, though not a citizen thereof, must pay a tax of one per centum annually upon his or her entire income in excess of $3,000 if single, or $4,000 if married.

"Where the income of a person is over $20,000 an additional graduated or surtax is charged. Various methods are provided for the collection of this tax.

"Every corporation, joint stock company, etc., no matter how created or organized is also subject to the income tax at the rate of one per cent. upon its entire net income arising or accruing from all sources during the preceding calendar year or during its fiscal year.

"Heavy penalties are prescribed by the law for refusal or failure to file return each year on or before March 1.

"Making false or fraudulent return or statement with intent to evade assessment is a misdemeanor, punishable by fine, or imprisonment, or both.

"Failure on the part of any person, persons or corporation to receive a blank form will not excuse either from making the return required or be relieved from any penalties prescribed.

"Persons or corporations or others who come within the jurisdiction of this new law residing or doing business in the First Collection District, which comprises Long Island and Staten Island, desiring information, blanks, etc., should communicate with William J. Maxwell, Collector, First District, Post Office Building, Brooklyn, New York."

Commenting upon the law in its application to physicians, there are some points of interest that should be emphasized, as a physician's income from his professional work differs somewhat from the income of a man in ordinary commercial pursuits. Just as the latter is permitted to credit the legitimate expenses of conducting his business against his gross income, so a physician is privileged to consider as legitimate expenses the up-keep, but not the original cost of an automobile; his expenses for telephone hire, for wages of an office assistant and, if his office be away from his home, for office rent. The question as to his right to charge a certain per cent. of his house rental as a proper running expense is one that is open to discussion. On the one hand it may be urged that having his office in his home does not entail any additional expense for office up-keep; on the other hand the average physician unquestionably pays a larger rental than does the ordinary citizen because he is in a measure compelled to keep up an appearance of prosperity for its effect as a business asset. It would seem only fair that he be permitted to regard at least a part of his rental if he rents, or a percentage upon the value of his property, if he owns, as a legitimate business expense. Salaries drawn from City, State or Federal employment are exempted in addition to the $3,000 allowed by the law.

The Editor has been too busy studying his own exemptions to moralize upon the probable affect of this added burden which the wisdom of the present administration has shifted from foreign to domestic shoulders, but he feels a shrewd suspicion that the Ananias Clubs will be inadequate and will probably be supplemented by a few Sapphira Sisterhoods.                    H. G. W.

## A VICIOUS DECISION.

A JURY in the Supreme Court on October 15th, awarded $7,000 damages to a nurse on the ground that in the year 1910 a boy ten years of age, under her care, struck her in the breast in a moment of anger and ten months later a malignant cancer developed from the blow. Counsel for the defendant contended that in the first place there was no evidence that she had been struck, and secondly denied that a blow was the cause of the cancer, but, nevertheless, the jury awarded the nurse $7,000 damages.

The case is of peculiar interest to physicians inasmuch as it goes to show, first the unsatisfactory state of medical testimony and next the authority that a lay jury may arrogate to itself in settling a question which has heretofore remained in doubt. A cursory examination of several text books on surgery, some of them containing articles upon cancer of the breast by men whose special study qualifies them to speak with authority, shows that there is still a divided opinion as to the traumatic origin of cancer. Our present ignorance of its etiology makes it impossible to deny that trauma may result in cancer, but at the most injury can only be a contributing cause, for otherwise every woman would likely develop mammary carcinoma, as it is doubtful whether a woman can be found who has not at some time of her life suffered some injury to the breast. The same holds good for cancer of the male breast. To argue that injury is the cause is at best to argue *post hoc propter hoc,* the most fallacious form of argument. The human tendency is ever to hark back to some particular occurrence which may explain a coincident happening. It is as fair to attribute birth marks to maternal impressions as to claim an injury as giving rise to cancer. Ten months, too, is a brief period in which a florid cancer may develop. It would seem that this view should be sufficiently logical to influence a jury in approaching such a subject in the light of common sense, but it was evidently insufficient to shake the public belief that cancer results from injury. Probably the contradictory expert testimony offered had much to do with the verdict and might well have been the real factor in the failure to carry conviction to the jury.

Until physicians can, as a whole, realize their duty to one another and can be made to testify, not from self interest but from motives of honor and unswervering fidelity to the spirit of truthfulness, we must expect to fail in any effort to carry conviction, even in cases where the truth seems evident.     H. G. W.

## THE OCTOBER MEETING.

THE Society is to be congratulated upon the quality and character of its recent meetings none of which has been more interesting and valuable than that of October 4th when we were the guests of the Commissioner of Public Charities at Blackwell's Island. Physicians in general are too little informed about the very things of which they should know most, and the generous opportunities which were offered the Society to inspect the work of the Charities Department in its various institutions cannot but be most helpful in arousing interest in the work which the City is conducting in its various charitable institutions.

It is not so very many years ago that the very name of the County Hospital and the Poor House caused a shudder in the unfortunate whose lack of means necessitated his becoming an inmate of one or the other. Today there are no better hospitals in equipment and medical and nursing service than the great hospitals conducted for the city poor. The policy of those to whom this work has been entrusted has been both broad and on a high plane. They have appreciated that efficiency depends not so much upon expenditure as upon the qualifications of the men to whom the working out of their plans must be entrusted and the results should cause a thrill of civic pride in every one who has had an opportunity to see what a city hospital should be. The lesson of efficient hospital management as worked out in the Department of Charities is one that may be well taken to heart by Boards of Managers of so-called private hospitals where too often the administration of the institution is placed in hands that are not qualified to appreciate the real needs of a hospital. A trained medical superintendent is as much an essential as a trained engineer is for a locomotive and without one the chances are all in favor of such an institution falling far below the limit of its capability.     H. G. W.

## A MEMORABLE ANNIVERSARY.

ON October 16, 1846, in the operating room of the Massachusetts General Hospital, Dr. Thomas Morton, before an audience of more than doubters, demonstrated for the first time that complete anæsthesia by means of ether was a safe and practical means of obviating the terrors that until then had surrounded surgery and opened the way for the marvels that we are apt today to consider as matters of course. It is most appropriate that this anniversary should be a matter of yearly celebration in the hospital where Morton's discovery was first demonstrated. We can now afford to forget the recrimination and heart burning and the disputes that arose as to priority of discovery. It was but a short time after that Sir James Y. Simpson demonstrated the anæsthetic properties of chloroform and about the same time Horace Wells introduced nitrous oxide into dental practice. There were giants in those days and among them the names of Morton, Simpson and Wells, two from New England and one from Edinborough, loom very large indeed.
     H. G. W.

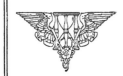 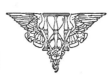

# Society Transactions

## TRANSACTIONS OF THE BROOKLYN PATHOLOGICAL SOCIETY.

*Stated Meeting of April* 10, 1913.

The President, Dr. P. M. Pilcher, in the Chair.

### The Pathology of the Ovary.

*(See pages* 419, 423 *and* 426.)

Dr. John O. Polak, in opening the discussion, said:—"It has been a rare privilege to listen to a discussion of this subject by men who have such experience and such definite opinions on the subject. It presents itself to us here frequently.

"Personally, I am very much in accord with all that has been said. I am going to confine myself to a few points that clinical observation impressed on me in my limited surgical work. In the first place, conservatism of the ovary, to my mind, is leaving that ovary alone—the true conservatism.

"I am very much in accord with Dr. Frank in the belief that the ovary, *per se*, is not the site of inflammatory disease; that it is in bad company we all know. It is presumably the tube which seems to be the conduit for all infections or a large number of them. Disease is localized in the peritoneum which again is a reservoir of a number of infections, places the ovary in a most embarrassing position, and yet that ovary will live, recover itself, and functionate. I speak of this particularly and want to impress on you one thing, and that is the necessity in the placing of an ovary or in the conservation of an ovary of securing its proper circulation and position. An ovary cannot work out of position. If it is out of position it has its circulation impaired. If it has its circulation impaired, we will notice coincidentally that there are varicosities in the broad ligaments on the side exactly similar to the varicocele in men, consequently the position of the ovary and its circulation have much to do with its function and whether it becomes microcystic or whether it has a thickened tunica.

"Now, when we have to do resection, which has been referred to tonight, and we have taken up this subject from many aspects in several series, we have about come to the conclusion that resection of the ovary should be confined to a certain definite class of tumors. We resect the ovarian cyst. I have resected only recently (I say recently, within a year), two large ovarian cysts, one as large as a man's head and the other as large as a child's head, from an ovary, leaving good ovaries behind, and have seen the woman become pregnant and have watched those ovaries up to the time of pregnancy. I cannot feel them now, as she is seven or eight months pregnant. The fibroid may be resected and healthy ovarian tissue left.

"I take exception to what Dr. Pool has said in regard to dermoids; that is, there are a large number of dermoids that can be resected from the ovary and the ovarian structure and functionating ovaries preserved.

"There is a class of cases that has been of very great interest to us lately, because, as you all know, we will have in a certain group of cases a series which will go along and present similar symptoms, a series of amenorrhœas have come to us with prolapse of both ovaries, varying from a year to fifteen or eighteen months. These cases have all presented one definite picture on exploration, and that is the large, smooth, white ovary with an extremely thickened tunica. It has been extremely interesting to notice that the resection of those ovaries down to nearly the hilum of the ovary has re-established menstruation and re-established functional ovaries.

"Another point to which I would call your attention is the tendency of a large number of men in tubal pregnancy to attack the ovaries without stripping them from their neighbors, that is, from their associations. The ovary is beneath a thickened mass, and because an ovary is a mass of material they sacrifice that individual ovary; and, again, because on the opposite ovary there has developed a corpus luteum cyst, they remove the ovary on the other side because it is cystic. That is a natural consequence of pregnancy. It will form a corpus luteum and it will become cystic in a large number of cases.

"Again, in resection, I want to call your attention to the fact that the ovary always swells as the result of resection. It sometimes takes three months for the ovary to return to its normal size, but if sufficient care is given to the patient that ovary will regain its activity and its proper function.

"One very interesting matter has been brought up here tonight, and that is the effects of castration. I find that castration in an analysis of a number of cases differs in different individuals under different circumstances, and we came to a few conclusions some two years ago. If you castrate women, taking the ovaries out, when you do an hysterectomy, the nervous symptoms are very much less marked as the result of castration when associated with inflammatory disease. You will further find that a woman in health will bear castration much more poorly than a woman who has been more or less exsanguinated and is regaining health and has a complete operation. Furthermore, a woman with a high blood pressure before operation has extremely marked neurasthenic symptoms as the result of castration, whereas a woman without a high blood pressure will not have as much nervous phenomena as will a woman with a high blood pressure. Those are simply some of the points one could wish to make as the result of a limited clinical experience in the resection of the ovary.

"In closing, I desire to say that surgery of the ovary itself is very insufficient and incomplete. All of the elements that contribute to the relation of that ovary so far as position and construction are concerned, such as fixations of the uterus, versions of the uterus and colonic stasis—all of those things bear a relation to the ultimate success of what you will do in any individual pelvis."

Dr. William J. Cruikshank, in discussion. said:—"I do not know why Dr. Pilcher should have had my name printed to discuss this question after the galaxy of stars that are doing ovarian surgical work all the time, and so the only excuse I presume I can offer is, that if I add anything on the subject, it will be from the standpoint of the man practicing general medicine.

"I observed that the keynote that has been struck this evening by every gentleman is that of conservatism in this question, and I couldn't help thinking, when I listened to that note being struck by every preceding gentleman, how much the surgeon is learning from the internist. It certainly is very interesting indeed.

"The literature on this subject and the whole question to those of us who have been through the post-radical period and those of us who have traveled along the line of the radical period and then the conservative, is certainly very interesting indeed. I think it was as far back as 1882 that Spencer Wells reported a thousand cases of ovarian operation for the purpose of demonstrating what has been said tonight by Dr. Pilcher and Dr. Polak and the other gentlemen. Following his suggestions along these lines came those of William H. Roke, who also made a strong plea for conservatism along this line as early as the Early Ages. Kelly, in referring to that question, says that it wasn't at all surprising to him that such tremendous radicalism should be used in ovarian surgery when we take into consideration the tremendous radicalism that was applied to surgery generally, and he refers, as an illustration, to a case which was brought into the hospital when he was an interne, of a bright, wise, healthy boy suffering from a perfectly clean compound fracture of the humerus and a perfectly clean, simple fracture of the radius and ulna upon the other side and an amputation of both extremities for the relief of the difficulty. That, Kelly says, was most amazing to him, but it was in perfect accord with what was being done with the surgery of the pelvis to the same extent, so I have concluded from Dr. Polak's remarks appertaining to the fact that the ovary was in bad company sometimes when it was lying in a mass of suppurated tissues perhaps, or close to it, that there was one other bad companion that the ovary could have, and that would be a young and inexperienced surgeon with great surgical aspirations.

"I feel, however, Mr. President and gentlemen, very much encouraged, I am sure, in speaking from the standpoint of the general practitioner, and I find Dr. Polak, Dr. Frank, Dr. Pool and Dr. Pilcher are in perfect accord with the feelings I have had for a great many years regarding the ovary, and I certainly feel I am in very good company. Those of us who have seen these cases that have passed out of the surgeon's hands after having been operated for these conditions, many of them now declared to have no specific pathological entity, and having attempted to relieve the psychic and other nervous conditions produced by the removal of the ovaries, certainly are very much impressed with the great importance of conserving the ovarian tissue. I learned something about that question from one of the most—said to be one of the most radical surgeons in Brooklyn—Dr. George R. Fowler. I remember having seen him operate on a case in which he left the merest sliver of ovary, and, turning to me, he said, 'Cruikshank, this little sliver will save you very many anxious thoughts and save the patient a great many uncomfortable experiences.' That patient is still a patient of mine and is perfectly well. That was twenty years ago, and I do not remember to have ever had to prescribe for her for any of the nervous conditions of which Dr. Pilcher has spoken so very nicely. I do not feel like taking up any further time in the discussion of this general question, and speaking again simply from the standpoint of the practitioner doing general medicine, 1 would say that this discussion is certainly a very happy one, in that it strikes the keynote of this whole question when it insists upon conservatism in the surgery of the ovary and when the discussion brings to the general practitioner's mind the fact that the ovary has more for its function than mere ovulation, but that it is an organ which has for its function besides that the development of an internal secretion which controls to some extent in conjunction with the other glands of that character, the entire metabolism."

DR. ROBERT T. FRANK, of Manhattan, in discussion, said:—"I will try to be brief. I was somewhat handicapped in what I said because I tried to keep from encroaching upon the field of the other speakers, especially the subject which Dr. Pool was to discuss. Evidently, in spite of my good intentions, I was not quite able to refrain from encroaching upon his ground.

"A few points have been brought out to which I would like to refer. Personally, I am unable to distinguish at the operating table whether an ovary is merely superficially affected by inflammatory processes. Of course, when, as Dr. Pool mentions, the entire ovary has become involved in the purulent process, that is, if we have an ovary changed into an abscess cavity, it is very easy to differentiate the condition, to recognize that the ovary has to be removed; but I am unable to distinguish, in the non-purulent inflammations, between the merely superficial and the deeper involvements of the gland, and would, even upon exploratory section of the ovary, be unable to do so.

"Unfortunately, physiological changes which might take place after castration in early childhood cannot be followed out to the later stages in a human being, because the operation is almost always performed for sarcomata, and these conditions invariably recur in two or three years; therefore, we have no data on this subject in the human being. In animal physiology, of course, Dr. Pilcher's remarks about the importance of the ovaries as glands of internal secretion are fully borne out.

"As to hyperovarianism in the human being, it is very difficult to recognize such a condition. Here again we have to turn to the animal kingdoms, and I must acknowledge that the veterinarians are many steps in advance of us. There is, for instance, a symptom-complex in mares; nymphomania is the term generally employed, and practically all the signs referred to by Dr. Pilcher as occurring in the human being are noticed in the animals. Here castration causes immediate and complete relief, but I do not, of course, recommend it in human beings where the psychical elements play such an important role."

DR. L. S. PILCHER:—"Are you aware whether in any of these animals a partial removal or an entire removal of the ovary has been done?"

DR. FRANK:—"I think entire removal has been the rule, but veterinary literature is so incomplete and thorough reports are so wanting that in my cursory examination of the subject I have been unable to find any very definite data except as to the symptomatology and effect of radical treatment."

DR. L. S. PILCHER:—"It would be very interesting to have veterinary surgeons' attention called to that and ask them to experiment to that end."

DR. FRANK:—"I was in communication with Dr. Williams, the obstetrician of the veterinary college at Ithaca, but he had such a press of work along other lines that he was unable to take up certain of these allied subjects.

"As to the polycystic ovary, the best illustration I know of to show that these polycystic conditions may be transitory, at least in certain instances (because no one in our present stage of knowledge can with justice give definite opinions on this subject), is furnished by the enlargement noticed in hydatid-mole and chorio-epithelioma of the uterus. Here, as a regular ocurrence, the ovaries enlarge immensely. We may have cystic tumors the size of a child's head. In former years it was the custom to remove these ovaries, even if they could be saved, when an hysterectomy was performed for uterine chorio-epithelioma. There are several cases on record where large tumors (particularly the cases reported by Fraenkel), consisting of these polycystic ovaries were seen at operation and were left in situ. Within the course of a year or less the ovaries returned to their normal size. This is the most exaggerated form of polycystic ovary and is purely a functional change.

"Referring to the amenorrhœas which Dr. Polak mentioned, here again we have to turn to the veterinarians for aid. In cows there is a condition called 'dumb rut.' These cows fail to rut, sometimes passing two to four periods. The veterinarians have become aware of the fact that in this condition one or both ovaries are enlarged. They resort, therefore, to a very crude procedure. They seize the enlarged ovary through the rectum and squeeze it out. What they do is to express a persistent corpus luteum. Within four weeks (I think the cycle of the cow is four weeks), menstruation is re-established and the fertility of the animal returns. I do not mean to imply thereby that all cases in the human are due to this same condition, but probably some are due to persistence of the corpus luteum.

"If I am not taking up too much of your time there are two or three other things to which I would like to refer. Personally, I feel that in doing resection of an ovary we lay the patient open to certain not always avoidable dangers; if, for instance, a portion of the ovary, during our manipulation, is made intraligamentous, intraligamentous cystic tumors may develop, which press upon the pelvic organs, and require removal on account of pain. I know of no operation which is technically more difficult than the removal of such a cystic remnant. They attach themselves most firmly to the entire course of the ureter and certainly give the operator who undertakes to remove them a bad half hour.

"In removing that 'bad companion' of the ovary, the tube, it is very important that we should not use a mass ligature. It is preferable to remove the tube by tying it off close to the edge of the tube itself and then to catch the bleeding vessels by whipping over the raw edge of the broad ligament; otherwise, the ovarian circulation is markedly interfered with.

"A cystic corpus luteum is considered a perfectly normal condition at a certain period of the involution of the corpus luteum.

"In conclusion, the most important thing to realize is that inflammatory conditions should be left alone until we have merely to deal with the residua of the inflammation; then we are in position to do conservative surgery.

"Lately I have resorted, with great success, to the X-ray in the menorrhagias and metrorrhagias due to ovarian inflammations. I invariably precede the X-ray treatment by a preliminary curettage in order to exclude any possibility of malignant uterine condition.

"Finally, I would like to repeat that in tumors we must be guided on the one hand by the factor of safety, and, therefore, it is most essential to be thoroughly familiar with the gross appearance of various kinds of tumors; and, on the other hand, we must sometimes be influenced by the expressed wishes of the patient in regard to future possibility of fertility."

DR. WM. P. POOL in closing the discussion, said:—"I have nothing to add except that I am in accord with those who have spoken of the danger of operating upon the ovary in the acute stage of inflammation. There can be no two opinions upon that point; and I also believe that it is much better to let the ovaries alone until one is absolutely convinced that the symptoms are caused by them and by nothing else. It should be our object to operate, when operation is necessary, not upon an inflammation, but upon the effects of inflammation."

DR. LEWIS S. PILCHER, in closing the discussion, said:—"I would like to take the opportunity, Mr. President, to simply say how greatly I have personally appreciated the remarks of our colleagues who have honored us by their presence here this evening, and to express my thanks for what they have done for us."

# TRANSACTIONS OF THE BROOKLYN SURGICAL SOCIETY.

*Stated Meeting, April* 3, 1913.

WALTER A. SHERWOOD, President, *pro tem,* in the Chair.

*(Continued from page* 418.)

### Review of 150 Cases Observed at the Mayo Clinic.

*By Dr. John A. Lee.*

DR. MATHIAS FIGUEIRA, in opening the discussion, said: "There is a point in regard to cancer of the rectum about which I would like to say a few words. It is not long ago (about a year) since I heard in this room a statement that surgery of the rectum was so complete that we did not have anything better to wish for. Well, it seems to me that this statement cannot be borne out, and Dr. Lee probably will agree with me if he looks back to what he saw at the Mayo clinic, and one class of cases that the doctor brought to my mind in speaking are those cases too far up to be reached from below and too far down to be reached from above. Now, cases of cancer of the descending colon and of the sigmoid that can be brought out and operated in two stages are all right enough; cases of the rectum that can be reached from below and be operated are good enough; but there is one variety of the recto-sigmoidal cancer, just at the junction of the upper part of the rectum with the sigmoid, that when you open the abdomen and try to reach them from above, they are fastened down and you cannot pull them, and you cannot get them out of the abdomen and do the anastomosis or two-stage operation, and, on the other hand, when you try to reach them from below, they are too far up and you cannot reach them very well, and when you excise them you have the anastomosis where the gut is not covered by peritoneum, and these are the cases where the trouble is and where the mortality is great, and Dr. Lee will bear me out, even at Mayo's clinic."

DR. R. P. SULLIVAN, in discussion, said: "Dr. Lee's report is one of personal observation; hence there is little room for discussion. However, when he mentioned that Dr. Mayo had reported 100 cases of gastroenterostomy which had been undone, Dr. Lee failed to bring out the point that these were patients who had the gastroenterostomy made at other hospitals and not at the Mayo clinic.

"Some of these cases were operated during my service at the Mayo clinic. The conditions which were found in some were chronic gall-bladder disease, chronic appendix, and one case I recall turned out to be one of diverticulitis of the sigmoid. In all the cases the gastroenterostomy was 'unhitched' and the proper surgical relief given. I recall one case which had been operated by Dr. Mayo and subsequent history led to the suspicion of a gastro-jejunal ulcer. At the second operation the gastro-jejunal opening was found patent, and at one angle a thickening, which was at first considered an ulcer. However, further exploration demonstrated an irritation due to a linen knot. This was excised and the anastomosis enlarged. The result has proved satisfactory ever since, the patient being a physician of Philadelphia.

"Dr. Lee, in speaking of the treatment of duodenal ulcer, failed to mention that Dr. Mayo has recently excised a number of these ulcers. During my term of service inversion of the ulcer and anastomosis was the rule, and I know this to be the method of treatment in a majority of cases at the present time. Of late, however, the Finney operation has been practised in a number of cases. Dr. Bogart will perhaps tell us more specifically the routine of today.

"As for the work in the operating room, you are all quite familiar with that now. You have seen a routine which is simplicity itself. The same thing may be said of the post-operative care. The routine treatment is established, and hence no frills and fancy. This is the reason why one can scarcely appreciate the stupendous amount of work accomplished.

"I recall one day when forty-two cases were operated. We started at 7.30 A. M. and finished at 2.45 P. M., and later in the day and evening Dr. Judd had four immediate acute cases. The great majority were major cases. It was simply a day when an overflow of cases had to be attended to in order that the standing list could be handled the following week.

"As regards the post-operative care of the patients, I have said that it was a simple routine. There is nothing done behind closed doors; inspection is open to all physicians. Each interne carries about forty cases a day on his list for dressings. He must look after his own supply of dressings, for nurses have no time to carry on the usual formality of preparing each case. The entire procedure is most simple. Each package contains sterile towels, gauze and cotton and paper bag for waste or soiled dressings. The work must be accomplished, and therefore the interne will have to hustle. Rounds are made at 7.05 A. M. and 6 P. M. by the attending surgeons and the internes must be ready. A big advantage is the fact that sterile water is on tap throughout the entire house. They do not use intravenous saline, considering subcutaneous the best. The saline can be made up in any part of the house, and I never saw infection follow its use.

"The diet is wholesome and very simple; the results are simply marvelous. If one could see the after-results as I did, I know all who saw would be just as enthusiastic."

DR. WALTER TRUSLOW, in discussion, said: "Could I ask the doctor to say in discussion how they avoid that which we all of us are more or less bothered with, where several cases are to be attended to, the waiting between cases which are to be operated, the going from one to another; does the surgeon finish the whole thing, or are there enough assistants to finish an operation?"

DR. R. P. SULLIVAN, in discussion, said: "The cases wait out in an anteroom; the majority of them walk in. If Dr. W. J. or Dr. C. H. Mayo or Dr. Judd are talking, generally the first assistant will go ahead and close up. It takes about five minutes to change the operating room and get another case in."

DR. J. B. BOGART, in discussion, said: "We see things with different eyes. Sometimes we see different things. Now, about sterile water. The water is passed through a boiler and is not sterilized in any other way. That will surprise Dr. Sullivan, I think, but I went into the matter very carefully with Dr. Wm. J. Mayo. He is continually insisting that we pay too much attention to aseptic frills.

"Anesthesia at this clinic is peculiar. Narcosis is very light. Very frequently during operation the patients are kicking their feet. They are thoroughly strapped down. The quantity of ether used, which is always given by a trained nurse with large experience, is surprisingly small and at the end of an operation the patient very promptly awakens. Dr. William J. told me that they have never had a death from ether at St. Mary's Hospital, and when you remember that the number of anesthesias is something over seven thousand a year, embracing all kinds of cases, this showing is pretty striking.

"They have tried out gas, gas and oxygen, and think that there is nothing in it and do not use it. They think Crile will soon get over his anoci-association.

"In regard to goiter operations, they are doing a great many one-vessel ligations as a sort of test of what the patient can stand. If the patient does not stand well ligature of one superior thyroid, they tie the vessel on the opposite side within a week and then send the patient home for three or four months before attempting to remove any of the gland. If a patient stands ligature of one vessel well, they remove a portion of the gland at the end of a week. In all bad goiter operations one of the first things they do is to divide the isthmus and uncover the trachea. They lay great stress on the fact that in goiter operations accidents are most often due to respiratory obstruction. They very quickly cover the capsule with forceps, which gives them a chance to lift up on the gland. In case of difficulty in respiration or hemorrhage, a simple lifting up will relieve the respiration and control the hemorrhage.

"In speaking of the goiter operation I was impressed by a remark which Dr. John B. Murphy made at his clinic. The chief requisites for the operation, he said, are the nerve of the operator, good light and plenty of artery clamps. In a goiter operation at St. Mary's Hospital they frequently use from seventy-five to a hundred pairs of forceps. They do a great many bilateral operations. In adenomata they frequently leave the middle portion of the gland with a small portion of one or both lobes.

"Coming to ulcer of the stomach and of the duodenum, Dr. Lee's and Dr. Mayo's views are quite at variance. I was very much impressed by the regularity with which stomach and duodenal ulcers are diagnosed in this clinic and when you take account of the different factors they have there is no wonder as to this. Their statistics prove that about fifty per cent. of the diagnoses are made from the history alone; then there is the careful physical examination, the X-ray and the test meal, which is always removed and examined by an expert. One man removes thousands of test meals and makes thousands

4

of examinations. That is very different from having an interne do this, as you never can tell whether he will recover the meal or not, but this one examiner has never failed.

"Stomach ulcers are either excised or else they are sewn in in a peculiar manner, which Dr. William J. has published, and which he believes practically cuts the ulcer out. The first through and through suture which completely surrounds the ulcer is covered again by others placed outside of it.

"I saw no duodenal ulcers excised except in one case, where a pylorectomy was done. The rule was to exclude the ulcer by sutures and then to cover it with an omental graft, at the same time temporarily occluding the pyloric orifice by a stitch or two of silk or linen, and doing a gastroenterostomy. At the present time Wm. J. is of the opinion that a gastroenterostomy should be done in all ulcer cases. Either excision or suture enclosure is apt to stir up trouble and the case is likely to do better if a gastroenterostomy is done.

"In regard to the diagnosis, they are making great use at the present time of the X-ray in screen work. I saw the report for the first quarter of the X-ray work alone. In that report, Dr. Carmen, the Röntgenologist for this department, stated that out of twenty-eight cases operated on in which a cancer of the stomach had been found, twenty-two had been diagnosed correctly by the X-ray; in four cases a diagnosis of cancer had been made by the X-ray in which none was present, and in two cases there was a cancer present which the X-ray had not revealed. He also made the statement that he thought those errors would be corrected by improvement in the technic and more attention to the interpretation of what had been seen. That practically says that all cancers of the stomach may be diagnosed by the X-ray when properly used.

"The reports of the work on cancer of the stomach are very gratifying indeed. They show, of 500 cases operated, 25 per cent. of five-year cures and 38.41 per cent. of three-year cures. I have seen as many as four duodenal ulcers in one morning in this clinic.

"Dr. William J. is removing the gall-bladder in almost all cases. When I visited the clinic three and a half years ago they were almost all drained. I asked him particularly whether he had settled the question in his own mind, and he said no; that they had done about 6,000 gall-bladder operations, but he was not satisfied whether to drain or take the gall-bladder out. He said he was taking the gall-bladder out and Charlie was draining, and that they would compare results. A great many of these cases had been operated on before, some a number of times. For common duct cases where the adhesions are universal and extremely dense, he is using a rectangular incision down the middle line to within an inch of the umbilicus and then across the rectus muscle as far to the right as is necessary in order to turn up a flap. It is a safe incision where you have dense adhesions or where the common duct lies deep. I have seen the results of suturing of the wound after this incision and the scar is in no way different from any other. There seems to be no objection to this incision and it is very useful in complicated cases.

"I do not see how it would be possible to compare the work we do with the work at the Mayo clinic because of the character of the cases that they get. I said to William J. one morning, after I had been there three weeks, that I had not seen a drop of pus. He said: 'I will show you some this morning,' and sure enough, in removing a gall-bladder there was a purulent discharge, so they do have pus at St. Mary's, but it must be remembered that they have from 25 to 40 cases a day. I understand that there had been some other pus cases during the three weeks, but I did not see them.

"There are very many other interesting features at this time that I would be glad to speak of, but time will not permit."

DR. L. W. PEARSON, in discussion, said: "I would like to ask one question relative to the diagnosis of cancer. Dr. Bogart said that twenty-two cases of cancer were diagnosed before operation. I would like to ask if these twenty-two cases were in the operable stage or, if not, what percentage of the cases were operable?"

DR. J. B. BOGART, in closing the discussion, said: "I could not tell you that. I think I saw two or three. I have heard Dr. William J. make the statement that about 75 per cent. of cases of cancer of the stomach that came into their clinic were in the operable stage."

### Adenocarcinoma of the Rectum.

*By Dr. F. W. Wunderlich.*

Ida R., single, age 64, native of Germany, came to my office August 24, 1912. She had always been in good health, had never any serious illness until about four months prior to her visit. Her sickness commenced with severe pain in the upper part of the abdomen and diarrhœa. She continued to have severe pain for about two weeks; since then she has been almost free from pain, but the diarrhœa has continued up to the present time. She complained that the food would pass through her rapidly. Half an hour after she had eaten she would have a stool, and the larger portion of the food would appear in it without having undergone any material change. She had noticed this first in April, and it has continued to act so since. She had been suffering with hemorrhoids about the same length of time. The patient had a good appetite, but she felt weak and had lost considerable weight. She had been under treatment, but the looseness of the bowels had never been controlled or checked.

Her complexion was sallow. Examination of the abdomen did not reveal anything abnormal, except a small mass in the lower left portion of the hypogastric and inguinal region, but she had no pain and no tenderness on pressure. Heart and lungs were normal. On examination of the anus, I found several hemorrhoids and a tumor with marks of malignancy. The finger detected a number of small nodules projecting into the lumen of the bowel, from the size of a small pea to that of a hazel-nut. The surface was smooth and not ulcerating. About two inches above the orifice a constricting ring was found.

*Treatment.*—Total abstinence from milk, coffee and tea. I prescribed R pulv. opii gr. vi bismuth, subcarb. one-half dram sacchar, albi one dram M. F. chartasxii S. A powder three times a day half-hour before meals.

She called again August 26th. The powders had given her much relief, the diarrhœa had been checked, and she felt much better.

The mass in the lower portion of the left hypogastric and inguinal region disappeared entirely after two good doses of ol. ricini had been given. To the sister of the patient I explained the nature of the disease, its probable course, and told her the only chance for a cure was in removal by operation; that the patient would lose the control of her bowels, and that it was impossible to tell whether the disease would return or not.

I sent the patient to Dr. L. G. Baldwin for examination. He concurred with my diagnosis and thought it was a case for operation.

Dr. Eastmond made a thorough X-ray examination to ascertain the presence or absence of any complications higher up in the intestines.

For a time the patient felt so much better, had so little pain and inconvenience, that she could not make up her mind to submit to an operation. However, in October the tumor commenced to ulcerate and she decided to have the operation performed. She entered the Skene Sanitarium October 18th, and the operation was done October 19th.

I made a free incision of the skin and turned it over the tumor with a pursestring suture, endeavoring to close the rectum and dissect the entire mass free until I could bring the healthy portion of the bowel down to the margin of the skin without infecting the operation wound. The dissection toward back progressed quite satisfactorily; however, difficulties arose when I attempted to carry the dissection through the perineum. Here the tumor had become soft, the outlines were obliterated, and I had the misfortune of breaking into it twice. I closed the rent immediately with sutures and carried the dissection higher up until I could bring down healthy bowel to the margin of the skin. The bleeding vessels were ligated as they were cut and the loss of blood was small.

Anteriorly, the peritoneal cavity was closed with a few catgut sutures. The diseased portion of the rectum was drawn down and a clamp applied above it. The portion above the clamp was cleared of fecal matter and another clamp applied to the healthy portion. The gut was cut close to the upper clamp and the stump was sterilized with the Paquelin cautery. Subsequently the margin of the rectum was sutured to the skin. The space behind the rectum was packed with gauze. After the wound had been carefully cleaned, a few catgut sutures were inserted anteriorly to bring the parts together. This was a mistake, because the wound had been infected and could not be thoroughly disinfected. Subsequently the sutures had to be removed and the wound packed with gauze. However, the infection was not serious. The temperature of the patient never rose above 101 F., and after the lapse of a few days became normal, yet the operation wound would have healed in a shorter time if infection had not occurred. The further progress of the case was uneventful. The patient left the sanitarium November 8th, and I attended her at her residence until the operation wound was healed. What the final result will be it is too early to say. There is no sign of return of the disease or metastasis at the present time. She has gained weight and strength.

## Hysteromyomectomy.
### *By Dr. F. W. Wunderlich.*

Mrs. S. M., age 35, married, born in the U. S., never had any serious illness until in the fourth month of her first pregnancy.

Prior to her marriage I had attended her for an enlargement of the thyroid gland and for muscular rheumatism. When Mrs. M. became pregnant she engaged Dr. A. A. Scouler, because she thought that she lived too far away for me to attend to her. In the middle of April she was seized with severe pain in the left side of the abdomen; she called on Dr. Scouler, he examined her and found that the pregnancy was complicated by the presence of a fibroid; the tumor gave rise to the pain. The doctor did not succeed in relieving the pain. April 24th he sent the patient to me with a note. The patient was very much emaciated and weakened by the continuous pain, nausea and sleepless nights. The tumor could be distinctly felt on the left side of the uterus; it was extremely painful on pressure. The patient had not only paroxysmal pains, but complained also of feeling chilly at times. Apparently the pain was caused by disturbance of the circulation in the tumor, owing to its rapid growth during pregnancy, and was due either to pressure or torsion. I agreed with Dr. Scouler's diagnosis of subserous fibroid and advised to give codein gr. ss. every two hours until pain was relieved. The pain was relieved for several days, but returned again. Dr. Scouler retired from the case.

May 15th the patient had acute pain. I made another examination, found no perceptible change. I gave her codein tablets gr. ss. to be taken every two hours until pain was relieved. She slept the following night, continued to take the tablets for four days, and the pain was entirely relieved and did not return. The relief was probably due to a change in the position of the tumor in some way more favorable for the circulation, because she had taken codein and morphine before with temporary relief only.

The patient entered Prospect Heights Hospital September 1st to await her confinement. Owing to a misunderstanding, I was not notified of her presence in the hospital until September 3rd. September 4th she had pains; I found the child in L. O. P. position; attempts to change the position to a L. O. A. position failed. The first stage was slow and protracted, owing to the persistent L. O. P. position; severe pains and no progress. After dilatation of the os I turned and delivered. Unfortunately the cord prolapsed, the child was stillborn and could not be resusticated after birth.

Bilateral lacerations of the cervix and the lacerated perineum were immediately repaired. She had normal puerperium; the swollen breasts gave her more pain and discomfort than the perineum. She left the hospital in good condition September 26th.

Mrs. M. improved rapidly. She was free from pain, and her condition was satisfactory until October 20th, when she was suddenly seized with acute pain in the tumor. The pain persisted, although codein and morphine were given. She entered the Prospect Heights Hospital October 24th and the operation was done on the 25th. I expected to find a subserous fibroid and contemplated to make a myomectomy, but found several small fibroids besides the large one, and made a hysteromyomectomy instead. Her recovery was uneventful, and she was discharged from the hospital November 9th. She has had no pain in her abdomen since and enjoys good health.

## Case of Fracture of the Lower End of the Humerus, with Displacement.
### *Reported by Dr. J. Sherman Wight.*

It is important to remember the following facts: The lower extremity of the humerus is flattened and presents on the ulnar side the internal condlye projecting nearly as far down anteriorly as the trochlea; on the radial the external condyle which is covered anteriorly by the capitellum. The internal condyle forms a groove posteriorly with the trochlea for the ulnar nerve. The inferior articular surface external to the internal condyle is subdivided by a low ridge into the trochlea and capitellum. Above the trochlea, on the anterior surface, is the coronoid fossa, and on the posterior surface the olecranon fossa. These fossæ are separated by a thin disc of bone. Above the capitellum, on the anterior surface, is a shallow fossa. The centers for the external condyle, the trochlea and the capitellum unite to form an epiphysis which fuses with the shaft at the seventeenth year. In fœtal life diaphyseal ossification proceeds through cartilage. Diaphyseal cartilage is a phase in bone formation. In adult life regeneration of bone takes place either through a transition stage of cartilage or by direct division of bone cells into osteoblasts. The cartilage cell is formed and ossification is retarded where the conditions are less favorable. The osteoblasts are directly formed from the bone cells and ossification is hastened where the conditions are most favorable, as in fractures freshly made, whose fragments are at once accurately coapted.

The diaphysis is largely compact, while the epiphysis is more cancellous bone, and the diaphysis has greater osteogenetic power. If, after injury, the epiphysis formed callus to the same extent as the diaphysis, the movements of joints would be seriously interfered with in fractures through the epiphysis. The fractures that produce ankylosis from large masses of callus involve the diaphyseal side of the bone, such as "T" fractures. The reproduction of bone is strictly limited if an excision keeps within the epiphyseal line. A separation of the lower end of the humerus strictly through the epiphyseal line is rare. The fracture line more commonly runs into the diaphysis. In order to prevent ankylosis of the joint, the fragments must be brought into the closest approximation with alinement and fixation of the fragments.

The case I have to present is an epiphyseal separation of the lower end of the humerus with a fracture line running into the diaphysis.

W. P., twelve years old, family history negative. He fractured his right humerus above the condyles in a fall during the summer of 1910; there was no displacement of the fragments, and they united with perfect function of the joint.

About September 1, 1911, he fell on his left arm, fracturing the humerus at the elbow. An X-ray picture was taken, an attempt made to reduce the deformity under an anæsthetic, and an anterior right angle splint was applied. He came to my office on September 6, 1911. I took an X-ray picture, which showed the lower fragment displaced backward and overridden by the lower end of the upper fragment. All attempts at reduction were unsuccessful.

Plate I shows the position of the fragments when the boy first came to me.

Plate II shows the position of the fragments after my attempt at reduction.

September 13, 1911, I sent him to the Long Island College Hospital and prepared his arm for operation. An incision was made along the back of the elbow and carried down to the bone, the tissues were separated from the bone on either side; the ulna nerve lifted from its groove; a chisel was placed between the fragments and the proximal fragment was raised and reduction effected. On account of obliquity of the fracture line, which ran from above downward and outward, the fragments would not remain in coaptation, so a Lane plate was secured to the posterior surface of the external condyle and the other end was secured to the shaft of the humerus, as shown in Plate III. The wound was closed and the arm put in a right angle splint. The boy left the hospital in three days and came to my office. At the end of two weeks the plate was removed under a local anæsthetic. At the end of three and a half weeks the splint was removed and passive motion was started. Massage and passive motion were continued until the middle of November; then there was some slight ankylosis of the joint and he was given an anæsthetic in the office and the arm fully extended. Passive motion was continued until the end of November, when he was discharged with a perfectly free elbow joint. Plate IV.

*Conclusions.*

The absence of an articular surface on the back of the external condyle makes this available for anchoring a very small distal fragment without damaging an articular surface.

In all cases of fracture at the joint it is important to get the closest approximation of the fragments so as to prevent ankylosis from encroaching bony masses. When close approximation is obtained in alinement union is hastened, as there is no intermediate stage of cartilage formation and no excessive callus.

DR. J. B. BOGART, in discussion, said: "I had the pleasure of seeing two similar cases at Dr. John B. Murphy's clinic in February. He also used the Lane plate after reducing the fracture, but accomplished the reduction in a little different way, which, it seems to me, has some advantages. He made an incision over the condyloid ridge on each side of the lower end of the humerus and then with a chisel raised the attachments of the muscles, and with them all the structures in front of the joint, and then reduced the fracture. That is a very easy way of getting at the fracture without taking any chance of injuring any important structure. I saw one of the cases operated upon and the other one some three weeks after operation. The result in that case was everything that could be desired. This is a class of cases in which we are going to do more of this work. One of the most striking evidences of this is the recent report of the conclusions of the Committee on the Treatment of Simple Fractures of the British Medical Association, which you have all read in the February number of Murphy's clinics.

"Dr. Wight made a very important point in regard to getting consent for these operations. It is astonishing what our judges and juries are doing and the verdicts that are being brought in. This question of malpractice suits is of such importance to the surgeon that it is not too much to make an effort to have a written consent for all these operations."

### Case of Tubercular Disease of the Red Marrow Treated With Partial Excision of Elbow Joint.

*Reported by Dr. J. Sherman Wight.*

It is necessary to become familiar with the functions of the various structures that enter into the formation of bones and joints. Bones are compact or cancellous. The canal of bone is filled with marrow. Bones, whether compact or cancellous, are filled with channels and spaces which contain the marrow. The marrow is either red or yellow; the former consists of connective tissue holding numbers of most diverse cells. The yellow marrow contains a good deal of fat and very few cells. The former is found in spongy bone and the latter in dense bone. The periosteum covers the bone and is composed of two layers—an inner cellular layer and an outer fibrous layer. The marrow and the periosteum communicate and both nourish the bone. The joint cartilage and the epiphyseal cartilage get their nourishment from the marrow and are passive like the bone itself, simply responding to the inflammatory changes that take place in the marrow and the periosteum. The synovia line the capsule of the joint and contain lymph spaces and blood vessels. They are continuous with the cartilage of the joint.

Tubercular disease attacks the red marrow of bone, the periosteum and the synovia. When it attacks the marrow of bone it exhibits tubercules. This shows active inflammation at times with engorgement of blood vessels, bacteria and pus. If the bone is denuded of its periosteum, it gets nourishment from the marrow. If the marrow becomes diseased and destroyed, the bone gets its nourishment from the periosteum. When both are destroyed the bone dies and separates; the cartilage suffers the same fate. Neither bone proper nor cartilage becomes infected; in fact, they restrain the onward march of infection.

The active tissues of the joint are continuous with one another and react in a similar way to disease. Disease may start in one and spread to another.

The second case that I have to present is one of extensive tubercular disease of the red marrow of the humerus and the upper end of the ulna and the synovial membrane of the elbow joint, with partial excision, resulting in recovery of the function of the elbow joint, followed by active tubercular processes in other parts of the body.

A. S., 21 years old, machinist's helper. Father died of an accident; mother alive and well; one brother died of consumption in 1910; previous personal history negative. Seven years ago he injured his left arm above the elbow in machinery. He suffered pain and swelling in that arm from that time on. It finally broke down and discharged. He was operated on at the Post-Graduate Hospital April 14, 1910, an incision made at the lower end of the left humerus and the bone scraped. This same operation was repeated September, 1911; the arm continued to discharge until I saw him October 9, 1911. I took the X-ray in Plate I; this shows a tubercular focus of the red marrow of the humerus at the middle third, another involving the lower end of that bone with an area of healthy bone between, and a focus in the upper end of the ulna.

I sent him to the Long Island College Hospital October 26, 1911, and excised the lower end of the humerus and the upper end of the ulna on a level with the head of the radius and curetted the humerus through a sinus in the middle third. The tubercular bacillus was recovered from the mass of bone removed. He left the hospital December 2, 1911, using his elbow-joint. December 15, 1911, an abscess appeared in his right calf and the whole calf was badly swollen. This was opened and drained. He was given two injections of tuberculin at the interval of a week, with considerable reaction; temperature rose to 103. The tuberculin was not repeated; he was given syrup of iodid of iron and kept out in the fresh air and sunshine. He improved after some time. Finally an abscess appeared at the root of the nose; I opened this February 20, 1913, and removed a considerable amount of dead bone. Since that time he has developed a swelling over the right parietal bone.

Plate II shows the change that has taken place in the elbow-joint. The articular end of the radius is free from any invasion, as well as the lower end of the humerus and the upper end of the ulna. There appears to be some osteoporosis of the middle third of the shaft of the humerus.

Comparing this with Plate I, it is fair to say that the red marrow in this region which was the seat of tubercular disease has been destroyed, and that it has disappeared. This is borne out by examination of the arm and explains the local cure.

Ely has asserted "that if the synovia and red marrow disappear from any locality, tubercular disease cannot exist. That without them there can be no such thing as joint tuberculosis." Attempts have been made to bring about this result by ankylosis or dislocation and thus effect a cure of this disease in the joint. This treatment has some value, especially when it is remembered that excisions of joints for tubercular disease are of little avail unless they remove every atom of the disease.

Dr. T. Wingate Todd presents a case in the March number of the *Annals of Surgery* which closely resembles mine, of old tubercular disease of the elbow cured by partial excision, the articular head of the radius being left. This patient had active tubercular lesions of bone in other parts of the body, particularly the frontal bone, which was necrotic on the right side and caused death through an abscess of mixed infection in that same area of the brain. This case would seem to contradict the law laid down by Ely "that without the synovia and the red marrow there can be no such thing as joint tuberculosis through an apparent corollary to this law that where tubercular disease has invaded the joint it cannot be eradicated without removing all the synovia and the red marrow entering into this joint."

On more careful consideration it will appear that this is not a corollary of the law laid down by Ely and is not borne out by the facts as appear in the cases cited.

*Conclusions.*

Tubercular disease of bones and points is confined to the red marrow, the periosteum and the synovia.

The obliteration of these arrests the disease whether by ankylosis, by excsion, or curettage of the bone.

If operation can remove every atom of the disease and still preserve some of the tissues which enter into the formation of the joint or of bone, the tubercular process will be locally arrested just the same.

---

# Medical Society of the County of Kings

## MONTHLY BULLETIN TO MEMBERS

### OCTOBER, 1913

MINUTES OF STATED MEETING, OCTOBER 21, 1913.

The President, Dr. James M. Winfield, in the chair.

There were 200 present.

The meeting was called to order at 8.30 P. M., and the minutes of the previous meeting were read and approved.

*Report of Council.*

The Council reported favorably upon the following applications for membership:

Louis Fisher, 318 Pennsylvania Ave.
Charles Goldman, 238 Nostrand Ave.
Frank D. Jennings, 53 Woodbine St.
R. S. Robertson, 271 Jefferson Ave.

## Election of Members.

The following, duly proposed and accepted by the Council, was declared elected to active membership:

Alfred C. Beck, L. I. College Hospital.
Geo. F. Buttschardt, 222 St. Nicholas Ave.
Harry Cleveland Harris, 25 Stuyvesant Ave.
Edward B. Haslam, 71 Oakland St.
Samuel Linder, 1780, St. Johns Pl.
Joseph Rosenthal, 572 Fifth St.
Carl Schumann, 116 Prospect Pl.
Walter T. Slevin, 65 Eighth Ave.
Alvarez H. Smith, 382 Carlton Ave.
Purvis Alex. Spain, 911 Greene Ave.
Wm. Alfred Sprenger, 1106 Bushwick Ave.

## Applications for Membership.

Applications for membership were received from the following:

Wm. Byron Agan, 981 E. 14th St.; P. & S., N. Y., 1912; proposed by G. H. Reichers; seconded by B. Harris.

Wm. Howard Barber, 905 Union St.; P. & S., N. Y., 1911; proposed by E. E. Cornwall; seconded by J. W. Fleming.

H. Wright Benoit, 442 Grand Ave.; McGill, 1909; proposed by E. E. Cornwall; seconded by Memb. Com.

Helen Dudley, 123 Joralemon St.; Cornell, 1911; proposed by E. A. Bruyn; seconded by Memb. Com.

David Feiner, 216 S. 3d St.; Univ. & Bell., 1912; proposed by H. A. Wade; seconded by E. E. Cornwall.

Frank Dormer Jennings, 53 Woodbine St.; P. & S., N. Y., 1902; proposed by J. E. Golding; seconded by J. G. Williams.

Thomas Bernard Kenny, 408 Westminster Road; Univ. Edinburgh, 1894; proposed by E. E. Cornwall; seconded by Memb. Com.

Henry John Kohlmann, 532 State St.; L. I. C. H., 1907; proposed by J. S. Read; seconded by A. L. Carroll.

Francis William Moore, 898 Sterling Pl.; P. & S., N. Y., 1910; proposed by J. M. Van Cott; seconded by J. C. MacEvitt.

Jacob Mauritz Morin, 1115 Bergen St.; L. I. C. H., 1899; proposed by J. H. Ohly; seconded by E. F. Luhrsen.

Wesley Grant Simmons, 956 Greene Ave.; Medico-Chir., Phila., 1898; proposed by W. P. Pool; seconded by W. A. Sprenger.

Milton I. Strahl, 164 S. 4th St.; Eclectic M. Coll., N. Y., 1912; proposed by E. E. Cornwall; seconded by Memb. Com.

## Executive Session.

Dr. Henry G. Webster, as Chairman of Legislative Committee, reported on the for the regulation of the distribution of cotics.

It was moved, seconded and carried, that following resolution be adopted:

Resolved, That the Medical Society of County of Kings heartily endorse the bill the regulation of the distribution of narco known as H. R. 6282, and urge its speedy actment and to this end direct the Secret of this Society to forward a copy of this r lution to each of the Senators and Mem of Congress from the State of New York

The President read the following necrolo

George Ransom Westbrook, M.D.   Mem 1879-1913.   Died July 19, 1913.

Robert Emory Moore, M.D.   Member 1 1913.   Died September 13, 1913.

John Randall Stivers, M.D.   Member 1 1913.   Died September 18, 1913.

Albert Thornton Birdsall, M.D.   Member 1 1913.   Died September 24, 1913.

William Henry Clowminzer, M.D.   Mem 1891-1895.   Died June 21, 1913.

James Lewis Watt, M.D.   Member 1895-1 Died June 24, 1913.

Henry Cushman Turner, M.D.   Member 18 1905.   Died August 16, 1913.

The President recommended that the S ety take some action in recognition of the de of the Treasurer, Dr. John R. Stivers.

Dr. Cox moved that the Society give a sta ing, silent vote as a mark of appreciation the honered service of Dr. Stivers and t deep regret of the loss to the Society in death.   Carried.

## Scientific Program.

1. Paper: "Conservation of the Pelvic Fl in Obstetric Delivery.'
   (a) By Supra-pelvic Manual Rotation Occipito-posterior Positions.
   (b) By Median Incision of the Disten Perineum.
   By Ralph H. Pomeroy, M.D.
2. Paper: "Cesarean and the Family Doct By O. Paul Humpstone, M.D.
3. Paper: "The Intra-Uterine Treatment the Interior of the Uterus in Post-part and Post-abortal Infection.'
   By John O. Polak, M.D.
   Discussed by Ralph M. Beach.
   Adjourned 10.30 P. M.

CLAUDE G. CRANE, Secretary

# LONG ISLAND MEDICAL JOURNAL

VOL. VII.          DECEMBER, 1913          No. 12

## Original Articles.

### THE MANAGEMENT OF THE INTERIOR OF THE UTERUS IN POST-ABORTAL AND POST-PARTUM INFECTION.*

By John Osborn Polak, M.Sc., M.D., F.C.S.,

of Brooklyn, N. Y.

PUERPERAL sepsis is not measured by its mortality, but rather by its morbidity, and this morbidity, we believe, has been largely due to meddlesome interference with the endometrium by surgical methods. Infection within the uterus, whether following an abortion or a full-time delivery, usually begins as an endometritis, and may extend by the lymphatics through the uterine wall, or reach the blood through the vessels of the placental site. Nature closes the uterine sinuses in the placental site by the formation of blood clots, which is a conservative process against extension of the infection from the endometrium to the blood stream.

A study of nearly 2,000 cases of puerperal infection has demonstrated that the endometrium should never be curetted in streptococcic infection, and that curettement of the placental site is a potent cause of thrombo-phlebitis of the pelvic veins. We have also observed that when the inside of the uterus is not disturbed by instrumental or digital exploration the infection is generally confined within the uterus, and that parametric and peritoneal complications are seldom noted. The infection may begin in a wound of the cervix, where the invasion is directly through the lymphatics, or blood channels, in the base of the broad ligaments, and a subperitoneal lymphangitis or bacteriemia promptly follows. When this has occurred no form of intra-uterine treatment can arrest its further advance.

It is generally admitted that puerperal infection is primarily a wound infection, due to the entrance of micro-organisms into wounds of the genital tract. These wounds are commonly found in the placental site, in the cervix, the lower uterine segment, and the vulvo-vaginal orifice. Consideration of the latter, however, does not come within the scope of this discussion.

---

* Read at International Congress, London, England, August 6, 1913, and by request before the Kings County Medical Society, October 21, 1913.

2

Infection of the uterus in mild cases is limited to the surface of the mucous membrane (an endometritis) and the placental site, and may be either of the putrid or septic variety. In the putrid form, the placental remains are invaded by saprophytes, and while the streptococcus and colon bacillus are frequently present, they are usually not of a virulent type. In the septic form, the streptococcus is the invader, and is found in pure culture in from 30 to 40 per cent., and in mixed culture in from 60 to 70 per cent.

In the putrid form, the uterus is bulky and flabby, there is an absence of muscular contraction, and the retraction of the uterus is arrested, the blood and lymph vessels within the uterine wall remain patent, and the lochia are abundant, dark, fetid and may even be mixed with pus.

Nature protects the organ against the invading organisms by the formation of a definite layer of leucocytes and small round tissue cells, which are deposited between the infected area and the underlying normal tissue. This layer is more or less well developed in all inflammations of the endometrium, except when the infecting organism is a streptococcus of the hemolytic type. When the organism is of this type it will pass through the walls of the uterus, either by the lymphatic channels or the blood vessels, with little or no local reaction, and reach the peritoneum or blood stream within a very few hours. Infection of such virulence cannot be checked by any form of intra-uterine treatment. These statements allow of no dispute; consequently, if we but stop for a moment to consider the analogy between the obstetric wound and wounds in other locations, it is hard to conceive how surgical intervention within the uterus has been so long countenanced. Any injured surface resists infection by the same process—*i.e.,* by the formation of a granulation zone; therefore, any intra-pelvic or intra-uterine manipulation made during the acute stage of a puerperal or post-abortal sepsis must always break down and disturb nature's protective barrier and permit the dissemination of the infection through freshly abraded or penetrated surfaces. For a moment, let us look at what is done by the curet; as is well known, the danger from curettage is increased as the period of pregnancy advances, because a large lax uterus cannot be emptied of its decidua, the protective wall of leucocytes is broken down and allows the streptococci to penetrate the uterine muscle through the patent lymphatics and extend the infection to the peritoneum and parametrium. It dislodges the clots in the mouths of the uterine sinuses and directly spreads the infection from the endometrium through the blood vessels. No one present has ever curetted a septic uterus without having the procedure followed by an immediate rise in temperature. It is also known that a relaxed uterus favors bacterial invasion through its patent lymphatic channels.

To limit the spread of infection, therefore, when the sepsis has begun within the uterus, it is necessary to meet certain definite indications which are based on our knowledge of the pathology—*i.e.,* first, to secure uterine drainage; second, to maintain uterine contraction and retraction, and, finally, to avoid interference in any way with nature's protective zone. The fulfillment of these general principles has been accomplished by the employment of postural drainage, the Fowler position, by the use of ergot and pituitrin in full doses in conjunction with ice-bags placed over the uterus, and by the avoidance of any form of intra-uterine manipulation or instrumentation, no matter what the uterine content may be. This treatment is supplemented by attention to the diet, the intestinal tract, the heart and blood changes, by general supportive measures, especially nourishment, fluids and fresh air.

Since January 1, 1912, we have had under our observation, in our gynecological and obstetrical wards, 104 cases of puerperal infection. Eighty-four followed full-term delivery, and twenty were of the post-abortal type. Of the full-term cases, fifty-nine had spontaneous deliveries, while twenty-five were operative cases; these include five craniotomies, ten forceps, five bougie inductions, and five versions.

A routine examination on admission was made on all of these patients, in which the following points were noted: the pulse rate and temperature, the condition of the tongue, of the heart, of the lungs, the amount of distention of the abdomen and its tension, the height and condition of the uterus, and notes made of any point or points of localized tenderness or intra-abdominal exudate. The examination was completed by taking a blood count and blood culture. In all except six of the cases making up this report repeated blood examinations were made. The vulva and vagina were then thoroughly cleansed and inspected for any injury or local focus of infection, and after the bladder was emptied a careful pelvic examination was proceeded with; this examination was performed under the strictest asepsis with the gloved hand. The following conditions are noted: the condition of the cervix, the degree of its patulousness, the height, contraction and retraction of the uterus; its mobility, the condition of the parametrium, and, finally, a bacteriological examination of the uterine secretion. It is needless to say, in such a company as this, that a well-contracted uterus, with a closed cervix, forbids exploration and is not entered, even for the introduction of a culture tube.

The points which we attempt to determine from this examination are—first, whether the infection is confined to the genital tract; second, what is the site of the local lesion—is it in the uterus or beyond the uterus? This is shown by the condition of the uterus, the parametrium, and the adjacent peritoneum; third, what is the form of the intoxication, and, finally, what natural resistance has the patient to combat the infection? This is shown by her general condition, and her hemoglobin, red and white cell counts. In this series the cultures from the interior of the uterus were reported as follows:

A hemolytic streptococcus was recovered thirty-four times, while a streptococcus of the non-hemolytic type in pure culture was recovered in ten cases. Pure streptococci not tested for hemolysis was found five times. Combined growths of the streptococcus and staphylococcus, ten times. In combination with colon bacillus, five. The saprophytic bacillus alone, five, and in combination with the streptococcus and colon bacillus, ten, times. The uterine culture showed no growth in ten of our cases. In fifteen patients the uterus was closed and no intra-uterine culture was made. Of this number, one hundred and one women recovered and three died, making the mortality of the series less than three per cent.

As has already been stated, blood cultures were made from all except six patients, with the following results: Thirty were negative on repeated examinations, twenty returned the staphylococcus aureus, twenty-nine showed the streptococcus longus in pure culture. Two were of the hemolytic variety, and seventeen returned a streptococcus brevis.

It is interesting to note that in the three fatal cases one failed to develop any organism from the blood; in another the streptococcus brevis was recovered, and in the third the bacteremia was due to the staphylococcus aureus. This fact is particularly impressive when we remember that a hemolytic streptococcus was recovered in thirty-four of the uterine culture. But these thirty-four women were not curetted.

The temperature on admission in these cases varied from 101 to 105.8, the pulse from 110 to 168. The highest temperature in this series was 106.8 Fahrenheit. Eighty ran a temperature of over 103 Fahrenheit. The duration of the persistence of temperature in this series varied from three to thirty-four days. The shortest stay of a patient in the hospital was eleven, the longest eighty-one, days. Of this number, twenty had a definite intra-uterine content on admission, with more or less persistent uterine hemorrhage; the bleeding in but one case was severe enough to need control: this was arrested by a firm cervico-vaginal pack of iodoform gauze, which was left in position for twenty-four hours, at the end of which time the patient passed a retained placenta and the bleeding ceased. All of these patients received one or more doses of vaccine. An autogenous vaccine was used in the patients from whom the streptococcus brevis and staphylococcus aureus were recovered. An injection of polyvalent stock vaccine of the staphylococcus, streptococcus, and colon bacillus was given to each patient on admission if the blood count showed less than 20,000 leucocytes.

From the foregoing we conclude:

First.—That each patient should be studied as to the clinical and bacteriological diagnosis.

Second.—That curettage, douches, or intra-uterine examinations, during the acute stage of a puerperal infection, break down the natural barriers, and that except in abortion cases of less than seven weeks, where the uterus is retroflexed, absolute non-interference with the inside of the uterine cavity in infections reduces the mortality and minimizes the morbidity.

Third.—That a uterus in its normal position, with its contents drained by posture, its muscle toned by ergot, pituitrin, and ice, will rid itself of its content and arrest bacterial invasion.


# THE INDICATIONS FOR CESAREAN SECTION FOUND IN A SERIES OF FORTY-FOUR CASES FROM THE GYNECOLOGICAL-OBSTETRICAL SERVICE OF THE BROOKLYN HOSPITAL.*

By Augustus Hussey, A.B., M.D.,
of Brooklyn, N. Y.

THE fortunate results of the Cesarean operation in the treatment of obstructed labor has led obstetricians to extend its indications. A search of recent literature will reveal reports of its successful use in almost every serious emergency of childbirth. The conservative physician views with distrust the seeming radicalism of this movement, and demands real and urgent reasons for the employment of a major operative procedure in the treatment of complications that have been handled in the past by

---

* Read before the Brooklyn Medical Society, October 17, 1913.

methods that appear to him less hazardous. The progressive physician, conscious of his increasing obligations to his obstetric patients and alive to the necessity of early recognition and prompt treatment of many conditions that were formerly temporized with, has been quick to realize and avail himself of the advantages offered by the surgical method of delivery.

With the hope of placing before both in compact and simple form the fundamentals on which the indications for Cesarean section are based, I present this review of the conditions for which we have operated at the Brooklyn Hospital. If the conservative shall find in it any justification for the operation, if the progressive physician shall find in it any suggestion that may increase his watchful and protective care of his obstetric patients, the writer will feel well repaid for his efforts.

Before taking up the indications for Cesarean section, however, I wish to speak of its contra-indications. The operation was devised in the interest of the baby. It was first done to remove from the womb of a woman dying in labor the unborn child in the hope of saving its life. To a great extent it is still employed in the interest of the baby. A careful analysis of reported cases will show that in the majority of these the mother might have been delivered by other methods at the sacrifice of the child.

Safeguarding the lives of unborn babies is one of the high ideals to which the operation is dedicated, but one should be reasonably sure that the baby has a life to be saved before one operates in its interest. There is a tendency to go too far in disregarding the interest of the mother. When there is any doubt of the viability of the child, one should not subject the mother to increased risk for sentimental reasons. Frequently, when the question of Cesarean section is raised, the baby's condition is such, either on account of the stress of prolonged labor or of damage done by injudicious attempts at delivery, that although alive it will not survive. Therefore, I would emphasize the point that Cesarean section is contra-indicated when the baby is not viable, unless there exist a condition that renders the operation imperative in the interest of the mother.

One of the chief reasons why patients upon whom this operation was performed before the era of aseptic surgery almost invariably died was that they were infected either before or during the operation, or both. To-day, infection is the great danger from which the woman about to be sectioned is to be protected, and the presence of infection must be regarded as a contra-indication to the operation unless there be no other recourse without the sacrifice of life.

Turning now to the indications for Cesarean section, I shall consider under nine different headings the conditions for which we have operated at the Brooklyn Hospital.

1. *Pelvic Deformity Obstructing Labor.*—Disproportion between the diameters of the head and those of the birth canal is the commonest indication for Cesarean section. In our series we have operated for this complication twenty-six times. The study of disproportion presents one of the most intricate and interesting problems of obstetrics. The factors which enter into the problem are—first, the size of the birth canal; second, the size, position, posture, and moldability of the head; third, the character of the

uterine contractions, and fourth, the general condition of the patients, mother and baby.

The degree of disproportion may for convenience of discussion be described as absolute or relative or apparent.

It is *absolute* when the difference between the diameters of the head in a favorable position and the diameters of the pelvis is so great that engagement cannot take place.

It is *relative* when the difference between the opposing diameters is such that engagement may or may not take place, according to the moldability of the head and the character of the labor.

It is *apparent* when an abnormal position or an imperfect flexion prevents the small diameters of the head from engaging with the small diameters of the pelvis. This should not be mistaken for actual disproportion, for it may be remedied by intrauterine manipulation.

An early diagnosis of disproportion is absolutely essential to successful treatment. Therefore, it is imperative to make a provisional diagnosis during pregnancy whenever the pelvic measurements are found to be below normal, and prove or disprove the diagnosis by a carefully conducted test of labor. In cases of major deformity—for example, in justominor pelves with a true conjugate of $7\frac{1}{2}$ cm. or less—a true diagnosis can be made at the end of pregnancy if the head is of normal size, and the test of labor is then unnecessary. In the majority of cases, however, the diagnosis can only be made after a test of labor.

The pelvic diameters that are most frequently at fault are the true conjugate, and the transverse and anteroposterior of the outlet. The indications for operating in obstructed labor cannot be based on centimeters of deformity. In a general way we may say that with a true conjugate of $7\frac{1}{2}$ cm. or less and a normal baby the indication for Cesarean is absolute; that with a larger conjugate the indication may or may not arise, according to the amount of disproportion that exists, the amount of molding that takes place, and the physical condition of the mother and child. Therefore, we must work out the indications for Cesarean section by comparing the size of the particular head and pelvis in question and determining the amount of disproportion; by noting the moldability of the head and estimating the power of the patient to mold it; and lastly, we must correct our reckoning by the viability of the child and the presence or absence of infection.

When a case is seen during pregnancy in which an absolute disproportion can be diagnosed Cesarean section is indicated at the onset of labor.

When a case is first seen after the onset of labor in which absolute disproportion can be diagnosed and the mother and baby are in good condition, section should be performed at the earliest possible moment.

When a case is not seen until the mother is in a desperate condition or the baby life has been compromised by injury or delay, section should only be performed when the deformity is so great that delivery cannot be safely accomplished by embryotomy.

When a preliminary diagnosis has been made during pregnancy, the case should be sent to a hospital for a test of labor.

Labor should be allowed to go into the second stage, when a vaginal examination is made under ether with the whole hand in the vagina. The pelvis is carefully explored, the head is palpated to determine its size, position, posture, and density. An effort is made to fit the head into the brim of the pelvis and to determine the degree of disproportion. If the disproportion is considerable, engagement cannot be expected to take place, and Cesarean section is indicated. If the head is soft and molding and the degree of disproportion is slight and the mother and baby are in good condition, the operation may be deferred; *but the fetal heart should be carefully watched, and the operation performed at the first indication of embarrassment of the fetal circulation.*

When the patient is not seen until after the onset of labor, the indications will be modified by two important factors, the viability of the child and the general condition of the mother. If the fetal heart is rapid and irregular in force and frequency, if the forceps have been applied to the head in an unsuccessful attempt to secure engagement, especially if the vaginal discharge is stained with meconium, the life of the child may be regarded as already compromised and its interest disregarded. Under such circumstances we should only operate when the deformity is so great that laparotomy becomes the safest procedure for the mother.

When a mother is undoubtedly infected and the child is still in good condition, the interest of the two patients clash. The operation becomes a dangerous one and must be followed by hysterectomy. It should therefore only be performed when the parents are willing to take the added risk in the interest of the child, unless the absolute indications for Cesarean exist.

Briefly, then, the indications are:

Section is indicated at the end of pregnancy *without* a test of labor when a diagnosis of absolute disproportion has been made.

Section is indicated *after a test of labor* when an examination under ether shows that the actual disproportion between the head and the pelvis is such that engagement or delivery cannot be expected without prolonging the labor to a degree that would jeopardize the life of the child.

Section may be deferred in deformities of minor degree if the examination shows that the head is molding and about to engage. But it should be performed without delay if a rising fetal heart rate gives notice of danger to the child.

Section is contra-indicated in the presence of a dead or dying baby, unless the deformity is such that delivery by embryotomy cannot be performed with safety.

Section is rendered dangerous by infection—*i.e.,* in cases that have been long in labor, frequently examined, or subjected to attempts at delivery under unfavorable conditions—and should only be performed when the interest of the child is paramount, unless the indication is absolute.

Group 2.

*Mechanical Obstruction by Diseased Conditions of the Pelvic Soft Parts.*—Tumors, new growths, cicatricial contractions, and inflammatory thickening of the pelvic soft parts occasionally offer serious obstruction and furnish indications for Cesarean section.

In this series we have operated for these conditions five times; twice for fibroid tumors of the supravaginal cervix; once for ovarian cyst; once for new growth of the upper rectum, and once for inflammatory contraction of the vagina due to vesico-vaginal fistula.

In general it may be said that Cesarean section will be indicated in the presence of a fixed pelvic tumor or new growth of such size and position as to block the descent of the fetus. It may be an operation of election if the obstruction of the soft parts is such that it can only be overcome at great risk of traumatism to the mother's tissues, provided the mother and child are in good condition.

The tumors most frequently seen are uterine fibroids, ovarian and broad-ligament cysts.

Fibroids only occasionally cause obstruction. Tumors situated above the cervical portion of the uterus may cause malposition of the fœtus, inertia uteri, or premature separation of the placenta, but do not often cause blockade. Fibroids in the cervix itself or in the broad ligament are not easily displaced from the pelvis by uterine retraction and will usually necessitate Cesarean section.

Ovarian cysts complicate labor about once in 3,000 cases. When present they will cause serious trouble during pregnancy, labor, or the puerperium in 25 per cent. of the cases. Hemorrhage into the cyst, twisting of the pedicle, rupture, or inflammation are some of the accidents to which they are liable. The danger does not end with the birth of the child. Complications may arise that necessitate laparotomy and removal of the cyst during the puerperium. Therefore, it seems the safest course to remove the cyst at the beginning of labor, or, if that is impossible, to do a Cesarean and then take out the tumor.

Group 3.

*Ventral or Vaginal Fixation Dystocia.*—Many reports of Cesarean section for dystocia due to ventral fixation have appeared in recent literature. The clinical findings have been a high posterior position of the cervix with a thick and undilating anterior lip, a dense anterior segment of the uterus fixed to the abdominal wall, and a much thinned out posterior wall and fundus.

The result of the condition is non-engagement and ineffective labor, with the possibility of death of the fetus or rupture of the uterus.

When these complications threaten Cesarean section is indicated. In less urgent cases relief may be given by other and simpler operations. Many of the cases should be amenable to treatment by anterior vaginal hysterotomy. Dickinson and Pomeroy have each relieved the situation by cutting the ligament that binds the fundus to the abdominal wall and allowing labor to proceed.

I have operated at the seventh month for threatened miscarriage due to this condition, released the adhesion, and later delivered the patient at term by a normal birth. Therefore, my judgment would be that in fixation dystocia Cesarean section is indicated only when a rapid termination of labor is necessary to the safety of the mother or child.

Group 4.

*Rupture of the Body of the Uterus.*—Intra-abdominal rupture of the uterus may occur late in labor in neglected cases of obstruction, or during pregnancy or early in labor when a previous operation has been performed upon the uterus. This is a serious complication and demands immediate operation. After the child is removed the uterus may be taken out or not, according to the conditions present. Two cases of rupture through old Cesarean scars have occurred in this series. Both occurred before the onset of true labor pains. The uterus was removed in both cases. The mothers recovered. The babies were dead when removed.

Group 5.

*Contraction Ring Dystocia.*—Occasionally a thick, firmly contracting ring forms above the cervix and below the head or shoulders of the fetus, blocking descent.

According to Dickinson, Cesarean section is indicated for this complication under the following conditions:

1. Child living and not definitely enfeebled by length of labor, long drainage of waters, or unskilled attempts at extraction.

2. Ring refusing to relax under morphia, or to yield to complete etherization, coupled with patient manual dilatation by a skilled obstetrician.

3. Mother in fair condition for a laparotomy and not infected.

4. Request by patient and husband that a somewhat increased risk to the mother be assumed for the sake of obtaining a living child, in lieu of embryotomy.

There are two operations in our series for this condition—one by Dickinson, one by Pomeroy.

Group 6.

*Inefficient Labor.*—Occasionally one may be justified in electing Cesarean section for the delivery of elderly primiparæ who are having prolonged and ineffective labors, where the condition of the soft parts is such that a forced vaginal delivery would be dangerous to the baby. Operation was done for this indication once in this series by Dr. Zimmermann.

Group 7.

*General Conditions of Mother Necessitating Rapid Delivery— —Eclampsia.*—The medical profession is divided into two opposing factions, waging bitter war over the treatment of eclampsia. Both admit that they do not know what eclampsia is, but each is sure that the condition is being wrongly treated by the other faction, and quote long lists of statistics to prove their contentions.

The conservatives would treat the patient with drugs and leave the uterus alone. The radicals would empty the uterus at the earliest possible moment and in the easiest possible way, and medicate the patient afterward, if necessary. On the theory that the uterus should be emptied in the easiest way, the indication for Cesarean section is based. The results obtained by section in the treatment of eclampsia have not been sufficiently favorable to induce one to try it as a general plan of treatment. But it is the opinion of many authorities that it may be indicated occasionally.

It has been done twice at the Brooklyn Hospital—once by

Dr. Zimmermann, once by myself. The indications for which we operated were severe eclampsia in a full term primipara with rigid soft parts, whose condition is favorable for a major operation, who is not infected, and whose baby is in good condition. In both instances mother and child made good recoveries.

My feeling at the present time is that the operation is occasionally justifiable; that it may be done in the interest of the child, providing the mother's condition is favorable, when there is good reason to suppose that the baby can be saved by it alone; that it should be done where there exists a condition that would necessitate its application in the interest of the mother irrespective of the eclampsia.

*Placenta Previa.*—The tendency here and abroad is to extend the indications for Cesarean section in placenta previa. The number of case reports is increasing, and the maternal mortality is being reduced by more careful selection of cases. It is not to be expected, however, that the maternal mortality by this method of treatment can be reduced sufficiently to compete with the Braxton Hicks version, or the bag method of treatment. The fetal mortality can undoubtedly be lowered by its use. And its chief application would appear to me to be to the severer forms of placenta previa, where the child is in good condition, the mother not infected, the period of utero gestation over eight months, and the condition of the pelvic soft parts such that easy delivery cannot be accomplished by the vaginal route.

I am not at all in accord with the view that placenta previa is an extra-uterine pregnancy and should be treated as such. There seems to me to be this material difference in the two conditions: the hemorrhage of placenta previa is so situated that it is a simple matter to control it in nine cases out of ten by the use of a bag or the breech to plug the cervix. The argument that this puts the life of the child in danger should be carefully scrutinized. Theoretically it is true, but practically we are not often called upon to treat cases of placenta previa when the child is of viable age or has any chance of living even if delivered alive.

For these reasons my judgment is that the operation should be limited to uninfected cases at or near term with living and viable babies, when the amount of placenta in front of the head or the condition of the soft parts is such that vaginal delivery would jeopardize the life of the child. The operation has been performed four times at the Brooklyn Hospital for this indication—twice by Dr. Pomeroy, once by Dr. Cary, and once by myself. All the mothers and two of the babies survived.

*Heart Disease.*—Valvular disease of the heart with broken compensation or myocarditis with dilatation occasionally present very serious complications to labor. The mortality is high if labor is allowed to proceed unassisted. The accepted treatment is to shorten labor as much as possible by the use of forceps. But it may happen that the patient's condition is so bad that she cannot stand the strain of even first-stage pains, and the cervix and vagina may be so rigid that forced delivery is impracticable. Under such conditions a rapid section may be the means of saving both mother and child.

I have operated once for this condition. Under morphine hyoscine narcosis, the patient was rapidly delivered. Her heart action improved during the operation. She made a smooth convalescence and left the hospital with a living baby.

*Conclusion.*—The tendency of the times is in the direction of humanitarianism, and we must follow its lead. The Cesarean section is humanitarian. It is designed to conserve life and health to mother and baby in emergencies where one or both are threatened. Its judicious use has done more to forward the progress of obstetrics than any innovation since the introduction of asepsis. Harm may be done by its injudicious use and the progress of our art retarded by its application to conditions that can be successfully met by simpler methods. But when the indications for it exist, we must recognize them promptly, and, having recognized them, it is our duty to earnestly and intelligently urge its claims, and to so handle our patients that, when the necessity arises, the operation may be done with the least possible risk. For we must remember that the results of the Cesarean operation lie not wholly in the hands of the operator, but largely in the hands of the man who has preceded him. Therefore, it is the duty of every one who confines women to keep in mind the indications for the operation, and especially its contra-indications, and to remember that the contra-indications are not, as a rule, inherent in the case itself, but arise through neglect in its early care.

## CESAREAN AND THE FAMILY DOCTOR.*

### By O. Paul Humpstone, M.D.,
of Brooklyn, N. Y.

" SUCCESSFUL surgery is usually the result of thoroughly organized team work." This precept of Reynolds, of Boston, seems true. There is an important member of the team, whose relation to the success is frequently overlooked—viz., the family doctor. It is this relation of the family doctor to this particular obstetric surgical procedure to which I direct your attention.

In the first place, concerning your acceptance of the practical usefulness of Cesarean. It does not seem possible, in the light of increasing reports of long series of patients, in which this operation has been performed in suitable cases, without fetal or maternal mortality, that any one can argue against this operation in favor of premature induction of labor, with its 20 to 30 per cent. fetal mortality and a maternal mortality of 1 to 2 per cent. and a maternal morbidity of even greater degree; or of high forceps on an unengaged head with fetal mortality of 15 to 60 per cent., and a maternal mortality of 2 to 4 per cent., and a maternal morbidity even greater than after induction; or of craniotomy on a living child. Never will I forget the look of satisfaction which came over the face of a fellow-practitioner after seeing a Cesarean done on a woman whom he had twice delivered by forceps, with great physical exertion, once of a dead baby, once of a baby that lived, but had a lasting mental defect. "Never again for me!" were his words. He had been converted to the use of the abdominal route in suitable cases. Furthermore, we must get away from the obsolete idea that

* Read before the Medical Society of the County of Kings, October 21, 1913.

Cesarean is an operation of last resort, and yet again we must not allow ourselves to become too radical and look upon Cesarean as an easy way out of every difficult labor. The American public is being educated by the press on medical questions to a degree exceeding that in any other country. Any advance in medicine is now heralded across the land without, in many cases, proper censorship. The public is now aware of the success in midwifery of the adoption of modern surgery. It is far more ready than formerly to recognize the advantage of hospital treatment in difficult cases of confinement, and to submit to the judgment of the doctor that such treatment is for its best interest. They expect and demand of their family physician that he tell them of the probability of a normal pregnancy and labor; that he examine the prospective mother more thoroughly than an occasional investigation of the urine.

He is far from being held blameless if a case of toxemia of pregnancy is treated as of little moment until it bursts forth in an eclamptic attack, or a warning bleeding at the sixth or seventh month is looked upon on lightly until there comes the terrific hemorrhage of placenta previa. Neither will they accept as providential the difficulties of the birth when a case has been allowed to go long over time on the excuse—"We must have miscalculated."

The public to-day demands of the family doctor (I quote Davis): "That he should be able to make a diagnosis of the most common abnormalities in obstetrics, and of the great and vital dangers to child-bearing women. In the interest of his patients, and for his own reputation and future practice, he should secure for complicated obstetric cases the same surgical attention given to appendicitis, ovarian tumor, uterine fibroids and ectopic gestation."

This leads me to my second point—how shall the family doctor diagnose the possibility of the practical usefulness of Cesarean in any given case?

The history of a multipara having had two or more difficult births with dead babies, or babies which died very shortly after birth, should always put one on guard. These patients seldom have the same doctor in succeeding pregnancies, feeling they may have "better luck" with a different doctor. Note that I say two or more difficult labors. While one such experience is suspicious, still the vast majority of first births that result in catastrophe to the child are due to faulty management of occipitoposterior positions, or too early or too late interference in normal presentations. In a primipara a history of rickets in childhood or of hip-joint disease affords a clue. In numerous cases a family history of difficult births suggests a family type of small pelvis.

By far the most important indication for Cesarean comes from disproportion between the size of the child and the pelvis; therefore, the thorough examination of the patient both as regards the size of the pelvis and the size of the baby is of first importance. External pelvimetry should always be employed, but the procedure is not to be given too much weight, because of its inaccuracy, unless the measurements are manifestly below what they should be. An external anteroposterior manifestly shortened with a measurement of the spines equalling or greater than the crests signifies at once a flat pelvis, but one should remember that nature accommodates the passenger to a flat pelvis better than any other type of contracted pelvis. A proportionate shortening of all the diameters, both of the inlet and of the outlet, is of more importance, indicating as it does a justominor pelvis, probably funnel in shape. You will recall how Williams has simplified our comprehension of the significance of the measurements of the outlet.

Of far more practical importance than external pelvimetry is the study with the examining hand of the inside of the pelvis. The depth of the symphisis, the curve of the sacrum, the prominence of the ischial spines and any irregularity of the development of the two lateral halves of the pelvis, the height of the promontory and its shape, and the estimation of the true conjugate by the measurement of the diagonal conjugate. If this observation shows a true conjugate of 7 cm. or less, the indication is absolute without any further discussion.

If the conjugate is between 7 and 9 cm. our indication is only relative, and bears a direct relation to the size of the baby and the powers of the uterus and abdominal muscles.

It is well to remember in this connection that the nearer term the examination is made, the more relaxed are the soft parts of the pelvis, and consequently the easier it is to judge accurately of the contour and size of the inside of the pelvis. One may wisely withhold any opinion of the ease of birth until the beginning of the ninth month. At this time it should be one's custom to make a most thorough examination.

It may be laid down as an axiom, that in any primipara in whom the head is floating at this time there is some disproportion. It is to be remembered that abnormal presentation is far more frequent in contracted pelvis than in the normal.

While it is possible with accuracy to judge of the size of the pelvis, the other two factors, the size of the baby and the driving force of the patient, are far more difficult to estimate. The size of the baby may be estimated by the measurements of the height of the fundus and the bimanual palpation of the head. One should note the degree of hardness of the bones, and the ease or difficulty with which the head can be fitted into the brim of the pelvis. The unengaged head may actually be measured in the occipitofrontal diameter through the abdominal and uterine walls. A child which is much over size can easily be recognized by these means.

By far the most difficult of the factors in all labors to judge beforehand is the power of the uterine muscle. There are some observations, however, which will aid one in an opinion. An aged primipara not only has a poor uterine muscle, but rigidity in all her soft parts. A woman who presents other stigmata of infantilism besides her small pelvis will have poor contractions of her uterus. The "hothouse type" of frail, highly neurotic girl is almost sure to have nagging, inefficient contractions, and will wear herself out struggling against the sensation of pain without accomplishing anything toward delivery. The pot-belly of rickets resulting in the pendulous abdomen of pregnancy points to an absolute uselessness of the abdominal muscles as a potent element in labor.

How often has the observation of one or more of these points during pregnancy made one worry a little as to the outcome of a given labor, and then, too late, has the thought been murmured to one's self—"this woman should have had a Cesarean."

This leads me to my third point—the management by the family physician of any case of obstetrics in which the possibility of the necessity of Cesarean arises in his mind after examination at the beginning of the ninth month.

If the examination has revealed an estimated true conjugate of 7 cm. or less, or a bony or soft tumor blocking the pelvis, the patient should be gently advised of the absolute necessity of Cesarean in a well-appointed hospital as an elective operation just after labor has begun. If the case is so-called "borderline," she should be told frankly that she may not be able to accomplish this birth by the natural way, that she will be given the opportunity to try when labor occurs, but that she should be in a hospital, because if she should fail the delay and exposure of removing her would count much against her, and the performance of the operation in the average house is not justifiable these days. Having accomplished these details when labor occurs, a trial of from five to ten hours is given her without any pelvic manipulation.

An examination at the end of this time revealing the head unengaged and an edematous two-finger dilated cervix, she should at once be submitted to Cesarean.

## MALIGNANT GROWTHS OF THE COLON, WITH ESPECIAL REFERENCE TO EARLY DIAGNOSIS AND TREATMENT.

### By Richard Ward Westbrook, M.D.,

of Brooklyn, N. Y.

CANCER of the small intestine is extremely rare. Cancer of the large intestine is common. Along with other surgeons, I am sure, I have met not infrequently with cases of advanced malignant disease of the colon, most of which were inoperable, or at best, only admitted of palliative relief. Some of these cases were in busy men, who could not, or would not, put themselves under observation for an indigestion which was new to them, but which they expected would pass off with time. Others were in individuals in the lower walks of life, who deferred seeking medical advice until forced to it by greatly reduced health or the sudden attack of intestinal obstruction. Others were cases who had been too long the victims of mistaken diagnoses, such as chronic appendicitis, colitis, movable kidney or pernicious anemia. The tendency of the profession not to suspect cancer of the bowel until a palpable tumor is present is exactly parallel with the delay in recognizing cancer of the stomach. Careful clinical observation of a patient at the cancer age with an unyielding indigestion of recent origin, whether it be of gastric or intestinal type, should either exclude or fix the suspicion of cancer. Then, with the diagnostic means now at our command, including exploratory incision if need be, a correct diagnosis might often be made before the period of palpable tumor.

There is in one respect a wide difference between cancer of the colon and cancer of the stomach. Excision of cancer in the colon, where the lymphatic supply is less rich, offers a much larger chance of permanent cure than does excision of cancer of the stomach. Many cases are recorded where no recurrence has taken place after excision of cancer of the colon where mesenteric glandular involvement was also present. And even in cases where recurrence has resulted, it has been of very slow development, making the surgical treatment in such instances distinctly worth while. Cancer of the colon, therefore, is relatively benign, and its early diagnosis and operative treatment offer special rewards. Recently I examined a patient from whom three years ago I removed the last four or five inches of the ileum, the cæcum and ascending colon for cancer of the cæcum with much glandular involvement of the mesentery. To my surprise there was no evidence of recurrence, although the patient was very anemic and emaciated at the time of operation. The enlarged glands seen in such cases are not all malignant, the outlying ones often containing no cancer cells.

DIAGNOSIS.

The question of early diagnosis, then, is the one of first importance in this phase of colon surgery. The same ideal should be aimed at as in stomach cancer,—to diagnose the case before a palpable tumor is present. This presents greater difficulty than in cancer of the stomach, as the latter has a fairly characteristic history and occurs more commonly after forty-five. Cancer of the colon occurs at an earlier age more often, and may also advance to the point of an acute intestinal obstruction without marked symptoms. It has no characteristic symptoms, but a carefully studied history, as in all other abdominal surgical diseases, may lead one to the point where an exploratory operation may be advised.

Tumors at the hepatic and splenic curvatures, and in the pelvic colon are difficult to detect at an early stage, or even in any part of the course of the colon in thick-walled abdomens. A recent exploratory operation revealed to me a mass in the cæcum which I could not palpate before operation, and neither could I detect it after the patient's recovery from an anastosmosis operation, it being also not tender, and the patient a muscular man.

The earliest sign is usually some irregularity of the bowels, usually toward constipation, and there may be attacks of diarrhœa rather frequently. Mucus is likely to appear. Pain of a colicky nature is an early symptom, or a constant sense of discomfort, of dull, dragging character. A good deal of weight has been attached to the symptom of "intestinal stiffening," a form of painless spasm of which the patient is aware in the early period of the disease. This may be the forerunner of a more marked peristaltic contraction of the bowel proximal to the growth, followed by gurgling, which is very apparent by palpitation after the growth is causing interference with the fecal current. As the patient expresses it, he can "feel the bowel rise up" under the hand. A desire to go to stool frequently, with the feeling that no adequate result has been accomplished, is a not uncommon symptom. Nausea or vomiting and a lack of appetite may be present, with weight loss.

It will be seen that the earliest symptoms of cancer of the colon are hardly more than those of colitis. As the disease progresses, a diagnosis can be made with certainty. Tumor may usually be made out sooner or later, varying from the size of a hickory nut to a child's head. In my experience blood in the stool has been usually noted at later stages of the disease, and occasionally as an early symptom. In one case of sarcoma of the splenic flexure, a profuse hemorrhage of the bowel was an early symptom, and later at intervals smaller quantities were passed. Profound anemia may be a symptom in the late cases, especially where hemorrhage is added to the toxemia produced by the growth itself. As the growth increases and encroaches upon the lumen of the bowel, symptoms of partial obstruction develop. Among the earlier of these are the exaggerated peristaltic phenomena of the titanic contractions with gas and gurgling, accompanied with colicky pain. Visible peristalsis may often be noticed through the abdominal wall. Complete obstruction may be brought about by a mass of hardened feces or other solid body occluding the narrowed lümen of the bowel. Otherwise complete obstruction is not common. Weight loss is not extreme, except quite late, or in the presence of protracted diarrhœa. Willy Meyer has made an interesting observation on four cases of cancer of the colon where many small pigmented spots and flat warts were present on the skin of the abdomen. This he regards as a significant diagnostic sign. I have recently noticed the same phenomenon in a case of inoperable cancer of the sigmoid with metastases in omentum and mesenteries, the patient being a woman of seventy. A large crop of flat, wartlike, blackish skin-growths formed a wide girdle over the upper abdomen. These spots varied in diameter from a quarter to half an inch, and Meyer has seen them disappear in one case after excision of a colon cancer had been done. I have had a similar case where the spots have greatly diminished during the year and a half since excision of a descending colon cancer. They are the manifestations of a trophoneurotic change in the skin of the abdomen due to chronic intra-abdominal disease, and while not pathognomonic of cancer, should strongly suggest advanced malignant disease.

While the symptoms of colon cancer present no characteristic course, and to make an early diagnosis requires familiarity with the function and diseases of the colon, it should be proper to place every case of recently developed disturbance of bowel habit, with pain or discomfort, constipation, gas, mucus and some weight loss under suspicion if the disturbance does not clear up with customary treatment. Two means might give important information at this stage—sigmoidoscopic examination and the X-ray. The sigmoidoscope is not difficult to use, and may reveal a growth in the sigmoid not readily detected otherwise. To be sure, only the pelvic colon can be thus inspected, but this is the part most commonly diseased. The X-ray is of undoubted value, and information more or less definite may be obtained with the help of the bismuth meal or enema. While the interpretation of the plate by the radiographist must not be taken too implicitly, it may strengthen or confirm other information, and prove of value in differential diagnosis. This kind of X-ray examination is difficult, and requires the best kind of apparatus. Examination under an anesthetic is a useful means of diagnosis. A bimanual examination through the rectum, with the patient on his back and the sphincter stretched to allow a higher reach, may reveal a sigmoidal growth. Palpation with the patient in different positions may reveal a movable growth.

### DIFFERENTIAL DIAGNOSIS.

The differential diagnosis of malignant growths of the colon has brought out some very interesting phases of the pathology of the colon in my experience. The most common seat of colon cancer, next to that of the sigmoid, is about the ileo-cecal valve, and here it is comparatively early accessible to palpation. Several instances have come to my notice where a diagnosis of chronic appendicitis has been made, a small mass being mistaken for a thickened appendix, with surrounding exudate. I have known a cancer of a very mobile cæcum to be diagnosed as movable kidney by a skilful surgeon. In one case of my own, that of a lady of 34, a movable tumor was present usually to the right of the umbilicus, but which at one time I found even to the left of the middle line. Aggravated symptoms of colitis, much tenderness, and severe cramping pain had been increasing over a period of several months. Operation revealed a mass in the cæcum, with inflamed colon wall and enlarged glands in the mesentery. The infiltration of the parts was not so dense as in the ordinary malignant case, but it seemed best to remove the cæcum and ascending colon and do a lateral anastomosis of ileum and transverse colon. An egg-shaped sessile growth within the cæcum proved to be a lipoma with ulcerating mucous membrane over it. The patient made a perfect recovery, with excellent function of the bowel remaining, when last seen after two years.

Cancer of the sigmoid is first in frequency of occurrence. Here an adherent mass may become confused with the several pelvic organs. A man was brought to me as a case of bladder disease, where an adherent malignant sigmoid was diagnosed, and I believe shown to be correct by autopsy. Several surgeons, including myself, recently diagnosed a mass in the cul-de-sac, adherent to the uterus, as a probable fibroma uteri. Incision showed it to be cancer of the sigmoid. The sigmoidoscope was neglected in this case, and a misleading history given undue weight. I have known chronic diverticulitis of the sigmoid to closely simulate cancer, and undoubtedly some of the brilliant results in cancer surgery in this region were upon cases which were not cancer at all. I have recently operated, with a colleague, on the case of a man near fifty, who had suffered for years past with a mucous colitis and obstructive symptoms in the later months. There was no history of ulcerative symptoms or confinement to bed. Anemia was marked. Operation disclosed a densely adherent sigmoid in the pelvis with thickened walls. An attempt to restore the bowel by the release of adhesions was only partially successful, and anastomosis seemed out of the question. An accidental rent in the bowel was closed, but reopened some days after operation, and the fecal fistula persisted for some months. The diagnosis seemed to point to a probable chronic diverticulitis, and the relief afforded by the fecal fistula and the operative attempt has brought the patient around to a much improved condition, and the bowels move normally.

In the transverse colon and at the hepatic and splenic flexures I have seen some half a dozen cases of malignant disease. In one case, that of a lady of sixty, the history showed colitis for ten years, accompanied with mucus and small quantities of blood, and soreness and a feeling of swelling in the right abdomen. Examination revealed an elongate tender mass in the line of the transverse colon leading from the hepatic flexure. An examination by a well-known stomach specialist in Buffalo a year before had shown the same conditions present then. In view of the long history, I made a diagnosis of a chronic inflammatory infiltration of the transverse colon—"pericolitis"—secondary to ulcer or diverticulitis. The patient was averse to any operative treatment, although suf-

8

fering much general distress. Her condition remained variable for another year, and while apparently improving during a stay in the country, she died suddenly after 24 hours of acute abdominal symptoms, evidently due to perforation. There was no autopsy. While this case was considered as cancer by a later observer in another town, I am inclined to think from the variable course and the probable perforation that my own diagnosis was correct. Either condition should have been subjected to operation.

A case of cancer near the splenic flexure was sent to me with the probable diagnosis of cancer of the cardiac portion of the stomach. Although the growth was largely surrounded by adhesions involving the stomach, the differential diagnosis was not difficult, as the symptoms were distinctly colonic. In another case, that of sarcoma at the splenic flexure, the diagnosis of pernicious anemia was thought probable by competent medical observers, and the small tumefaction felt was considered the left kidney. The history of this case, however, showed marked constipation beginning nearly a year before, and blood in the stool. He was treated, so he said, in a large Manhattan hospital four months before I saw him under the diagnosis of constipation merely. The small tumor was often not tender, but fairly so at other times. Soon after coming under my observation the hemoglobin diminished to 17 per cent. Acceding to the request to do a palliative operation, I made an anastomosis between the transverse colon and upper sigmoid, which the patient apparently stood well. His strength later failed, however, and he died of inanition within a week. Autopsy showed the growth to be a sarcoma, a very rare form of colonic malignancy. The patient was twenty-two years of age and the symptoms had persisted over a year. Metastasis was present in the liver. Mummery, of London, could find records of but seven cases of sarcoma of the colon. In sixty-one cases of malignant disease of the colon, operated on by Mayo, only one proved to be sarcoma.

### OPERATIVE TREATMENT.

In discussing the operative treatment of cancer of the colon, I would like to emphasize two opinions. The first is that cases will not be brought to operation early enough for radical cure in considerable percentage unless exploratory laparotomy be resorted to where there is good reason to suspect cancer. There will be cases where symptoms point to a lesion in the colon, but where its character and exact location cannot be determined without exploratory laparotomy.

My second point to emphasize is the value of operation in fairly advanced cases. I have already cited one case with advanced tumor and glandular involvement who is still well three years after free excision. Also, in cases hopeless of cure, an anastomosis is often distinctly worth while. This was recently shown in a woman of 50, the mother of a growing family of children, who was suffering with distention, cramping pain, and the aggravated constipation of chronic obstruction at the splenic flexure. She could eat little and was losing ground rapidly, although very anxious to live as long as possible for her children's sake. A palliative anastomosis gave her great relief, and although she is now failing after eight or nine months, the increased period of comparatively comfortable and useful existence has been worth much to her.

Of the radical operations on the colon, resection with lateral anastomosis of remaining segments at one sitting is the ideal procedure. In the presence of acute obstruction, or considerable degree of chronic obstruction, it will be unwise to attempt anything like a complete operation, and to confine one's attention solely to the immediate relief of the obstruction. Statistics indicate that the mortality in the presence of obstruction in resection and anastomosis in one stage is twice that where the operation is done in two stages. Artificial anus should be first established by means of colostomy and the growth removed at a later sitting. Or Paul's operation may be done, removing the growth, and stitching glass tubes into the two segments of gut for drainage of fecal contents, and later closing the artificial anus. Or the three-stage operation of von Mikulicz may be done, first mobilizing the gut with the growth and bringing it outside the incision, suturing the parietal peritoneum to the loop of gut and closing the wound around the outlying loop, after 12 to 24 hours cutting away the growth with the cautery, and closing the remaining artificial anus at a third sitting. Von Mikulicz reported 11 recoveries out of 12 cases done in this manner. I have recently had a recovery in a gentleman of 82 by this method. The disadvantage of this operation is the inability to do such careful dissection of the lymphatics, on the part of the operator, and the tiresome convalescence on the part of the patient.

In the ideal operation in one sitting, it is important to mobilize the bowel thoroughly by dividing the upper peritoneal reflection of the mesentery to the abdominal wall, thus freeing the part so as to allow it to be brought outside the abdomen, where the remainder of the work may be completed. After excision, the method of anastomosis to be preferred is the lateral, with the clamp. This is technically not difficult, and the results are excellent. End to end anastomosis is difficult and more likely to complicate the recovery and healing. It is wise to make a liberal excision of bowel and mesentery, as this insures a better chance of cure, and the loss of large portions of the colon leaves the patient no worse off. The mortality risk in operations on the colon will diminish. Mayo advises removing not less than 6 inches of the ileum in excision of the cecum to remove the ileo-cecal group of glands with the ileo-cecal mesentery.

Of palliative operations, lateral anastomosis with the clamp is the most desirable. The anastomosis may be made between portions of colon which come into easy contact and lie at sufficient distance from the growth, or between ileum and colon. The danger of infection being far greater in opening the colon than in similar work upon the upper intestine, it is always my custom to leave at least a cigarette drain down to the anastomosis as a precaution.

The establishment of an artificial anus becomes necessary in certain otherwise inoperable cases, but fortunately this is made less often necessary than formerly, with earlier diagnosis and treatment.

In conclusion, I would like to emphasize again the fact of the relatively benign character of cancer of the colon, and the considerable field for the cure of cancer which is opened up with the increasing improvement in the technic of colon surgery. And also, to urge the necessity of a better attempt at early diagnosis of colon cancer on the part of the profession as a whole.

# GASTRIC ULCER.*

## By Russell S. Fowler, M.D.,

of Brooklyn, N. Y.

THE main indication in the treatment of gastric ulcer medically considered is stomach rest. Paradoxical as it may seem this is best achieved through surgical measures. Years ago jejunal feeding was practiced by the German surgeons in fecal fistulas involving the jejunum but attempts to maintain nutrition by these measures were ineffectual for the most part on account of the retro-peristalsis set up and the character of the opening in the intestine. More recently Mayo Robson† devised an operation upon the jejunum by which stomach rest could be secured and jejunal feeding practised with certainty. Independently of the above the operation has been elaborated by Mayo‡. Briefly, the operation consists in a laparotomy, bringing up a loop of jejunum to the surface and doing a Witzel operation with a rubber catheter size 16 E or thereabouts and attaching the loop of jejunum to the parietal peritoneum. Patients can be easily nourished through such an opening and upon withdrawal of the catheter the jejunal opening readily closes. I have performed this operation eight times for ulcer of the stomach in cases in which the condition of the patient did not warrant a more radical operation: Four of these cases were cured while four in which the ulcer had perforated before the operation and to which a plastic operation on the ulcer was added to the above, died as the result of the diffuse septic peritonitis already existing prior to the operation.

In three cases of inoperable carcinoma of the stomach jejunostomy has been done and feeding practised to maintain stomach rest. These cases have gone about their business after a period of rest of two or three weeks and the tumor of the stomach shrunk so materially in one case that a second radical operation was advised but refused on account of the comfort which the patient had.

A second method to secure stomach rest may be employed by means of a special tube passed to the first part of the duodenum (Einhorn).

Of the two methods, however, jejunal feeding is preferable on account of the ease with which it can be carried out by the patient and the inconvenience of maintaining the tube in the duodenum passed per os as in the Einhorn method.

The treatment of ulcer of the stomach, whether medical or surgical, is not as yet upon truly scientific lines since the cause is not definitely known.

---

* Discussion of Dr. Edward E. Cornwall's paper, "The Non-Surgical Treatment of Gastric Ulcer," read before the Brooklyn Medical Society, February 21, 1913.

† Mayo Robson: *British Med. Journ.,* January 6, 1912.

‡ Mayo: *Am. Journ. of Med. Sciences,* April, 1912.

# A POINT IN THE TREATMENT OF DIABETES MELLITUS.*

## By Edward E. Cornwall, M.D.,
of Brooklyn, N. Y.

I WISH to call attention to a point in the treatment of diabetes which seems to have been overlooked (at least, I do not remember finding mention of it in medical literature), but which I believe to be a point of fundamental importance. It is this: That the diet in diabetes should be arranged so as to make as easy as possible the processes involved in protein metabolism; that insufficiency of protein metabolism should be considered in the treatment of diabetes just as much as insufficiency of storage and combustion of carbohydrates.

The dietetic treatments for diabetes which are in vogue look only to the restriction and selection of carbohydrates; they fail to regard or favor nitrogenous metabolism; worse than that, they impose unnecessary burdens on nitrogenous metabolism by giving protein in excess, and also by giving it largely in a form whose metabolism is comparatively difficult—viz., animal tissues. Protein in that form puts on the liver, already incapable of properly performing its carbohydrate-metabolic duties, the work of breaking up the purin substances directly introduced with it, and the products of its putrefaction by the saprophytic bacteria in the intestines. The instability of the liver as regards its glycogenic function is, we would naturally expect, increased by such treatment; and it may be that the reason why extreme limitation of carbohydrates has seemed necessary in certain cases can be found—partly, at least—in such overworking of the protein-metabolic function of the liver.

The argument which I am advancing receives support from the fact that a large proportion of cases of diabetes occur in families in which gout, obesity, chronic arthritis, chronic nephritis, apoplexy and cardiovascular diseases are prevalent. It was in treating persistent glycosuria occurring in such patients, whose nitrogenous metabolism was obviously insufficient, that my attention was drawn to the therapeutic value of an "easy" nitrogenous diet in diabetes.

To illustrate my point, let me report briefly a few sample cases.

A man thirty-three years old, apparently robust and healthy, with a lithemic family history, was refused insurance because a little sugar was found in his urine. I put him on a diet in which the quantity of his various food elements was limited to the needs of his body, but in which their normal ratio was not disturbed, and in which his protein was supplied from articles that were purin free and comparatively insusceptible to putrefaction in his intestinal tract. His glycosuria promptly disappeared.

A man now sixty years old, of a gouty tendency, during the fifteen years ending five years ago, always showed a trace of sugar in his urine. Five ears ago I put him, like the patient mentioned above, on what I call the "easy diet;" that is, one which

*Part of a discussion before the Medical Association of Greater New York, October 20, 1913.

supplied him a sufficient but not excessive quantity of food, of kinds which would least tax his nitrogenous metabolsm, which meant one consisting almost exclusively of milk and its products, cereals, fruits and vegetables. Since then his urine has been free from sugar.

A woman, forty-three years old, obese, with a lithemic family history, about two years ago developed glycosuria to the extent of five per cent., with polyuria and other symptoms belonging to the glycosuric syndrome. I put her on a moderately severe non-putrefactive diet, allowing a generous quantity of selected carbohydrates. In four weeks her urine was clear. Lately, after indiscretion in eating during her summer vacation, the glycosuria reappeared. A similar diet reduced the sugar in her urine from four per cent. to nothing in nine days.

The therapeutic principle to which I have made allusion in these remarks is not limited in its application to diabetes. It has a wider application. It may be formulated thus: In any condition in which the body is laboring under one particular burden of disease, relief of other burdens, physiological or pathological, enables it better to bear and to throw off the particular burden. In the case of diabetes, making easier the burden of nitrogenous metabolism facilitates the rectification of carbohydrate metabolism.

# THE ANNUAL MEETING

## OF THE

# Associated Physicians of Long Island

### WILL BE HELD ON

## SATURDAY, JANUARY 31, 1914

# EDITORIAL

## DOCTOR AND DRUGGIST.

THE attention of the JOURNAL has been recently called to the bill now before Congress regulating inter-State traffic in narcotic drugs. Investigation seems to show that the ultimate factor in at least one recent outbreak between negroes and whites in Louisiana was cocaine. Unquestionably the using of this drug as an intoxicant has spread widely among a certain class in our large cities. It is known to be smuggled into prisons, where, in one instance, at least, its sale netted a profit of $500 in one month, and it is logical to believe that the legitimate use of the drug has fallen far behind its sales for purposes of debauchery. H. R. 6282 seems to be a bill drawn with sufficient breadth and care to accomplish much in tracing sales, of cocaine in particular, that seem by their size to indicate their unlawful purpose. Quoting from Bulletin No. 1 of the American Association of Pharmaceutical Chemists, the requirements of the bill are summarized as follows:

The first section of the bill requires every person who produces, imports, manufactures, compounds, deals in, dispenses, sells, distributes or gives away any opium or coca leaves or any of their derivatives, compounds, manufactures, salts, or preparations, to register his name, etc., with the collector of internal revenue of the district where he carries on his business; and also to pay a special tax of $1 per annum. It further provides that it shall be unlawful for any person to do business of this nature without having registered and paid the special tax. It also provides that the Commissioner of Internal Revenue, with the approval of the Secretary of the Treasury, shall make all *needful* rules and regulations for carrying the provisions of this act into effect. *The power to regulate is properly limited and such regulations can neither add to nor take away from the express provisions of the Act.*

Section 2 provides that it shall be unlawful for any person to sell, barter, exchange or give away any of these drugs except in pursuance of a written order of the purchaser or person to whom such article is given on a form to be issued in blank for that purpose by the Commissioner of Internal Revenue; and requires the seller to keep such order for a period of two years, so that it may be accessible for inspection by Federal and State officials. The purchaser who makes out this order blank must keep a duplicate in a similar manner. The buyer and seller have, therefore, duplicate copies of every order of sale. *This method of duplicate order blanks, however, is expressly made not to apply to the dispensing or distribution of these drugs to a patient by a physician, dentist, or veterinary surgeon registered under this act in the course of his professional practice only: Provided, however, that such physician, dentist, or veterinary surgeon shall personally attend upon such patient.* This method of duplicate order blanks is expressly made not to apply, also, to the sale, dispensing or distribution of these drugs by a pharmacist to a consumer upon a written prescription of a registered physician, dentist or veterinary surgeon, provided the prescription is dated and signed by the physician, etc., and preserved by the pharmacist for two years; nor to the exportation of drugs. The duplicate order blanks are to be prepared and sold by the Internal Revenue Department for a nominal sum.

Section 3 provides that any person registered under this act may be required by the collector of internal revenue to render a statement, verified by affidavit, setting forth (a) quantity of these drugs received during a period not exceeding three months prior to the demand of the collector, (b) the names of the persons from whom the drugs were received, (c) and the quantity and date in each instance. *It will be noted that the duplicate order form required to be retained by the seller by the provisions of section 2 serves as the record of all sales. The statement required by section 3 refers to receipts and defines the record of such receipts which must be kept in addition to retaining the duplicate order forms indicating purchases.*

Section 4 makes it unlawful for any person who shall not have registered and paid the special tax to transport or send any of these drugs from State to State, except in the case of common carriers, written prescriptions of physicians, etc.

Section 5 makes accessible to the Federal and State officials the duplicate order forms and prescriptions preserved by the provisions of section 2 and the statements required by the provisions of section 3. It further provides that the collectors of internal revenue shall furnish upon written request, to any person, a certified copy of the names of any or all persons who may be listed in their respective collection districts as special-tax payers under the provisions of this act upon payment of a fee of $1 for each 100 names or fraction thereof.

Section 6 exempts preparations and remedies which do not contain more than 2 grains of opium, or more than $\frac{1}{4}$ grain of morphine or more than 1-12 grain of heroin, or more than 1 grain of codeine or any salt derivative of them in a fluid or avoirdupois ounce; liniments, ointments or other preparations for external use only, except such as contain cocaine or any of its salts or alpha or beta eucaine or any of their salts or any synthetic substitute for them; decocainized coca leaves or preparations made therefrom or other preparations of coca leaves which do not contain cocaine.

Section 7 makes applicable laws relating to the collection of internal revenue taxes, and especially section 3229 of the Revised Statutes permitting compromises and remission of fines by the Commissioner of Internal Revenue upon the advice of the Secretary of the Treasury and Attorney General.

Section 8 makes it unlawful for any person not registered and who has not paid the special tax to have any of these drugs in his possession or under his control, and such possession or control is made presumptive evidence of violation; exceptions are made for drugs prescribed by physicians, etc.

Section 9 provides the penalty of a fine of not more than $2,000, imprisonment for not more than 5 years, or both.

Sections 10 and 11 are administrative provisions.

Section 12 provides that this act shall not repeal the pure food law and exclusive act of 1909.

**This Law, if enacted, will go into effect on January 1, 1914.**

It will be noted, therefore, that physicians, under this act, need only (1) register and (2) pay the special tax of $1 per year and (3) make out the duplicate order form (obtained from the Internal Revenue officials), sending the original to the manufacturer, wholesaler, or retailer, and retaining for two years the duplicate order form. The duplicate order forms will indicate the receipts and so provide, if the date of receipt is added, the record resuired by section 3. The dispensing and distributing by the registered physician to his patient in the course of his professional practice and when he personally attends upon the patient is entirely free and unrestricted.

The manufacturer, wholesaler or retailer is required:

1. To register and pay the annual tax of $1.

2. To preserve for the period of two years the duplicate order forms received—*indicating the sales.* The duplicate order forms are not required in the case of the sale, dispensing or distribution by the pharmacist to the consumer upon prescription as set forth in section 2. The pharmacist must in that case preserve the prescription for two years.

3. To keep a record of the quantities of these drugs received, the names of the persons from whom received and the quantity and date in each instance—*indicating the receipts.* The purchases must also be indicated by preserving the duplicate order forms for two years.

The purpose of the act is clear—to trace the line of distribution from the importer and manufacturer down to the ultimate purchaser. Undue purchases will be apparent. Free from the usual burdensome and complicated provisions of revenue measures this bill is extremely simple in its requirements.

It is quite important that the trade and medical profession lend their active support to this commendable measure, dealing with an evil apparent to all, as this law will serve as the model for similar uniform State laws.

The bill as originally drawn was the result of co-operation on the part of the American Association of Pharmaceutical Chemists and the American Medical Association, and was concurred in by the National Association of Retail Druggists. Its passage through Congress seemed assured until the last-named organization suddenly withdrew its support and substituted active opposition. Light is thrown on the reason for this change of attitude by some very frank remarks reported to come from its former President, in the course of which exception was taken to the latitude allowed physicians by the bill, the only practical restrictions to which they are subjected being the requirement for purchasing the necessary blanks from the Treasury department. If we interpret correctly the stand which seems to have been taken by a portion of the retail druggists' national organization, we seem to see an ulterior purpose to prevent physicians in general practice from dispensing their own drugs, and conversation with certain well-informed drug_ gists bears out this view. In point of fact, certain Western States have already passed legislation so drastic as to make it practically essential that a physician shall provide his patients with drugs on pre- scription only, thus constituting a virtual monopoly for the retail druggist. To be a little more explicit, in one State at least, the law requires that if a physician supplies his patients personally with cer- tain drugs or narcotics, he must at the same time provide the patient with a prescription such as he would submit to a druggist, and must keep on file a copy of same; at certain specified times this must be submitted to the State Board of Pharmacy. Furthermore, should the patient die, the physician is forbidden to provide a death cer- tificate, which can only be issued under these circumstances by the district medical officer. The result is, of course, to place the physi- cian absolutely at the mercy of the retail druggist. It seems evi- dent that the standard set by this State will be used as a model for subsequent legislation in others, an end that would be difficult to obtain should the sensible provisions of the present Federal bill become effective.

The attitude of the National Association of Retail Druggists evidently grows out of the habit of dispensing tablets and other drugs that has sprung up among physicians in recent years. The proportions to which this practice has grown are emphasized by the large number of concerns now in the field that trade almost exclusively with the physician direct. It is probable that the cus- tom is much more extensive in the rural districts, where conven- ience of dispensing directly to the patient is evident because of the scarcity of pharmacies, while hospitals and sanitaria are also large purchasers. The claim is made that such purchasers are by no means exacting in the quality of the goods they buy, being apt to make cheapness the important consideration; and, as is always the case, cheapness is known to mean inferior quality ,and competition only tends to increase the evil. Could the druggist feel that the dispensing physician is always careful to choose none but goods of approved quality, his objection to office dispensing would neces- sarily be.a business consideration only. But where he knows of undisputed instances in which inferior goods are purchased and dispensed, he rightly feels that such competition is unfair. The average practicing physician has no way of determining the quality of the tablet he buys except the reputation of the manu- facturer, and unscrupulous dealers might readily supply him with the poorest of drugs for the sake of profit. It is just here that the dispensing physician is vulnerable in claiming his right to dispense drugs if he be so disposed. The pharmacist is supposed to be trained in the preparation, identification and compounding of medicinal sub- stances. The physician, while trained in theapeusis, knows noth- ing, as a rule, of the commercial side of the pharmacist's training. If he wishes to compete with the pharmacist, he ought at least to be assured that his preparations, like Cæsar's wife, are above suspicion.

There is an evident trend toward legislative control in prac- tically every calling, and the profession of medicine, if it has not already done so,, must awaken to the evident faults that, unless corrected, will speedily be taken up by the people, who are the court of last resort, and set its house in order before it is too late.

That a physician is qualified to hand to his patient the appropriate drug that may be indicated at the time is beyond question, provided he is sure that the dose and quality are unquestionaby correct. The physician or institution that deals in cheap drugs cannot be certain of these two essentials, and by so doing is playing directly into the hands of those druggists who rejoice at the opportunity of putting a complete and permanent end to the doctors' privilege of dispensing, and incidentally gain for themselves a control over the drug business that sooner or later will bring about a most embarrassing situation for the physician who will find himself absolutely controlled by the retail drug trade.

The lack of unity among physicians, the shortsightedness and pettiness that so many display, is more than emphasized by the methods of such organizations as have been quoted. How many physicians in the State of New York are aware of the legislation that is introduced each year affecting their profession? The custom that prevails at present in our loose organization is primitive in the extreme. The County Society, which is the unit of organization, at its annual meeting selects a legislative committee who are usually men of some years' experience, who are generally busy and always unpaid. Upon them falls the burden of watching the Legislature in the interests of all their brother practitioners, who not infrequently are only too willing to hold up their failure, if they have failed, to censure and never say even "thank you" if they succeed in defeating pernicious legislation. Usually those who are most dissatisfied are the ones who take the least active interest in their society. Compare with this archaic situation the thorough organization which prevails in the business world; every railroad, every trade, even the labor unions, maintain a paid central bureau and publish comprehensive bulletins to each one of their members, who stand ready to contribute time, effort and money to see that their rights are maintained. Is it not time that the physicians of this country adopt similar means to see that the profession to which they belong is properly represented and effectively handled, so that instead of indignant protest that comes too late we may employ efficient prevision and put to practical use the method of prevention which we recognize as so essential in our calling?

H. G. W.

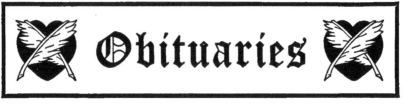

## JOHN RANDALL STIVERS, M.D.

DR. STIVERS was born May 16, 1870, at Ridgebury, N. Y., and died September 18, 1913, at Brooklyn, N. Y. He was the son of Randall Stivers and Ellen J. Hulse, both of New Jersey.

His early education was received at Willkill Academy, his medical education was under the direction of Frank D. Myers, M.D., receiv-the degree of M.D. from the Long Island College Hospital, class of 1894, followed by a term as interne of the Kings County Hospital. During his professional life for a number of years was physician to the Kings County Hospital, and physician-in-chief of the Samaritan Hospital.

He was a member of the Medical Society County of Kings, from 1896; associate treasurer from 1900 to 1906, and treasurer from 1907 to the time of his death; American Medical Association, Long Island Medical Society, Brooklyn Pathological Society, of which he was president in 1911; Kings County Hospital Club, president in 1899; Alumni Association of the Long Island College Hospital, president in 1913; Acanthus Lodge No. 719, F. & A. M., of which he was master in 1906. Instructor in Physical Diagnosis at the Long Island College Hospital 1902 to 1904.

His medical papers were as follows: "Renal Calculus Passed Through the Urethra," "Prognosis of Meningitis," "Article in the Twentieth Century Practice of Medicine," "Some Points in the Diagnosis and Treatment of Pneumonia," "Typhoid Fever," "Prognosis of Meningitis," "Some Observations from Cases of Sudden Death."

Dr. Stivers is survived by his widow, Susan M. Havens and two daughters, Cristina and Gladys. W. S., SR.

---

## ROBERT EMORY MOORE, A.B., M.D.

DR. MOORE was born in Baltimore, Md., January 10, 1880, and died at Saranac Lake, N. Y., on September 18, 1913. His father was William H. Moore, and his mother, Alice S. Burch, both of Baltimore.

He was educated at the Baltimore City College—an A.B. from Johns Hopkins University in 1902, receiving the degree of M.D. from the same university in 1906. This was followed with a term as interne at the Kings County Hospital, a member of the Medical Society, County of Kings, from 1909; American Medical Association, Brooklyn Pathological Society, Brooklyn Surgical Society, New York Society of Anæsthetists, Society of ex-Internes of the Kings County Hospital, Bunker Hill Lodge, No. 136, I. O. O. F.; Montauk Camp, No. 12859, M. W. of A., and the University Club. He is survived by his widow, Mrs. Ida Henry, of Baltimore. W. S., SR.

## DANIEL ALOYSIUS SHAY, M.D.

DR. SHAY died at Marlborough, N. Y., on August 21, 1913. He was born in New York City, October 21, 1875.

His medical education was received at the University of Baltimore, where the degree of M.D. was conferred upon him in 1901.

He practiced medicine in the Bay Ridge section of our city. He is survived by his widow, Mary Grace Bush, and one son.

W. S., SR..

## EMMA T. P. ALLEN, M.D.

DR. ALLEN was born in Bath, Me., in 1845, and died in Brooklyn, N. Y., August 9, 1913. She was graduated in 1892 from the Medical College and Hospital for Women, a member of the County and State Homœopathic Medical Society, and the American Institute of Homœopathy.

W. S., SR.

## HENRY CUSHMAN TURNER, M.D.

DR. TURNER died at Washington, Conn., on August 16, 1913; born in Brooklyn, N. Y., December 30, 1844. He was the son of Joseph Mott Turner, M.D., his mother was Sophia Cushman.

His medical education was received at the College of Physicians and Surgeons, N. Y., where he was graduated in the class of 1867.

For a number of years he was physician to the Norwegian Hospital, and from 1867 to 1905 a member of the Medical Society County of Kings. He practiced medicine n Brooklyn, N. Y., during his professional life. He was an elder in the Westminster Presbyterian Church, where the funeral services were conducted.     W. S., SR.

## GEORGE DRURY, M.D.

DR. DRURY was born in Morrisania, N. Y., on April 14, 1857, and died in Brooklyn, N. Y., October 20, 1913. He was the son of Alfred T. Drury, M.D., and Henrietta H. King, both of England. He was educated in the private schools, his medical education was under the direction of his father, receiving the degree of M.D. from the Long Island College Hospital in the class of 1878.

From 1880 to 1886 he was assistant to the Chair of Practice of Medicine in the same institution.

Dr. Drury married Mary A. Packard, April 27, 1881. His children are Alfred Thomas Drury; Irene, wife of Dr. Woolley; Florence L., wife of Mr. Ramsey, and Miss Marguerite Henrietta Drury.

He was a member of the Medical Society, County of Kings, from 1879 to 1903; Brooklyn Pathological Society, Associated Physicians of Long Island from 1905 to 1913, Commonwealth Lodge, No. 409, F. & A. M.; Orient Chapter, No. 138, R. A. M.; Clinton Commandery, No. 14, K. T.; Union Leage, and the Dyker Heights Golf Clubs.     W. S., SR.

## ALFRED THORNTON BIRDSALL, M.D.

DR. BIRDSALL was born in the city of Brooklyn, 43 years ago, where he died on September 24, 1913. He was educated in the public schools and the University of Minnesota, where he received his degree of M. D., in 1896. A few years later he came to Brooklyn, where he remained during his professional life.

He was a member of the Medical Society, County of Kings, from 1900, and physician to the Tubercular Clinic.

He leaves his widow, Virginia Field, and a son, Daniel T. Birdsall. W. S., Sr.

## S. S. HUBER, M.D.

Dr. Huber was born in Chambersburg, Pa., in 1836, and died in Brooklyn, N. Y., October 16, 1913. He received the degree of M.D. from the Jefferson Medical College in 1865, and served in the hospital department during the Civil War. He was for a number of years in practice in this city. He leaves a widow, Amelia, and two sons, Ralph and Frank. W. S., Sr.

## JOHN DUTTON BRUNDAGE, M.D.

Dr. Brundage was born at Brookfield, Conn., January 17, 1835, and died at Torrington, Conn., October 22, 1913. His father was Alfred M. Brundage, of New Jersey, and his mother, Lucy Parker, of Connecticut.

Dr. Brundage was married to Delia G. Higgins, April 6, 1864. The children born of this union were Minnie G., Mary E., Marion L. and Estha W. Brundage.

He received his education in the public and high schools, and the study of medicine under the direction of Amos L. Williams, M.D., of Conneticut, graduating from Yale Medical College in 1864.

He was a member of the Associated Physicians of Long Island from 1906. W. S., Sr.

## GOTTHARD HIRSEMAN, M.D.

Dr. Hirseman was for many years a practicing physician in this city. He died at Highland Mills, N. Y., on October 6, 1913. He was a graduate of the Long Island College Hospital in the class of 1888. He leaves a son, Walter G. Hirseman, M.D. W. S., Sr.

## CARL WILLICH, M.D.

Dr. Willich was born in Germany, July 23, 1851, and died in Brooklyn, N. Y., September 23, 1913. He received the degree of M.D. from Bellevue Hospital Medical College in 1893. He is survived by his widow, Helen, and two children, Helen and Carl. W. S., Sr.

## WILLIAM ANDERSON MITCHELL, M.D.

Dr. Mitchell died in Brooklyn, N. Y., September 26, 1913. He was an A.B. from Columbia, and M.D. from Yale University in 1867. He was a veteran of the Civil War, and a member of Tefft Post, G. A. R. W. S., Sr.

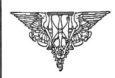 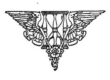

## TRANSACTIONS OF THE BROOKLYN GYNECOLOGICAL SOCIETY.

*Stated Meeting of April* 4, 1913.

The President, CARROLL CHASE, M.D., in the Chair.

### Presentation of Specimens.

DR. VICTOR A. ROBERTSON presented a specimen of arteriosclerosis and fibrosis of the uterus.

DR. ROBERTSON :—"This specimen illustrates a condition that must always be thought of in considering diseases of the uterus. The patient was a virgin fifty years of age who had suffered from a persistent menorrhagia for several years, and the flow was so great at times as to create a condition almost of extremis. Medical treatment was of no avail. Examination showed no displacement, no neoplasm, and no disease of the adnexa, but the uterus was somewhat enlarged, much firmer and denser in consistency than normal, not painful to pressure. Curettage gave temporary relief. Hysterectomy was advised and consented to three years ago, and since the operation the patient has been in perfect health. The diagnosis was made by exclusion, cancer, fibroid, and uterine polypus being considered. The uterus was regular in shape and showed no nodular masses, and the scrapings revealed merely a fungoid endometritis which often accompanies this condition. She also showed no signs of general vascular change. The cervix was normal in appearance and did not bleed on touch; the condition seemed to be confined to the uterine body." Dr. Robertson then read the following pathological tissue report of the case by Dr. William McKimmie Higgins, of New York:

"Patient, Miss E. The length of the virgin uterus is about 3 inches, width 1½ to 2 inches, thickness about 1 inch; that is 3 inches by 1½ to 2 inches by 1 inch. Its walls are on the average ⅜ of an inch. In the specimen submitted the length is four inches, the width 2¼ inches, and in thickness it is 1¾ inches. The wall on the average is ⅞ of an inch through. It is about an inch longer than the virgin uterus, quite a little wider, and thicker by almost an inch. In outline the organ is normal, though less flattened than usual, but is considerably hypertrophied. The uterus, however, after fifty, should become atrophied. Taking the size of uteri in multipara that have undergone simple hypertrophy, the degree of enlargement in this case would be considered moderate. The tissue is much firmer than usual and cuts less readily than that of the normal uterus. Microscopically, the mucous membrane is normal; the connective tissue is seen in about the usual proportion, and the glands are short, simple, tubular, and not increased in number. As a whole, throughout the section the muscle bands are a little broader and coarser than is usually seen. While the connective tissue is also increased, the increase is more noticeable in the outer half of the organ. There are no places where there is any decided increase of the fibrous tissue or replacement of the normal tissue, but throughout the sections the fibrous bands running between the muscle bundles and the muscle fibres are thicker than usual, so that on the whole there is quite a degree of fibrous increase, more marked in the outer half. The elastic tissue is very small in amount. There is no scar tissue, and no appearance of any inflammatory reaction. Once in a while there is a very small area, especially in the neighborhood of the blood vessels, that is apparently undergoing hyaline degeneration. The blood vessels, for uterine tissue, are neither numerous nor very large. They might be considered a little more numerous than usual, but the increase is not at all marked. As a rule, they are either small or of moderate size. The lumina are open, the intima is normal, while the other two coats are hypertrophied. Of the two latter the media or muscle coats show the greatest degree of enlargement, but the adventitia is also wider than usual. Towards the outer half there are several groups of very large vessels which show the same abnormalities in the relative proportion of the different coats. Most of the blood vessels are open, though the lumina are not widely distended; the tendency of the blood vessels to remain open and their appearance of rigidity is more marked in the vessels of moderate size than in the larger ones, which appear to be more readily collapsible. The increase in the size of the arteries is not a very marked one, but seems to be general throughout the organ. The increase in fibrous tissue in the uterus is not confined to any particular part, though more marked in the outer half, but seems to be general throughout the organ. The hypertrophy of the uterus is due also, in part, to increase in the amount of muscle tissue. Although not extensive, the sum total of increase makes the amount of connective tissue relatively much greater, as compared with the muscle tissue, than is seen in the normal organ. The specimen may be considered, therefore, a case of hyper-trophy due to a general increase in both the muscle and fibrous tissue, but especially in the tissue of the latter type."

DR. JUDD:—"I do not know of any class of cases that come to us that are so uncertain as these cases of fibrosis of the uterus. Most of them have been curetted many times with temporary relief. I should like to ask Dr. Robertson if there was any special reason for the removal of both ovaries in this case; they seem to be normal."

DR. W. B. CHASE:—"I did not follow the analysis closely. Was the condition due to any characteristic lesion in the blood vessels themselves or to an increase in the fibrous structure?"

DR. ROBERTSON:—"This woman was fifty years of age, past the physiological menopause, and it occurred to me that the ovaries were of no further value after removal of the uterus and there was no reason why they should remain. The ovaries in the specimen are shrunken by being kept in formalin solution; they were cystic on removal. In answer to Dr. Chase's question I would say that the tissue report shows a thickening and hyperplasia of the walls of the blood vessels with fibrous bands running between and replacing the muscle bundles, which would affect the contractile power of these vessels and thus account for the persistent menorrhagia."

DR. ALBERT M. JUDD presented a specimen of hydatidiform mole, or cystic degeneration of the chorionic villi. This patient was PARA XII ..............
Her last previous labor was in June, 1911. Her last menstrual period was in November, 1912, exact date not known. She was admitted to the Kings County Hospital with the uterus the size of a seven or eight months' pregnancy. There was a history of spotting one month ago, with hemorrhage again one week ago. Examination at the hospital did not disclose any fœtal parts, and no fœtal heart could be found. You have here a history of a typical case of hydatidiform mole. There was rapid enlargement, lack of fœtal parts, with hemorrhages. The house obstetrician made a diagnosis of placenta previa, and he could hardly be blamed for the error, as there was a clot of blood at the os that felt very much like the condition found in placenta previa. The uterus was emptied manually, and here is the specimen.

"I wish to put on record a modification of the Coffey method of plication of the broad ligaments which I did at the Jewish Hospital recently. The operation is done as follows: Before starting in the ordinary plication, you separate the bladder from the uterus at the uterovesical junction in the same manner as for a hysterectomy. This method I have used, and felt it was applicable for cases of retroversion presenting cystocele. After the separation of the bladder and lifting it up, to go on with the plication, you proceed as in the Coffey method, with this exception, that you start lower down on the broad ligaments and plicate in front of the cervix and form a sling to throw the fundus forward, finishing above as Coffey suggests; then the bladder is brought up and attached as high on the uterus as necessary to overcome the fall of that organ and the occurrence of a cystocele.

"I wish to make a preliminary report on some cases in which a Wassermann was done antepartum in some and postpartum in others. We all see many cases of probable syphilis among our private cases of which we feel that we must not speak too freely. I have a woman who is to be married this month with this condition. It has seemed to me that if we insist upon this test as a part of the examination of pregnant women we might in some cases save fœtal life. These cases are as follows:

"CASE 1. Halloran. Primipara, strong, robust female. Received 606 in September, 1912, and January, 1913, following positive Wassermann's, which were negative on our service, to which she was admitted January 28, 1913. Baby born March 13, 1913, showing no evidence of syphilis beyond slight snuffles. Mother has nursed her babe, which is thriving.

"Case 2. Wormsen. Stout, robust female of 24; para III.; first child born alive four years ago; second pregnancy resulted in an abortion at the second month. Wassermann positive on admission to our service early in January, about seven months' pregnant. She received semi-weekly inunctions from January 17 to date of delivery on March 16. Beyond a slight vaginal hemorrhage, such as is seen in many new-born female babies, her child is perfectly normal.

"Case 3. Fanning. Thin, anemic girl. Wassermann positive, and she received inunctions instead of 606 because of cardiac and nephritic insufficiency. She delivered herself of a premature and dead fœtus.

"Case 4. Mott. Large, obese and healthy woman with a positive Wassermann. At time of admission had an eruption which, because of a positive W., was regarded with suspicion; it had been pronounced scabies by dermatologists. Received inunctions of Hg. and delivered herself of a living and apparently healthy babe.

"Case 5. Abert. Robust female. First child born alive, then followed three miscarriages, all at six to seven months, then this delivery, for which she came to our service in labor, and was delivered of a six weeks' premature and macerated fœtus. Wassermann taken postpartum was XX. Instructed on discharge to begin treatment, especially as she is anxious to have another child.

"Case 6. Smith. Admitted with multiple condylomata, very large; growths found to be specific and Wassermann positive. Para I. Received Hg. salicylate intramuscularly instead of 606, because of a recurring toxemia of pregnancy of nephritic type. Baby is at present alive and due in a few weeks. (Since delivered of an apparently normal child.)"

"The other series of cases are as follows:

"Case 1A. Kane. Age, 26, para IV.; thin, weak, and anemic. First child born alive in August, 1908; second pregnancy aborted in 1910 at 2½ months; third pregnancy aborted in September, 1911, at 3 months. Last menstruation August, 1912, and admitted to our service about seven months pregnant with a live fœtus in utero. Condylomata developed one month before admission, and Wassermann found positive. Received two injections of 606 and baby is at present alive; due in May.

"Case 2A. Cook. One child born alive three years ago; no miscarriages. Admitted seven months pregnant with no evidences of syphilis beyond positive Wassermann. Baby is alive at present. No treatment for purposes of control.

"Case 3A. Palase. Para VIII. Thin, weak Italian; in Kings County Hospital March 1911, for syphilitic ascites, and at that time had positive Noguchi. She was pregnant then and was delivered of a premature dead fœtus. Received injections of Hg. Salicylate and left hospital with positive Noguchi. Admitted to our service about two months ago and Wassermann found positive. Baby is at present alive and patient is receiving no treatment for purposes of control and observation.

"Of the above patients four were discovered only by routine examination of the blood for Wassermann test of every antepartem case. There were no other evidences of syphilis. The value of this routine in saving the then growing fœtus, or in saving the future babies is apparent. How many of our former cases of stillbirths would have shown positive Wassermanns can only be conjectured. The one patient (Fanning) who delivered herself of a dead child in spite of persistent treatment can be explained by the frequent occurrence of this mishap in nephritis, which here complicated her syphilis.

"The observance of any symptoms beyond the positive Wassermanns is merely stated, not explained.

"I hope the doctors will take up this matter and advise the use of the Wassermann test as a routine measure in pregnancy."

In answer to a question Dr. Judd stated that the case of hydatidiform mole was operated on only a week ago.

Dr. Cummiskey asked if the Wassermann test had been used on the new-born babies, and said that sometimes the mother would not show a positive Wassermann, yet the test would be positive in the baby.

Dr. Humpstone was pleased to hear that Dr. Judd was investigating the Wassermann reaction in pregnancy, labor, the puerperium. There are many factors in connection with this question, which we do not know much about, as yet. For example, why a new-born baby should show a positive Wassermann, while the mother had been negative all during her pregnancy, and three weeks postpartum develop a positive reaction.

The examination of pregnant women for syphilis is quite likely to become a part of the routine investigation of the specialist in obstetrics. We shall co-operate with Dr. Judd in investigating a long series of cases and then study the results.

DR. JUDD:—"I am glad Dr. Cummiskey brought up the question of examination of the babies. No Wassermann has been done on the children in the cases I have recorded. Referring to Dr. Humpstone's remarks, I would say that the authorities state that the Wassermann is sometimes negative in a woman at one time and positive at another time. I hope to have all the cases tested in the genitourinary service. I think also it is essential to have the placental blood tested as well as the mother's blood."

DR. WILLIAM P. POOL then read the paper of the evening: Some Phases of Pelvic Infection. 1. Indications and Limitations of Surgical Treatment. 2. Differentiation of Infections. 3. Most Favorable Time and Method of Operation.

DR. HOLDEN:—"I am sure the Society is indebted to Dr. Pool for his splendid paper and it is too bad that Societies of general practitioners do not have such papers brought to their attention. Men who are doing hospital work see the results of the general practitioners' methods in these cases, and the effects of their work. All I have to say on the papers is to refer to the conservative methods advocated by Dr. Pool. During the past year I have seen cases, with the history of pelvic infection, treated conservatively, and when subsequently operated upon for other conditions have had the pleasure of finding absence of adhesions or other evidence of previous troubles, showing that nature will do a great deal. In the last six months at the Long Island Hospital under Dr. Polak's service in our cases with retained secundines we have waited. Last year we would have considered it conservative treatment to explore the uterus and pack it with iodine gauze. In the last six months we have not entered a uterus except for hemorrhage which was persistent, otherwise we have not made any such examination, and we have had a very low morbidity. I have also insisted upon turning the patients upon the abdomen for a few minutes and from side to side, and have advocated hygenic treatment, and fresh air, even taking the patients to the roof while in bed to aid in convalescence."

DR. HYDE:—"It has always seemed to me that true pelvic cellulitis is never gonorrhœal but usually obstetrical. It is unilateral, in distinction from gonorrhœal salpingitis. The point that Dr. Pool makes that gonorrhœal tubes are usually sterile, is not difficult to understand. These tubes become occluded at the fimbriated ends either by salpingitic closure, or peritonitic closure, and the gonoccoccus dies because of no new nutrient medium in which to live. It actually starves to death. Very different from gonococci in the vagina and urethra, where they flourish well and practically never die. These sterile tubes have made some operators careless. Having operated on some cases and ruptured the tube during enucleation and seeing no bad results follow—(although there had been a free escape of pus into the pelvic cavity)—they possibly feel that all pus tubes, when ruptured, will never produce any infection (peritonitis). But some pus tubes with a mixed infection, or in the early stage before sterilization, when ruptured, are capable of establishing a most virulent infection of the peritoneum. Acute gonorrhœal peritonitis is not common. Kelly has reported a few cases.

"I was interested, recently, in reading an English gynecology, in which the routine treatment advocated for opening pelvic abscesses, was by an incision above Poupart's ligament, extraperitoneally. I have had but two cases where I employed this incision and was interested to note the great disproportion between the size of the mass and the amount of pus evacuated, hardly more than an ounce, yet the mass, in both instances, was well above the pelvic brim. The size of the mass would lead the operator to think that there was a large collection of pus.

"In accute infection with pus formation, drain from below. In acute streptococcic or staphylococcic, never go above. But after all has been said regarding etiology and treatment, there is another side of the question of pelvic infection which interests us as gynecologists, namely, the pain, sterility, menstrual disturbances, the neurasthenias, which follow in the wake of pelvic infection. It is these conditions which should engage our attention, as gynecologists, quite as much."

DR. KNIGHT:—"I want to endorse everything that has been said by Dr. Pool. I am convinced, however, that in the severe streptococcus infections we should make a simple posterior vaginal section and insert a small gauze drain into the cul-de-sac. I have seen these patients doing badly, but after draining them improvement began and very little shock to the patient was produced."

DR. ROBERTSON:—"I can speak confirmatory of the statements of Dr.

Pool and Dr. Hyde as to the innocuousness of pus that has been retained in tubal infections. Ten years ago with the late Dr. Wilson, of the Hoagland Laboratory, I examined many specimens of pus from such conditions and we were surprised at the number that were sterile. All I can further say is merely in corroboration as to the wisdom of conservatism in the treatment of postpartum conditions. I have seen in hospital service women who had been dreadfully infected by midwives and physicians, do well under wise and conservative treatment. I make no examinations except for hemorrhage, and let the uterus entirely alone. In the treatment of streptococcic infection in the cul-de-sac I have seen irrigation tried after opening the pus collection and I think it unwise. In regard to incising the cul-de-sac in the absence of pointing I think an opening can at times be made sooner than the writer says, even when we get only an œdematous feeling. Such cases have always done well in my hands even when I have not waited for focalization of the pus. The cul-de-sac can be opened with perfect freedom from bad results in these cases."

Dr. Judd:—"Dr. Pool's conclusions are the same as my own. A few years ago I listened to a paper at Bellevue College, New York, on when to operate on gonorrhœal infected tubes. The writer took the stand that all cases should be examined carefully and where there were gonococci in the cervix secretions the operation should be deferred. I have tried to carry out his plan at various times. In my work during the past winter I have been surprised where I have advocated interference in cases of pus tubes at the number where the pathologists have found gonococci, and yet there has been very slight post-operative reaction. I have not found a method whereby I may know when to operate or when not to operate. When you do interfere you must be radical. Taking up the subject of streptococcic infection in postpartem cases my method is extremely conservative. I make one examination with the gloved finger and the patient is left in bed in the Fowler position, with the use of fuchsin, externally, sometimes, as a placebo. The method of treatment of gonococcic infection advocated by Dr. Knight I condemned some years ago, and I do not agree with Dr. Robertson in the method of opening through the cul-de-sac in such cases. I believe you do not help the case and at times you may do incalculable injury. One statement made by Dr. Pool I wish to take issue with. He has said that he does not believe in stenosis of the cervix; I presume he refers to occlusion of the cervix by flexion. I have felt that such conditions do appear and with a sudden rise of temperature, and passing of the finger up to straighten the cervix will result in a dropping of the temperature."

Dr. Pool:—"Dr. Hyde's reference to mixed infections brings up an interesting subject, and one that is somewhat speculative—mixed infections undoubtedly occur, but so far as our present knowledge goes, the different organisms do not infect at the same time or in the same way.

An early attempt at drainage in parametrial inflamation is, I believe, unwise. In the first place the disease may get well without operation, and also the extensive traumatism which is likely to be done in searching for a pus focus furnishes a broad avenue for the further absorption of infection. It is a common thing to have a sharp rise in temperature following the simplest drainage operation, which means that more toxines are dumped into the circulation. The same thing happens sometimes at the result of a forcible examination. If the inflamation remain local the patient's life is not in danger and nothing is lost by waiting, and if infection have become general nothing is gained by operation. Therefore, it seems wiser to me to wait until there is a well-developed and walled-in focus to attack."

The method suggested by Dr. Judd of determining the presence of gonococci in the tubes by the presence of those germs in the cervix seems to me to be somewhat inaccurate, because gonococci will live much longer in the cervix than when shut up in a tubal abcess. One advantage of such a calculation might be that some cases would be given time to recover while we are waiting for a suitable time to operate.

As to stenosis of the cervix my belief is that when there is any narrowing of the cause it is due to a flexed uterus and not to any actual constriction of the cervical tissues.

I have faithfully vaccinated all my septic cases for a number of years. The results in some have apparently been brilliant; in others nil. The best results have been obtained in localized stophylococcic infections, and gonococcic infections have also been helped without question. But I have never been able to convince myself that a streptococcic process, local or general, has been materially modified by this form of treatment."

# TRANSACTIONS OF THE BROOKLYN SURGICAL SOCIETY.

*Stated Meeting, May 1, 1913.*

The President, DR. RICHARD W. WESTBROOK, in the Chair.

**Paper: "Cancer of the Colon" with Report of Cases.**

*By Dr. Onslow A. Gordon.*

It is not the purpose of the writer to occupy the time of a scientific body like this with a long paper upon a subject which is well within the grasp of every member, but rather to relate abbreviated histories of a few cases that have recently come under my care.

Much has been written and said concerning cancer of the colon, but the number of patients suffering from conditions beyond hope of relief as a result of procrastination and disregard of the danger signals seems not to have diminished.

In none of the cases that have been referred to me during the past year had a diagnosis of malignancy been considered, although all gave a history that should excite suspicion.

CASE 1.—A man of fifty years was seen after several days of obstruction with fecal vomiting, distention and in a state of shock. Operation was advised and relucantly accepted. Upon opening the abdomen a hard, nodular mass, the size of an orange, was found in the ascending colon. Owing to the exhausted state of the patient a resection was considered inadvisable at the time and a colostomy was done which afforded relief for a few hours only. The patient succumbed on the second day following operation.

CASE 2.—Male, sixty-seven years of age. Gave a history extending over several years which pointed to gradual narrowing of the lumen of the intestine. His abdomen was enormously distended and he was vomiting constantly and in every way presented a most unfavorable outlook. The gravity of the situation was explained to his family and an exploratory operation suggested as the only possible hope of relief. This was accepted and when the abdomen was opened a large quantity of fluid mixed with intestinal contents escaped. A nodular mass was found in the sigmoid, which had perforated. A rubber tube was hastily stitched into the opening and a large quantity of fluid feces and gas escaped through the tube. The abdomen was washed out with normal saline solution and closed with through and through sutures. He died about ten hours after the operation, which did not consume more than twenty-five minutes.

CASE 3.—A woman forty-seven years of age, married, mother of three children; gave a history which was characteristic of an intestinal growth. Came from up the state to be operated for supposed pelvic trouble. She was emaciated and septic and was suffering pain and vomiting; peristalsis was visible through the thin abdominal wall; a large fluctuating mass was easily palpated in the left iliac region, which was opened extra-peritoneally and about a quart of foul smelling pus evacuated. It was found that the cavity communicated with the large bowel, drainage was provided and the patient experienced great relief for a time, a probable diagnosis of malignant growth of the sigmoid was made, but owing to the presence of suppuration, further operation was considered contraindicated. She lived about four weeks, dying from exhaustion. At autopsy a hard annular growth was found in the upper portion of the sigmoid, which had perforated extra-peritoneally. The growth was so located that a resection might have been done easily had the trouble been discovered before perforation. Dr. Hulst reported that the tumor was an adenocarcinoma.

CASE 4.—One of the first in the series, a female, married, mother of three children; referred to me one year ago; gave a characteristic group of symptoms covering two or more years; loss of appetite and flesh; impaired digestion; increasing constipation; intermittent diarrhœa, colic and anæmia.

In the light of present knowledge of her case her symptoms pointed very decidedly to partial obstruction. They were, however, interpreted by different physicians (and not without some ground for justification) as being due to gall stones or possibly appendical in origin. Owing to quite thick abdominal walls, the tumor was not easily palpated. Exploratory laparotomy was advised and accepted. When the abdominal cavity was opened a large tumor involving the cecum and first portion of the ascending colon was readily located. A resection was done, the stumps of the ileum and ascending colon inverted and lateral anastomosis of the ileum and ascending colon made. The operation was easily done. The patient reacted promptly and made an uneventful recovery, since which time (lacking but a few days of a year) her bowels have acted normally and she has gained forty pounds in weight. While it is too soon to claim a cure, we have prolonged her life and she is living in comfort. As will be seen by an examination of the tumor, the ileo-cecal orifice will barely admit a lead pencil.

Dr. Hulst reported the growth to be adenocarcinoma. When patients are convinced that it is safer to submit to exploratory laparotomy whenever suspicion points to a possible growth, than to run the risk of waiting for positive evidence (such as palpable tumor, complete obstruction or perforation) and when the profession fully realizes the importance of such a procedure, then may we hope for a reduction in the mortality from intestinal cancer. If the early exploration reveals a growth, the advantages to the patient are obvious. If the disturbance is due to some minor pathological condition which can be relieved with less operative danger, the operation will be justified. In the writer's opinion, exploratory laparotomy should be advised whenever the following danger signals are present: Increasing constipation, colicky pain, frequent and unsatisfactory stools and intermittent diarrhœa, steady loss of flesh and gradually increasing anemia. The operative mortality from simple exploratory laparotomy is practically nil; from resection for cancer about 14%; from non-interference 100%. When we consider that there is a fair chance that some may be cured, many lives prolonged in comfort, and those less fortunate saved from the horrors of death from obstruction, is it not our duty to urge the acceptance of the only procedure that offers a chance?

## Case of Chronic Osteomyelitis, etc.
### By Dr. W. B. Brinsmade.
### Discussion.

Dr. CHARLES EASTMOND in interpreting the radiographs in the above case said: The condition is purely one of the diaphysis. The changes in the right humerus consist of a general enlargement of the affected part from overgrowth of the cortex, together with more or less obliteration of the medullary canal from the same cause. It is with the greatest difficulty that the medulla can be outlined or, in fact, any trace of it seen.

In determining the question of diagnosis, two conditions must be taken into account:

Chronic osteomyelitis and syphilis.—As an aid in differentiating these, several regions of the body were examined to discover whether or not changes were present elsewhere.

In the knees, the margins are perfectly clear, the medullary canal is clear and even the articular surfaces are sharp, showing that they are perfectly normal. The plate of the left knee presents no changes of any kind. The right knee is likewise negative, both in the joint and in the adjoining portions of the bone.

Next the pelvis, hip-joints and femora were covered and those regions found to be also perfectly normal.

When the man came in first the complaint was of the left shoulder, and on the first plate taken the outer portion of the clavicle appears perfectly distinct, but the inner portion appears very much enlarged with loss of bone substance centrally.

The left clavicle is a little higher than the corresponding portion of the acromion process at the acromio-clavicular articulation, and there has evidently been a relaxation at that point.

Going still further over the body, plates were taken of both hands. In the long bones, the phalanges and metacarpals, there was found to be some minute changes in the general outline. They are perfectly smooth, but some of them are a little enlarged. The fifth, on the right hand, for example, is a trifle enlarged and there are changes in the medullary canal, which do not have the normal striated appearance. It appears also through the proximal row of the phalanges, and with that there is also a slight thickening of the cortex. In discussing this with Dr. Brinsmade, I told him that the only condition I could think of which would present that appearance would be syphilis, one of either a late tertiary or a congenital type.

To return to the arm.

What diseased condition has produced that form of bone? I do not believe that syphilis can be blamed entirely for it, although the condition of the hands, and the fact that the opposite clavicle is affected might lead to that conclusion. I have seen a similar condition only once before, and that was in a person who was non-syphilitic, so far as we could determine, and I believe that the condition is a low-grade chronic osteomyelitis. The infection which was probably hematogonous was not sufficiently virulent to produce necrosis, but as fast as the bone was broken down through disease it was absorbed, and regeneration took place until we finally have the present condition.

There certainly is no evidence of active disease now.

### A Case of Chronic Indurated Ulcer of the Stomach with Malignant Degeneration. Presentation of Patient.

#### *Reported By Dr. W. B. Brinsmade.*

DR. J. D. SULLIVAN, in opening the discussion, said: "Did I understand Dr. Brinsmade to say that the pain was relieved by eating in this case?"

DR. W. B. BRINSMADE, in answer to Dr. Sullivan's question, said: "Yes sir."

### A Case of Chronic Osteomyelitis, with Changes in the Right Humerus and Digits of Both Hands. Subcoracoid Dislocation on Left Side. Radiographs and Presentation of Patient.

#### *By W. B. Brinsmade, M. D.*

DR. J. D. SULLIVAN, in discussion, said: "It appears to me that this case is hardly demonstrated to be one of osteomyelitis. It looks to me more like a case of pure osteitis without the myelitis, a case in which there has been an infection and a low grade of inflammation in the osseous tissue alone, just like we get in a chronic inflammation of the fibrous tissue in any other organ—as cirrhosis of the liver or any of these chronic fibrous inflammations—a sclerotic osteitis. I think it is a fact that we can have a pure simple osteitis of a progressive or proliferative type without any inflammation of the marrow of the bone. If it were an osteomyelitis he would have had suppuration somewhere in his system and certainly in the marrow of the bone. In this case there has been no suppuration, but the lumen of the medullary canal is diminished by the hypertrophic osteitis."

DR. MATHIAS FIGUEIRA, in discussion, said: "Did he not have some inflammation in some other bone besides the humerus?"

DR. W. B. BRINSMADE, answering Dr. Figueira's question, said: "The right humerus and left clavicle show in the picture, but he was never conscious of it."

DR. MATHIAS FIGUEIRA, in discussion, said: "I asked if he did not have some inflammation in some other bone besides the humerus."

DR. W. B. BRINSMADE, answering Dr. Figueira's question, said: "Yes, sir."

DR. MATHIAS FIGUEIRA, in discussion, said: "I think that we have here a man presenting symptoms affecting the body in various places. In this case, if I remember rightly, not only does he have deformity in the right humerus, but also on the left clavicle and pain in one knee and induration of his testicles and that seems to point to something more than a local trouble. It seems to point to something back of the local trouble. Though it centered itself in one bone, it seems to point to a general infection.

"We know that there are two things to which we may attribute this condition, namely, syphilis or tuberculosis. It may be primary or it may be inherited. Both diseases can be transmitted from the parents. In the case of syphilis, the germ itself is transmitted. In the case of tuberculosis, only the tendency to the disease is inherited. I do believe that some of these cases of diseases of the bone, and many other forms of chronic diseases are to be accounted for by syphilis and tuberculosis in the parent, though in this case it is not clear and we are at a disadvantage, because we do not happen to have a clear history of the man's antecedents, the family history in regard to meningitis, joint diseases, miscarriages, and other points that may lead to the conclusion that he is suffering from inherited syphilis or tubercular trouble, or both combined."

DR. J. D. SULLIVAN, in discussion, said: 'I think I omitted to say, Mr. President, that I think the cause of this trouble was of a hematogenous origin; that is, the infection has set up the inflammatory process in the bone, with the result that it has obliterated the canaliculae, increased its size and density, producing an ivory condition, an ebonization of the bone. The early stage of this low grade of chronic osteitis are usually attended with considerable pain, which according to my experience, is more or less intermittent in character."

DR. WILLIAM LINDER, in discussion, said: "Was a Wassermann taken on this fellow?

DR. JOSEPH P. MURPHY. in discussion, said: "In regard to those obscure conditions of the bones, might not the condition be due to some cerebral disturbance, as in the pituitary body or pineal gland?"

DR. J. D. SULLIVAN, in discussing the question put up by Dr. Murphy, said: "I do not think that would be painful."

### By Dr. O. A. Gordon.

Dr. MATHIAS FIGUEIRA, in discussion, said: "I think Dr. Brinsmade's statement should not be allowed to pass without comment.

"With full knowledge of the resources and progress of modern surgery, to tell a person with an abdominal surgical disease, even so advanced, to go home and die without giving him the chance of an exploratory operation, is to do something which I do not see we are warranted in doing. We all know that it is impossible to judge of the chances such a case may have before we open the peritoneal cavity and look at it. The case might look desperate, but when the abdominal cavity is open one may find that something in the way of an operation can be done that may cure or relieve it.

"Dr. Sullivan presented such a case here last year. It was a large tumor of the abdominal cavity in a man. He had been refused operation and given up to die. Dr. Sullivan took the case and operated and it got well. He presented the patient and the tumor here. So it is with many other cases which we see.

"In carcinoma of the stomach, I have seen cases hardly able to walk, in which there was a large tumor of the stomach, in which there was marked cachexia, yet a gastro-enterostomy was done and although it looked desperate and the chance was very small indeed, yet when the operation was over he recovered and enjoyed six months of comparatively easy life and died without the suffering that these cases die with, if not operated. The same way with many other cases of abdominal disease that the surgeon is able to relieve. I think that in all cases it is nothing but proper to look and see what can be done. Suppose we do operate on a case like the doctor did and the case dies. The case would have died anyway. Suppose the doctor hastened the woman's death. He saved her hours and days of misery and suffering. If by chance a man operates in a thousand cases of this kind and they all die, and in the thousandth and one he is able to do some good, he is justified in doing it."

### By Dr. O. A. Gordon.

Dr. H. B. DELATOUR, in discussion, said: "It is certainly an interesting subject and the discussion is getting more interesting. I quite agree with Dr. Brinsmade in the class of cases I understand he is talking of. There is a class of cases that comes to us in the very last hours and anything we attempt to do can hardly be considered more than an ante mortem post mortem. These cases on the very face of them will not recover from any procedure we may undertake, and in these I feel with Dr. Brinsmade that it is not a wise thing to interfere, even to make an exploratory operation or simply an artificial anus. I believe there is some harm done to surgery by operations followed by death in a few hours.

"As Dr. Figueira has said, many a case that is given up to die by a number of men subsequently falls into the hands of some one else who is fortunate enough to operate and bring the case through and get a fine recovery, but that does not fit with cases of this sort. Even the cases of carcinoma of the stomach or intestines that are so weak they cannot even get out of bed, are not in the condition Dr. Brinsmade refers to where you have complete obstruction that has existed for days, an immense distention of the abdomen, constant fecal vomiting and a pulse that is almost unaccountable.

"Now, as to carcinoma of the various parts of the intestine. I think we will find if we look back over the cases we have had that there is a decided difference in the malignancy of apparently the same growth in different parts of the large intestine. I have a patient living now about five years, in whom I did the same operation Dr. Gordon described to-night, for a carcinoma of the cecum. I believe I have three cases in which I did a resection of the cecum for carcinoma apparently well advanced, and even had to take out a number of large glands and do a resection between the small intestine and the transverse colon. Those cases do well. They do not show much tendency to recurrence. Carcinoma in the lower part of the rectum show more tendency to recurrence than those a little higher up (those in the sigmoid), so we can feel more hope in operating in those carcinomas of the large intestine the further away we get from the rectum. At least that has been my experiecne.

Dr. MATHIAS FIGUEIRA, in discussion, said: "When I spoke I did not speak of cases that were dead or dying. These gentlemen that have talked that way are simply hedging, see? They see that they have no argument and they are hedging, that is all. I spoke of cases that were not dead or dying. These cases that the doctor operated on were not dead and were not dying at all."

*(Concluded in January.)*

# Medical Society of the County of King

## MONTHLY BULLETIN TO MEMBERS

MINUTES OF STATED MEETING,

NOVEMBER 18, 1913.

The President, Dr. James M. Winfield, in the chair.

There were about 75 present.

The meeting was called to order at 8.45 P. M., and the minutes of the previous meeting were read and approved.

### Election of Members.

The following, duly proposed and accepted by the Council, were declared elected to active membership:

Louis Fisher, 318 Pennsylvania Ave.
Charles Goldman, 238 Nostrand Ave.
Frank D. Jennings, 53 Woodbine St.
R. S. Robertson, 271 Jefferson Ave.

### Applications for Membership.

Applications for membership were received from the following:

Gerhard William Heuser, 560 McDonough St.; Cornell University Medical College, 1904; proposed by J. W. Stevens; seconded by J. A. Ferguson.

Leon E. Lesser, 28 Douglas St.; L. I. C. H., 1911; proposed by T. Howard; seconded by Memb. Com.

Marcus F. Searle, 775 Washington Ave.; Cleveland Hom. Medical College, 1909; proposed by Calvin F. Barger; seconded by Memb. Com.

John H. Schall, 119 St. Marks Ave.; Hahnemann, Phila., 1893; proposed by E. A. Bruyn; seconded by Memb. Com.

Wesley G. Simmons, 956 Greene Ave.; Med.-Chir., Phila., 1898; proposed by W. P. Pool; seconded by W. A. Sprenger.

### Executive Session.

#### Nominations.

Nominations for officers and delegates for the ensuing year were then made as follows:

For President—James M. Winfield;* J. Richard Kevin.

For Vice-President—Henry G. Webster; Russell S. Fowler.

For Secretary—Burton Harris; C. Euge Lack; Claude G. Crane.*

For Associate Secretary—Charles E. S field.

For Treasurer—Sylvester J. MacNama Stephen H. Lutz.

For Associate Treasurer—Robert L. Mo head; James P. Glynn.

For Directing Librarian—Frederick Tilne

For Trustees—James M. Winfield.

Five Censors—Henry A. Wade, Earl Mayne, Eliza M. Mosher, Sigfried Block, B D. Harrington, John G. Williams, John Lee, Charles Eastmond, John Sturdivant Re Walter A. Sherwood.

For Delegate to the State Society, 1914, expired term of Algernon T. Bristow—Cha E. Scofield.

For Eleven Delegates to the State Soci 1914-1915—Claude G. Crane, Henry M. Sm Edwin A. Griffin, Martha J. Peebles, James Winfield, Walter D. Ludlum, George R. H ley, William Browning, Albert M. Judd, J C. MacEvitt, Edward E. Cornwall, Leo J Commiskey, Louis C. Ager, William J. Cr shank, James W. Ingalls.

For Twenty-three Alternate Delegates the State Society for 1914.

It was moved, seconded and carried, the Council be empowered to select twe three Alternate Delegates.

### Scientific Program.

1. Paper: "Bacteriological Diagnosis."
   By Horace Greeley, M.D.

2. Paper: "The Possibilities of Immun Milk in Disease (A Preliminary Report).'
   By Benjamin F. Corwin, M.D.

3. Paper: "The Common Ground of Opht mology and General Medicine."
   By Henry Mitchell Smith, M.D.
   Discussed by Nelson L. North, John Ohly, Henry R. Price, Horace G ley, Benjamin M. Briggs.
   Closed by Henry M. Smith, M.D.

Adjourned 10.15 P. M.

CLAUDE G. CRANE, *Secretar*

* Declined nomination.

498

Lightning Source UK Ltd.
Milton Keynes UK
UKHW012029040119
334856UK00003B/226/P